Sunlight, Vitamin D and Skin Cancer

ADVANCES IN EXPERIMENTAL MEDICINE AND BIOLOGY

Sunlight, Vitamin D and Skin Cancer

Edited by

Jörg Reichrath

Clinic for Dermatology, Venerology and Allergology, The Saarland University Hospital, Homburg/Saar, Germany

Springer Science+Business Media, LLC
Landes Bioscience

Springer Science+Business Media, LLC
Landes Bioscience

Printed in the U.S.A.

Springer Science+Business Media, LLC, 233 Spring Street, New York, New York 10013, U.S.A.

Please address all inquiries to the publishers:
Landes Bioscience, 1002 West Avenue, 2nd Floor, Austin, Texas 78701, U.S.A.
Phone: 512/ 637 5060; FAX: 512/ 637 6079
http://www.landesbioscience.com

Sunlight, Vitamin D and Skin Cancer, edited by Jörg Reichrath, Landes Bioscience / Springer Science+Business Media, LLC dual imprint / Springer series: Advances in Experimental Medicine and Biology.

ISBN: 978-0-387-77573-9

Library of Congress Cataloging-in-Publication Data

Sunlight, vitamin D, and skin cancer / edited by Jörg Reichrath.
    p. ; cm. -- (Advances in experimental medicine and biology ; v. 624)
  Includes bibliographical references and index.
  ISBN 978-0-387-77573-9
  1. Skin--Cancer. 2. Sunshine. 3. Vitamin D--Therapeutic use. I. Reichrath, J. (Jörg), 1962- II. Series.
  [DNLM: 1. Skin Neoplasms--prevention & control. 2. Sunlight. 3. Vitamin D--therapeutic use. W1 AD559 v.624 2008 / WR 500 S958 2008]
  RC280.S5S86 2008
  616.99'477--dc22
                        2007049792

DEDICATION

I dedicate this book to Michael Holick and Wolfgang Tilgen, my teachers in vitamin D and dermato-oncology.

PREFACE

UV-exposure represents the most important risk factor for the development of nonmelanoma skin cancer. Additionally, assessment of sun exposure parameters has consistently shown an association between the development of malignant melanoma and short-term, intense UV-exposure, particularly burning in childhood. As a consequence, protection of the skin from UV-exposure is an integral part of skin cancer prevention programs. However, more chronic, less intense UV-exposure has not been found to be a risk factor for melanoma and in fact has been found in some studies to be protective. Moreover, 90% of all requisite vitamin D is formed within the skin through the action of the sun—a serious problem—for a connection between vitamin D deficiency and various types of cancer (e.g., colon, prostate and breast cancers) has been demonstrated in a large number of studies. Hence, the association between vitamin D deficiency and various internal malignancies has now opened a debate among dermatologists and other clinicians how to balance between positive and negative effects of solar and artificial UV-exposure.

The goal of this volume is to provide a comprehensive, highly readable overview of our present knowledge of positive and negative effects of UV-exposure, with a focus on vitamin D and skin cancer. Topics that are discussed in-depth by leading researchers and clinicians range from the newest findings in endocrinology, epidemiology, histology, photobiology, immunology, cytogenetics and molecular pathology to new concepts for prophylaxis and treatment. Experts in the field as well as health care professionals not intimately involved in these specialized areas are provided with the most significant and timely information related to these topics. It is the aim of this book to summarize essential up-to-date information for every clinician or scientist interested in how to balance between positive and negative effects of UV-exposure to minimize the risks of developing vitamin D deficiency and skin cancer.

All the chapters are written by authors who are experts in their respective research areas, and I am grateful for their willingness to contribute to this book. I would also like to express my thanks to Ron Landes, Cynthia Conomos, Megan Klein, Sara Lord and all the other members of the Landes Bioscience staff for their expertise, diligence and patience in helping me complete this work.

Jörg Reichrath, Ph.D.

ABOUT THE EDITOR...

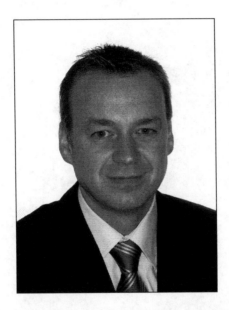

JÖRG REICHRATH is Professor for Dermatology and Deputy Director of the Clinic for Dermatology, Allergology and Venerology at the Saarland University Hospital in Homburg/Saar, Germany. His main research interests include photobiology, dermato-endocrinology and dermato-oncology. He is a member of numerous national and international scientific organisations, including the German Dermatological Society (DDG), the Deutsche Krebsgesellschaft (DKG), the German Dermatologic Co-operative Oncology Group (DeCOG), and the European Society of Dermatological Research (ESDR). He has been awarded numerous prices including the Arnold-Rikli-Prize 2006. Jörg Reichrath received his academic degrees (Dr. med., venia legendi) from the Saarland University, Germany.

PARTICIPANTS

Honnavara N. Ananthaswamy
Department of Immunology
The University of Texas M.D. Anderson
    Cancer Center
Houston, Texas
U.S.A.

Elma D. Baron
Department of Dermatology
University Hospitals of Cleveland
Case Western Reserve University
and
Dermatology Department
Cleveland Veterans Affairs Medical
    Center
Cleveland, Ohio
U.S.A.

Cara L. Benjamin
Department of Immunology
The University of Texas M.D. Anderson
    Cancer Center
Houston, Texas
U.S.A.

Guido Bens
Clermont-Ferrand University Hospital
Department of Dermatology
    Hôtel-Dieu
Clermont-Ferrand
France

Marianne Berwick
Department of Internal Medicine
University of New Mexico Cancer
    Center
Albuquerque, New Mexico
U.S.A.

Heike A. Bischoff-Ferrari
Department of Rheumatology
    and Institute of Physical Medicine
University Hospital Zurich
Zurich
Switzerland

Eckhard W. Breitbart
Center of Dermatology
Elbenkliniken Stade/Buxtehude
Center of Dermatology
Buxtehude
Germany

Melanie A. Carless
Department of Genetics
Southwest Foundation for Biomedical
    Research
San Antonio, Texas
U.S.A.

Arne Dahlback
Department of Physics
University of Oslo
Oslo
Norway

Ola Engelsen
Norwegian Institute for Air Research
Polar Environment Centre
Tromso, Norway

Peter Erb
Institute for Medical Microbiology
University of Basel
Basel
Switzerland

Claus Garbe
Division of Dermatoloncology
Department of Dermatology
University Medical Center
Tuebingen
Germany

Edward Giovannucci
Departments of Nutrition
 and Epidemiology
Harvard School of Public Health
and
Channing Laboratory
Department of Medicine
Harvard Medical School
and
Brigham and Women's Hospital
Boston, Massachusetts
U.S.A.

William B. Grant
Sunlight, Nutrition, and Health
 Research Center
San Francisco, California
U.S.A.

Rüdiger Greinert
Center of Dermatology
Elbenkliniken Stade/Buxtehude
Center of Dermatology
Buxtehude
Germany

Lyn R. Griffiths
Genomics Research Centre
School of Health Science
Griffith University Gold Coast
Bundall
Australia

Ulrich R. Hengge
Department of Dermatology
Heinrich-Heine-University
Düsseldorf
Germany

Michael F. Holick
Department of Medicine
Section of Endocrinology, Nutrition,
 and Diabetes
Vitamin D, Skin and Bone Research
 Laboratory
Boston University Medical Center
Boston, Massachusetts
U.S.A.

Jingmin Ji
Institute for Medical Microbiology
University of Basel
Basel
Switzerland

Erwin Kump
Institute for Medical Microbiology
University of Basel
Basel
Switzerland

Anne Lachiewicz
Department of Internal Medicine
University of New Mexico Cancer
 Center
Albuquerque, New Mexico
U.S.A.

Ulrike Leiter
Division of Dermatooncology
Department of Dermatology
University Medical Center
Eberhard Karls-University
 of Tuebingen
Tuebingen
Germany

Pablo Mancheño-Corvo
Instituto de Investigaciones
 Biomédicas Alberto Sols
Departamento de Biotecnología
Universidad Francisco de Vitoria
Madrid
Spain

Pilar Martín-Duque
Instituto de Investigaciones Biomédicas
    Alberto Sols
Departamento de Biotecnología
Universidad Francisco de Vitoria
Madrid
Spain

Vladislava O. Melnikova
Department of Cancer Biology
The University of Texas M.D. Anderson
    Cancer Center
Houston, Texas
U.S.A.

Ainhoa Mielgo
University of California San Diego
Moores Cancer Center
La Jolla, California
U.S.A.

Johan Moan
Department of Radiation Biology
Institute for Cancer Research
Montebello
and
Department of Physics
University of Oslo
Oslo
Norway

Peter Mohr
Center of Dermatology
Elbenkliniken Stade/Buxtehude
Center of Dermatology
Buxtehude
Germany

Cornelia S.L. Mueller
The Saarland University Hospital
Dermatology Clinic Kirrbergerstr
Homburg/Saar
Germany

Bernd Nürnberg
Clinic for Dermatology, Venerology
    and Allergology
The Saarland University Hospital
Homburg/Saar
Germany

Claire Pestak
Department of Internal Medicine
University of New Mexico Cancer
    Center
Albuquerque, New Mexico
U.S.A.

Mar Pons
Instituto de Investigaciones Biomédicas
    Alberto Sols
Departamento de Biotecnología
Universidad Francisco de Vitoria
Madrid
Spain

Alina Carmen Porojnicu
Department of Radiation Biology
Institute for Cancer Research
Montebello, Oslo
Norway

Miguel Quintanilla
Instituto de Investigaciones
    Biomédicas Alberto Sols
SCIC-UAM
Madrid
Spain

Knuth Rass
The Saarland University Hospital
Dermatology Clinic
Homburg/Saar
Germany

Jörg Reichrath
Clinic for Dermatology, Venerology
    and Allergology
The Saarland University Hospital
Homburg/Saar
Germany

Diana Santo Domingo
Department of Dermatology
University Hospitals of Cleveland
Case Western Reserve University
Cleveland, Ohio
U.S.A.

Nancy Thomas
Department of Internal Medicine
University of New Mexico Cancer
    Center
Albuquerque, New Mexico
U.S.A.

Wolfgang Tilgen
Clinic for Dermatology, Venerology
    and Allergology
The Saarland University Hospital
Homburg/Saar
Germany

Beate Volkmer
Center of Dermatology
Elbenkliniken Stade/Buxtehude
Center of Dermatology
Buxtehude
Germany

Ann R. Webb
Centre for Atmospheric Sciences
School of Earth Atmospheric
    and Environmental Sciences
University of Manchester
Manchester
U.K.

Marion Wernli
Institute for Medical Microbiology
University of Basel
Basel
Switzerland

Jingwu Xie
Department of Pharmacology
    and Toxicology
Sealy Center for Cancer Cell Biology
University of Texas Medical Branch
Galveston, Texas
U.S.A.

CONTENTS

13. UV DAMAGE AND DNA REPAIR IN MALIGNANT MELANOMA AND NONMELANOMA SKIN CANCER 162

Knuth Rass and Jörg Reichrath

14. ROLE OF VIRUSES IN THE DEVELOPMENT OF SQUAMOUS CELL CANCER AND MELANOMA 179

Ulrich R. Hengge

15. MELANOMA AND NONMELANOMA SKIN CANCERS AND THE IMMUNE SYSTEM 187

Diana Santo Domingo and Elma D. Baron

16. SOLAR UV-RADIATION, VITAMIN D AND SKIN CANCER SURVEILLANCE IN ORGAN TRANSPLANT RECIPIENTS (OTRS).. 203

Jörg Reichrath and Bernd Nürnberg

17. HISTOLOGY OF MELANOMA AND NONMELANOMA SKIN CANCER... 215

Cornelia S.L. Mueller and Jörg Reichrath

22. APOPTOSIS AND PATHOGENESIS OF MELANOMA AND NONMELANOMA SKIN CANCER... 283

Peter Erb, Jingmin Ji, Erwin Kump, Ainhoa Mielgo and Marion Wernli

23. TREATMENT OF MELANOMA AND NONMELANOMA SKIN CANCER.. 296

Knuth Rass and Wolfgang Tilgen

CHAPTER 1

Sunlight, UV-Radiation, Vitamin D and Skin Cancer:
How Much Sunlight Do We Need?

Michael F. Holick*

Abstract

Vitamin D is the sunshine vitamin for good reason. During exposure to sunlight, the ultraviolet B photons enter the skin and photolyze 7-dehydrocholesterol to previtamin D_3 which in turn is isomerized by the body's temperature to vitamin D_3. Most humans have depended on sun for their vitamin D requirement. Skin pigment, sunscreen use, aging, time of day, season and latitude dramatically affect previtamin D_3 synthesis. Vitamin D deficiency was thought to have been conquered, but it is now recognized that more than 50% of the world's population is at risk for vitamin D deficiency. This deficiency is in part due to the inadequate fortification of foods with vitamin D and the misconception that a healthy diet contains an adequate amount of vitamin D. Vitamin D deficiency causes growth retardation and rickets in children and will precipitate and exacerbate osteopenia, osteoporosis and increase risk of fracture in adults. The vitamin D deficiency has been associated pandemic with other serious consequences including increased risk of common cancers, autoimmune diseases, infectious diseases and cardiovascular disease. There needs to be a renewed appreciation of the beneficial effect of moderate sunlight for providing all humans with their vitamin D requirement for health.

Prehistorical and Historic Perspectives

The major source of vitamin D for most land vertebrates, including humans, comes from exposure to sunlight. From a prehistoric perspective, some of the earliest unicellular organisms that evolved in the oceans including phytoplankton produced vitamin D when exposed to sunlight.[1,2] Vertebrates that evolved in the ocean took advantage of their high calcium environment and used it effectively for developing a mineralized endoskeleton. When vertebrates ventured onto land, they needed to adapt to the calcium poor environment by increasing their efficiency for intestinal absorption of dietary calcium. They took with them the ability to photosynthesize vitamin D_3 in their skin which became essential for enhancing intestinal calcium absorption and maintaining serum calcium levels in most land vertebrates including homosapiens.[1,2]

In the mid-1600s Whistler and Glissen reported that children living in industrialized cities in Great Britain had short stature and deformities of their skeleton especially their lower legs.[3] This scourge of the industrialization of Europe and North America persisted for more than 250 years. Even though Sniadecki[4] suggested in 1822 that the most likely reason for why his young patients who lived in Warsaw had a high incidence of rickets while the children whom he cared for living in the countryside did not was due to lack of sun exposure. It would take 100 years to appreciate this insightful observation. Palm in 1889[5] also recognized that "sunbathing" was

*Michael F. Holick—Department of Medicine, Section of Endocrinology, Nutrition and Diabetes. Vitamin D, Skin and Bone Research Laboratory, Boston University Medical Center, 715 Albany Street, M-1013, Boston, MA 02118, U.S.A. Email: mfholick@bu.edu

Sunlight, Vitamin D and Skin Cancer, edited by Jörg Reichrath. ©2008 Landes Bioscience and Springer Science+Business Media.

important for preventing rickets based on reports from his colleagues who saw children living in the most squalid conditions in India and Asia who were not afflicted with rickets whereas it was epidemic in the industrialized cities in Great Britain. By the turn of the 20th century upwards of 90% of children living in Leyden, The Netherlands and in Boston and New York City were afflicted with this bone deforming disease and suffered its long term consequences. In 1903 Finsen received the Nobel Prize for his insightful observations that exposure to sunlight cured a variety of diseases including lupus vulgaris (skin infected with tuberculosis).[6] Finally, in 1919, Huldschinski[7] reported that exposure of children to radiation from a mercury arc lamp was an effective means of treating rickets. This was quickly followed by the observation of Hess and Unger[8] that exposure of children to sunlight on the roof of a New York City hospital was an effective means of treating rickets.

The recognition that exposure of both people and animals to ultraviolet radiation was effective in preventing and treating rickets prompted Hess and Weinstock[9] and Steenbock and Black[10] to irradiate with ultraviolet radiation a wide variety of substances including lettuce, grasses and corn, olive and cotton seed oils. Before the irradiation, none of the substances had antirachitic activity, but after the irradiation, they were effective in preventing rickets in rodents. It was also known at that time that cod liver oil was an effective method for preventing and treating rickets and it was Park[11] who demonstrated that rachitic rats could be cured of their bone disease by either cod liver oil or by ultraviolet irradiation suggesting that the two were related. Steenbock[12] appreciated the practical benefit of these observations when he reported that the irradiation of cow's milk imparted antirachitic activity and, thus, would be an ideal way of preventing rickets in children.

By the early 1930s it was appreciated throughout Europe and in the northeastern United States that exposing children to sensible and adequate sunlight without causing sunburn was an effective method of preventing rickets in children. The United States set up an agency in the US Government that promoted sensible sun exposure to parents as a means of preventing their children from developing rickets.[3,13]

Photoproduction of Vitamin D$_3$

When the skin is exposed to sunlight, the ultraviolet B radiation (UVB) that is able to penetrate through the ozone layer with energies 290-315 nm (Fig. 1) is absorbed by 7-dehydrocholesterol in the epidermis and dermis.[2,14,15] This absorption causes the double bonds to be excited causing the B-ring to open making the rigid steroid structure into a more flexible molecule known as previtamin D$_3$ (Fig. 2). Previtamin D$_3$ exists in two conformations. It is the thermodynamically less favorable cis, cis form that converts to vitamin D$_3$. Thus, when previtamin D$_3$ was made in an isotropic organic solution such as hexane or ethanol, it would take several days for it to convert to vitamin D$_3$ at 37°C. To enhance the thermal induced isomerization of previtamin D$_3$ to vitamin D$_3$, 7-dehydrocholesterol is incorporated within the fatty acid hydrocarbon side chain and polar head group of the triglycerides in the plasma membrane. When exposed to sunlight, 7-dehydrocholesterol is efficiently converted to the cis, cis conformer which rapidly isomerizes to vitamin D$_3$ (Fig. 2). Vitamin D$_3$ is ejected out of the plasma membrane into the extracellular space where it enters the dermal capillary bed bound to the vitamin D binding protein.[16]

There has been a lot of debate as to whether dietary vitamin D$_3$ is equivalent to vitamin D$_3$ made in the skin. Although both have the same biologic activity once they are metabolized, the half-life of vitamin D$_3$ produced in the skin is prolonged in the circulation because 100% is bound to the vitamin D binding protein whereas when vitamin D$_3$ is ingested, only about 60% is bound to the vitamin D binding protein and 40% is rapidly cleared in the lipoprotein bound fraction.[17]

Factors Controlling Cutaneous Vitamin D Synthesis

Melanin evolved as a sunscreen that absorbed UVB and ultraviolet A (320-400 nm) radiation protecting the UV absorbing macromolecules including DNA, RNA and proteins from the damaging effects from excessive exposure to UVR. However, as people migrated north and south

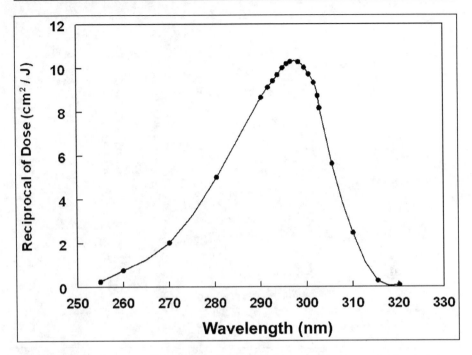

Figure 1. Action spectrum of 7-dehydrocholesterol to previtamin D_3 conversion in human skin. Holick copyright 2007 with permission.

of the equator, they needed to quickly mutate their skin pigment gene in order to have the ability to make enough vitamin D_3 to sustain their calcium and bone metabolism.[18]

Melanin is so efficient in absorbing UVB radiation that it markedly reduces the cutaneous photosynthesis of vitamin D_3. The dark melanin pigment of Africans and African Americans with skin types 5 and 6 (never burns, always tans) is so efficient in absorbing UVB radiation that it reduces the capacity of the skin to produce previtamin D_3 by 95 to 99% when compared to a Caucasian with skin type 2 (always burns, sometimes tans).[19]

The application of a sunscreen with a sun protection factor of 15 absorbs approximately 99% of UVB radiation and, thus, reduces the skin's capacity to produce previtamin D_3 by 99%.[20] The angle at which the sun's rays hit the earth's surface has a dramatic effect on the cutaneous production of previtamin D_3. As the angle of the sun becomes more oblique to the earth's surface, the UVB photons have to travel a longer path through ozone which efficiently absorbs them. Thus, season, latitude, time of day, as well as weather conditions dramatically affect the cutaneous production of previtamin D_3[21] (Fig. 3). Living above and below approximately 35° latitude, children and adults are able to produce an adequate amount of vitamin D_3 in their skin during the spring, summer and fall. However, essentially all of the UVB photons are absorbed during the winter months, thus either completely eliminating or markedly reducing the capacity of the skin to produce vitamin D_3. This is the explanation for why there is a seasonal variation in circulating levels of 25-hydroxyvitamin D_3 [25(OH)D] which is considered to be the major circulating form of vitamin D[22] (Fig. 4). Similarly, early in the morning and late in the afternoon, the sun's rays are more oblique and as a result, most of if not all of the UVB photons are absorbed by the ozone layer. Thus, even in the summer in the early morning and late afternoon little, if any, vitamin D_3 is produced in the skin (Fig. 3).

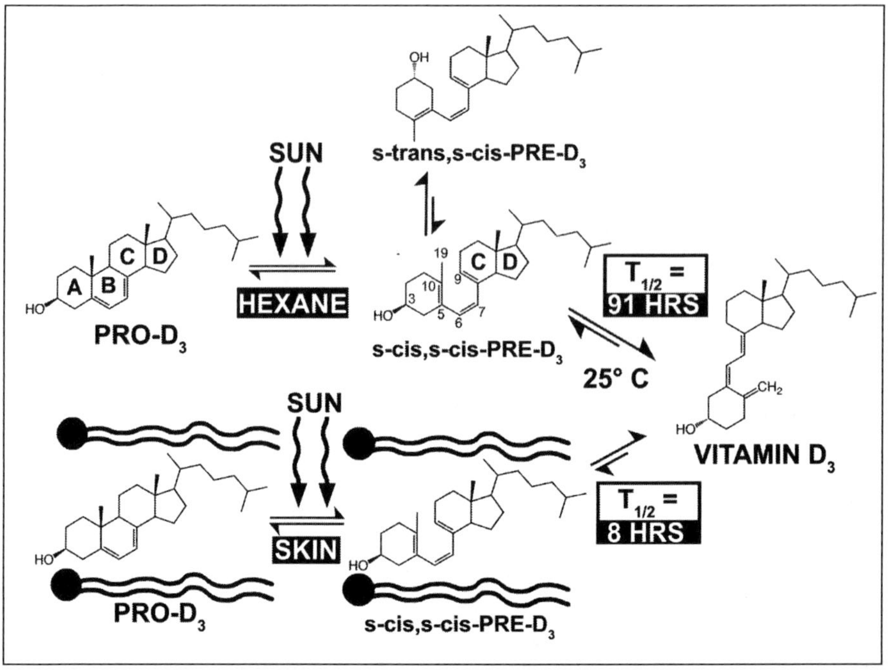

Figure 2. Photolysis of provitamin D_3 (pro-D_3; 7-dehydrocholesterol) into previtamin D_3 (pre D_3) and its thermal isomerization to vitamin D_3 in hexane and in lizard skin. In hexane is pro-D_3 photolyzed to *s-cis,s-cis*-preD$_3$. Once formed, this energetically unstable conformation undergoes a conformational change to the *s-trans,s-cis*-preD$_3$. Only the *s-cis,s-cis*-preD$_3$ can undergo thermal isomerization to vitamin D_3. The *s-cis,s-cis* conformer of preD$_3$ is stabilized in the phospholipid bilayer by hydrophilic interactions between the 3β-hydroxl group and the polar head of the lipids, as well as by the van der Waals interactions between the steroid ring and side-chain structure and the hydrophobic tail of the lipids. These interactions significantly decrease the conversion of the *s-cis,s-cis* conformer to the *s-trans,s-cis* conformer, thereby facilitating the thermal isomerization of *s-cis,s-cis*-preD$_3$ to vitamin D_3. Reproduced with permission,[15] copyright 1995 National Academy of Sciences, U.S.A.

Sources and Metabolism of Vitamin D

The major source of vitamin D (D represents D_2 or D_3) for most humans is exposure to sunlight. Very few foods naturally contain vitamin D. These include oily fish such as salmon, cod liver oil which contains vitamin D_3 and sun dried mushrooms which contains vitamin D_2. Vitamin D_3 is 2 to 3 times more effective in raising blood levels of 25(OH)D compared to the same dose of vitamin D_2.[23] Some foods are fortified with vitamin D including milk and some juice products in the United States and Canada and some breads, margarines, cereals in the United States, Canada and Europe. Sweden and Finland now fortify milk with vitamin D. Typically there is 100 IU (10 micrograms) of vitamin D in a serving such as 8 ounces of milk or orange juice.[3,23]

Once vitamin D is made in the skin or ingested from the diet, it must metabolize in the liver to 25(OH)D[24-26] (Fig. 5). The metabolite is biologically inactive, however, it is the major circulating form of vitamin D that is used by physicians to determine a patient's vitamin D status. 25(OH)D undergoes an obligate hydroxylation by the 25-hydroxyvitamin D-1α-hydroxylase (CYP27B1; 1-OHase) in the kidneys to form the biologically active form 1,25-dihydroxyvitamin D (1,25(OH)$_2$D). 1,25(OH)$_2$D, a steroid like hormone, interacts with its nuclear vitamin D receptor (VDR) in target tissues including the small intestine, osteoblasts in bone and in the renal tubular

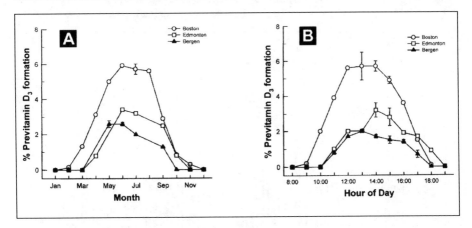

Figure 3. Influence of season, time of day in July and latitude on the synthesis of previtamin D_3 in Boston (42°N)-o-, Edmonton (52°N)-□-, Bergen (60°) -▲-. The hour is the end of the one hour exposure time in July. Holick copyright 2007 with permission.

cells in the kidneys. $1,25(OH)_2D$ is responsible for the maintenance of calcium homeostasis and bone health by increasing the efficiency of intestinal calcium absorption, stimulating osteoblast function and increase bone calcium resorption. It also enhances the tubular resorption of calcium in the kidneys (Fig. 5).

$1,25(OH)_2D$ is such a potent regulator of calcium metabolism that in order to control its own actions, it induces its own destruction by enhancing the expression of the 25-hydroxyvitamin D-24-hydroxylase (CYP24).[23-26] CYP24 causes oxidation on carbons 24 and 23 leading to the formation of a C23 acid known as calcitroic acid. This water soluble inactive metabolite is excreted in the bile (Fig. 5).

Role of Vitamin D in the Prevention of Chronic Diseases

Most tissues and cells in the body including brain, skin, breast, prostate, colon and activated T and B lymphocytes possess a VDR.[23-27] It is now recognized that $1,25(OH)_2D$ is one of the most potent hormones for regulating cell growth and maturation. It is estimated that more than 200 genes are either directly or indirectly influenced by $1,25(OH)_2D$.[28]

There have been numerous studies that have implicated living at higher latitudes and being at increased risk of vitamin D deficiency with many serious and chronic and deadly diseases including cancers of the colon, prostate and breast, autoimmune diseases including multiple sclerosis, type I diabetes and rheumatoid arthritis, infectious diseases including tuberculosis and influenza and hypertension and heart disease.[23,29-46]

What has been perplexing is the fact that exposure to sunlight results in an increase of circulating levels of $25(OH)D$ but not $1,25(OH)_2D$. The reason is that parathyroid hormone, calcium and phosphorus and fiberblast growth factor 23 tightly control the production of $1,25(OH)_2D$ in the kidneys[23] (Fig. 5). Since $25(OH)D$ is incapable of altering vitamin D responsive gene expression at physiologic concentrations, there needed to be another explanation for the sunlight-vitamin D health connection.

It has been recognized for more than 30 years that activated macrophages, placenta and skin expressed the 1-OHase.[47-49] In the late 1990's, there were numerous reports of various cell culture systems that expressed the 1-OHase that were capable of converting $25(OH)D_3$ to $1,25(OH)_2D_3$ including colon, prostate, breast and lung cell cultures.[50-54] It was also observed that normal prostate cells obtained from prostate biopsies and both normal and colon cancer cells obtained at the time of surgery expressed the 1-OHase and had the capacity to make $1,25(OH)_2D$.[50-52] These observations have led to the hypothesis that by raising blood levels of $25(OH)D$, there is enough substrate

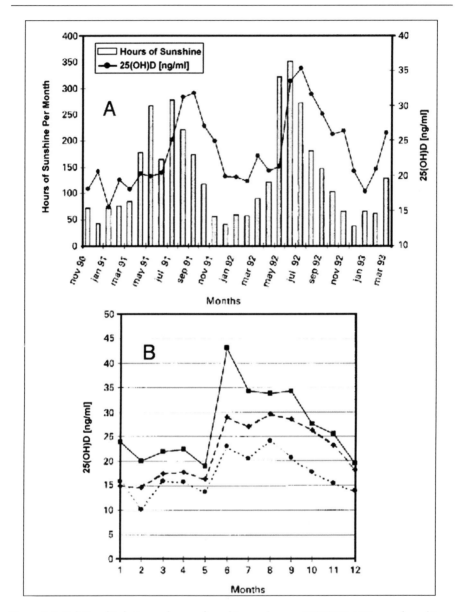

Figure 4. A: Relationship between hours of sunshine and serum 25(OH)D. ■ Hours of sunshine;
• 25(OH)D (ng/ml). B: Seasonal fluctuation of serum 25(OH)D according to frequency of
sun exposure. ■ Regular sun exposure; ♦ Occasional sun exposure; • Avoiding direct sun
exposure. Reproduced with permission,[22] copyright 2001 British Journal of Nutrition.

for many tissues and cells in the body that express the 1-OHase to produce locally $1,25(OH)_2D$.
It's believed that the local production of $1,25(OH)_2D$ is important for regulating cell growth and
maturation and, thus, is able to prevent cells from becoming malignant. $1,25(OH)_2D_3$ accomplishes this by either restoring the cell to its normal proliferative state or by inducing its death by

apoptosis. If the cell becomes malignant, an additional strategy for $1,25(OH)_2D^{15}$ is to inhibit angiogenesis to the malignant cells.[55]

$1,25(OH)_2D$ locally produced by macrophages is important for innate immunity in humans. $1,25(OH)_2D$ enhances the production of the bacteriocidal protein cathelicidin which was shown to be effective in killing infective agents including Microbacterium tuberculosis.[44] $1,25(OH)_2D$ is also an effective immunomodulator which may be the explanation for why the local production of $1,25(OH)_2D$ by activated macrophages may be important for reducing risk of developing multiple sclerosis, rheumatoid arthritis and Crohn's disease.[23] In addition, $1,25(OH)_2D$ enhances the production of insulin and, thus, may play an important role in type II diabetes[56] and metabolic syndrome[57] and inhibits the production of renin[58] which is important for blood pressure regulation.

Vitamin D Deficiency Pandemic

It is estimated that one billion people world-wide are at risk of vitamin D deficiency.[23] Upwards of 30-50% of both children and adults in the United States, Europe, South America, Middle East and Far East are at risk.[59-75] The major cause for this pandemic is the lack of appreciation of the beneficial effect of sunlight in producing vitamin D.[3,23,75] In the sunniest areas of the world, vitamin D deficiency is common because of lack of adequate sun exposure.[70-72]

It has been previously thought that the adequate intake for vitamin D to satisfy the body's requirement is 200 IU for all children and adults up to the age of 50 years, 400 IU for adults 51 to 70 years and 600 IU of vitamin D for adults over the age of 70.[76] However, it is now recognized that a 25(OH)D should be at least 30 ng/ml to have the full benefits of vitamin D for overall health and welfare.[3,25,77,78] In order to attain a level above 30 ng/ml, 800 to 1,000 IU of vitamin D/d is required from dietary sources or from exposure to sunlight.[3,23,75,79] Since diets that include vitamin D supplemented foods are only able to satisfy between 10 and 40% of this requirement, it is not at all surprising that vitamin D deficiency is probably one of the most common medical conditions world-wide.

The consequences of vitamin D deficiency are often silent, but insidious in nature. For children, it may prevent them from attaining their peak height and bone mineral density.[3,80] Adults are at increase risk of developing osteopenia, osteoporosis and increase risk of fracture.[23,75,78] In addition, vitamin D deficiency increases risk of a wide variety of chronic diseases (Fig. 6).

Sunlight, Vitamin D and the Skin Cancer Conundrum

Humans evolved in sunlight and their skin pigment gene has evolved in order to protect the skin from the damaging effects from excessive exposure to sunlight, but permitting enough UVB radiation to enter the skin to produce an adequate amount of vitamin D to sustain health. The pigment gene has rapidly mutated to decrease skin pigmentation[18] in order to permit humans to survive in environments where there is markedly reduced UVB irradiation and, thus, vitamin D_3 synthesis.

The skin has a large capacity to make vitamin D_3.[3,23] When young and middle aged adults were exposed one time to one minimal erythemal dose of ultraviolet B radiation, the circulating levels of vitamin D that were observed 24 hours after the exposure were similar to adults who ingested between 10,000 and 25,000 IU of vitamin D_2[81] (Fig. 7). Thus, only minimum suberythemal exposure to sunlight is often adequate to satisfy the body's vitamin D requirement.[82,83]

It is well documented that excessive exposure to sunlight will increase risk of nonmelanoma skin cancers.[84] However, it is also known that occupational sun exposure decreases the risk of the most deadly form of skin cancer, melanoma.[84,85]

People of color who live near the equator and are exposed to sunlight on a daily basis sustain blood levels of 25(OH)D of 40-60 ng/ml.[86] Their skin was designed to produce an adequate amount of vitamin D and the melanin pigmentation prevents the damaging effects minimizing risk of nonmelanoma skin cancer.

As skin pigment devolved in order to permit humans to produce an adequate amount of vitamin D_3, the skin was perfectly designed to take advantage of the beneficial effect of sun exposure

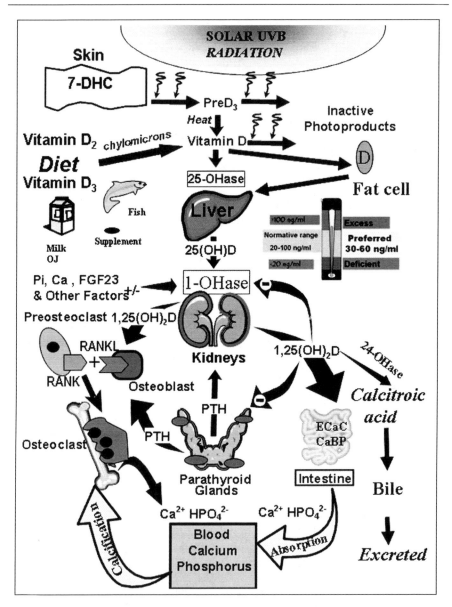

Figure 5. Schematic representation of the synthesis and metabolism of vitamin D for regulating calcium, phosphorus and bone metabolism. During exposure to sunlight 7-dehydrocholesterol (7-DHC) in the skin is converted to previtamin D_3 (preD_3). PreD_3 immediately converts by a heat dependent process to vitamin D_3. Excessive exposure to sunlight degrades previtamin D_3 and vitamin D_3 into inactive photoproducts. Vitamin D_2 and vitamin D_3 from dietary sources are incorporated into chylomicrons, transported by the lymphatic system into the venous circulation. Vitamin D (D represents D_2 or D_3) made in the skin or ingested in the diet can be stored in and then released from fat cells. Vitamin D in the circulation is bound to the vitamin D binding protein which transports it to the liver where vitamin D is converted by the vitamin D-25-hydroxylase (25-OHase) to 25-hydroxyvitamin D [25(OH)D]. Figure legend continued on next page.

Figure 5, continued from previous page. This is the major circulating form of vitamin D that is used by clinicians to measure vitamin D status (although most reference laboratories report the normal range to be 20-100 ng/ml, the preferred healthful range is 30-60 ng/ml). 25(OH)D is biologically inactive and must be converted in the kidneys by the 25-hydroxyvitamin D-1α-hydroxylase (1-OHase) to its biologically active form 1,25-dihydroxyvitamin D [1,25(OH)$_2$D]. Serum phosphorus, calcium, fibroblast growth factor (FGF-23) and other factors can either increase (+) or decrease (-) the renal production of 1,25(OH)$_2$D. 1,25(OH)$_2$D feedback regulates its own synthesis and decreases the synthesis and secretion of parathyroid hormone (PTH) in the parathyroid glands. 1,25(OH)$_2$D increases the expression of the 25-hydroxyvitamin D-24-hydroxylase (24-OHase) to catabolize 1,25(OH)$_2$D and 25(OH)D to the water soluble biologically inactive calcitroic acid which is excreted in the bile. 1,25(OH)$_2$D enhances intestinal calcium absorption in the small intestine by stimulating the expression of the epithelial calcium channel (ECaC; also known as transient receptor potential cation channel sub family V member 6; TRPV6)) and the calbindin 9K (calcium binding protein; CaBP). 1,25(OH)$_2$D is recognized by its receptor in osteoblasts causing an increase in the expression of receptor activator of NFκB ligand (RANKL). Its receptor RANK on the preosteoclast binds RANKL which induces the preosteoclast to become a mature osteoclast. The mature osteoclast removes calcium and phosphorus from the bone to maintain blood calcium and phosphorus levels. Adequate calcium and phosphorus levels promote the mineralization of the skeleton and maintain neuromuscular function. Holick copyright 2007 with permission.

while minimizing the damaging effects. A study in people who frequent a tanning bed at least once a week at the end of the winter had robust levels of 25(OH)D of approximately 40-50 ng/ml which was comparable to people of color being exposed to sunlight on almost a daily basis living near the equator[87] (Fig. 8).

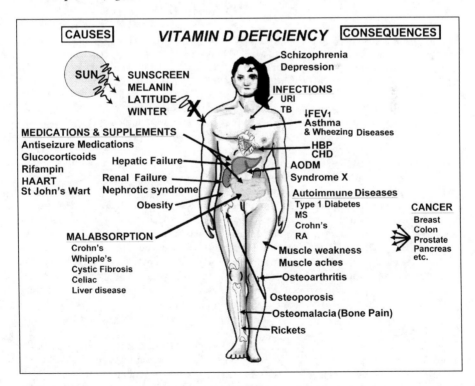

Figure 6. A schematic representation of the major causes for vitamin D deficiency and potential health consequences. Holick copyright 2007 with permission.

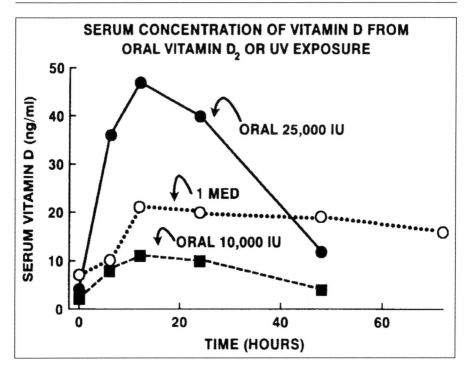

Figure 7. Comparison of serum vitamin D_3 levels after a whole-body (in a bathing suit; trunks for men, bikini for women) exposure to 1 MED (minimal erythemal dose) of simulated sunlight compared with a single oral dose of either 10,000 or 25,000 IU of vitamin D_2. Reproduced with permission,[81] copyright 2002 Current Opinion in Endocrinology and Diabetes.

Aging will dramatically affect the amount of 7-dehydrocholesterol in human skin.[88] As a result, a 70 year old has about 25% of the capacity to produce vitamin D_3 in their skin compared to a young adult. However, because the skin has such a large capacity to produce vitamin D_3, elders exposed to either sunlight,[3,23,56] a tanning bed[87] or other UVB emitting devices[89] are able to raise their blood levels of 25(OH)D often above 30 ng/ml.

How long should a person be exposed to sunlight to satisfy their vitamin D requirement? It depends on time of day, season of year, latitude, weather conditions and the person's degree of skin pigmentation. Typically for a Caucasian's skin type II living at approximately 42° N in June at noon-time, exposure of arms and legs to sunlight on a clear day between the hours of 10 and 3 pm for approximately 5-15 minutes, two to three times a week is adequate to satisfy the body's vitamin D requirement. The use of sun protection of the face is reasonable since it is often the face that is most sun exposed and sun damaged and relative to the rest of the body based on surface area provides only a minimum amount of vitamin D_3. After the 5-15 minutes of sun exposure, the application of a sunscreen with a SPF of at least 15 is then recommended if the person stays outside for a longer period of time in order to prevent sun burning and the damaging effects due to excessive exposure to sunlight.

Conclusion

Humans have always depended on sun for their vitamin D requirement. It is curious that the same UVB radiation that is so beneficial for making vitamin D_3 is also the major cause of nonmelanoma skin cancer. It is excessive exposure to sunlight and the number of sunburns that is responsible for the alarming increase in nonmelanoma skin cancer.[84] The fact that most melanomas occur on the least sun exposed areas at least raises the question whether moderate sun exposure is at all

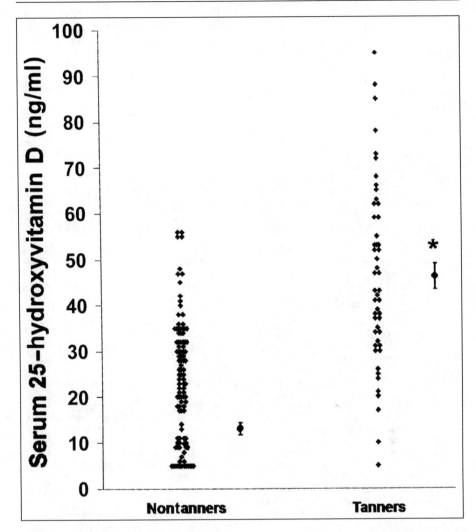

Figure 8. Mean (±SEM) serum 25-hydroxyvitamin D concentrations in tanners and nontanners. Single points for each category are means ± SEMS. *Significantly different from nontanners, P <0.001. Reproduced with permission,[87] copyright 2004, American Society for Nutrition.

related to an increase risk of this deadly disease. Two reports suggest that moderate sun exposure decreases the risk.[84,85] It is also worth noting that children and young adults who had moderate sun exposure had a decreased mortality if they developed melanoma[90] and a 40% reduced risk of developing nonHodgkin's lyumphoma.[91]

It's unfortunate that the sun has been demonized for more than thirty years by those who have been poorly informed or lack knowledge about the beneficial effect of sunlight[92] that our forefathers had appreciated more than 100 years ago. Most experts agree that at least 800-1,000 IU of vitamin D/d is needed for all children and adults to help sustain healthful blood levels of 25(OH)D of >30 ng/ml. It is very difficult if not impossible to obtain this amount of vitamin D from dietary sources. It is also unrealistic to recommend that all humans on the planet increase their vitamin D intake to 1,000 IU of vitamin D/d and to avoid all direct sun exposure. There needs to be moderation in the recommendation regarding sensible sun exposure and increasing the awareness of the vitamin D deficiency pandemic. Increased food fortification with vitamin D and encouraging both children and adults to increase their vitamin D intake from a vitamin D supplement of 1,000 IU/d is also needed.

Acknowledgements

This work was supported in part by NIH grants M01RR00533 and AR36963 and the UV Foundation.

References

1. Holick MF. Phylogenetic and evolutionary aspects of vitamin D from phytoplankton to humans. In: Pang PKT, Schreibman MP, eds. Vertebrate Endocrinology: Fundamentals and Biomedical Implications, Vol 3. Orlando: Academic Press, 1989:7-43.
2. Holick MF. Vitamin D: A millennium perspective. J Cell Biochem 2003; 88:296-307.
3. Holick MF. Resurrection of vitamin D deficiency and rickets. J Clin Invest 2006; 116(8):2062-2072.
4. Sniadecki J. Jerdrzej Sniadecki (1768-1838) on the cure of rickets. (1840) Cited by W. Mozolowski. Nature 1939; 143:121-124.
5. Palm TA. The geographical distribution and aetiology of rickets. The Practitioner 1890; XLV[4]:270-342.
6. Holick MF. Biologic effects of light: historical and new perspectives. In: Holick MF, Jung EG, eds. Biologic Effects of Light 1998. Proceedings of a Symposium Basel, Switzerland 1998. Boston: Kluwer Academic Publishers, 1999:10-32.
7. Huldschinsky K. Heilung von Rachitis durch Kunstliche Hohensonne. Deutsche Med Wochenschr 1919; 45:712-713.
8. Hess AF, Unger LJ. The cure of infantile rickets by sunlight. JAMA 1921; 77:39-41.
9. Hess AF, Weinstock M. Antirachitic properties imparted to inert fluids and to green vegetables by ultraviolet irradiation. J Biol Chem 1924; 62:301-313.
10. Steenbock H, Black A. The reduction of growth-promoting and calcifying properties in a ration by exposure to ultraviolet light. J Biol Chem 1924; 61:408-422.
11. Park EA. The etiology of rickets. Physiol Rev 1923; 3:106-163.
12. Steenbock H. The induction of growth-prompting and calcifying properties in a ration exposed to light. Science 1924; 60:224-225.
13. Hess AF. Rickets including osteomalacia and tetany. Pennsylvania: Lea J. Febiger, 1929:401-429.
14. Holick MF, MacLaughlin JA, Clark MB et al. Photosynthesis of previtamin D_3 in human skin and the physiologic consequences. Science 1980; 210:203-205.
15. Holick MF, Tian XQ, Allen M. Evolutionary importance for the membrane enhancement of the production of vitamin D_3 in the skin of poikilothermic animals. Proc Natl Acad Sci 1995; 92:3124-3126.
16. Haddad JG, Walgate J, Miyyn C et al. Vitamin D metabolite-binding proteins in human tissue. Biochem Biophys Acta 1976; 444:921-925.
17. Haddad JG, Matsuoka LY, Hollis BW et al. Human plasma transport of vitamin D after its endogenous synthesis. J Clin Invest 1993; 91:2552-2555.
18. Lamason RL, Mohideen MAPK, Mest JR et al. SLC24A5, a putative cation exchanger, affects pigmentation in zebrafish and humans. Science 2005; 310(5755):1782-1786.
19. Clemens TL, Henderson SL, Adams JS et al. Increased skin pigment reduces the capacity of skin to synthesis vitamin D_3. Lancet 1982; 74-76.
20. Matsuoka LY, Ide L, Wortsman J et al. Sunscreens suppress cutaneous vitamin D_3 synthesis. J Clin Endocrinol Metab 1987; 64:1165-1168.
21. Webb AR, Kline L, Holick MF. Influence of season and latitude on the cutaneous synthesis of vitamin D_3: Exposure to winter sunlight in Boston and Edmonton will not promote vitamin D_3 synthesis in human skin. J Clin Endocrinol Metab 1988; 67:373-378.
22. Brot C, Vestergaad P, Kolthoff N et al. Vitamin D status and its adequacy in healthy Danish premenopausal women: relationships to dietary intake, sun exposure and serum parathyroid hormone 40. British Journal of Nutrition 2001; 86(1):S97-103.
23. Holick MF. Vitamin D Deficiency. N Eng J Med 2007; 357:266-281.
24. Bouillon R. Vitamin D: From photosynthesis, metabolism and action to clinical applications. In: DeGroot LJ, Jameson JL, eds. Endocrinology. Philadelphia: WB Saunders, 2001; 1009-1028.
25. DeLuca H. Overview of general physiologic features and functions of vitamin D. Am J Clin Nutr 2004; 80(Suppl):1689S-96S.
26. Holick MF, Garabedian M. Vitamin D: photobiology, metabolism, mechanism of action, and clinical applications. In: Favus MJ, ed. Primer on the Metabolic Bone Diseases and Disorders of Mineral Metabolism, Sixth Edition. Washington, DC: American Society for Bone and Mineral Research, 2006; 129-37.

27. Stumpf WE, Sar M, Reid FA et al. Target cells for 1,25-dihydroxyvitamin D_3 in intestinal tract, stomach, kidney, skin, pituitary and parathyroid. Science 1979; 206:1188-1190.
28. Nagpal S, Na S, Rathnachalam R. Noncalcemic actions of vitamin D receptor ligands. Endocr Rev 2005; 26:662-87.
29. Apperly FL. The relation of solar radiation to cancer mortality in North America. Cancer Res 1941; 1:191-195.
30. Gorham ED, Garland CF, Garland FC et al. Vitamin D and prevention of colorectal cancer. J Steroid Biochem Mol Biol 2005; 97(1-2):179-194.
31. Hanchette CL, Schwartz GG. Geographic patterns of prostate cancer mortality. Cancer 1992; 70:2861-2869.
32. Grant WB. An estimate of premature cancer mortality in the US due to inadequate doses of solar ultraviolet-B radiation. Cancer 2002; 70:2861-2869.
33. Garland C, Garland F, Gorham E et al. The role of vitamin D in prevention of cancer—analytic essay forum 112. Am J Public Health 2006; 96(2):252-261.
34. Cantorna MT, Zhu Y, Froicu M et al. Vitamin D status, 1,25-dihydroxyvitamin D_3 and the immune system. Am J Clin Nutr 2004; 80(suppl):1717S-1720S.
35. Ponsonby A-L, McMichael A, van der Mei I. Ultraviolet radiation and autoimmune disease: insights from epidemiological research. Toxocology 2002; 181-182:71-78.
36. Rostand SG. Ultraviolet light may contribute to geographic and racial blood pressure differences. Hypertension 1979; 30:150-156.
37. Krause R, Buhring M, Hopfenmuller W et al. Ultraviolet B and blood pressure. Lancet 1998; 352:709-710.
38. Zittermann A, Schleithoff SS, Tenderich G et al. Low vitamin D status: a contributing factor in the pathogenesis of congestive heart failure? J Am Coll Cardiol 2003; 41:105-12.
39. McGrath J, Selten JP, Chant D. Long-term trends in sunshine duration and its association with schizophrenia birth rates and age at first registration—data from Australia and the Netherlands. Schizophr Res 2002; 54:199-212.
40. Ahonen MH, Tenkanen L, Teppo L et al. Prostate cancer risk and prediagnostic serum 25-hydroxyvitamin D levels (Finland). Cancer Causes Control 2000; 11:847-52.
41. Feskanich JM, Fuchs CS, Kirkner GJ et al. Plasma vitamin D metabolites and risk of colorectal cancer in women. Cancer Epidemiol Biomarkers Prev 2004; 13(9):1502-1508.
42. Giovannucci E, Liu Y, Rimm EB et al. Prospective Study of Predictors of Vitamin D Status and Cancer Incidence and Mortality in Men. Journal of the National Cancer Institute 2006; 98:451-459.
43. Chiu KC, Chu A, Go VLW et al. Hypovitaminosis D is associated with insulin resistance and β cell dysfunction. Am J Clin Nutr 2004; 79:820-825.
44. Liu PT, Stenger S, Li H et al. Toll-like receptor triggering of a vitamin D-mediated human antimicrobial response. Sciencexpress 2006; 3:1770-1773.
45. Cannell JJ, Vieth R, Umhau JC et al. Epidemic influenza and vitamin D. Epidemiol Infect 2006; 134(6):1129-40.
46. Camargo Jr CA, Rifas-Shiman SL, Litonjua AA et al. Maternal intake of vitamin D during pregnancy and risk of recurrent wheeze in children at 3 y of age. Am J Clin Nutr 2007; 85(3)788-795.
47. Bikle DD. Vitamin D: Role in skin and hair. In: Feldman et al, eds. Vitamin D. New Jersey: Elsevier Academic Press, 2005:609-630.
48. Zerwekh JE, Breslau NA. Human placental production of 1α,25-dihydroxyvitamin D_3: Biochemical characterization and production in normal subjects and patents with pseudohypoparathyroidism. J Clin Endocrinol Metab 1986; 62(1):192-196.
49. Adams JS, Hewison M. Hypercalcemia caused by granuloma-forming disorders. In: Favus, MJ, ed, Primer on the Metabolic Bone Diseases and Disorders of Mineral Metabolism, Sixth Edition. Washington, DC: American Society for Bone and Mineral Research, 2006:200-202.
50. Schwartz GG, Whitlatch LW, Chen TC et al. Human prostate cells synthesize 1,25-dihydroxyvitamin D_3 from 25-hydroxyvitamin D_3. Cancer Epidemiol Biomarkers Prev 1998; 7:391-395.
51. Tangpricha V, Flanagan JN, Whitlatch LW et al. 25-hydroxyvitamin D-1α-hydroxylase in normal and malignant colon tissue. Lancet 2001; 357:1673-1674.
52. Cross HS, Bareis P, Hofer H et al. 25- Hydroxyvitamin D_3-1-hydroxylase and vitamin D receptor gene expression in human colonic mucosa is elevated during early cancerogenesis. Steroids 2001; 66:287-292.
53. Mawer EB, Hayes ME, Heys SE et al. Constitutive synthesis of 1,25-dihydroxyvitamin D_3 by a human small cell lung cell line. J Clin Endocrinol Metab 1994; 79:554-560.
54. Feldman D, Zha, XY, Krishnan AV. Editorial/Mini-review: Vitamin D and prostate cancer. Endocrinology 2000; 141:5-9.
55. Mantell DJ, Owens PE, Bundred NJ et al. 1α,25-dihydroxyvitamin D_3 inhibits angiogenesis in vitro and in vivo. Circ Res 2000; 87:214-220.

56. Pittas AG, Dawson-Hughes B, Li T et al. Vitamin D and calcium intake in relation to type 2 diabetes in women. Diabetes Care 2006; 29:650-56.
57. Chiu KC, Chu A, Go VLW et al. Hypovitaminosis D is associated with insulin resistance and β cell dysfunction. Am J Clin Nutr 2004; 79:820-825.
58. Li YC. Vitamin D regulation of the renin-angiotensin system. J Cell Biochem 2003; 88:327-331.
59. Lips P. Vitamin D status and nutrition in Europe and Asia. J Steroid Biochem Mol Biol 2007; 103(3-5):620-625.
60. Chapuy MC, Schott AM, Garnero P et al. Healthy elderly French women living at home have secondary hyperparathyroidism and high bone turnover in winter. J Clin Endocrinol Metab 1996; 81:1129-1133.
61. Malabanan A, Veronikis IE, Holick MF. Redefining vitamin D insufficiency. Lancet 1998; 351:805-806.
62. Holick MF, Siris ES, Binkley N et al. Prevalence of vitamin D inadequacy among postmenopausal North American women receiving osteoporosis therapy. J Clin Endocrinol Metab 2005; 90:3215-3224.
63. Dawson-Hughes B, Dallal GE, Krall EZ et al. Effect of vitamin D supplementation on wintertime and overall bone loss in healthy postmenopausal women. Ann Intern Med 1991; 115:505-512.
64. Bakhtiyarova S, Lesnyak O, Kyznesova N et al. Vitamin D status among patients with hip fracture and elderly control subjects in Yekaterinburg, Russia. Osteoporos Int 2006; 17:441-46.
65. Boonen S, Bischoff-Ferrari A, Cooper C et al. Addressing the musculoskeletal components of fracture risk with calcium and vitamin D: a review of the evidence. Calcif Tissue Int 2006; 78:257-70.
66. Gloth III FM; Gundberg CM, Hollis BW et al. Vitamin D deficiency in homebound elderly persons. JAMA 1995; 274(21):1683-1686.
67. Sullivan SS, Rosen CJ, Halteman WA et al. Adolescent girls in Maine at risk for vitamin D insufficiency. J Am Diet Assoc 2005; 105:971-974.
68. Tangpricha V, Pearce EN, Chen TC et al. Vitamin D insufficiency among free-living healthy young adults. Am J Med 2002; 112(8):659-662.
69. Gordon CM, DePeter KC, Estherann G et al. Prevalance of vitamin D deficiency among healthy adolescents. Arch Pediatr Adolesc Med 2004; 158:531-537.
70. El-Hajj Fuleihan G, Nabulsi M, Choucair M et al. Hypovitaminosis D in healthy school children. Pediatrics 2001; 107:E53.
71. Marwaha RK, Tandon N, Reddy D et al. Vitamin D and bone mineral density status of healthy school-children in northern India. Am J Clin Nutr 2005; 82:477-482.
72. Sedrani SH. Low 25-hydroxyvitamin D and normal serum calcium concentrations in Saudi Arabia: Riyadh region. Ann Nutr Metab 1984; 28:181-185.
73. Lee JM, Smith JR, Philipp BL et al. Vitamin D deficiency in a healthy group of mothers and newborn infants. Clin Pediatr 2007; 46:42-44.
74. Bodnar LM, Simhan HN, Powers RW et al. High prevalence of vitamin D insufficiency in black and white pregnant women residing in the northern United States and their neonates. J Nutr 2007; 137:447-452.
75. Holick MF. High prevalence of vitamin D inadequacy and implications for health. Mayo Clin Proc 2006; 81(3):353-373.
76. Standing committee on the scientific evaluation of dietary reference intakes food and nutrition board institute of medicine 1997 Vitamin D. In: Dietary Reference Intakes for Calcium, Phosphorus, Magnesium, Vitamin D and Fluoride. National Academy Press: Washington, DC, 1999:250-287.
77. Heaney RP, Dowell MS, Hale CA et al. Calcium absorption varies within the reference range for serum 25-hydroxyvitamin D. J Am Coll Nutr 2003; 22(2):142-146.
78. Bischoff-Ferrari HA, Giovannucci E, Willett WC et al. Estimation of optimal serum concentrations of 25-hydroxyvitamin D for multiple health outcomes. Am J Clin Nutr 2006; 84:18-28.
79. Tangpricha V, Koutkia P, Rieke SM et al. Fortification or orange juice with vitamin D: a novel approach to enhance vitamin D nutritional health. Am J Clin Nutr 2003; 77:1478-1483.
80. Cooper C, Javaid K, Westlake S et al. Developmental origins of osteoporotic fracture: the role of maternal vitamin D insufficiency. J Nutr 2005; 135:2728S-2734S.
81. Holick MF. Vitamin D: The underappreciated D-lightful hormone that is important for skeletal and cellular health. Current opinion in endocrinology and diabetes 2002; 9:87-98.
82. Reid IR, Gallagher DJA, Bosworth J. Prophylaxis against vitamin D deficiency in the elderly by regular sunlight exposure. Age Ageing 1985; 15:35-40.
83. Holick MF. Vitamin D and skin physiology: A D-lightful story. JBMR, in press.
84. Kennedy C, Bajdik CD, Willemze R et al. The influence of painful sunburns and lifetime of sun exposure on the risk of actinic keratoses, seborrheic warts, melanocytic nevi, atypical nevi and skin cancer. J Invest Dermatol 2003; 120(6):1087-1093.
85. Garland FC, Garland CF. Occupational sunlight exposure and melanoma in the US Navy. Arch Env Health 1990; 45:261-267.

86. Vieth R, Garland C, Heaney R et al. The urgent need to reconsider recommendations for vitamin D nutrition intake. Am J of Clin Nutr 2007; 85:649-650.
87. Tangpricha V, Turner A, Spina C et al. Tanning is associated with optimal vitamin D status (serum 25-hydroxyvitamin D concentration) and higher bone mineral density. Am J Clin Nutr 2004; 80:1645-1649.
88. MacLaughlin J, Holick MF. Aging decreases the capacity of human skin to produce vitamin D_3. J Clin Invest 1985; 76:1536-1538.
89. Chuck A, Todd J, Diffey B. Subliminal ultraviolet-B irradiation for the prevention of vitamin D deficiency in the elderly: a feasibility study. Photochem Photoimmun Photomed 2001; 17(4):168-171.
91. Berwick M, Armstrong BK, Ben-Porat L et al. Sun exposure and mortality from melanoma. J Natl Cancer Inst 2005; 97:195-199.
92. Chang ET, Smedby KE, Hjalgrim H et al. Family history of hematopoietic malignancy and risk of lymphoma. J Natl Cancer Inst 2005; 97:1466-74.
93. Wolpowitz D, Gilchrest BA. The vitamin D questions: how much do you need and how should you get it? J Am Acad Dermatol 2006; 54:301-317.

CHAPTER 2

Solar Ultraviolet Irradiance and Cancer Incidence and Mortality

William B. Grant*

Introduction

R ates for many cancers are generally higher with increased distance from the equator. The first paper positing a link between sunlight and reduced risk of cancer was published in 1937.[1] Persons in the US Navy with greater "skin irritation" (actinic keratosis and skin cancer) had lower risk of internal cancers. A second paper appeared then reported that residents of sunnier states had lower cancer risk.[1] Although many studies have tried to explain these geographic variations, including differences in dietary factors and socioeconomic status, the most promising is that solar ultraviolet-B (UVB) (290-315 nm), through production of vitamin D, reduces the risk of cancer incidence and increases survival chances. Data at the World Health Organization[3] indicated large latitudinal gradients in cancer mortality rates recorded as early as 1955 for breast, colon, intestinal, lung, prostate, rectal and renal cancer. However, rates were also low for countries where much fish was consumed, such as Iceland and Japan and in countries where animal products were a small fraction of the total energy supply, such as Egypt. Thus, it would have taken a clever researcher to suggest that solar UVB and fish were important sources of vitamin D and could explain much of the variance.

This chapter reviews the observational support for the UVB/vitamin D/cancer theory, outlines the supporting evidence and discusses the level of certainty for the theory. It also presents the evidence for beneficial effects of UVB and vitamin D for other diseases and conditions.

Cancer

Solar UVB of Geographic Location as the Index of Vitamin D Production—Single-Country Studies

The solar UVB/vitamin D/cancer theory was proposed in 1980 by Cedric and Frank Garland, then associated with the Johns Hopkins School of Public Health. They heard a lecture on the geographic variation of cancer mortality rates in the United States that was based on the Atlas of Cancer Mortality for US Counties: *1950-1969*.[4] Maps had age-adjusted mortality rates for various cancers displayed in color for five categories:

- significantly high, in highest decile;
- significantly high, not in highest decile;
- in highest decile, not significant;
- not significantly different from the United States; and
- significantly lower than the United States.

For most of the cancers, the color for "not significantly different from the US" dominated the atlas. However, for large-intestine-except-rectum cancer for males, Arizona, southern California

*William B. Grant—Sunlight, Nutrition and Health Research Center (SUNARC), San Francisco, CA, U.S.A. Email: wbgrant@infionline.net

Sunlight, Vitamin D and Skin Cancer, edited by Jörg Reichrath. ©2008 Landes Bioscience and Springer Science+Business Media.

and New Mexico were colored "significantly lower than the US," as were parts of the southern states east of the Mississippi River, whereas the northeast had the highest rates. They knew that it was sunny in the southwest and hypothesized that since the most important physiological effect of solar radiation was the production of vitamin D, vitamin D levels must be higher in the southwest. Vitamin D, they posited, reduced the risk of cancer mortality. They did an ecologic study of colon cancer mortality rates for 17 metropolitan and 32 nonmetropolitan states[5] with respect to annual hours of solar radiation on the basis of cancer data in Lilienfeld et al.[6]

Their work was slowly extended over the next two decades. They showed that dietary vitamin D and calcium were inversely correlated with colorectal cancer[7] and that serum 25-hydroxyvitamin D (calcidiol) levels were inversely correlated with colon cancer.[8] They also extended their ecologic studies to include breast[9,10] and ovarian cancer.[11] Their account of their work on vitamin D was recently published as a commentary[12] along with the republication of their seminal paper in the International Journal of Epidemiology,[13] along with commentaries by others on the progress and status of the understanding of the roles of UVB and vitamin D in cancer risk reduction.[14-18] Schwartz and coworkers added prostate cancer to the list of vitamin D-sensitive cancers in the 1990s as well.[19,20] Freedman added nonHodgkin's lymphoma (NHL) in 1997 through a study of residential and occupational exposure to sunlight and mortality.[21]

However, the 1990s saw little progress on the UVB/vitamin D/cancer theory, partly because the ecologic approach was considered only a hypothesis-generating approach[22] and since the case-control and cohort studies designed to test the hypothesis were based primarily on dietary vitamin D. Diet provides about 250-300 international units (IU) (6-8 µg) of vitamin D per day in the United States, primarily from vitamin D3-fortified foods such as dairy.[23] Dietary sources of vitamin D are too low to have an easily discernible effect on colorectal cancer risk since it takes about 1,000-1,500 IU/day to reduce the risk by about 50%.[24-26] Supplements could provide that much, but the US recommended daily allowance is about 400 IU/day and both vitamin D2 (ergocalciferol) and vitamin D3 (cholecalciferol) are used in US supplements. Vitamin D2 is much less effective than vitamin D3,[27] and most researchers did not consider whether the vitamin D used was D2 or D3. Thus, there was little support provided for the theory for about two decades.

Two ongoing concerns: 1) many think that UV irradiance is associated primarily with risk of skin cancer and cutaneous malignant melanoma (CMM) and 2) market-based economic systems have little incentive to promote solar UVB irradiance and oral vitamin D consumption to reduce the burden of disease. However, the risk of skin cancer and CMM should generally be of much less concern than the health benefits of vitamin D for most people.

The case for the UVB/vitamin D/cancer theory was bolstered in 2002 when I, then working in atmospheric sciences at the NASA Langley Research Center in Hampton, Virginia, published a paper identifying 14 UVB/vitamin D-sensitive cancers [Grant, 2002b] (Tables 1 and 2). After publishing a few ecologic studies of dietary links to Alzheimer's disease,[28] heart disease,[29] prostate cancer,[30] and rheumatoid arthritis,[31] I focused on cancer in the United States after the more recent *Atlas of Cancer Mortality in the United States, 1950-94*,[32] became available. After determining that dietary factors could not explain the up to a factor-of-two variation in mortality rates between the southwest and northeast, I posed two questions: how many cancers were UVB sensitive and how many Americans died prematurely from cancer annually because of insufficient UVB and vitamin D. Since my position at NASA dealt with stratospheric ozone, I knew about the surface solar UVB map for July 1992 derived from the NASA Total Ozone Mapping Spectrometer (TOMS) satellite instrument.[33] The overall variation of the UVB doses seemed to match the maps in the Atlas, with highest UVB in the southwest, lowest in the northeast and intermediate elsewhere. I digitized the map to provide values to use with the approximately 500 state economic areas of cancer mortality rate data. I omitted some states from the analysis since some of the high cancer rates near the Mexican border were apparently unrelated to solar UVB and other cancer risk-modifying factors were not included in the analysis. The finding in this study was that about 14 cancers were UVB/vitamin D sensitive and that 17,000-23,000 Americans died prematurely from cancer annually.[34] This study prompted others on the role of solar UVB and vitamin D in reducing cancer risk.

Table 1. *Vitamin D-sensitive cancers with strong support*

Cancer	Mortality Rate, 1970-94[32] M,F*	North America	Europe	Asia	Multi-Continent	Australia	Second Cancer after NMSC	Other Studies
Bladder	6.56, 1.87	34, 38, 39						
Breast	0.25, 26.89	9, 10, 34, 35, 37, 38, 39	66, 72, 67, 56					95
Colon	20.13, 14.97	5, 34, 35, 37, 38, 39, 98	66, 67, 56	92	77		62	7, 8, 25, 26
Esophageal	4.80, 1.24	34, 37, 38, 39, 98	56	92			62	
Gallbladder	0.57, 1.10	38, 39		92			62	
Gastric	7.33, 3.41	34, 37, 38, 39		92			62	
Hodgkin's lymphoma	1.10, 0.67	38, 39	45, 56					
Melanoma	2.96, 1.61		56					83, 85
NHL	7.03, 4.76	34, 38, 39	66, 45, 56		77	44		
Ovarian	—, 8.38	11, 34, 35, 38, 39	66, 67, 56		77, 79			
Pancreatic	10.21, 6.84	34, 38, 39, 98	66, 67, 56					96
Prostate	22.01, —	19, 34, 35, 38, 39	66, 67	92	73, 75		63, 64	
Rectal	4.40, 2.54	34, 37, 38, 39, 98	67,56	92			62	
Renal	4.90, 2.24	34, 38, 39	66		77,78		62	
Uterine corpus	—, 3.72	34, 38, 39	56					
Totals		14	11	6	5	1	6	

*deaths/100,000/year in the United States

Table 2. Vitamin D-sensitive cancers with moderate support

Cancer	Mortality Rate, 1970-94[32] M,F	North America	Europe
Leukemia	8.80, 5.16	39, 98	
Lung	69.4, 23.93	34, 37	
Multiple myeloma	3.10, 2.08	39	66, 67, 56
Oral	3.99, 1.41	38, 98	
Ocular melanoma, uveal		121	
Small intestine		39	
Thyroid	0.33, 0.42	39	56
Totals		7	2

*deaths/100,000/year in the United States

Soon, Freedman reported her findings regarding sunlight and mortality from breast, ovarian, colon, prostate and nonmelanoma skin cancer (NMSC) on the basis of a composite death certificate-based case-control study.[35] Only female breast and colon cancer, however, also showed significant negative associations with jobs with the highest occupational exposure to sunlight (odds ratio [OR], 0.82 (95% confidence interval [CI], 0.70-0.97) for female breast cancer; OR 0.90 (95% CI, 0.86-0.94) for colon cancer). NMSC was directly correlated with sunlight, yielding evidence that the index of solar UVB was reasonable.

Since the ecologic study using the TOMS UVB doses did not include data for other cancer risk-modifying factors, more studies were conducted in which such factors were included. Lung cancer mortality rate was used as the index of the health effects of smoking, based on an analysis of lung cancer mortality rates with respect to other cancer mortality rates for black American males.[36] Other factors included alcohol consumption per capita rates, fraction of the population living below the poverty level, fraction of the population living in urban regions and ethnic background. Mortality rate data in the United States are divided into those for white and black Americans, white Americans including Hispanics. Thus, the data for black Americans could be treated separately, whereas for Hispanic heritage, the fraction of the population with Hispanic heritage was used as a factor. Since the data for several of these factors was most readily available by state, the state was adopted as the geographical unit in these studies.

Fifteen types of cancer were then identified as UVB/vitamin D sensitive[37,38] (Tables 1 and 2). Three minor cancers, gallbladder and oral cancer and Hodgkin's lymphoma, were added to that list. They could be added because 1) by using state-averaged data, the statistical uncertainties were reduced and 2) by including the other factors, their effects on the geographic variations could be accounted for. Three cancers reported as having significant correlations with UVB—cervical, laryngeal and pancreatic cancer—were later determined to have a spurious correlation due to an interaction with other factors rather than an effect of solar UVB. The correlations with other risk-modifying factors other than the poverty index generally agreed with the journal literature. However, it was recently realized that the criterion for statistical significance at the 95% confidence level ($p < 0.05$) is valid only for univariate regressions; in multiple linear regression analyses, the correct value is $0.05/n$, where n is the number of factors in the model. Thus, many of the factors identified in boldface font in Refs. 37 and 38 as statistically significant at the 95% confidence level but with $p > 0.009$ were found not to be significant in a later analysis that also included dietary factors [Grant, in preparation]. The poverty index was no longer correlated with cancer risk when dietary factors were included.

More recently, Boscoe and Shymura[39] did an ecologic study of US cancer incidence and mortality rates. They used data from a set of 3.1 million incident cancer cases and 3.1 million cancer deaths from the North American Association of Central Cancer Registries[40] and the National Cancer Institute's SEER*Stat database.[41] They processed TOMS UVB data to obtain annual average data with a 1-degree by 1-degree (approximately 100 km × 100 km) grid. They found strong inverse correlations with cancers at 12 sites, weaker inverse correlations for eight sites and inverse correlations for three cancers that were different for the sexes. For some cancers, mortality rates had a higher correlation with UVB than did incidence rates: bladder, colon, other biliary, ovarian, rectal, renal, soft tissue, uterine corpus and vulvar cancer and NHL, whereas for others, the situation was reversed: gastric, pancreatic and prostate cancer, leukemia and multiple myeloma. The effect of vitamin D may be apparently stronger with respect to mortality rates than with incidence rates since cancer initiation and progression is affected by many factors, whereas metastasis may be affected by fewer factors and vitamin D reduces metastasis. Also, some of the cancer screening programs such as mammography often identify types of cancer that might not become life threatening if left untreated.

Diet is also important in cancer etiology. In previous work, I assumed that dietary macro- and micronutrients were too uniformly consumed in the United States to determine their effect. However, I recently found dietary data for the four quadrants of the United States for 1988-94[42,43] and included these data in the analysis of US cancer mortality rates for 1970-94. Dietary zinc was inversely correlated with 12 types of cancer, whereas dietary iron was directly correlated with 10 and solar UVB was inversely correlated with 11 cancers for which the iron and/or zinc index was significantly correlated [Grant, in preparation]. Thus, adding more factors to the ecologic study did not eliminate solar UVB as a risk reduction factor for US cancer. However, the dietary sources of zinc include whole grains, beans/legumes, red meat and seafood, whereas the primary dietary source of iron is red meat. Many components of the dietary sources probably contribute to cancer risk modification, so taking zinc supplements to try to reduce the risk of cancer would be premature.

Two case-control studies found NHL inversely correlated with solar UVB. An Australian study found odds ratios (ORs) of 0.5-0.6 for increased solar irradiance, with greater benefit correlated with nonworkday exposures.[44] A Swedish study found ORs of 0.6-0.7 for the highest levels of solar irradiance.[45] Interestingly, both countries have many light-skinned white people who live in countries with near highest and lowest solar UVB doses. However, a recent study conducted in Connecticut, USA, found direct correlations between several measures of solar UV irradiance and risk of NHL.[46] In addition, it was noted that several other papers had reported similar results. It could be the case that UVB, through production of vitamin D, reduces the risk of NHL, while UVA, through other mechanisms, increases the risk of NHL. Further research is clearly indicated.

Five independent reviews of single-country ecologic studies of solar UVB irradiance and cancer risk have been conducted recently. Two were from those actively developing and extending the theory.[47,48] Two others were from some who have devoted most of their careers to studying the ill effects of solar UV irradiance such as a risk factor for CMM and NMSC.[49,50] Another was from a group with little investment either way.[51] All five reviews agreed that, at least for some cancers, there is reasonably strong evidence for a beneficial effect.

Critique of Geographic Location as the Index of Solar UVB Irradiance
Despite the general agreement among these three US ecologic studies, the concerns have been raised that either UVB irradiances are not well correlated with UVB doses or that in summer, vitamin D production rates from solar UVB irradiance are practically independent of latitude.[52] Kimlin et al's objection is surprising in light of the large variation of US solar UVB doses in July,[33] as well as a recent estimate of vitamin D production rates as a function of latitude in Australia, finding a strong latitudinal gradient.[53] The US July variation is due primarily to two factors: 1) higher surface elevation from the Rocky Mountains to the west and 2) lower stratospheric ozone column over the western United States because of the prevailing westerly winds pushing the tropopause height upward as the air masses prepare to cross the Rocky Mountains.

NMSC as the Index of Vitamin D Production
Several studies have addressed the first objection by using NMSC incidence or mortality rate as the index of UVB irradiance at the population level. For fair-skinned individuals, approximately

80% of NMSC deaths are due to squamous cell carcinoma (SCC).[54] The most important risk factor for SCC is integrated lifetime UVB irradiance.[55]

I recently used NMSC mortality rates as the index of UVB irradiance at the population level in an ecologic study of cancer morality rates in Spain.[56] In a country such as Spain, where the inhabitants descended from people who have lived there long enough that their skin phenotype has adapted to normal UV doses, they are fairly well protected against skin cancer and CMM.[57] Thus, NMSC mortality rates should reflect UVB irradiance rather than merely being related to latitude, as it is in countries such as the United States, where most inhabitants have skin phenotypes that are not well suited for the usual UV doses in the southern portion of the country. Lung cancer mortality rates were used for the effects of smoking and both latitude and CMM mortality rates were used in an exploratory fashion. Age-adjusted mortality rates for various cancers for 48 continental provinces for 1978-92 were used. Seventeen cancers had mortality rates inversely correlated with NMSC mortality rates,[56] including both lung cancer and CMM. UVA irradiance appears to be the primary risk factor for CMM in association with light pigmentation, whereas UVB and vitamin D reduce the risk. Latitude was not as useful an index for UVB as was NMSC in this case.

A second study was a meta-analysis of discovery of a second cancer after diagnosis of NMSC. The data for each type of second cancer had to be adjusted for smoking rates for each population by using lung cancer rates since smoking is a risk factor for basal cell carcinoma (BCC)[58] and SCC[59] but a risk reduction factor for CMM.[60,61] Several cancers were found to have rates significantly less than 1.00 for average lung cancer rates: for a diagnosis of SCC, risk ratios for subsequent colon, gastric and rectal cancers were significantly reduced, with that for renal cancer being marginally insignificant. For NMSC, risk ratios for cervical, esophageal, gastric and rectal cancer were significantly reduced; those for colon and gallbladder cancer were marginally insignificant, whereas those for female breast, laryngeal, ovarian, renal and uterine corpus cancers were insignificantly reduced.[62]

Several other studies correlated diagnosis of NMSC with reduced risk of other cancers. A study in The Netherlands found that skin cancer patients were at decreased risk of developing prostate cancer compared with the general population (standardized incidence ratio [SIR], 0.89, 95% CI, 0.78-0.99), especially shortly after diagnosis.[63] The risk of advanced prostate cancer was significantly decreased (SIR, 0.73, 95% CI, 0.56-0.94), indicating a possible antiprogression effect of ultraviolet radiation. A UK study correlated all measures of solar UVB irradiance (e.g., skin phenotype, childhood sunburning and sunbathing) with reduced risk of prostate cancer.[64] Although reduced risk of prostate cancer was always correlated with increased risk of BCC, this seems a small price to pay, especially since BCC is easy to treat and when similar effects would be expected for many UK cancers. Thus, the studies involving diagnosis of or death from NMSC strongly support the UVB/vitamin D/cancer theory.

Solar UVB Doses or Geographic Location as the Index of Vitamin D Production—Multicountry Studies

Single-country ecologic studies prove that cancer incidence and mortality rates often increase with increasing latitude. This phenomenon can also be seen in a comparison of cancer mortality rates versus latitude for common cancers in several countries. However, there is not a good correlation of cancer rate with latitude per se for such data since many factors affect cancer risk in addition to solar UVB. Thus, other factors such as diet,[65] smoking rates and alcohol consumption should be included in the model for multicountry ecologic studies. A second challenge is to find an appropriate index for solar UVB. Latitude is the easiest index to use, but better indices are based on either UVB measurements or models to estimate UVB doses on the basis of latitude, stratospheric ozone, cloud cover and perhaps surface elevation. The third challenge is that health care systems differ in screening and treatment for cancer and other diseases. Including countries with similar health care systems or including as many countries as possible to overcome the effect of different health care systems is one solution.

I presented the first multicountry study to investigate the role of UVB in reducing the risk of cancer.[66,67] I used cancer mortality rates for 1989-91 for 16 Western European countries in an ecologic study. The first study used latitude as the index of solar UVB doses, whereas the second used annual average solar UVB doses from the European Light Dosimeter Network.[68] Dietary supply factors including alcohol for 1974-76 or 1979-81[69] were used for the effects of diet. It takes about 15-20 years for cancer to go from initiation to discovery or death,[70] so there should be a similar lag between dietary supply data and cancer rates. Eight cancers had significant correlations with increasing latitude (Tables 1 and 2). Latitude or solar UVB doses were not a good index for vitamin D for the Nordic countries, where fish and supplements provide much of the vitamin D.[71]

I conducted an ecologic study of breast cancer by using mortality rates for 1989-96, dietary supply data from 1974-76 and 1979-81 and latitude from 35 countries.[72] The countries were studied as all, all less Asian and all less Asian and Latin American countries. The fraction of energy derived from animal products (risk) combined with that from vegetable products (risk reduction), followed by solar UV-B radiation and, to a lesser extent, energy derived from alcohol (risk) and fish intake (risk reduction), explained 80% of the variance of breast carcinoma mortality rates. The dietary factors identified in this study are now generally accepted as important for breast cancer risk.

There have been a few multicountry ecologic studies of prostate cancer with respect to solar UVB. In one study, mortality rates in 32 countries with white people as the predominant population were used with latitude and dietary supply factors.[73] Latitude was not a significant factor in a multiple linear regression analysis. In the second study, mortality rate data for 71 countries in 2000 were used with UVB data that were obtained from the Tropospheric Emission Monitoring Internet Service,[74] and dietary factors were obtained from the FAO.[69,75] The normalized correlation coefficient for the UVB index was –0.27 (95% CI, –0.58 to 0.04). Thus, this study found UVB to be marginally insignificantly inversely correlated with prostate cancer mortality rates.

Cancer incidence and mortality rates for 17 Western developed countries in 2002[76] were recently used in a multicountry study with latitude and maximum temperature used as UVB indices, along with dietary supply factors for 1985, fraction of energy derived from animal products, alcohol, fruit and sweeteners (added sugar).[77] Interestingly, for breast cancer, the UVB index was important for mortality rates but not incidence rates, possibly reflecting the effect of mammographic screening on incidence rates. For NHL and renal cancer, the adjusted R^2 was higher for mortality rates than for incidence rates. Perhaps more factors affect cancer incidence than cancer mortality, so that the UVB/vitamin D effect is more pronounced for mortality rates.

The multicountry ecologic approach is now being applied to cancer incidence rates on a truly global scale by the group at UC-San Diego led by Garland. They developed a UVB index based on solar UVB at the top of the atmosphere, the angle with respect to the surface and either cloud cover in winter[78] or stratospheric ozone amount.[79] For renal cancer, solar UVB was significantly inversely correlated with incidence rates, as was fraction of dietary energy derived from animal products, whereas cloud cover was inversely correlated.[78] For ovarian cancer, solar UVB and fertility rate were inversely correlated with incidence rates, whereas ozone was directly correlated.[79] More investigations using this approach are under way.

CMM

Several studies indicate that CMM is also a vitamin D-sensitive cancer. Sunscreen use was linked to CMM risk in the 1990s.[80] The reason proposed was that sunscreen in widespread use at the time blocked UVB well but not UVA. Diffey essentially conceded that point when pointing out that modern sunscreen formulations should provide good protection against CMM.[81] A study reported that risk of CMM among fair-skinned people living at different latitudes changes more slowly than that for SCC and BCC.[82] The difference is attributed to the slower latitudinal variation of UVA than UVB. Osborne and Hutchinson[83] reviewed the evidence for vitamin D. Another study reported that CMM rates in a multicountry study were correlated with the ratio of UVA to UVB.[84] A dietary study found that risk of CMM was inversely correlated with oral vitamin D.[85] The finding of the ecologic study in Spain that CMM mortality rates were inversely correlated with NMSC further indicates a beneficial role of UVB.[56]

UVB is considered an important risk factor for CMM partly because CMM rates are strongly correlated with solar UV doses where fair-skinned white people live in countries considerably equatorward of their Northern European ancestral homelands and little effort is made to separate the effects of UVA and UVB. However, inspection of data in the Atlas of Cancer Mortality in the United States, 1950-94,[32] provides more evidence for the role of UVA, not UVB, in the etiology of CMM. First, between 1950-69 and 1970-94, mortality rates for NMSC decreased by 31% for white males and 47% for white females, whereas the corresponding changes for CMM were increases of 89% and 42%, respectively. Second, in an ecologic study of cancers that includes such factors as smoking, poverty and dietary data, CMM rates are linked to latitude, whereas NMSC rates are linked to solar UVB doses for July [Grant, submitted]. Latitude here is assumed to be an index for solar UVA doses since UVA is much less affected by surface elevation than UVB and is not affected by ozone.

Causality

Most evidence supporting a beneficial role of solar UVB for cancer is observational and generally ecologic. Thus, examining the ecologic approach's validity and determining whether the criteria for causality in a biological system are generally satisfied is worthwhile.

Ecologic Approach

The ecologic approach has long been used. A famous early work was John Snow's use of a map of cholera cases in London to identify the Broad Street well as source of the outbreak and take effective action, even though the mechanism of transmission was unknown.[86] A well-known ecologic study of the relation between diet and various forms of cancer appeared in 1975.[65] Many types of cancer were found correlated with animal fat in a multicountry ecologic study, providing the strongest evidence up to that time of diet's importance in cancer risk. However, a paper by one of the same authors later suggested that ecologic studies could be used only for generating hypotheses, not in proving links.[22] Ecologic studies are considered prone to overlook confounding factors that more likely explain the correlations identified. The ecologic approach has been held in low regard for many years partly because seemingly well-designed cohort studies could not confirm the findings of the ecologic studies.[87] However, when overall dietary patterns were considered, the cohort studies identified that the Western diet was associated with colorectal cancer risk.[88] A case-control study found meat directly correlated and fish inversely correlated with breast cancer incidence.[89] The vegetable to meat consumption ratio was a relevant factor in cancer studies.[90] Thus, systematic problems with the cohort studies may sometimes be used to downplay ecologic study results. One limitation is that many of those in the cohort have similar dietary patterns. This effect was recently highlighted in the Women's Health Initiative study of a "low-fat diet" and risk of colorectal cancer; the low-fat diet had the women consuming about 30%-32% of their energy in the form of fat compared with 40% in the control group or at the start of the study;[91] no significant risk reduction was found.

Another way to judge the effectiveness of ecologic studies is to look for ecologic studies that first identified the link between a risk factor and a disease. Some examples from my work include the first study to link dietary factors to risk of Alzheimer's disease (total fat and total energy as risk factors, fish and cereals/grains as risk reduction factors),[28] sugar as a risk factor for coronary heart disease for women,[29] meat as a risk factor for the expression of rheumatoid arthritis,[31] and the addition of nine cancers to the list of UVB/vitamin D-sensitive cancers.[34] All these findings have been well supported in subsequent observational studies.

Yet another way to judge the validity of a hypothesis or theory is to examine whether predictions based on the model can be verified. There are several ways this has been done for the UVB/vitamin D/cancer theory:

- Determining whether oral vitamin D reduced the risk of cancer. This prediction was satisfied for colorectal cancer[7,25,26] and breast cancer.[95]

- Determining whether serum calcidiol is inversely correlated with cancer risk, which it is.[8]
- Determining whether cancer rates correlate inversely with indices for solar UVB irradiance in individual countries. This assertion has been found true for Japan,[92] Australia,[44] Norway,[45] Spain,[56] China [Grant, submitted] and France [Grant, submitted].

Criteria for Causality

Hill laid out causality criteria for a biological system in his Presidential Address to the Royal Medical Society in 1965.[93] They were based on those postulated by Robert Koch in 1882, which Koch had used to help justify his finding that a bacterium caused tuberculosis.[94] Criteria are useful because cause-effect relations in biology do not generally have tight equations as they do for physics and engineering.

The primary criteria for diseases such as cancer are strength of association, reproducibility in different populations, a generally linear dose-response relation, identification of mechanisms, accounting for confounding factors and experimental verification.

Strength of Association

Strong inverse correlations have been found for many cancers with respect to solar UVB doses or irradiances (Tables 1 and 2).

Reproducibility

The ecologic study results have been repeated in many populations and under many different conditions, as indicated in Tables 1 and 2. Some earlier studies on dietary vitamin D or serum calcidiol failed to find a significant effect on cancer risk reduction because the amounts considered in the study were generally too low, often because the contributions from solar UVB irradiance were overlooked.[38] However, there are some puzzling results in the literature, such as for pancreatic cancer. The data from two cohorts in the United States found a statistically significant risk reduction with respect to dietary vitamin D.[96] However, a study of male Finnish smokers found that higher prediagnostic serum calcidiol was associated with a threefold increased risk of pancreatic cancer.[97]

Dose-Response Relation

Dose-response relations are generally linear, although there may be some saturation at the higher doses.[34] Meta-analyses of studies of oral intake of vitamin D and serum calcidiol have estimated the dose-response relations for colorectal cancer, with 1,000-1,500 IU/day required for a 50% reduction[25,26] and breast cancer (4,000 IU/day for a 50% reduction).[95] Giovannucci et al[98] estimated that 1,500 IU/day would reduce male cancer mortality rate by 29%.

However, several studies have questioned the dose-response relation for prostate cancer. The most recent, one in the Nordic countries,[99] found that both low and high levels of serum calcidiol were associated with increased risk for prostate cancer. This finding is still being investigated.

Mechanisms

The well-known mechanisms whereby vitamin D reduces the risk of cancer include increased cellular differentiation and apoptosis, increased calcium absorption, attenuation of growth signals, reduced angiogenesis around tumors and reduced metastasis.[100-102]

Accounting for Confounding Factors

Recent studies of solar UVB and cancer mortality rates have included several other risk-modifying factors such as smoking, alcohol consumption, ethnic background,[37,38] and diet.[67,77,78]

Experimental Verification

Lack of experimental verification in a prospective double-blind, randomized, placebo-controlled study is the primary weakness in linking solar UVB and vitamin D to cancer risk reduction. The health systems used to qualify synthetic pharmaceutical drugs for disease treatment and generally require such a study showing effectiveness before drugs can be marketed. There has been at least one prospective double-blind study on vitamin D plus calcium supplementation and colorectal adenoma, a precursor to colorectal cancer,[103] which found a beneficial effect of the two substances combined. The largest related trial to date, the Women's Health Initiative study,[104] had the participants take only 400 IU of vitamin D3/day and found no effect on risk of either colon cancer or hip fracture rate. This amount was too low to have a pronounced effect. However, those women with higher oral intake of vitamin D before starting the study had a 40% reduced colorectal cancer risk.[105]

In summary, the UVB/vitamin D/cancer theory generally satisfies the criteria for causality, lacking only a well-designed and conducted double-blind study. I believe that such a study would readily provide the desired experimental verification.

Other Diseases for Which Solar UVB and Vitamin D Are Beneficial/Protective

Although solar UVB and vitamin D are hot topics in cancer risk reduction, these factors are also beneficial for other problems, including bone conditions and diseases, muscles and neuromuscular control, autoimmune diseases and infectious diseases. Table 3 summarizes these conditions and diseases and the strength of the evidence for the beneficial effect of solar UVB and/or vitamin D. There are also several recent reviews on the health benefits of vitamin D.[122-129]

Summary and Conclusion

Evidence supporting the UVB/vitamin D/cancer theory continues to mount with little detraction, although there are some inconsistent results, such as some from Nordic countries, with respect to serum calcidiol levels. Also, studies designed and conducted before it was realized that dietary sources are largely inadequate to have a pronounced effect on cancer risk were largely unable to confirm a beneficial role for vitamin D in reducing the risk of cancer.[24]

The analysis of the economic burden of solar UVB irradiance and vitamin D deficiencies compared to excess solar UV irradiance for the United States yielded interesting findings. One was that the US economic burden due to vitamin D insufficiency from inadequate exposure to solar UVB irradiance, diet and supplements was estimated at $40 billion to $56 billion in 2004, whereas the economic burden for excess UV irradiance was estimated at $6 billion to $7 billion.[130] These findings are probably still approximately correct, if not on the low side, with respect to vitamin D because of the additional benefits found recently, such as protection against infectious diseases.

Table 3. Conditions and diseases for which solar UVB and/or vitamin D are beneficial

Condition or Disease	Hypothesis	Latitudinal Studies	Case-Control, Cohort Studies	Mechanisms
Bone health				107, 108
Muscle pain avoidance			109	
Hypertension		110		
Periodontal disease			111	
Parkinson's disease	112			
Multiple sclerosis		113, 114		115, 116
Type 1 diabetes mellitus		117	118	
HIV	119			
Influenza	120			

References

1. Peller S, Stephenson CS. Skin irritation and cancer in the United states Navy. Am J Med Sci 1937; 194:326-333.
2. Apperly FL. The relation of solar radiation to cancer mortality in North America. Cancer Res 1941; 1:191-5.
3. World Health Organization (WHO). WHO Mortality Database. http://www-dep.iarc.fr/ (accessed 2007).
4. Mason TJ, McKay FW, Hoover R et al. Atlas of Cancer Mortality for US Counties: 1950-69. US Dept. of Health, Education and Welfare. DHEW Pub. No. 75-780, 1975.
5. Garland CF, Garland FC. Do sunlight and vitamin D reduce the likelihood of colon cancer? Int J Epidemiol 1980; 9:227-31.
6. Lilienfeld AM, Levin ML, Kesler II. Cancer in the United States. Harvard Univ., Cambridge 1972:467-72.
7. Garland C, Shekelle RB, Barrett-Connor E et al. Dietary vitamin D and calcium and risk of colorectal cancer: a 19-year prospective study in men. Lancet 1985; 1:307-9.
8. Garland CF, Comstock GW, Garland FC et al. Serum 25-hydroxyvitamin D and colon cancer: eight-year prospective study. Lancet 1989; 2:1176-8.
9. Gorham ED, Garland CF, Garland FC. Acid haze air pollution and breast and colon cancer mortality in 20 Canadian cities. Can J Public Health 1989; 80:96-100.
10. Garland FC, Garland CF, Gorham ED et al. Geographic variation in breast cancer mortality in the United States: a hypothesis involving exposure to solar radiation. Prev Med 1990; 19:614-22.
11. Lefkowitz ES, Garland CF. Sunlight, vitamin D and ovarian cancer mortality rates in US women. Int J Epidemiol 1994; 23:1133-6.
12. Garland CF, Garland FC. Commentary: progress of a paradigm. Int J Epidemiol 2006; 35:220-2.
13. Garland CF, Garland FC. Do sunlight and vitamin D reduce the likelihood of colon cancer? Int J Epidemiol 2006; 35:217-20.
14. Cross HS. Commentary: from epidemiology to molecular biology—vitamin D and colorectal cancer prevention. Int J Epidemiol 2006; 35:225-7.
15. Egan KM. Commentary: sunlight, vitamin D and the cancer connection revisited. Int J Epidemiol 2006; 35:227-30.
16. Giovannucci E. Commentary: vitamin D and colorectal cancer—twenty-five years later. Int J Epidemiol 2006; 35:222-4.
17. Grant WB, Gorham ED. Commentary: time for public health action on vitamin D for cancer risk reduction. Int J Epidemiol 2006; 35:224-5.
18. Kricker A, Armstrong B. Does sunlight have a beneficial influence on certain cancers? Prog Biophys Mol Biol 2006; 92:132-9.
19. Schwartz GG, Hulka BS. Is vitamin D deficiency a risk factor for prostate cancer? (Hypothesis). Anticancer Res 1990; 10:1307-11.
20. Hanchette CL, Schwartz GG. Geographic patterns of prostate cancer mortality. Evidence for a protective effect of ultraviolet radiation. Cancer 1992; 70:2861-9.
21. Freedman DM, Zahm SH, Dosemeci M. Residential and occupational exposure to sunlight and mortality from nonHodgkin's lymphoma: composite (threefold) case-control study. BMJ 1997; 314:1451-5.
22. Doll R, Peto R. The causes of cancer: quantitative estimates of avoidable risks of cancer in the United States today. J Natl Cancer Inst 1981; 66:1191-308.
23. Calvo MS, Whiting SJ, Barton CN. Vitamin D fortification in the United States and Canada: current status and data needs. Am J Clin Nutr 2004; 80:1710S-6S.
24. Grant WB, Garland CF. A critical review of studies on vitamin D in relation to colorectal cancer. Nutr Cancer 2004; 48:115-23.
25. Gorham ED, Garland CF, Garland FC et al. Vitamin D and prevention of colorectal cancer. J Steroid Biochem Mol Biol 2005; 97:179-94.
26. Gorham ED, Garland CF, Garland FC et al. Optimal vitamin D status for colorectal cancer prevention a quantitative meta analysis. Am J Prev Med 2007; 32:210-6.
27. Houghton LA, Vieth R. The case against ergocalciferol (vitamin D2) as a vitamin supplement. Am J Clin Nutr 2006; 84:694-7.
28. Grant WB. Dietary links to Alzheimer's disease. Alz Dis Rev 1997; 2:42-55 (http://www.sunarc.org/JAD97.pdf)
29. Grant WB. Milk and other dietary influences on coronary heart disease. Altern Med Rev 1998; 3:281-94.
30. Grant WB. An ecologic study of dietary links to prostate cancer. Altern Med Rev 1999; 4:162-169.
31. Grant WB. The role of meat in the expression of rheumatoid arthritis. Brit J Nutr 2000; 85:589-95.

32. Devesa SS, Grauman DJ, Blot WJ et al. Atlas of Cancer Mortality in the United States, 1950-1994. NIH Publication 99-4564, 1999. http://cancer.gov/atlasplus/new.html (accessed 2007).
33. Leffell DJ, Brash DE. Sunlight and skin cancer. Sci Am 1996; 275:52-3, 56-9. http://toms.gsfc.nasa.gov/ery_uv/dna_exp.gif (accessed 2007).
34. Grant WB. An estimate of premature cancer mortality in the US due to inadequate doses of solar ultraviolet-B radiation. Cancer 2002; 94:1867-75.
35. Freedman DM, Dosemeci M, McGlynn K. Sunlight and mortality from breast, ovarian, colon, prostate and nonmelanoma skin cancer: a composite death certificate based case-control study. Occup Environ Med 2002; 59:257-62.
36. Leistikow B. Lung cancer rates as an index of tobacco smoke exposures: validation against black male approximate nonlung cancer death rates, 1969-2000. Prev Med 2004; 38:511-5.
37. Grant WB. Lower vitamin-D production from solar ultraviolet-B irradiance may explain some differences in cancer survival rates. J Natl Med Assoc 2006; 98:357-64.
38. Grant WB, Garland CF. The association of solar ultraviolet B (UVB) with reducing risk of cancer: multifactorial ecologic analysis of geographic variation in age-adjusted cancer mortality rates. Anticancer Res 2006; 26:2687-99.
39. Boscoe FP, Schymura MJ. Solar ultraviolet-B exposure and cancer incidence and mortality in the United States, 1993-2000. BMC Cancer 2006; 6:264.
40. North American Association of Central Cancer Registries: SEER*Stat Database: NAACCR Incidence—CiNA Analytic File, 1995-2002, NHIA Origin, Boscoe—Solar Radiation (project-specific file). Springfield, IL: North American Association of Central Cancer Registries, 2005.
41. Surveillance Epidemiology and End Results (SEER) Program: SEER*Stat Database: Mortality—All COD, Public-Use With County, Total US (1969-2002). [http://www.seer.cancer.gov] Bethesda, MD: National Cancer Institute, DCCPS, Surveillance Research Program, Cancer Statistics Branch, 2005.
42. National Center for Health Statistics. Plan and Operation of the Third National Health and Nutrition Survey, 1988-1994. National Center for Health Statistics, Hyattsville, MD. Vital Health Stat, 1994; 32:1-407.
43. Hajjar I, Kotchen T. Regional variations of blood pressure in the United States are associated with regional variations in dietary intakes: the NHANES-III data. J Nutr 2003; 133:211-4.
44. Hughes AM, Armstrong BK, Vajdic CM et al. Sun exposure may protect against nonHodgkin lymphoma: a case-control study. Int J Cancer 2004; 112:865-71.
45. Smedby KE, Hjalgrim H, Melbye M et al. Ultraviolet radiation exposure and risk of malignant lymphomas. J Natl Cancer Inst 2005; 97:199-209.
46. Zhang Y, Holford TR, Leaderer B et al. Ultraviolet Radiation Exposure and Risk of nonHodgkin's Lymphoma. Am J Epidemiol 2007 [Epub ahead of print].
47. Garland CF, Garland FC, Gorham ED et al. The role of vitamin D in cancer prevention. Am J Public Health 2006; 96:252-61.
48. Grant WB. Epidemiology of disease risks in relation to vitamin D insufficiency. Prog Biophys Mol Biol 2006; 92:65-79.
49. Kricker A, Armstrong B. Does sunlight have a beneficial influence on certain cancers? Prog Biophys Mol Biol 2006; 92:132-9.
50. van der Rhee HJ, de Vries E, Coebergh JW. Does sunlight prevent cancer? A systematic review. Eur J Cancer 2006; 42:2222-32.
51. Krause R, Matulla-Nolte B, Essers M et al. UV radiation and cancer prevention: what is the evidence? Anticancer Res 2006; 26:2723-7.
52. Kimlin MG, Olds WJ, Moore MR. Location and Vitamin D synthesis: Is the hypothesis validated by geophysical data? J Photochem Photobiol B 2007; 86:234-9.
53. Samanek AJ, Croager EJ, Gies P et al. Estimates of beneficial and harmful sun exposure times during the year for major Australian population centres. Med J Aust 2006; 184:338-41.
54. Lewis KG, Weinstock MA. Nonmelanoma skin cancer mortality (1988-2000): the Rhode Island follow-back study. Arch Dermatol 2004; 140:837-42.
55. Kennedy C, Bajdik CD, Willemze R et al. Leiden Skin Cancer Study. The influence of painful sunburns and lifetime sun exposure on the risk of actinic keratoses, seborrheic warts, melanocytic nevi, atypical nevi and skin cancer. J Invest Dermatol 2003; 120:1087-93.
56. Grant WB. An ecologic study of cancer mortality rates in Spain with respect to indices of solar UV irradiance and smoking. Int J Cancer 2007; 120:1123-7.
57. Jablonski NG, Chaplin G. The evolution of human skin coloration. J Hum Evol 2000; 39:57-106.
58. Milan T, Verkasalo PK, Kaprio J et al. Lifestyle differences in twin pairs discordant for basal cell carcinoma of the skin. Br J Dermatol 2003; 149:115-23.
59. De Hertog SA, Wensveen CA, Bastiaens MT et al. Relation between smoking and skin cancer. J Clin Oncol 2001; 19:231-8.

60. Freedman DM, Sigurdson A, Doody MM et al. Risk of melanoma in relation to smoking, alcohol intake and other factors in a large occupational cohort. Cancer Causes Control 2003; 14:847-57.
61. Odenbro A, Gillgren P, Bellocco R et al. The risk for cutaneous malignant melanoma, melanoma in situ and intraocular malignant melanoma in relation to tobacco use and body mass index. Br J Dermatol 2007; 156:99-105.
62. Grant WB. A meta-analysis of second cancers after a diagnosis of nonmelanoma skin cancer: additional evidence that solar ultraviolet-B irradiance reduces the risk of internal cancers. J Steroid Biochem Mol 2007;103:668-74.
63. de Vries E, Soerjomataram I, Houterman S et al. Decreased Risk of Prostate Cancer after Skin Cancer Diagnosis: A Protective Role of Ultraviolet Radiation? Am J Epidemiol 2007;165: 966-72.
64. Rukin NJ, Zeegers MP, Ramachandran S et al. A comparison of sunlight exposure in men with prostate cancer and basal cell carcinoma. Br J Cancer 2007; 96:523-8.
65. Armstrong B, Doll R. Environmental factors and cancer incidence and mortality in different countries, with special reference to dietary practices. Int J Cancer 1975; 15:617-31.
66. Grant WB. An ecologic study of the role of solar UV-B radiation in reducing the risk of cancer using cancer mortality data, dietary supply data and latitude for European countries, In; Holick MF, ed. Biologic Effects of Light 2001, Proceedings of the Biologic Effects of Light Symposium, Boston, USA, Massachusetts, 2001, 2002:267-76.
67. Grant WB. Ecologic studies of solar UV-B radiation and cancer mortality rates. Recent Results Cancer Res 2003; 164:371-7.
68. Lebert M, Schuster M, Hader DP. The European Light Dosimeter Network: four years of measurements. J Photochem Photobiol B 2002; 66:81-7.
69. Food and Agriculture Organization (FAO) of the United Nations. Food Balance Sheets, 1992-94 Average. FAO, Rome, 1996.
70. Harashima E, Nakagawa Y, Urata G et al. Time-lag estimate between dietary intake and breast cancer mortality in Japan. Asia Pac J Clin Nutr 2007; 16:193-198.
71. Tylavsky FA, Cheng S, Lyytikainen A et al. Strategies to improve vitamin D status in northern European children: exploring the merits of vitamin D fortification and supplementation. J Nutr 2006; 136:1130-4.
72. Grant WB. An ecologic study of dietary and solar ultraviolet-B links to breast carcinoma mortality rates. Cancer 2002; 94:272-81.
73. Grant WB. A multicountry ecologic study of risk and risk reduction factors for prostate cancer mortality. Eur Urol 2004; 45:371-9.
74. European Space Agency. Erythemal UV Index-Yearly average (2000). Tropospheric Emission Monitoring Internet Service. http://www.temis.nl/uvradiation/GOME/ (accessed 2007).
75. Colli JL, Colli A. International comparisons of prostate cancer mortality rates with dietary practices and sunlight levels. Urol Oncol 2006; 24:184-94.
76. Ferlay J, Bray F, Pisani P et al. GLOBOCAN 2002: Cancer Incidence, Mortality and Prevalence Worldwide IARC CancerBase No. 5. version 2.0, IARCPress, Lyon, 2004. http://www-dep.iarc.fr/ (accessed 2007).
77. Grant WB. The likely role of vitamin D from solar ultraviolet-B irradiance in increasing cancer survival. Anticancer Res 2006; 26:2605-14.
78. Mohr SB, Gorham ED, Garland CF et al. Are low ultraviolet B and high animal protein intake associated with risk of renal cancer? Int J Cancer 2006; 119:2705-9.
79. Garland CF, Mohr SB, Gorham ED et al. Role of ultraviolet-B irradiance and vitamin D in the prevention of ovarian cancer. Am J Prev Med 2006; 31:512-4.
80. Garland CF, Garland FC, Gorham ED. Rising trends in melanoma. An hypothesis concerning sunscreen effectiveness. Ann Epidemiol 1993; 3:103-10.
81. Diffey BL. Sunscreens and melanoma: the future looks bright. Br J Dermatol 2005; 153:378-81.
82. Moan J, Dahlback A, Setlow RB. Epidemiological support for an hypothesis for melanoma induction indicating a role for UVA radiation. Photochem Photobiol 1999; 70:243-7.
83. Osborne JE, Hutchinson PE. Vitamin D and systemic cancer: is this relevant to malignant melanoma? Br J Dermatol 2002; 147:197-213.
84. Garland CF, Garland FC, Gorham ED. Epidemiologic evidence for different roles of ultraviolet A and B radiation in melanoma mortality rates. Ann Epidemiol 2003; 13:395-404.
85. Millen AE, Tucker MA, Hartge P et al. Diet and melanoma in a case-control study. Cancer Epidemiol Biomarkers Prev 2004; 13:1042-51.
86. Newsom SW. Pioneers in infection control: John Snow, Henry Whitehead, the Broad Street pump and the beginnings of geographical epidemiology. J Hosp Infect 2006; 64:210-6.
87. Willett WC. Dietary fat intake and cancer risk: a controversial and instructive story. Semin Cancer Biol 1998; 8:245-53.

88. Fung T, Hu FB, Fuchs C et al. Major dietary patterns and the risk of colorectal cancer in women. Arch Intern Med 2003; 163:309-14.
89. Shannon J, Cook LS, Stanford JL. Dietary intake and risk of postmenopausal breast cancer (United States). Cancer Causes Control 2003; 14:19-27.
90. Kapiszewska M. A vegetable to meat consumption ratio as a relevant factor determining cancer preventive diet. The Mediterranean versus other European countries. Forum Nutr 2006; 59:130-53.
91. Beresford SA, Johnson KC, Ritenbaugh C et al. Low-fat dietary pattern and risk of colorectal cancer: the Women's Health Initiative Randomized Controlled Dietary Modification Trial. JAMA 2006; 295:643-54.
92. Mizoue T. Ecological study of solar radiation and cancer mortality in Japan. Health Phys 2004; 87:532-8.
93. Hill AB. The environment and disease: association or causation? Proc R Soc Med 1965; 58:295-300.
94. Koch R. Classics in infectious diseases. The etiology of tuberculosis: Robert Koch. Berlin, Germany 1882. Rev Infect Dis 1982; 4:1270-4.
95. Garland CF, Gorham ED, Mohr SB et al. Vitamin D and prevention of breast cancer: Pooled analysis. J Steoid Biochem Mol Biol. 2007; 103:708-11.
96. Skinner HG, Michaud DS, Giovannucci E et al. Vitamin D intake and the risk of pancreatic cancer in two cohort studies. Cancer Epidemiol Biomarkers Prevention 2006; 15:1688-95.
97. Stolzenberg-Solomon RZ, Vieth R, Azad A et al. A prospective nested case-control study of vitamin d status and pancreatic cancer risk in male smokers. Cancer Res 2006; 66:10213-9.
98. Giovannucci E, Liu Y, Rimm EB et al. Prospective study of predictors of vitamin D status and cancer incidence and mortality in men. JNCI 2006; 98:451-9.
99. Tuohimaa P, Tenkanen L, Ahonen M et al. Both high and low levels of blood vitamin D are associated with a higher prostate cancer risk: a longitudinal, nested case-control study in the Nordic countries. Int J Cancer 2004; 108:104-8.
100. van den Bemd GJ, Chang GT. Vitamin D and vitamin D analogs in cancer treatment. Curr Drug Targets 2002; 3:85-94.
101. Krishnan AV, Peehl DM, Feldman D. Inhibition of prostate cancer growth by vitamin D: Regulation of target gene expression. J Cell Biochem 2003; 88:363-71.
102. Lamprecht SA, Lipkin M. Chemoprevention of colon cancer by calcium, vitamin D and folate: molecular mechanisms. Nat Rev Cancer 2003; 3:601-14.
103. Grau MV, Baron JA, Sandler RS et al. Vitamin D, calcium supplementation and colorectal adenomas: results of a randomized trial. J Natl Cancer Inst 2003; 95:1765-71.
104. Wactawski-Wende J, Kotchen JM, Anderson GL et al. Calcium plus vitamin D supplementation and the risk of colorectal cancer. N Engl J Med 2006; 354:684-96.
105. Holick MF. Calcium plus vitamin D and the risk of colorectal cancer. N Engl J Med 2006; 354:2287-8; author reply 2287-8.
106. Holick MF. The role of vitamin D for bone health and fracture prevention. Curr 107. Osteoporos Rep 2006; 4:96-102.
108. Heaney RP. Bone health. Am J Clin Nutr 2007; 85:300S-3S.
109. Plotnikoff GA, Quigley JM. Prevalence of severe hypovitaminosis D in patients with persistent, nonspecific musculoskeletal pain. Mayo Clin Proc 2003; 78:1463-70.
110. Rostand SG. Ultraviolet light may contribute to geographic and racial blood pressure differences. Hypertension 1997; 30:150-6.
111. Dietrich T, Joshipura KJ, Dawson-Hughes B et al. Association between serum concentrations of 25-hydroxyvitamin D3 and periodontal disease in the US population. Am J Clin Nutr 2004; 80:108-13.
112. Newmark HL, Newmark J. Vitamin D and Parkinson's disease-A hypothesis. Mov Disord 2007 [Epub ahead of print].
113. Kurtzke JF, Beebe GW, Norman JE Jr. Epidemiology of multiple sclerosis in US veterans: 1. Race, sex and geographic distribution. Neurology 1979; 29:1228-35.
114. van der Mei IA, Ponsonby AL, Blizzard L et al. Regional variation in multiple sclerosis prevalence in Australia and its association with ambient ultraviolet radiation. Neuroepidemiology 2001; 20:168-74.
115. Cantorna MT, Mahon BD. Mounting evidence for vitamin D as an environmental factor affecting autoimmune disease prevalence. Exp Biol Med (Maywood) 2004; 229:1136-42.
116. Cantorna MT. Vitamin D and its role in immunology: multiple sclerosis and inflammatory bowel disease. Prog Biophys Mol Biol 2006; 92:60-4.
117. Staples JA, Ponsonby AL, Lim LL et al. Ecologic analysis of some immune-related disorders, including type 1 diabetes, in Australia: latitude, regional ultraviolet radiation and disease prevalence. Environ Health Perspect 2003; 111:518-23.
118. Hypponen E, Laara E, Reunanen A et al. Intake of vitamin D and risk of type 1 diabetes: a birth-cohort study. Lancet 2001; 358:1500-3.

119. Villamor E. A potential role for vitamin D on HIV infection? Nutr Rev 2006; 64:226-33.
120. Cannell JJ, Vieth R, Umhau JC et al. Epidemic influenza and vitamin D. Epidemiol Infect 2006;
     134:1129-40.
121. Yu GP, Hu DN, McCormick SA. Latitude and Incidence of Ocular Melanoma. Photochem Photobiol
     2006; 82:1621-6.
122. Zittermann A. Vitamin D in preventive medicine: are we ignoring the evidence? Br J Nutr 2003;
     89:552-72.
123. Holick MF. Vitamin D: importance in the prevention of cancers, type 1 diabetes, heart disease and
     osteoporosis. Am J Clin Nutr 2004; 79:362-71.
124. Peterlik M, Cross HS. Vitamin D and calcium deficits predispose for multiple chronic diseases. Eur J
     Clin Invest 2005; 35:290-304.
125. Grant WB, Holick MF. Benefits and requirements of vitamin D for optimal health: a review. Altern
     Med Rev 2005; 10:94-111.
126. Zittermann A, Schleithoff SS, Koerfer R. Putting cardiovascular disease and vitamin D insufficiency into
     perspective. Br J Nutr 2005; 94:483-92.
127. Holick MF. High prevalence of vitamin D inadequacy and implications for health. Mayo Clin Proc
     2006; 81:353-73.
128. Zittermann A. Vitamin D and disease prevention with special reference to cardiovascular disease. Prog
     Biophys Mol Biol 2006; 92:39-48.
129. Bouillon R, Eelen G, Verlinden L et al. Vitamin D and cancer. J Steroid Biochem Mol Biol 2006;
     102:156-62.
130. Grant WB, Garland CF, Holick MF. Comparisons of estimated economic burdens due to insufficient solar
     ultraviolet irradiance and vitamin D and excess solar UV irradiance for the United States. Photochem
     Photobiol 2005; 81:1276-86.

CHAPTER 3

Vitamin D Status and Cancer Incidence and Mortality

Edward Giovannucci*

Introduction

The role of excessive sun exposure in increasing risk of skin cancers is well established. Less known, less established and more controversial is the potential role of sun exposure in reducing risk of several types of internal cancers. The hypothesis that sunlight may be beneficial against several types of cancer extends back almost seven decades. Initially, Peller and Stephenson observed higher rates of skin cancer, but lower rates of other malignancies in United States Navy personnel in the 1930s.[1] Based on this observation, Peller and Stephenson hypothesized that acquiring skin cancer conferred immunity against other cancers. Several years later, Apperly observed an association between latitude and cancer mortality rate, which led him to state that "The presence of skin cancer is really an occasional accompaniment of a relative cancer immunity in some way related to the exposure to solar radiation".[2] However, no plausible mechanism was proffered and these observations were essentially ignored for about four decades. In 1980, Garland and colleagues hypothesized that the potential benefit of sun exposure was attributed to vitamin D.[3] Initially, the hypothesis was centered on colon cancer,[3] but later it was extended to breast cancer,[4] ovarian cancer,[5] prostate cancer,[6,7] and to multiple cancer types.[8]

When Garland and colleagues hypothesized a role of vitamin D, the hypothesis was premised on the fact that sun exposure increases vitamin D levels, but the varied actions of vitamin D were not well understood at the time. Subsequently, the potential benefit of vitamin D on cancer risk has received substantial experimental support. These laboratory studies have suggested the following model: many cells types, normal as well as neoplastic, express vitamin D receptors, express 1-α-hydroxylase which can convert 25(OH)D to the active 1,25(OH)$_2$D and activation of the vitamin D receptor induces a number of anti-cancer properties, including reduced proliferation, invasiveness, angiogenesis and metastatic potential and increased differentiation and apoptosis.[9] Such data suggest that autocrine or paracrine influences of 25(OH)D could potentially help retard cancer causation or progression in some tissues. If the 25(OH)D level is rate limiting for these actions, associations with indicators of vitamin D status and cancer incidence and mortality should be observable in human populations, depending on the dose-response relation and on the range of vitamin D status in the specific population considered.

Since Garland's initial hypothesis, a number of epidemiologic studies have generated evidence regarding the role of sun exposure or vitamin D on risk of various cancers. In these studies, the measurement of sun exposure is assumed to be a determinant of vitamin D status. The basis of this assumption is that the vast majority of vitamin D in most human populations is made through exposure to solar UV-B radiation. However, it is possible that sun exposure has other yet to be identified effects. Limited randomized trial data to test the vitamin D-cancer hypothesis are currently available. This chapter provides a review and synthesis of these studies, focusing on the

*Edward Giovannucci—Harvard School of Public Health and Brigham and Women's Hospital, Boston, MA 02115, U.S.A. Email: egiovann@hsph.harvard.edu

Sunlight, Vitamin D and Skin Cancer, edited by Jörg Reichrath. ©2008 Landes Bioscience and Springer Science+Business Media.

relative strengths and limitations of the various approaches that have been utilized to evaluate the relationship between vitamin D status and cancer occurrence or progression.

Ecologic Studies of Sun Exposure

Latitude or region UV-B radiation has been examined in relation to various cancers.[3-8,10] In general, lower incidence and mortality rates of various cancer have been noted in regions with greater solar UV-B exposure. For example, Grant showed that regional UV-B radiation in the United States correlated inversely with mortality rates of numerous cancers, especially for cancers of digestive organs.[8] In Grant's analysis, the strongest associations were observed for cancers of the colon and rectum; out of all the preventable cancers estimated attributable to living in a low sun area, 60% were due to colorectal cancer in men; in women, 35% were due to colorectal cancer and 42% were attributable to breast cancer. In total, at least 15 types of cancers have been correlated with low sun exposure.[11] Those of the colorectum and breast appear to be most important quantitatively.

An important limitation of these ecologic studies is that other potentially confounding factors related to regional differences in solar UV-B radiation could account for the associations; thus, a cause-effect association is not secure. However, corroborating evidence that an inverse association between regional solar UV-B exposure and cancer risk may be causal is that this association is observed in regions outside of the United States. Indeed, similar relationships have been observed in diverse populations such as in Japan for digestive organ cancers (esophagus, stomach, colon, rectum, pancreas and gallbladder and bile ducts)[10] and Spain.[12] Thus, a putative confounding factor would have to have similar relationships with regional solar UV-B exposure in diverse populations such as in the United, Spain and Japan. This possibility cannot be excluded, but appears somewhat remote.

The capability of region to act as a surrogate of solar UV-B radiation and vitamin D status is prone to a number of complexities. These include increasing urbanization over time and more time spent indoors, winter vacations to sunny climates and altered sun exposure behavior such as sun avoidance or use of sun-screen. These factors could vary among populations and could change over time within the same population. Of note, in a study in Spain,[12] the rates a number of cancers correlated inversely with rates of nonmelanoma skin cancer. This finding confirms that region is a good surrogate of actual UV-B exposure, at least in some circumstances, because rates of nonmelanoma skin cancer (especially squamous cell cancer) are very likely associated with cumulative sun exposure. A potential strength of ecologic studies is that they may provide some indication of sun exposure during childhood and adolescence; such an assessment may be difficult in typical cancer cohort or case-control studies, which are usually conducted in adulthood. Even cancers that are diagnosed in middle-aged or elderly individuals may have been initiated during childhood.

Case-Control and Cohort Studies of Sun Exposure

Ecologic data examine hypotheses at the population level. Case-control and cohort studies, called analytic epidemiologic studies, assess exposure and outcome at the individual level. In principle, confounding may be better controlled because typically more detailed information can be assessed on other covariates in analytic studies. In addition, the study population may be relatively homogenous, which may reduce the potential for residual or uncontrolled confounding that may not be captured by multivariate analysis. An additional strength of such studies is that exposure is actually assessed for the individual, whereas in ecologic studies exposure is inferred—for example, presumably living in sunnier regions may allow for greater opportunity for sun exposure, but actual exposure will depend on the individuals' behaviors. Because the strengths and potential limitations of ecologic and analytic epidemiologic studies differ, these two sources of data can be considered complementary.

Several case-control and cohort studies have assessed surrogates of sun exposure in relation to cancer risk. Prostate cancer appears to be the most studied cancer through this method. In a cohort study of 3414 white men, among whom 153 developed prostate cancer based on NHANES I data, residence in the South at baseline (relative risk (RR) = 0.68), state of longest residence in the South (RR = 0.62) and high solar radiation in the state of birth (RR = 0.49) were associated with significant reductions in prostate cancer risk.[13] In a recent population-based cohort study conducted in the Netherlands, male skin cancer patients diagnosed since 1970 (2,620 squamous cell carcinomas, 9,501 basal cell carcinomas and 1,420 cutaneous malignant melanomas) were followed up for incidence of invasive prostate cancer until 2005.[14] Skin cancer patients had an 11% reduction in total prostate cancer and a 27% reduction in advanced prostate cancer relative to expected population rates. The reduction was especially seen in patients with skin cancers that were located in the chronically ultraviolet radiation-exposed head and neck area.

An innovative approach has been to use a reflectometer to measure constitutive skin pigmentation on the upper underarm (a sun-protected site) and facultative pigmentation on the forehead (a sun-exposed site) to calculate a sun exposure index.[15] The difference between facultative skin pigmentation and constitutive pigmentation is a function of overall sun exposure, at least on the forehead. This measurement predicted risk of advanced prostate cancer in a case-control study. Specifically, a reduced risk of advanced prostate cancer was associated with high sun exposure determined by reflectometry (RR = 0.51) and high occupational outdoor activity level (RR = 0.73). Others have used factors such as childhood sunburns, holidays in a hot climate and skin type in case-control studies to predict prostate cancer risk. In a study in the United Kingdom, subgroups stratified by childhood sunburns, holidays in a hot climate and skin type displayed a remarkable 13-fold gradient in prostate cancer risk across extremes of sun and skin type exposure.[16,17]

Freedman et al[18] conducted a large death certificate based case-control study of mortality from five cancers: female breast, ovarian, colon, prostate and nonmelanoma skin cancer as a positive control to examine associations with residential and occupational exposure to sunlight. The cases consisted of all deaths from these cancers between 1984 and 1995 in 24 states of the United States. The controls were age frequency matched to a series of cases and excluded deaths from cancer and certain neurological diseases because of possible relationships with sun exposure. The investigators found that residential exposure to sunlight was inversely associated with mortality from female breast, ovarian, prostate and colon cancer. However, only female breast and colon cancer also were significantly inversely associated with jobs with the highest occupational exposure to sunlight (RR = 0.82 for breast cancer and RR = 0.90 for colon cancer). For both of these cancers, the inverse association with occupational sunlight was greatest in the geographical region of highest exposure to sunlight. Also, these associations were independent of occupational physical activity level. Nonmelanoma skin cancer, acting as a "positive control", was positively associated with both residential and occupational sunlight.

In the Health Professionals Follow-Up Study, men living in the northeastern and mid-Atlantic states had a statistically significant 24% higher rate of cancers of the digestive system compared to those living in the southern states.[19] This result was adjusted for multiple cancer risk factors, including age, tobacco use, body weight, physical activity, various dietary factors and alcohol. In a sample of the cohort, men living in these states were shown to have lower levels of 25(OH)D by 6.4 nmol/L compared to men living in the South. In a United States population-based case-control study of colon cancer limited to Northern California, Utah and Minnesota, estimated sun exposure by residence was only weakly and non-significantly associated with a reduced cancer risk (RR = 0.9).[20]

Prospective Studies of Circulating 25(OH)vitamin D and Cancer Risk

A relatively small number of studies have examined plasma or serum 25(OH) level in relation to cancer risk, especially for colorectal cancer and for prostate cancer. The circulating 25(OH)D level accounts not only for skin exposure to UV-B radiation, but also for total vitamin D intake and for factors such as skin pigmentation that all affect vitamin D status. 25(OH)D has a relatively long half-life ($t_{1/2}$) in the circulation of about 2-3 weeks and thus can provide a fairly good albeit imperfect indicator of long-term vitamin D status. For example, in one study of middle-aged to elderly men, the correlation of two 25(OH)D measures approximately three years apart was 0.7[21] In epidemiologic studies, circulating 25(OH)D has typically been based on a measure in archived blood samples in a nested case-control study. Because the sample is taken before the diagnosis of cancer, in some cases over a decade before, it is unlikely that any association observed is spuriously due to the cancer influencing the blood level, a phenomenon referred to as reverse causation. Several studies have been based on the measurement of 25(OH)D in individuals already diagnosed with cancer; these studies need to be interpreted very cautiously because of the potential for the phenomenon of reverse causation. Results for studies of colorectal cancer, prostate cancer and breast cancer are briefly reviewed here.

Studies that have examined 25(OH)D levels prospectively in relation to risk of colorectal cancer or adenoma have generally supported an inverse association.[22-29] In a recent systematic review of the colorectal cancer studies, individuals with ≥33 ng/mL (82 nmol/L) serum 25-hydroxyvitamin D had 50% lower incidence of colorectal cancer ($p < 0.01$) compared to those with relatively low values of less than or equal to 12 ng/mL (30 nmol/L).[30] The total number of colorectal cancer cases was 535. The two largest studies were based on the Nurses' Health Study (NHS) and the Women's Health Initiative (WHI) In the NHS,[24] the multivariable RR, controlling for the known risk factors for colorectal cancer, decreased monotonically across quintiles of plasma 25(OH)D concentration, with an RR of about 0.5 for those with the highest compared to the lowest levels of 25(OH)D. In the WHI, a similar inverse association was observed between baseline 25(OH)D level and colorectal cancer risk. The WHI was primarily a randomized placebo-controlled trial of 400 IU vitamin D plus 1,000 mg a day of calcium in 36,282 postmenopausal women; however, as discussed below, the interventional component of this study did not support a protective role of vitamin D intake.[29] A similar reduced risk of colorectal cancer has been confirmed in the Health Professionals Follow-Up Study (submitted manuscript). Thus, based on multiple studies of circulating 25(OH)D and colorectal cancer risk, individuals in the high quartile or quintile of 25(OH)D had about half the risk of colorectal cancer as did those in the lowest group. The dose-response appears fairly linear up to a 25(OH)D level of at least 35-40 ng/mL and controlling for multiple covariates have had little influence on the findings.

Although ecologic studies of regional UV-B exposure and of sun exposure in case-control studies tend to support an association for sun exposure and prostate cancer risk, higher 25(OH)D level has not been clearly associated with a reduced risk for prostate, although some of the studies suggest weak inverse associations.[31-36] In addition, four studies that have evaluated dietary or supplemental vitamin D have not found substantial protection for prostate cancer.[37-40] Only two studies,[41,42] which were conducted in Nordic countries, supported an inverse association for 25(OH)D. However, one of these studies also found an increased risk in men with the highest 25(OH)D values.[42] Although $1,25(OH)_2D$ that is produced intracellularly is believed to be more important than circulating $1,25(OH)_2D$, several studies found supportive[32] or suggestive[33] inverse associations for circulating 25(OH)D and aggressive prostate cancer, particularly in older men. With further follow-up in the Physicians' Health Study, men with both low 25(OH)D and $1,25(OH)_2D$ were at higher risk of aggressive prostate cancer (RR = 1.9).[43] In the Health Professionals Follow-up Study, both lower 25(OH)D and $1,25(OH)_2D$ appeared to be associated surprisingly with lower (mostly early stage) prostate cancer risk[35] but possibly with higher risk of advanced prostate cancer, although numbers of advanced cases were limited (n = 60).[35] Thus, overall the studies of circulating 25(OH)D have been equivocal for prostate cancer; the association has not been as clear as that for colorectal cancer.

In one study, breast cancer cases had lower 25(OH)D levels than did controls.[44] Another study found that serum levels of 25(OH)D were significantly higher in patients with early-stage breast cancer than in women with locally advanced or metastatic disease.[45] However, the possibility of reverse causation cannot be ruled out in these two studies because 25(OH)D levels were assessed in women who already had breast cancer. In the Nurses' Health Study, stored plasma samples were assessed in 701 breast cancer cases and 724 controls.[46] Cases had a lower mean 25(OH)D level than controls (P = 0.01) and women in the highest quintile of 25(OH)D had a RR of 0.73 (P trend = 0.06) compared with those in the lowest quintile. The association was stronger in women ages

60 years and older, suggesting that vitamin D may be more important for postmenopausal breast cancer. There have been no other prospective studies of 25(OH)D level and breast cancer risk.

There is one report of a prospective study of serum 25(OH)D in relation to pancreatic cancer risk. This study was based on the Finnish Alpha-Tocopherol, Beta-Carotene Cancer Prevention cohort of male Finnish smokers.[47] Contrary to expectation, this study found a significant positive association between higher 25(OH)D levels and increased risk of pancreatic cancer. This association persisted in multivariate analysis and after excluding cases early in follow-up (to avoid reverse causation).

One analysis based on the Health Professionals Follow-up Study used a surrogate of 25(OH)D to examine risk of total cancer.[19] The analysis was based on a two-stage approach. First, in a sample of 1,095 men in this cohort circulating 25(OH)D levels were measured. Then, geographical region, skin pigmentation, dietary intake, supplement intake, body mass index and leisure-time physical activity (a surrogate of potential exposure to sunlight UV-B) were used to develop a predicted 25(OH)D score using multiple linear regression. This score can be interpreted as an estimate of 25(OH)D level. Secondly, the score was calculated for each of approximately 47,000 cohort members and then this variable was examined in relation to subsequent risk of cancer incidence and mortality using multivariate analysis. In the cohort analysis, a 25 nmol/L increment in predicted 25(OH)D was associated with a 17% reduction in total cancer incidence and an even greater 29% reduction in total cancer mortality. Additionally, digestive cancers (colorectal, pancreatic, stomach and esophageal cancers) were considered as a group, as these had been considered a priori to be most likely to be "vitamin D sensitive" based on ecologic geographic data in the United States and in Japan.[8,10] The risk reduction of total cancer incidence and mortality was largely though not solely due to a the reduction in digestive organ cancers; specifically, a 43% reduction in incidence and 45% reduction in mortality for these cancers was associated with a 25 nmol/L increment in 25(OH)D. A strong inverse association overall was also found for oral/pharyngeal cancers and for leukemias. Multivariate analysis of the major known risk factors for cancer risk had little influence on the findings.

The predicted 25(OH)D approach may have some advantages and disadvantages compared to the use of a single measurement of circulating 25(OH)D in epidemiologic studies. The measurement of 25(OH)D is more direct, intuitive and encompasses some of the sources of variability of 25(OH)D not taken into account by the score. The most important of these is actual sun exposure behaviors, such as type of clothing and use of sunscreen. However, in some aspects, the predicted 25(OH)D measure may provide a comparable or superior estimate of long-term vitamin D status over a single measurement of circulating 25(OH)D. Most importantly, some factors accounted by the predicted 25(OH)D score are immutable (skin color) or relatively stable (region of residence, body mass index). In contrast, circulating 25(OH)D level has a half-life of two to three weeks and thus a substantial proportion of variability picked up by a single blood measure would likely be due to relatively recent exposures that are not necessarily representative of long-term exposure. Of interest, in the Health Professionals Follow-Up Study, for colon and advanced prostate cancer, an actual measure of 25(OH)D and the score provide similar (approximately 40-50% reduction in colon cancer risk and suggestive but nonsignificant 20% reductions in advanced prostate cancer risk. These finding suggest that as a measure of long-term vitamin D status, presumably the exposure of interest, the predicted score provides a comparable assessment as does a single measurement of circulating 25(OH)D.

Studies of Vitamin D Intake

Vitamin D intakes are relatively low in general and in most populations much more vitamin D is made from sun exposure than is ingested. Nonetheless, vitamin D intake is an important contributor to 25(OH)D levels, especially in winter months in regions at high latitudes when it may be the sole contributor. A number of case-control and cohort studies have examined vitamin D intake in relation to risk of colorectal cancer or adenoma. These studies, which have been reviewed in detail previously, have generally found an inverse association between vitamin

D intake and risk of colorectal cancer or adenoma.[9,48,49] Many of the studies controlled for known or suspected risk factors for colorectal cancer. However, because calcium and vitamin D intakes tend to be correlated, the independent effects of vitamin D and calcium intakes may be difficult to separate entirely. The magnitudes of the risk reductions have been relatively modest in the range of 20 to 30% reductions in studies in the United States, where supplement use is higher and milk is fortified with vitamin D. Yet, even with added vitamin D from supplementation and fortification, vitamin D intake at typical levels currently do not raise 25(OH)D levels substantially and most variability in populations comes generally from sun exposure.

In contrast to colorectal cancer, studies of vitamin D intake and prostate cancer risk have generally not supported an association with prostate cancer incidence.[37-40] One report, which combined data from the Nurses' Health Study and the Health Professionals Follow-Up Study examined total vitamin D intake (from diet and supplements) in relation to pancreatic cancer risk based on 365 incident cases over 16 years of follow-up.[50] This study found a linear inverse association, with a significant 41 percent reduction in risk comparing high (≥600 IU/day) to low total vitamin D intake (<150 IU/day). There is some suggestive but limited evidence of a potential relationship between higher vitamin D intake and lower risk of breast cancer. [51-53]

Randomized Trial of Vitamin D Intake and Colorectal Cancer

Only one adequately powered randomized controlled trial has examined vitamin D intake in relation to cancer risk, specifically colorectal cancer. The WHI, a randomized placebo-controlled trial of 400 IU vitamin D plus 1000 mg a day of calcium in 36,282 postmenopausal women, did not support a protective role of calcium and vitamin D over a period of seven years, with 332 colorectal cancer cases diagnosed.[30] However, this study likely had important limitations. First, the vitamin D dose of 400 IU/day was probably inadequate to yield a substantial contrast between the treated and the control groups. Specifically, the expected increase of serum 25(OH)D level following an increment of 400 IU/day would be approximately 3 ng/ml. In comparison, in the epidemiologic studies of 25(OH)D, the contrast between the high and low quintiles was generally at least 20 ng/mL. This wide range is likely due primarily to differences in sun exposure. Further, the adherence was sub-optimal and a high percentage of women took nonstudy supplements, so the actual contrast of 25(OH)D tested between the treated and the placebo group in the intent-to-treat analysis was further reduced. An additional factor is that it is unclear if the duration of seven years was sufficiently long to show an effect. In fact, the epidemiologic data on duration, although limited, suggest that any influence of calcium and vitamin D intakes may require at least 10 years to emerge for colorectal cancer as the endpoint.[54] Thus, this WHI trial was probably not a robust test of the hypothesis that improving vitamin D status would lower the incidence of colorectal cancer.

Solar Radiation, Vitamin D and Survival Rate of Colon Cancer

Some recent studies have examined seasonal variation of the time of cancer diagnosis and treatment in relation cancer prognosis. The populations studied were in areas of high latitude, where vitamin D production does not occur during the winter months. The first study was conducted in Norway, where all cancer diagnoses since 1953 have been registered in the Cancer Registry. The investigators examined the influence of season of diagnosis on survival from colon, prostate and breast cancers.[55,56] No significant annual variation in the incidence rates of these cancers was found, suggesting that there was no seasonal bias in the diagnosis of cancers. The death rates at 18 months, 36 months and 45 months were 20 to 30% lower in the cancers diagnosed in autumn months compared with those diagnosed in the winter months. The findings were very statistically robust, being based on over 40,000 breast, colon and prostate cancer cases. Subsequently, some potential benefit of autumn season of diagnosis was observed for lung cancer with an approximately 15% lower case fatality for young male patients diagnosed during autumn versus winter.[57] Finally, in this population, season of diagnosis was examined in relation to survival from Hodgkin's lymphoma.[58] A 22% improved survival was observed for autumn versus winter diagnosis and a 63% improved survival was noted for patients younger than 30 years.

A study of surgery season and vitamin D intake with recurrence-free survival in 456 early-stage nonsmall cell lung cancer patients was conducted in Boston, Massachusetts.[59] Patients who had surgery in the summer had a better recurrence-free survival than those who had surgery in the winter (adjusted hazard ratio, 0.75), with 5-year recurrence-free survival rates of 53% and 40%, respectively. Furthermore, patients who had surgery during summer with the highest vitamin D intake had better recurrence-free survival (adjusted hazard ratio, 0.33) than those who had surgery during winter with the lowest vitamin D intake, with the 5-year recurrence-free survival rates of 56% and 23%, respectively. Surgery season and vitamin D intake were similarly associated with overall survival. Subsequently, levels of 25(OH)D at the time of surgery were taken for these patients and similar results suggesting a survival benefit associated with high 25(OH)D levels was found.[60]

Recently, a large study of season of diagnosis and sunlight exposure in cancer survival for cancers of the breast, colorectum, lung, prostate and at all sites combined was conducted of over a million cancer patients from the United Kingdom.[61] The investigators found evidence of substantial seasonality in cancer survival, with diagnosis in summer and autumn associated with improved survival compared with that in winter, although the associations tended to be weaker than those observed in the Norwegian study. Reductions in the hazards ratio were observed for female breast cancer patients (hazard ratio, 0.86) and both male and female lung cancer patients (hazard ratio, 0.95). Cumulative sunlight exposure in the months preceding diagnosis was also a predictor of subsequent survival, although season of diagnosis was a stronger predictor than cumulative sunlight exposure.

The findings from these three studies indicate that summer/autumn season of diagnosis may improve survival for multiple cancers. The mechanism behind this influence of season is unclear, but could possibly relate to vitamin D status. In the late summer in Norway, 25(OH)D levels are about 50% higher than that in late winter. Wintertime vitamin D production is also minimal in Boston and in the United Kingdom, where the other studies were conducted. Effects of vitamin D in late carcinogenesis stages such as reduction in metastases are observed in numerous animal models. In some animal studies, vitamin D may improve tumor control by radiation treatment, possibly by promoting apoptosis.[62]

Vitamin D and Cancer Rates in United States Black Men

Melanin efficiently blocks UV-B induced production of vitamin D in the skin. Not surprisingly, darker skinned individuals, such as African-Americans, have been documented to have markedly lower vitamin D levels.[63-68] In African-Americans, low levels of vitamin D had been hypothesized to account for their higher prostate cancer rates,[6] more aggressive prostate and breast cancer,[69] and higher total cancer incidence and mortality.[9] In addition, an inverse association between regional solar UV-B radiation and mortality rate of breast, colon, esophageal and gastric cancers was demonstrated for African-Americans in one study.[70] In the Health Professionals Follow-Up Study cohort, a prospective study which consists of highly educated, generally health conscious male health professionals, even after adjusting for multiple dietary, lifestyle and medical risk factors, Black men were at 32% higher risk of total cancer incidence and 89% higher risk of total cancer mortality compared to Whites.[71] In multivariate analyses, Black men also had especially high risk of digestive organ malignancies (colon, rectum, oral cavity, esophagus, stomach and pancreas), the group of cancers that had been identified most strongly associated with low predicted vitamin D by other studies. The increased risk of these cancers in Black men was especially marked if they had additional risk factors for vitamin D deficiency, such as low vitamin D intake or living in the northeastern part of the United States.

The higher rates of these cancers in Blacks do not prove a cause and effect relationship because other factors could be relevant. Nonetheless, one cannot ignore that that African-Americans have a particularly high prevalence of hypovitaminosis D and they have higher rates of the types of malignancies that appear to be most associated with low sun exposure or vitamin D levels. Moreover, the relationships appear stronger for mortality than for incidence. These patterns suggest that the high prevalence of vitamin D deficiency in African-Americans could potentially contribute to their substantially higher rates of cancer mortality.

Synthesis of Evidence Regarding Sun Exposure, Vitamin D and Cancer Incidence and Mortality

Since Garland and Garland initiated the hypothesis that vitamin D reduces cancer incidence and mortality in 1980, a number of epidemiologic and mechanistic studies have been conducted to test this hypothesis. This chapter has reviewed the major studies that have examined the vitamin D-cancer hypothesis. Many of the initial studies were based on correlation between incidence or mortality rates of various cancers with estimations of solar UV-B by region. In addition, a number of case-control and cohort studies have found that individuals with higher exposure to sun (measured in a variety of ways) have a reduction in cancer incidence and cancer mortality rates. Quantitatively, malignancies of the large bowel and breast appear to be the most important.

There are two major limitations in interpreting these studies; first, a confounding factor may account for the association with solar UV-B radiation and second, if one assumes the association is real, a factor other than vitamin D could be the causal protective factor. Confounding could occur if regions with more solar UV-B have a higher prevalence of a protective factor and/or a lower prevalence of a causal risk factor. Some of the ecologic analyses have accounted for some of the likely major confounding factors for cancer incidence (e.g., tobacco use, alcohol) and these do not seem to account for the association. Perhaps the strongest argument against confounding is that these associations have been observed in diverse populations, such as in the United States, Japan and Spain. It is not impossible, but appears unlikely that a consistent confounding factor would be operative in all these diverse populations. The second consideration is whether vitamin D does indeed account for the association. This is impossible to prove through such studies, though the mechanistic evidence for vitamin D appears strong and no other strong candidates for cancer protective effects of sunlight have been offered. Other lines of evidence are required to evaluate whether vitamin D is the causal agent.

Probably the most direct evidence for a role of vitamin D is from serum or plasma based studies of vitamin D status. To date, colorectal cancer and prostate cancer have received the most study. The studies have been relatively consistent for colorectal cancer and support about a doubling of risk of this malignancy associated with low levels of 25(OH)D. For prostate cancer, the data on circulating 25(OH)D have been equivocal, suggesting no association, or at least an association of a much weaker magnitude as has been observed for colorectal cancer. It is plausible that for prostate cancer, vitamin D level much longer before the time of diagnosis is most relevant, consistent with the notion that the process of prostate carcinogenesis encompasses a very long time period. Prostate cancer cells appear to lose 1-alpha-hydroxylase activity early in carcinogenesis, so it is plausible that exposure to vitamin D early in life is most relevant. In addition, determinants of prostate cancer incidence may differ from prostate cancer progression and ultimately mortality and most of the available data have assessed incident prostate cancer, as opposed to aggressive or fatal prostate cancer.

In the plasma- or serum-based studies, the best single indicator of vitamin D status, 25(OH)D, is assessed at the individual level and examined in relation to subsequent risk of cancer. Potentially confounding factors such as body mass index and physical activity are accounted for in the statistical analyses. A limitation is that although the $t_{1/2}$ in the circulation is only about 2-3 weeks, studies have been based on a single measurement throughout the year and the correlation with long-term (for example, over decades) vitamin D status is unclear. An important feature of these studies is that they are conducted in a single region or controlled for region so the variation in 25(OH)D levels is completely independent of region. This fact is critically important because if an association with cancer is shown, these results can be considered as completely independent supporting evidence from the studies based on regional solar UV-B level. It is unlikely that the same confounding factors would occur for region UV-B and for individual vitamin D levels in individuals in the same region. At the ecologic level, the overall potential for sun exposure is assessed based on how much UV-B radiation is falling in that region. At the individual level within a specified region, this variable in not variant and behaviors and skin pigmentation determine actual exposure.

In regards to dietary studies, it is important to understand that in most populations diet contributes a relatively small proportion to vitamin D stores. For example, a glass of fortified milk, though generally perceived as being a good source of vitamin D contains only 100 IU vitamin D, whereas being exposed to enough UV-B radiation to cause a slight pinkness to the skin with most of the skin uncovered (1 minimal erythemal dose) produces vitamin D equivalent to an oral dose of 20,000 IU vitamin D.[72,73] On the other hand, in higher latitudes during the winter months no vitamin D is made from sun exposure so diets and supplements become relatively more important sources. One important issue is that ergocalciferol (D2) is often used in supplements and ergocalciferol has been estimated to be only one-fourth as potent as cholecalciferol (D3) in raising 25(OH)D.[74] Only colorectal cancers and adenomas have been reasonable well studied in relation to vitamin D intake and as a whole, the literature is suggestive of a moderate inverse association associated with higher intakes (i.e., about a 20 to 25% risk reduction). From epidemiologic studies, it has not been possible to study the effects of intakes above 600 IU per day, because few individuals have had such high intakes in the populations that have been studied to date. In addition, adequate calcium intake is a likely protective factor for colorectal cancer and in populations that fortify milk with vitamin D and that consume abundant milk products, calcium intake will tend to be correlated with vitamin D intake. Thus, it has not been possible to disentangle the independent effect of vitamin D from these studies.

In the past several years, some studies have found that prognosis of various cancers, including colon, breast, lung, prostate and Hodgkin's lymphoma may be better in those diagnosed and presumably treated in the summer months than in the winter months. These studies were conducted in northern latitudes (Norway, United Kingdom, northeastern United States) in which 25(OH)D levels differ markedly between summer and winter months. It is possible that a confounding factor accounts for these results, but they suggest the intriguing possibility that vitamin D status at the time of treatment may influence outcome of various cancers. Given that many patients are vitamin D deficient at the time of diagnosis, randomized intervention trials can be feasibly conducted in which high doses or vitamin D are provided to the randomized subjects to rapidly increase vitamin D stores at the time shortly before treatment.

Implications for Future Research

The data on vitamin D and cancer incidence or mortality are intriguing, but many important questions remain. Although not definitive at this point, the epidemiologic and supporting mechanistic and animal evidence indicate that vitamin D may have a role in reducing cancer incidence and progression. The "gold standard" study would be a randomized intervention that unequivocally demonstrates a reduction in cancer risk. The only relevant randomized study to date, the WHI, did not show a benefit of vitamin D, but several important limitations of that study cannot be ignored. Based on hypotheses suggested by the current evidence, several types of trials may be considered. A primary prevention trial with the endpoint of cancer incidence may be most difficult to achieve, because the time period needed and the required dose are unknown. Doses much higher than 400 IU/day of vitamin D and periods longer than seven years may be required to observe an effect. Trials of established intermediate endpoints, such as colorectal adenoma recurrence, may be useful. One such trial is currently being conducted (Baron J, personal communication). Other intermediate endpoints, such as cell proliferation and apoptosis in specific tissues would not be definitive, but such studies could provide useful complementary mechanistic evidence. Probably the most feasible trial design would be to enhance vitamin D status at the time of cancer diagnosis with high doses of vitamin D to test the hypothesis that vitamin D status may favorably interact with treatment. Such a trial may achieve a result within a relatively short time frame.

Beyond randomized trials, further observational studies would be useful in testing the hypothesis that vitamin D may help prevent cancer. Serum or plasma-based studies of a wider spectrum of cancers than has been studied would be useful. Such studies could help establish the dose-response, what level of 25(OH)D is optimal and what intakes of vitamin D would be required to achieve this level. These studies can also help establish the role modifying factors, such as genetic variants in the vitamin D pathway and other factors such as retinol intake, which may antagonize the actions of vitamin D. In addition, the evidence for a causal association between sun exposure or enhanced vitamin D status and cancer risk can be fortified if these relationships are observed in a variety of diverse populations worldwide. If a relevant genetic polymorphism in the vitamin D pathway were consistently associated with a cancer, the evidence for causality would be increased. To date, only the vitamin D receptor has received substantial study and the functionality of polymorphisms studied have been unclear. Thus, perhaps not surprisingly, the results have been equivocal.

Confirming that vitamin D reduces risk of cancer incidence or mortality is critical because current health recommendations typically do not encourage high intakes of vitamin D and they tend to discourage sun exposure. Current dietary recommendations are geared only to prevent quite low vitamin D levels and if the association between vitamin D and reduced cancer risk is causal, such levels are almost definitely inadequate. While messages to avoid excessive sun exposure, which may cause skin aging and cancer, are appropriate, one cannot ignore that extreme avoidance of sun exposure, if not countered by relatively high intakes of vitamin D, may be associated with hypovitaminosis D, a potential risk factor for numerous cancers. Defining what are optimal levels of vitamin D for general health status remains a challenge and further study should be a high priority because of the great potential for cancer prevention achievable through vitamin D.

References

1. Peller S, Stephenson CS. Skin irritation and cancer in the United States Navy. Am J Med Sci 1937; 194:326-333.
2. Apperly FL. The relation of solar radiation to cancer mortality in North American. Cancer Res 1941; 1:191-195.
3. Garland CF, Garland FC. Do sunlight and vitamin D reduce the likelihood of colon cancer? Int J Epidemiol 1980; 9:227-231.
4. Garland FC, Garland CF, Gorham ED et al. Geographic variation in breast cancer mortality in the United States: a hypothesis involving exposure to solar radiation. Prev Med 1990; 19:614-622.
5. Lefkowitz ES, Garland CF. Sunlight, vitamin D and ovarian cancer mortality rates in US women. Int J Epidemiol 1994; 23:1133-1136.
6. Schwartz GG, Hulka BS. Is vitamin D deficiency a risk factor for prostate cancer? (Hypothesis). Anticancer Res 1990; 10:1307-1311.
7. Hanchette CL, Schwartz GG. Geographic patterns of prostate cancer mortality. Cancer 1992; 70: 2861-2869.
8. Grant WB. An estimate of premature cancer mortality in the US due to inadequate doses of solar ultraviolet-B radiation. Cancer 2002; 94(6):1867-1875.
9. Giovannucci E. The epidemiology of vitamin D and cancer incidence and mortality: a review (United States). Cancer Causes Control 2005; 16(2):83-95.
10. Mizoue T. Ecological study of solar radiation and cancer mortality in Japan. Health Phys 2004; 87(5): 532-538.
11. Grant WB, Garland CF. The association of solar ultraviolet B (UVB) with reducing risk of cancer: multifactorial ecologic analysis of geographic variation in age-adjusted cancer mortality rates. Anticancer Res 2006; 26(4A):2687-2699.
12. Grant WB. An ecologic study of cancer mortality rates in Spain with respect to indices of solar UVB irradiance and smoking. Int J Cancer 2007; 120(5):1123-1128.
13. John EM, Dreon DM, Koo J et al. Residential sunlight exposure is associated with a decreased risk of prostate cancer. J Steroid Biochem Mol Biol 2004:89-90, 549-552.
14. de Vries E, Soerjomataram I, Houterman S et al. Decreased risk of prostate cancer after skin cancer diagnosis: a protective role of ultraviolet radiation? Am J Epidemiol 2007; PMID:17255116.
15. John EM, Schwartz GG, Koo J et al. Sun exposure, vitamin D receptor gene polymorphisms and risk of advanced prostate cancer. Cancer Res 2005; 65(12):5470-5479.
16. Luscombe CJ, Fryer AA, French ME et al. Exposure to ultraviolet radiation: association with susceptibility and age at presentation with prostate cancer. Lancet 2001; 358(9282):641-642.
17. Bodiwala D, Luscombe CJ, French ME et al. Associations between prostate cancer susceptibility and parameters of exposure to ultraviolet radiation. Cancer Lett 2003; 200(2):141-148.

18. Freedman DM, Dosemeci M, McGlynn K. Sunlight and mortality from breast, ovarian, colon, prostate and nonmelanoma skin cancer: a composite death certificate based case-control study. Occup Environ Med 2002; 59(4):257-262.
19. Giovannucci E, Liu Y, Rimm EB et al. Prospective study of predictors of vitamin D status and cancer incidence and mortality in men. J Natl Cancer Inst 2006; 98(7):451-459.
20. Kampman E, Slattery ML, Caan B et al. Calcium, vitamin D, sunshine exposures, dairy products and colon cancer risk (United States). Cancer Causes Control 2000; 11:459-466.
21. Platz EA, Rimm EB, Willett WC et al. Racial variation in prostate cancer incidence and in hormonal system markers among male health professionals. J Natl Cancer Inst 2000; 92:2009-2017.
22. Garland CF, Comstock GW, Garland FC et al. Serum 25-hydroxyvitamin D and colon cancer: eight-year prospective study. Lancet 1989; 2:1176-1178.
23. Tangrea J, Helzlsouer K, Pietinen P et al. Serum levels of vitamin D metabolites and the subsequent risk of colon and rectal cancer in Finnish men. Cancer Causes Control 1997; 8:615-625.
24. Feskanich D, Ma J, Fuchs CS et al. Plasma vitamin D metabolites and risk of colorectal cancer in women. Cancer Epidemiol Biomarkers Prev 2004; 13(9):1502-1508.
25. Levine AJ, Harper JM, Ervin CM et al. Serum 25-hydroxyvitamin D, dietary calcium in take and distal colorectal adenoma risk. Nutr Cancer 2001; 39:35-41.
26. Peters U, McGlynn KA, Chatterjee N et al. Vitamin D, calcium and vitamin D receptor polymorphism in colorectal adenomas. Cancer Epidemiol Biomarkers Prev 2001; 10:1267-1274.
27. Platz EA, Hankinson SE, Hollis BW et al. Plasma 1,25-dihydroxy-and 25-hydroxyvitamin D and adenomatous polyps of the distal colorectum. Cancer Epidemiol Biomarkers Prev 2000; 9:1059-1065.
28. Grau MV, Baron JA, Sandler RS et al. Vitamin D, calcium supplementation and colorectal adenomas: results of a randomized trail. J Natl Cancer Inst 2003; 95:1765-1771.
29. Wactawski-Wende J, Kotchen JM anderson GL et al. Calcium plus vitamin D supplementation and the risk of colorectal cancer. N Engl J Med 2006; 354(7):684-696.
30. Gorham ED, Garland CF, Garland FC et al. Optimal vitamin D status for colorectal cancer prevention. A quantitative meta analysis. Am J Prev Med 2007; 32(3):210-216.
31. Braun MM, Helzlsouer KJ, Hollis BW et al. Prostate cancer and prediagnostic levels of serum vitamin D metabolites (Maryland, United States). Cancer Causes Control 1995; 6:235-239.
32. Corder EH, Guess HA, Hulka BS et al. Vitamin D and prostate cancer: a prediagnostic study with stored sera. Cancer Epidemiol Biomarkers Prev 1993; 2:467-472.
33. Gann PH, Ma J, Hennekens CH et al. Circulating vitamin D metabolites in relation to subsequent development of prostate cancer. Cancer Epidemiol Biomarkers Prev 1996; 5:121-126.
34. Nomura AM, Stemmermann GN, Lee J et al. Serum vitamin D metabolite levels and the subsequent development of prostate cancer. Cancer Causes Control 1998; 9:425-432.
35. Platz EA, Leitzmann MF, Hollis BW et al. Plasma 1,25-dihydroxy- and 25-hydroxyvitamin D and subsequent risk of prostate cancer. Cancer Causes Control 2004; 15:255-265.
36. Jacobs ET, Giuliano AR, Martinez ME et al. Plasma levels of 25-hydroxyvitamin D, 1,25-dihydroxyvitamin D and the risk of prostate cancer. J Steroid Biochem Mol Biol 2004; 89-90:533-537.
37. Giovannucci E, Rimm EB, Wolk A et al. Calcium and fructose intake in relation to risk of prostate cancer. Cancer Res 1998; 58:442-447.
38. Chan JM, Giovannucci E andersson SO et al. Dairy products, calcium, phosphorous, vitamin D and risk of prostate cancer. Cancer Causes Control 1998; 9:559-566.
39. Chan JM, Pietinen P, Virtanen M et al. Diet and prostate cancer risk in a cohort of smokers, with a specific focus on calcium and phosphorus (Finland). Cancer Causes Control 2000; 11:859-867.
40. Kristal AR, Cohen JH, Qu P et al. Associations of energy, fat, calcium and vitamin D with prostate cancer risk. Cancer Epidemiol Biomarkers Prev 2002; 11:719-725.
41. Ahonen MH, Tenkanen L, Teppo L et al. Prostate cancer risk and prediagnostic serum 25-hydroxyvitamin D levels (Finland). Cancer Causes Control 2000; 11:847-852.
42. Tuohimaa P, Tenkanen L, Ahonen M et al. Both high and low levels of blood vitamin D are associated with a higher prostate cancer risk: a longitudinal, nested case-control study in the Nordic countries. Int J Cancer 2004; 108(1):104-108.
43. Li H, Stampfer MJ, Hollis BW et al. A prospective study of plasma vitamin D metabolites, vitamin D receptor polymorphisms and prostate cancer. PLoS Medicine 2007; 4(3):e103.
44. Colston KW, Lowe LC, Mansi JL et al. Vitamin D status and breast cancer risk. Anticancer Res 2006; 26(4A):2573-2580.
45. Palmieri C, MacGregor T, Girgis S et al. Serum 25-hydroxyvitamin D levels in early and advanced breast cancer. J Clin Pathol 2006; 59(12):1334-1336.
46. Bertone-Johnson E, Chen WY, Holick MF et al. Plasma 25-hydroxyvitamin D and 1,25-dihydroxyvitamin D and risk of breast cancer. Cancer Epidemiol Biomarkers Prev 2005; 14(8):1991-1997.

47. Stolzenberg-Solomon RZ, Vieth R, Azad A et al. A prospective nested case-control study of vitamin D status and pancreatic cancer risk in male smokers. Cancer Res 2006; 66(20):10213-10219.
48. Grant WB, Garland CF. A critical review of studies on vitamin D in relation to colorectal cancer. Nutr Cancer 2004; 48(2):115-123.
49. Gorham ED, Garland CF, Garland FC et al. Vitamin D and prevention of colorectal cancer. J Steroid Biochem Mol Biol 2005; 97(1-2):179-194.
50. Skinner HG, Michaud DS, Giovannucci E et al. Vitamin D intake and the risk for pancreatic cancer in two cohort studies. Cancer Epidemiol Biomarkers Prev 2006; 15(9):1688-1695.
51. John EM, Schwartz GG, Dreon DM et al. Vitamin D and breast cancer risk: the NHANES I Epidemiologic follow-up study, 1971-1975 to 1992. National Health and Nutrition Examination Survey. Cancer Epidemiol Biomarkers Prev 1999; 8(5):399-406.
52. Shin MH, Holmes MD, Hankinson SE et al. Intake of dairy products, calcium and vitamin D and risk of breast cancer. J Natl Cancer Inst 2002; 94(17):1301-1310.
53. McCullough ML, Rodriguez C, Diver WR et al. Dairy, calcium and vitamin D intake and postmenopausal breast cancer risk in the Cancer Prevention Study II Nutrition Cohort. Cancer Epidemiol Biomarkers Prev 2005; 14(12):2898-2904.
54. Martinez ME, Giovannucci EL, Colditz GA et al. Calcium, vitamin D and the occurrence of colorectal cancer among women. J Natl Cancer Inst 1996; 88:1375-1382.
55. Robsahm TE, Tretli S, Dahlback A et al. Vitamin D3 from sunlight may improve the prognosis of breast-, colon- and prostate cancer (Norway). Cancer Causes Control 2004; 15(2):149-158.
56. Porojnicu AC, Lagunova Z, Robsahm TE et al. Changes in risk of death from breast cancer with season and latitude: Sun exposure and breast cancer survival in Norway. Breast Cancer Res Treat 2007; PMID: 17028983 [2006; Epub ahead of print].
57. Porojnicu AC, Robsahm TE, Dahlback A et al. Seasonal and geographical variations in lung cancer prognosis in Norway. Does Vitamin D from the sun play a role? Lung Cancer 2007; PMID:17207891 [2007; Epub ahead of print].
58. Porojnicu AC, Robsahm TE, Ree AH et al. Season of diagnosis is a prognostic factor in Hodgkin's lymphoma: a possible role of sun-induced vitamin D. Br J Cancer 2005; 93(5):571-574.
59. Zhou W, Suk R, Liu G et al. Vitamin D is associated with overall survival in early stage nonsmall cell lung cancer patients. Cancer Epidemiol Biomarkers Prev 2005; 14(10):2303-2309.
60. Zhou W, Heist RS, Liu G et al. Circulating 25-hydroxyvitamin d levels predict survival in early-stage nonsmall-cell lung cancer patients. J Clin Oncol 2007; 25(5):479-485.
61. Lim HS, Roychoudhuri R, Peto J et al. Cancer survival is dependent on season of diagnosis and sunlight exposure. Int J Cancer 2006; 119(7):1530-1536.
62. DeMasters GA, Gupta MS, Jones KR et al. Potentiation of cell killing by fractionated radiation and suppression of proliferative recovery in MCF-7 breast tumor cells by the Vitamin D3 analog EB 1089. J Steroid Biochem Mol Biol 2004; 92(5):365-374.
63. Matsuoka LY, Wortsman J, Chen TC et al. Compensation for the interracial variance in the cutaneous synthesis of vitamin D. J Lab Clin Med 1995; 126(5):452-457.
64. Harris SS, Dawson-Hughes B. Seasonal changes in plasma 25-hydroxyvitamin D concentrations of young American black and white women. Am J Clin Nutr 1998; 67(6):1232-1236.
65. Looker AC, Dawson-Hughes B, Calvo MS et al. Serum 25-hydroxyvitamin D status of adolescents and adults in two seasonal subpopulations from NHANES III. Bone 2002; 30(5):771-777.
66. Harris SS, Soteriades E, Coolidge JA et al. Vitamin D insufficiency and hyperparathyroidism in a low income, multiracial, elderly population. J Clin Endocrinol Metab 2000; 85(11):4125-4130.
67. Clemens TL, Adams JS, Henderson SL et al. Increased skin pigment reduces the capacity of skin to synthesise vitamin D3. Lancet 1982; 1(8263):74-76.
68. Nesby-O'Dell S, Scanlon KS, Cogswell ME et al. Hypovitaminosis D prevalence and determinants among African American and white women of reproductive age: third National Health and Nutrition Examination Survey, 1988-1994. Am J Clin Nutr 2002; 76(1):187-192.
69. Studzinski GP, Moore DC. Sunlight—can it prevent as well as cause cancer? Cancer Res 1995; 55(18):4014-4022.
70. Grant WB. Lower vitamin-D production from solar ultraviolet-B irradiance may explain some differences in cancer survival rates. J Natl Med Assoc 2006; 98(3):357-364.
71. Giovannucci E, Liu Y, Willett WC. Cancer incidence and mortality and vitamin D in Black and White male health professionals. Cancer Epidemiol Biomarkers Prev 2006; 15(12):2445-2452.
72. Holick MF. Vitamin D: importance in the prevention of cancers, type 1 diabetes, heart disease and osteoporosis. Am J Clin Nutr 2004; 79(3):362-371.
73. Hollis BW. Circulating 25-hydroxyvitamin D levels indicative of vitamin D sufficiency: implications for establishing a new effective dietary intake recommendation for vitamin D. J Nutr 2005; 135(2):317-322.
74. Vieth R. The pharmacology of vitamin D, including fortification strategies. In: Feldman D, Pike JW, Glorieux FH, editors. Vitamin D, Second Edition. Amsterdam: Elsevier Academic Press, 2005:995-1015.

CHAPTER 4

Sun Exposure and Cancer Survival in Norway:
Changes in the Risk of Death with Season of Diagnosis and Latitude

Alina Carmen Porojnicu,* Arne Dahlback and Johan Moan

Abstract

Epidemiological and experimental studies suggest that derivatives of vitamin D may improve prognosis of a number of cancer types. Sun is our most important source of vitamin D. Seasonal variations and latitudinal gradients of calcidiol (the marker of vitamin D status) have been reported. We wanted to investigate if season and latitude play any role for survival from seven different cancer types in Norway. Seasonal and geographical variations of vitamin D were estimated by calculations and were compared with clinical data. For the survival analyses, 249373 cancer patients were followed for three years after diagnosis and the risk of death was analyzed separately for summer- and winter diagnosis, as well as for two geographical regions with different UV exposures. We found a 15-25 % better survival for patients diagnosed during summer and a slight beneficial effect for residents of the high UV region for some of the cancer forms investigated.

Based on our results we suggest that calcidiol concentration at the time of cancer diagnosis is related to survival and discuss briefly ways to improve the vitamin D levels in the general population.

Introduction

Solar radiation, a recognized skin carcinogen,[1] may also reduce mortality from internal cancers. This intriguing suggestion was first published by Apperly in 1941.[2] He observed that cancer patients living at high latitudes in USA had a higher mortality risk compared with those living in the south. Later, in 1980, Garland and Garland[3] surveyed the association between solar exposure and risk of dying from colon cancer and hypothesized that the negative association between these two may be related to the level of vitamin D. A number of similar ecological studies were carried out in the following years, most of them supporting the proposed association.[4-9] The level of solar exposure were either approximated by using latitude, UV satellite measurements, UV indexes (the case of ecological work), assessed through records of personal history of sun exposure or estimated by structural changes in the skin.[10] A number of cancers were investigated throughout this period and in a recent publication fifteen cancer types were found to be sun-sensitive with respect to progression.[11]

A north-south gradient seems to be present in USA as well as in Europe[12,13] and even in Japan.[14]

*Corresponding Author: Alina Carmen Porojnicu—Deparment of Radiation Biology, Institute for Cancer Research, Montebello, Oslo, Norway. Email: a.c.porojnicu@usit.uio.no

Sunlight, Vitamin D and Skin Cancer, edited by Jörg Reichrath. ©2008 Landes Bioscience and Springer Science+Business Media.

These epidemiological observations triggered experimental work aimed at understanding the mechanistic background. As suggested by Garland and Garland a possible link between the level of solar exposure and cancer mortality is vitamin D.[3] It is well known that sun is our main source of vitamin D. Our epidermis and dermis contain 7-dehydrocholesterol (7-DHC), a precursor of both vitamin D and cholesterol.[15] When UVB (ultraviolet B, 280-320 nm) photons from the sun or from artificial sources, hit the skin, 7-DHC absorbs energy and is structurally changed to previtamin D which is unstable and isomerizes in a temperature dependent process to vitamin D. Vitamin D is transported by the blood flow, bound to DBP (vitamin D protein), first to the liver and then to the kidneys. The molecule undergoes steps of enzyme-catalyzed hydroxylation, resulting in the formation of 25 hydroxyvitamin D (calcidiol) in the liver and 1,25 dihydroxyvitamin D (calcitriol) in the kidneys.[15] Calcidiol is used in the clinical vitamin D monitoring, since its formation is not tightly regulated. Therefore it is reflecting the vitamin D status.

The serum level of UV-induced calcidiol is influenced by several factors that modify the biosynthetic pathway. Among these, the level of UVB reaching the ground, the skin properties (pigmentation, thickness), the function of liver and kidneys as primary sources of active vitamin D as well as BMI (body mass index) and possibly hormonal status are the main predictors.[16-19]

The seasonal variation of calcidiol is a well documented fact. In a healthy, adult population living in Norway the percent increase from winter to summer is 15-50%.[20-24] From October to April solar vitamin D synthesis does not take place in this part of the world[25] and vitamin D deficiency will become manifest unless adequate amounts of the vitamin are ingested. The maximal serum levels of calcidiol are usually achieved during the months September-October, reflecting a delay from the maximal solar UVB fluence rate midsummer.

Materials and Methods

The purpose of our work was to study the association between the level of solar exposure and cancer prognosis in Norway. The exposure level changes with season and residential region. Outcome was calculated using Cox proportional hazards regression model and expressed as relative risk of death (RR). The category with the lowest solar exposure was chosen as reference and set to 1. Analyses were adjusted for a number of possible confounders, as outlined below.

Cancer Database

In our study we used data from The National Cancer Registry of Norway, a population-based registry that since 1953 collects data on cancer incidence and survival. Information is obtained from three sources: diagnosing physician, pathology laboratories and Statistics Central Bureau and this assures a high degree of reliability. The Registry records information on patients characteristics (date of birth, sex, residence), date of diagnosis, primary tumor site, stage of diagnosis and follow up for vital status.

After 1960, each Norwegian inhabitant received a unique identification number. This allowed us to link the Cancer Database to The Population Registry whenever we were interested in obtaining further socio-demographic information.

In our work we included all patients diagnosed with prostate-, breast -, colon -, lung-, ovarian- and bladder cancer, as well as with Hodgkin lymphoma. Description of the period of inclusion, number of cases and number of deaths from cancer is presented in Table 1.

Using the date of diagnosis, the season of diagnosis was defined as follows: winter (December 1-May 31) and summer (June 1-November 30).

Solar Exposure in Norway

The main factors influencing the ultraviolet (UV) irradiances at ground level are solar zenith angle (variable with season, latitude and time of day), cloud and snow cover and the thickness of the ozone layer.[26]

In this study, the global solar UV irradiance was calculated using a radiative transfer model.[27,28] Total ozone amounts used in this model were measured by TOMS satellite instruments. The daily cloud cover varies in Norway, with coastal regions being cloudier than the inland regions. The

Table 1. Description of population included

Cancer Type	Period of Inclusion	No Cases	Mean Age ± Std	No Deaths
Prostate cancer	1964-1992	46205	74 ± 8	10090
Breast cancer	1964-1992	49821	62 ± 14	6615
Colon cancer	1964-1992	38541	70 ± 11	14221
Lung cancer	1960-2001	45681	66 ± 10	29856
Ovarian cancer	1964-2000	42096	59 ± 14	7112
Bladder cancer	1964-2000	23890	68 ± 11	5864
Hogkin lymphoma	1964-2000	3139	44 ± 19	769

magnitude of this was estimated for each of the Norwegians counties, from measured reflectivities from an ozone-insensitive channel of the same satellite instruments. The effect of snow cover was estimated by comparing the calculations with UV measurements from the Norwegian UV monitoring network. The calculated annual UV exposures are based on available satellite measurements in the period 1980-2000.

Seasonal UV Doses

The results are partly presented as erythemally effective UV doses (CIE) measured in units of $J/m.^2$ In some of the analyses we used the efficiency spectrum for vitamin D production giving the relative effectiveness of solar radiation at different wavelengths in converting 7-DHC to previtamin D. Briefly, an efficiency spectrum is calculated by multiplying the intensity of the solar radiation (wavelength by wavelength) with the action spectrum for the vitamin D production for the corresponding wavelength. The vitamin D action spectrum was measured by MacLaughlin et al in ex vivo skin specimens.[29]

Regional UV Doses

The Norwegian mainland covers 13° of latitude, from 58° N to more than 71° N (Fig. 1). In the present study we have investigated the mean annual UV irradiances in each of the Norwegian counties and attempted to correlate them with cancer survival. Additionally, to control for the real UV exposure obtained by different populations, we have plotted the incidence rates (IR) of squamous cell carcinoma of the skin (SCC) vs the calculated UV dose in each of the Norwegian counties, since it is widely accepted that UV from the sun is the main risk factor for SCC.[1] The incidence rates were age-adjusted and the plotted values represent an average of the period 1960-2004. Log—log plots are usually used for incidence—annual UV—dose relationships in the case of skin cancer.[30] The reason for this is that the relationship is not linear, but closer to quadratic. In fact, in most cases it follows the equation log (incidence) = A_b log (Dose), where A_b is the so-called biological amplification factor.[30] The largest city, Oslo, was excluded from all analyses, to reduce errors that may arise from different sun-exposure habits and high immigration rate. Oslo has the highest proportion of immigrants with 18% of its population being of nonwestern origin.[31]

Statistical Analyses

The data were analysed in a multivariate Cox regression model using SPSS Version 10 (SPSS Inc, USA). The dependent variable was death from cancer within 36 months after diagnosis (or 18 months in the case of lung cancer). As independent variables we included in most analyses: age, sex (were relevant), birth cohort, stage of disease and a UV index based on season of diagnosis and residential region. Additionally, for prostate, breast and colon cancer, attention has been paid to the level of education, profession and parity as described elsewhere.[32] Since these adjustments did not significantly change the estimates, we did not include them in the analyses of the other cancer forms.

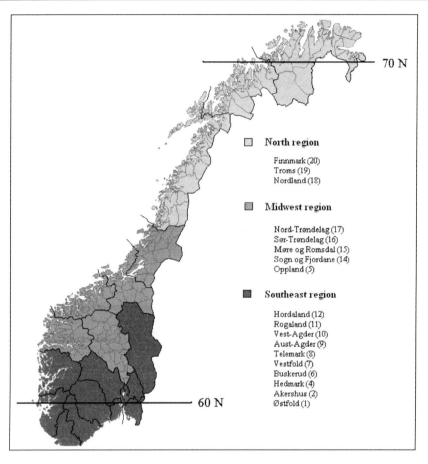

Figure 1. A map of Norway showing its latitude and division into counties. The three different tones of color denote the three regions shown in Figure 5.

In this paper we present the effect of season of diagnosis and/or residential region on the relative risk of death (RR death) from cancer. Concerning the seasonal comparisons, winter (the season with lowest UV doses and the lowest vitamin D levels) was chosen as the reference group. When we included the combined UV variable that took into account both season of diagnosis and residential region, diagnosis in the winter in the midwest region was chosen as the reference category.

Dependency of Survival on Season of Diagnosis

Figure 2 presents the seasonal variation of calculated production of vitamin D in human skin at two geographical locations: north Norway and south Norway.

Seasonal variation of UV doses may be relevant for cancer survival and we hypothesized that the effect may be mediated through vitamin D synthesis in the skin. Figure 3 summarizes the relative risk of death by season of diagnosis for all cancer types included. Significantly reduced RR_s (relative risk) of deaths were found in the summer for cancers of prostate (0,76), breast (0,75) colon (0,79) and Hodgkins lymphoma (0,84). The mortality from ovary-, bladder- and lung cancer showed no seasonal variation.

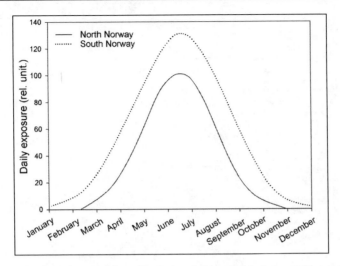

Figure 2. Calculated production of vitamin D (in relative units) in human skin at two different geographical locations in Norway.

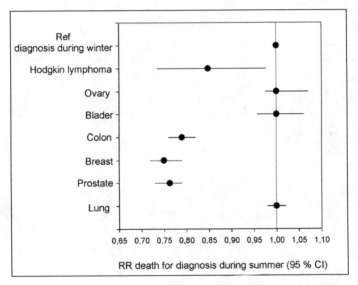

Figure 3. RR death within 36 months after cancer diagnosis for cases diagnosed during summer. Diagnosis during winter is the reference category and is set to 1.

Dependency of Survival on Residential Region

The Norwegian mainland covers 13° of latitude, from 58° N to more than 71° N (Fig. 1) and the UV level decreases with increasing latitude (Fig. 4). The UV exposure rate is roughly 30% higher at 56° N than at 70° N in the middle of the summer (Fig. 2).

The UV exposure at ground level does not necessarily reflect the exposure achieved by the population. To check the significance of this, we grouped the Norwegian counties according to the incidence rate of SCC, which is known to be strongly correlated with the accumulated UV exposure. When we have plotted the age adjusted incidence rates of SCC in each of the counties against the calculated UV dose, three regions with different UV exposure patterns can

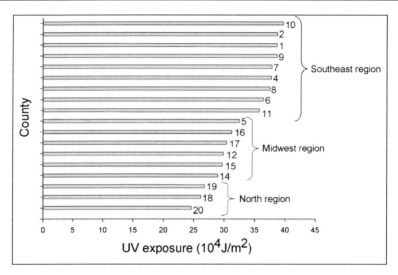

Figure 4. The UV exposure from the sun in Norway, adjusted according to the CIE reference spectrum of erythema. The number in the brackets gives the county's number.

be identified: the northern region (counties 18-20); the midwest region (counties 5, 12, 14-17) and the southeast region (counties 1, 2, 4, 6-11) (Fig. 5). A complicating factor in the regional analyses,is the difference in the level of vitamin D intake. People living in the northern region, are exposed to low UV doses but consume high quantities of vitamin D through fat fish.[33] According to Brustad et al[20] the level of fish intake in the north does not show any seasonal variation. Inhabitants of the midwest region receive moderately high doses of both UV and vitamin D through food while those living in the southeast are exposed to high UV doses and have a low vitamin D intake (Table 2).

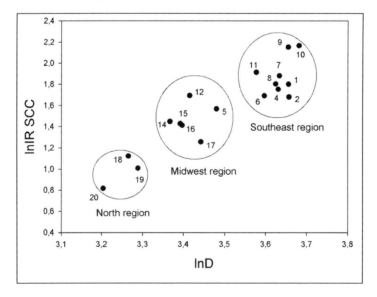

Figure 5. Annual ambient UV exposure (D) vs age adjusted rate of squamous cell carcinoma (R) in Norway (1960-2004). The relationship is described by the relationship lnR = A*lnD, where A is the amplification factor.[30]

Table 2. *Relative values for the annual synthesis of vitamin D and the daily intake of vitamin D and fish in the three regions*

	North Region	Midwest Region	Southeast Region
Annual vitamin D formation in skin (rel. unit)[25]	1	1,2	1,5
Vitamin D intake (µg/day)[33]	5,4	5	4,7
Fish intake (g/day)[33]	90	72	59

Table 3. *Relative risk of death at 36 months after diagnosis for summer and winter diagnosis in two different regions marked in Figure 2*

	Midwest, Winter (Ref)	Midwest, Summer	Southeast, Winter	Southeast, Summer
Prostate cancer	1	0,8 (0,7-0,84)*	1 (0,99-1,1)	0,8 (0,75-0,85)*
Breast cancer	1	0,76 (0,7-0,8)*	0,97 (0,9-1,05)	0,75 (0,7-0,8)*
Colon cancer	1	0,82 (0,7-0,86)*	1 (0,9-1,07)	0,79 (0,7-0,84)*
Lung cancer**	1	1 (0,96-1)	0,93 (0,89-0,96)*	0,93 (0,89-0,96)*
Ovarian cancer	1	1 (0,8-1,3)	1 (0,8-1,3)	1 (0,6-1)
Bladder cancer	1	1 (0,9-1,1)	0,9 (0,8-1)	0,9 (0,9-1)
Hodgkin lymphoma	1	1 (0,9-1,1)	1 (0,9-1)	0,8 (0,9-1,1)

*indicates statistical significance, $p < 0,05$
**follow-up was restricted at 18 months
The death rate for winter diagnosis in the midwest region is set to unity. Overall data for all ages and both sexes are presented. Values in parentheses indicate 95% confidence intervals.

In the multivariate analyses of prognosis we have not included data from the northern region because of the high intake of vitamin D and the relatively low population number. Furthermore, we have created a combined variable that accounts for both season of diagnosis and residential region. We consider four categories: winter diagnosis in the midwest region (reference); summer diagnosis in the midwest region; winter diagnosis in the southeast region and summer diagnosis in the southeast region.

Table 3 shows the results of the multivariate regression analyses. The relative risk of death seems to be slightly lower in the southeast region (i.e., high UV doses) for breast-, colon- and lung cancers, while no regional effect is observed for the other cancer types.

Discussion

Our results can be summarized as follows: For prostate-, breast-, colon cancer and Hodgkin lymphoma, patients diagnosed during the summer have a 15-25% reduced risk of death during the first 36 months after diagnosis, compared with those diagnosed during the winter. In addition, residing in southeast Norway seems to add an extra beneficial effect to the improved summer prognosis for breast- and colon cancer and makes apparent a slight protective effect for lung cancer. No seasonal or latitudinal gradient was observed for bladder and ovary cancer.

It is well established that season is an important predictor of the vitamin D level. The seasonal calcidiol variation in humans has been investigated in a number of Norwegian studies and the results show a winter to summer increase of 15-50%.[20-24] which is in accordance with our calculated vitamin D production (Fig. 2).

The fact that the incidence rates of SCC decrease monotonously with increasing latitude (Fig. 5) indicates that the UV exposures achieved by the population can be approximated by calculated or measured ambient UV fluences, as earlier done.[34,35] Unfortunately, no comparison of measured calcidiol levels in north and south Norway has been performed. However, one can make a rough analysis, based on the knowledge of the yield of calcidiol from skin synthesis and that from intake. Following similar calculations as described in[25] we found that a 15% higher vitamin D intake in the fish region (Table 2) is balanced by the 50% larger annual UV fluence in the south (Table 2). Furthermore, the mid-summer photosynthesis of vitamin D is only 30% larger in the south than in the north according to our calculations (Fig. 2) and the real differences in calcidiol levels are likely to be smaller, since large UV fluences degrade vitamin D in skin.[15] Moreover, whole body exposure to one MED (minimal erythema dose) gives a high increase in the vitamin D concentration but only a moderate increase in the serum calcidiol level.[15] Comparisons of our calculation with measured calcidiol levels in Scandinavia confirm that calcidiol concentrations in the south of Scandinavia are not significantly higher than those in the north.[20,24,36,37]

The cancer sites that have been most extensively examined in relation to vitamin D status are colorectal, breast and prostate cancers.[38] For other internal cancers, evidence is limited and comes mostly from ecologic investigations.[9,11,12]

Our study indicates that cancer survival may be affected by the level of UV exposure close to the time of cancer diagnosis in five out of seven cancers types investigated (Table 3). We have suggested that this may be explained in terms of vitamin D-photosynthesis. According to our hypothesis, patients with high levels of calcidiol at the time of diagnosis (summer diagnosis) have a greater chance to survive compared with patients with low levels of calcidiol (winter diagnosis). High calcidiol concentrations in the serum would provide the cancer cells with the precursor for local synthesis of calcitriol, or, alternatively, calcidiol itself may be bind directly to the VDR (vitamin D receptor) and act anticarcinogenic.

The anticarcinogenic effects of vitamin D are indicated by a number of experimental investigations with cell lines and animal models. In the case of breast cancer an important amount of research, thoroughly reviewed by Colston et al[39] shows that calcitriol is able to regulate cell cycle progression, induce apoptosis, modulate cell signalling through growth factors and reduce invasiveness and angiogenic activity in breast cancer models.[35] A number of preclinical studies have proven that calcitriol derivatives enhance the effect of established chemotherapeutics for breast cancer treatment.[40-44] Cancer of the prostate also responds to vitamin D therapies presumably by similar molecular mechanisms.[45-48] The same is true for colon cancer.[49,50] In vitro studies, performed with lung-cancer cell lines, have shown that vitamin D derivatives inhibit cell-growth and proliferation[51] Animal studies have demonstrated the capability of these compounds to suppress invasion, metastasis and angiogenesis in vivo.[52-54]

Controversy still exists as to whether only calcitriol, or both calcidiol and calcitriol, have biological functions in humans. Each of these derivatives binds specifically to the VDR receptor (member of the nuclear receptor superfamily), the affinity of calcitriol beeing 600-700 higher than that of calcidiol.[55] On the other hand calcidiol is present in an approximately 1000 times larger concentration in serum and is therefore more bioavailable than calcitriol. Beside the well described role of calcitriol in maintaining calcium homeostasis through processes in the intestine, bones and kidneys, calcitriol and/or calcidiol may act in other normal or pathologic tissues.[56] The effect may either be from the systemic pool or from local ones in tissue, since most tissues are able to produce their own calcitriol.[56] The concentrations at which calcitriol is active in vivo appear to be higher than what has been assumed physiological concentrations, i.e., above 100 pmol/l. However, this effect may at least partly be mediated by locally produced calcitriol or directly by calcidiol taken up from the blood.

Our epidemiological data from Norway point to the importance of calcidiol.[57]

Conclusions

The vitamin D level in serum of Norwegians is 15-50% higher in summer than in winter. Recently, our group hypothesised for the first time that this may be of significance for the prognosis of major cancer forms, like prostate cancer, breast cancer, colon cancer, lung cancer and lymphomas.[25,32,34,58] The relative risk of death three years after diagnosis and start of therapy is estimated to be 15-25% higher for summer diagnosis than for winter diagnosis. A recent study involving over a million cancer patients in the United Kingdom gave similar results.[57] The action mechanism has almost equivocally been attributed to vitamin D production by UV and this view is supported by cell and animal experiments as reviewed in the present chapter.

The health effects of ultraviolet radiation from the sun are now being debated worldwide.[59] Focus of this debate is an understanding that UV has both negative health effects, namely induction of skin cancer[1] and beneficial health effects through induction of vitamin D.[60] Solar UV is a well-established skin carcinogen being responsible for more than half of all cancers and causing about 250 deaths per year in Norway.[61] Large sun-safety campaigns have been launched, which seems to have had a significant impact since the increasing trend of skin cancer incidence rates observed from 1960 or earlier is reversed for young persons after about 1990 (for more details, see chapter by Leiter and Garbe). However, in the same time period, i.e., after 1990, vitamin D deficiency has developed in many populations. Since solar UV is a main source of vitamin D, this deficiency may, at least partly, be due to reduced sun exposure. Another important source of vitamin D is supplemental/dietary intake. From evolutionary, epidemiological and experimental perspectives, the optimal nutritional intake vitamin D may be defined as the amount equivalent to what an adult can acquire through exposing the whole skin surface to summer sunshine.[62] Based on this, a physiologic intake of vitamin D for an adult might range up to 250 μg/day (i.e., 50 times the daily recommended dose in Norway).[63]

Implementation of public health policies to optimise the vitamin D nutritional status would be relatively inexpensive but would meet various limiting factors such as: risk of toxicity in susceptible populations (infants, individuals suffering from hyperparathyroidism, sarcoidosis, tuberculosis, lymphomas, William's syndrome, etc), inability to reach vulnerable populations with different dietary preferences or aversions against specific foods such as milk, higher prevalence of lactose intolerance and low milk consumption in African-Americans (population at high risk of vitamin D deficiency), need for thorough labelling of all food items containing vitamin D. Any public health strategy requires both safety- and efficacy-testing.[64] Controlled use of UV exposure might be evaluated as a supplemental and safe source of vitamin D. Due to the seriousness of both vitamin D deficiency and skin cancer induction, more research is needed on the topic of UV and health.

Acknowledgement

The present work was supported by Sigval Bergesen D.Y. og hustru Nankis Foundation and by Helse Sør Medical Enterprise. The TOMS data were provided by NASA/GSFC. We thank Trude Eid Robsahm and Steinar Tretli at Norwegian Cancer Registry for assistance in obtaining and analyzing cancer data.

References

1. Armstrong BK, Kricker A, English DR. Sun exposure and skin cancer. Australas J Dermatol 1997; 38 Suppl 1:S1-S6.
2. Apperly FL. The relation of solar radiation to cancer mortality in North America. Cancer Res 1941; 191-195.
3. Garland CF, Garland FC. Do sunlight and vitamin D reduce the likelihood of colon cancer? Int J Epidemiol 1980; 9:227-231.
4. Garland FC, Garland CF, Gorham ED et al. Geographic variation in breast cancer mortality in the United States: a hypothesis involving exposure to solar radiation. Prev Med 1990; 19:614-622.
5. Schwartz GG, Hulka BS. Is vitamin D deficiency a risk factor for prostate cancer? (Hypothesis). Anticancer Res 1990; 10:1307-1311.
6. Hanchette CL, Schwartz GG. Geographic patterns of prostate cancer mortality. Evidence for a protective effect of ultraviolet radiation. Cancer 1992; 70:2861-2869.

7. Lefkowitz ES, Garland CF. Sunlight, vitamin D and ovarian cancer mortality rates in US women. Int J Epidemiol 1994; 23:1133-1136.
8. Grant WB. An estimate of premature cancer mortality in the US due to inadequate doses of solar ultraviolet-B radiation. Cancer 2002; 94:1867-1875.
9. Freedman DM, Dosemeci M, McGlynn K. Sunlight and mortality from breast, ovarian, colon, prostate and nonmelanoma skin cancer: a composite death certificate based case-control study. Occup Environ Med 2002; 59:257-262.
10. Berwick M, Armstrong BK, Ben Porat L et al. Sun exposure and mortality from melanoma. J Natl Cancer Inst 2005; 97:195-199.
11. Grant WB, Garland CF. The association of solar ultraviolet B (UVB) with reducing risk of cancer: multifactorial ecologic analysis of geographic variation in age-adjusted cancer mortality rates. Anticancer Res 2006; 26:2687-2699.
12. Grant WB. The likely role of vitamin D from solar ultraviolet-B irradiance in increasing cancer survival. Anticancer Res 2006; 26:2605-2614.
13. Grant WB. An ecologic study of cancer mortality rates in Spain with respect to indices of solar UVB irradiance and smoking. Int J Cancer 2007; 120:1123-1128.
14. Mizoue T. Ecological study of solar radiation and cancer mortality in Japan. Health Phys 2004; 87:532-538.
15. Holick MF. Vitamin D: photobiology, metabolism and clinical application. In: Arias IM, Boyer JL, Fausto N et al, eds. The liver: biology and photobiology. New York: Raven Press 1994; 543-62.
16. Panidis D, Balaris C, Farmakiotis D et al. Serum parathyroid hormone concentrations are increased in women with polycystic ovary syndrome. Clin Chem 2005; 51:1691-1697.
17. Bischof MG, Heinze G, Vierhapper H. Vitamin D status and its relation to age and body mass index. Horm Res 2006; 66:211-215.
18. Hahn S, Haselhorst U, Tan S et al. Low serum 25-hydroxyvitamin D concentrations are associated with insulin resistance and obesity in women with polycystic ovary syndrome. Exp Clin Endocrinol Diabetes 2006; 114:577-583.
19. Hagenfeldt Y, Carlstrom K, Berlin T et al. Effects of orchidectomy and different modes of high dose estrogen treatment on circulating free and total 1,25-dihydroxyvitamin D in patients with prostatic cancer. J Steroid Biochem Mol Biol 1991; 39:155-159.
20. Brustad M, Alsaker E, Engelsen O et al. Vitamin D status of middle-aged women at 65-71 degrees N in relation to dietary intake and exposure to ultraviolet radiation. Public Health Nutr 2004; 7:327-335.
21. Meyer HE, Falch JA, Sogaard AJ et al. Vitamin D deficiency and secondary hyperparathyroidism and the association with bone mineral density in persons with Pakistani and Norwegian background living in Oslo, Norway, The Oslo Health Study. Bone 2004; 35:412-417.
22. Mowe M, Bohmer T, Haug E. Vitamin D deficiency among hospitalized and home-bound elderly. Tidsskr Nor Laegeforen 1998; 118:3929-3931.
23. Sem SW, Sjoen RJ, Trygg K et al. Vitamin D status of two groups of elderly in Oslo: living in old people's homes and living in own homes. Compr Gerontol [A] 1987; 1:126-130.
24. Vik T, Try K, Stromme JH. The vitamin D status of man at 70 degrees north. Scand J Clin Lab Invest 1980; 40:227-232.
25. Moan J, Porojnicu AC, Robsahm TE et al. Solar radiation, vitamin D and survival rate of colon cancer in Norway. J Photochem Photobiol B 2005; 78:189-193.
26. Madronich S, McKenzie RL, Bjorn LO et al. Changes in biologically active ultraviolet radiation reaching the Earth's surface. J Photochem Photobiol B 1998; 46:5-19.
27. Stamnes K, Tsay SC, Wiscombe W et al. Numerically stable algorithm for discrete-ordinate-method for radiative transfer in multiple scattering and emitting layered media. Appl Opt 1988:2502-2509.
28. Dahlback A, Stamnes K. A new spherical model for computing the radiation field available for photolysis and heating rate at twilight. Planet Space Sci 1991:671-683.
29. MacLaughlin JA, Anderson RR, Holick MF. Spectral character of sunlight modulates photosynthesis of previtamin D3 and its photoisomers in human skin. Science 1982; 216:1001-1003.
30. Moan J, Dahlback A, Henriksen T et al. Biological amplification factor for sunlight-induced nonmelanoma skin cancer at high latitudes. Cancer Res 1989; 49:5207-5212.
31. Statistics Norway. http://www.ssb.no/english/subjects/02/01/10/innvbef_en/ . 24-11-2005 (Accessed on February 2007).
32. Robsahm TE, Tretli S, Dahlback A et al. Vitamin D3 from sunlight may improve the prognosis of breast-, colon- and prostate cancer (Norway). Cancer Causes Control 2004; 15:149-158.
33. Johansson L, Solvoll K. Norkost 1997 Norwegian National Dietary Survey 45. 1999. Oslo, Statens råd for ernæring of fysisk aktivitet. Ref Type: Report

34. Porojnicu AC, Robsahm TE, Dahlback A et al. Seasonal and geographical variations in lung cancer prognosis in Norway. Does vitamin D from the sun play a role? Lung Cancer 2005. DOI: 10.1016/J lungcan 2006:11-013.
35. Porojnicu AC, Lagunova Z, Robsahm TE et al. Changes in risk of death from breast cancer with season and latitude: Sun exposure and breast cancer survival in Norway. Breast Cancer Res Treat 2007; 102:323-328.
36. Brot C, Vestergaard P, Kolthoff N et al. Vitamin D status and its adequacy in healthy Danish perimenopausal women: relationships to dietary intake, sun exposure and serum parathyroid hormone. Br J Nutr 2001; 86 Suppl 1:S97-103.
37. Lund B, Sorensen OH. Measurement of 25-hydroxyvitamin D in serum and its relation to sunshine, age and vitamin D intake in the Danish population. Scand J Clin Lab Invest 1979; 39:23-30.
38. Giovannucci E. The epidemiology of vitamin D and cancer incidence and mortality: A review (United States). Cancer Causes Control 2005; 16:83-95.
39. Colston KW, Hansen CM. Mechanisms implicated in the growth regulatory effects of vitamin D in breast cancer. Endocr Relat Cancer 2002; 9:45-59.
40. Gewirtz DA, Sundaram S, Magnet KJ. Influence of topoisomerase II inhibitors and ionizing radiation on growth arrest and cell death pathways in the breast tumor cell. Cell Biochem Biophys 2000; 33:19-31.
41. James SY, Mackay AG, Colston KW. Vitamin D derivatives in combination with 9-cis retinoic acid promote active cell death in breast cancer cells. J Mol Endocrinol 1995; 14:391-394.
42. Ravid A, Rocker D, Machlenkin A et al. 1,25-Dihydroxyvitamin D3 enhances the susceptibility of breast cancer cells to doxorubicin-induced oxidative damage. Cancer Res 1999; 59:862-867.
43. Vink-van Wijngaarden T, Pols HA, Buurman CJ et al. Inhibition of breast cancer cell growth by combined treatment with vitamin D3 analogues and tamoxifen. Cancer Res 1994; 54:5711-5717.
44. Wang Q, Yang W, Uytingco MS et al. 1,25-Dihydroxyvitamin D3 and all-trans-retinoic acid sensitize breast cancer cells to chemotherapy-induced cell death. Cancer Res 2000; 60:2040-2048.
45. Polek TC, Weigel NL. Vitamin D and prostate cancer. J Androl 2002; 23:9-17.
46. Ting HJ, Hsu J, Bao BY et al. Docetaxel-induced growth inhibition and apoptosis in androgen independent prostate cancer cells are enhanced by 1alpha, 25-dihydroxyvitamin D(3). Cancer Lett 2007; 247:122-129.
47. Bao BY, Yao J, Lee YF. 1alpha, 25-dihydroxyvitamin D3 suppresses interleukin-8-mediated prostate cancer cell angiogenesis. Carcinogenesis 2006; 27:1883-1893.
48. Bao BY, Yeh SD, Lee YF. 1alpha, 25-dihydroxyvitamin D3 inhibits prostate cancer cell invasion via modulation of selective proteases. Carcinogenesis 2006; 27:32-42.
49. Gonzalez-Sancho JM, Larriba MJ, Ordonez-Moran P et al. Effects of 1alpha,25-dihydroxyvitamin D3 in human colon cancer cells. Anticancer Res 2006; 26:2669-2681.
50. Cross HS, Bises G, Lechner D et al. The Vitamin D endocrine system of the gut—its possible role in colorectal cancer prevention. J Steroid Biochem Mol Biol 2005; 97:121-128.
51. Guzey M, Sattler C, DeLuca HF. Combinational effects of vitamin D3 and retinoic acid (all trans and 9 cis) on proliferation, differentiation and programmed cell death in two small cell lung carcinoma cell lines. Biochem Biophys Res Commun 1998; 249:735-744.
52. Nakagawa K, Kawaura A, Kato S et al. Metastatic growth of lung cancer cells is extremely reduced in Vitamin D receptor knockout mice. J Steroid Biochem Mol Biol 2004; 89-90:545-547.
53. Nakagawa K, Kawaura A, Kato S et al. 1 alpha,25-Dihydroxyvitamin D(3) is a preventive factor in the metastasis of lung cancer. Carcinogenesis 2005; 26:429-440.
54. Nakagawa K, Sasaki Y, Kato S et al. 22-Oxa-1alpha,25-dihydroxyvitamin D3 inhibits metastasis and angiogenesis in lung cancer. Carcinogenesis 2005; 26:1044-1054.
55. DeLuca HF, Schnoes HK. Metabolism and mechanism of action of vitamin D. Annu Rev Biochem 1976; 45:631-66.:631-666.
56. Zehnder D, Bland R, Williams MC et al. Extrarenal expression of 25-hydroxyvitamin d(3)-1 alpha-hydroxylase. J Clin Endocrinol Metab 2001; 86:888-894.
57. Lim HS, Roychoudhuri R, Peto J et al. Cancer survival is dependent on season of diagnosis and sunlight exposure. Int J Cancer 2006; 119:1530-1536.
58. Porojnicu AC, Robsahm TE, Hansen Ree A et al. Season of diagnosis is a prognostic factor in Hodgkin lymphoma. A possible role of sun-induced vitamin D. Br J Cancer 2005; 93:571-574.
59. Reichrath J. The challenge resulting from positive and negative effects of sunlight: How much solar UV exposure is appropriate to balance between risks of vitamin D deficiency and skin cancer? Prog Biophys Mol Biol 2006; 92:9-16.
60. Holick MF. Vitamin D: importance in the prevention of cancers, type 1 diabetes, heart disease and osteoporosis. Am J Clin Nutr 2004; 79:362-371.

61. Hansen S, Norstein J, Næss, A. Cancer in Norway 2001. Cancer Registry in Norway. Oslo 2004; 36-37.
62. Vieth R. Why the optimal requirement for Vitamin D3 is probably much higher than what is officially recommended for adults. J Steroid Biochem Mol Biol 2004; 89-90:575-579.
63. Vieth R. Critique of the considerations for establishing the tolerable upper intake level for vitamin D: critical need for revision upwards. J Nutr 2006; 136:1117-1122.
64. Calvo MS, Whiting SJ. Public health strategies to overcome barriers to optimal vitamin D status in populations with special needs. J Nutr 2006; 136:1135-1139.

Chapter 5

Optimal Serum 25-Hydroxyvitamin D Levels for Multiple Health Outcomes

Heike A. Bischoff-Ferrari*

Abstract

Recent evidence suggests that higher vitamin D intakes beyond current recommendations may be associated with better health outcomes. In this chapter, evidence is summarized from different studies that evaluate threshold levels for serum 25(OH)D levels in relation to bone mineral density (BMD), lower extremity function, dental health, risk of falls, admission to nursing home, fractures, cancer prevention and incident hypertension. For all endpoints, the most advantageous serum levels for 25(OH)D appeared to be at least 75 nmol/l (30 ng/ml) and for cancer prevention, desirable 25(OH)D levels are between 90-120 nmol/l (36-48 ng/ml). An intake of no less than 1000 IU (25 mcg) of vitamin D3 (cholecalciferol) per day for all adults may bring at least 50% of the population up to 75 nmol/l. Thus, higher doses of vitamin D are needed to bring most individuals into the desired range. While estimates suggest that 2000 IU vitamin D3 per day may successfully and safely achieve this goal, the implications of 2000 IU or higher doses for the total adult population need to be addressed in future studies.

Introduction

Current efforts to assess optimal levels of serum 25(OH)D levels generally focus on bone health in older Caucasian persons and the common means to define optimal 25(OH)D has been the level that maximally suppresses serum parathyroid hormone (PTH). This is a useful criterion because PTH promotes bone loss, but concerns related to this approach are several, such as fluctuations related to diet,[2,3] time of day,[4] renal function[2] and physical activity.[5] Estimates of optimal 25(OH)D levels using PTH suppression vary widely from 20 to 110 nmol/l (9 to 38 ng/ml)[6-11] and a consensus has not been reached.

Thus, this chapter examines several alternative endpoints to the maximal suppression of PTH for bone health, including BMD in younger and older adults of different racial/ethnic backgrounds and antifracture efficacy based on a recent meta-analysis of double-blind randomized controlled trials (RCTs).[12] In addition, optimal 25(OH)D levels for nonskeletal outcomes of public health significance are evaluated, including lower extremity function and falls, nursing home admission, dental health, cancer prevention and hypertension. Finally, the optimal 25(OH)D levels and corresponding vitamin D intakes throughout adult life that best enhance health are discussed.[13]

25(OH)D Levels and Bone Health

Background

BMD may be a better endpoint than serum PTH for the estimation of optimal 25(OH)D levels in regard to bone health for a large part of the population, including younger individuals

*Heike A. Bischoff-Ferrari—Deptartment of Rheumatology and Institute of Physical Medicine, University Hospital Zurich, Zurich, Switzerland. Email: heike.bischoff@usz.ch

Sunlight, Vitamin D and Skin Cancer, edited by Jörg Reichrath. ©2008 Landes Bioscience and Springer Science+Business Media.

and nonCaucasian ethnicities. In the elderly, BMD is a strong predictor of fracture risk[14] and evidence from several RCTs suggest a positive effect of vitamin D supplementation on BMD.[15-17] Furthermore, BMD integrates the lifetime impact of many influences on the skeleton, including PTH.

Optimal 25(OH)D Levels for BMD

A threshold for optimal 25(OH)D and hip BMD has been addressed among 13,432 individuals of NHANES III (The Third National Health and Nutrition Examination Survey) including both younger (20-49 years) and older (50+ years) individuals with different ethnic racial background.[18] Compared to the lowest quintile of 25(OH)D the highest quintile had higher mean BMD by 4.1% in younger whites (test for trend; p < 0.0001), by 4.8% in older whites (p < 0.0001), by 1.8% in younger Mexican Americans (p = 0.004), by 3.6% in older Mexican Americans (p = 0.01), by 1.2% in younger blacks (p = 0.08) and by 2.5% in older blacks (p = 0.03). In the regression plots higher serum 25(OH)D levels were associated with higher BMD throughout the reference range of 22.5 to 94 nmol/l in all subgroups (Figs. 1A and B). In younger whites and younger Mexican Americans, higher 25(OH)D was associated with higher BMD even beyond 100 nmol/l.

Optimal 25(OH)D Levels for Fracture Prevention Efficacy

A meta-analysis of primary prevention high-quality RCTs published in 2005, evaluated the antifracture efficacy of oral vitamin D supplementation in older persons (all trials used chole-calciferol).[12] Five RCTs for hip fracture (n = 9294) and seven RCTs for nonvertebral fracture risk (n = 9820) were included. There was heterogeneity among studies for both hip fracture and nonvertebral fracture prevention, which disappeared after pooling RCTs with low dose vitamin D (400 IU/day, 10 mcg/day) and higher dose vitamin D (700-800 IU/day; 17.5-20 mcg/day) separately. 700-800 IU vitamin D per day reduced the relative risk (RR) of hip fracture by 26% (pooled RR = 0.74; 95% CI [0.61,0.88]) and any nonvertebral fracture by 23% (pooled RR = 0.77; 95% CI [0.68,0.87]) compared to calcium or placebo. No significant benefit was observed for RCTs with 400 IU vitamin D per day (pooled RR for hip fracture was 1.15; 95% CI [0.88,1.50] and for any nonvertebral fracture 1.03; 95% CI [0.86,1.24]). The most recent Women's Health Initiative (WHI) trial comparing 400 IU vitamin D plus 1000 mg calcium to placebo among 36,282 postmenopausal women confirm the findings of the earlier meta-analysis indicating no benefit of low dose vitamin D on hip fracture risk (RR = 0.88; 95% CI [0.72,1.08]).[19]

From left to right, Figures 2 A and B indicate increased antifracture efficacy with higher achieved 25(OH)D levels in the treatment group for both hip (2A) and any nonvertebral fracture (2B), which reached significance in meta-regression analyses. From Figures 2 A and B optimal fracture prevention appeared to occur in trials with achieved mean 25(OH)D levels of at least 74 nmol/l. This level was reached only in trials that gave 700-800 IU cholecalciferol starting from mean baseline levels between 44 to 77 nmol/l. Thus optimal fracture prevention may require more than 700-800 IU vitamin D in populations with baseline 25(OH)D levels below 44 nmol/l and baseline levels may depend on latitude,[20] type of dwelling)[21,22] and fortification of dairy products with vitamin D.[23] Low baseline levels plus low compliance may in part explain why two recent trials from the UK, which were not included in the 2005 meta-analysis, did not achieve antifracture efficacy with 800 IU cholecalciferol per day.[24,25]

In the Record Trial, starting from a mean of 38 nmol/l (15.2 ng/ml), the achieved mean 25(OH)D levels were 62 nmol/l in the vitamin D treatment group. This is, according to the 2005 meta-analysis, not enough for fracture prevention. The small increase in 25(OH)D levels despite the 800 IU vitamin D intervention dose may be explained by the low compliance in the trial: 60% at 12 months and 47% at 24 months among persons who returned the 4-monthly questionnaire and even lower if all participants were considered. In the second UK trial 800 IU vitamin D by Porthouse and colleagues 25(OH)D levels were not reported.[25] Limitations of the Porthouse trial were the open design plus low compliance. In addition, instructions given to the control group regarding adequate calcium and vitamin D intake may have biased the result towards the null. Still, the authors report an effect size for hip fracture prevention with vitamin D that is similar to

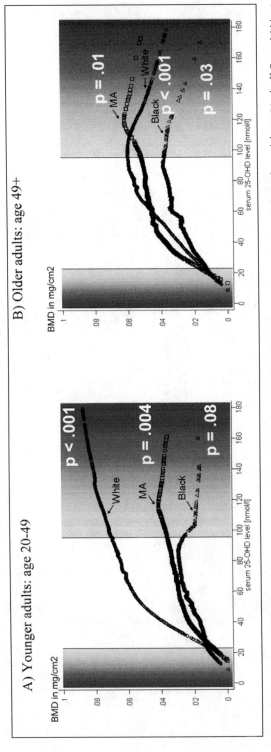

Figures 1A and B. Association between 25(OH)D serum levels and total hip bone mineral density. Figure 1 is adapted from Bischoff-Ferrari HA et al. "Positive association between 25-hydroxy vitamin d levels and bone mineral density: a population-based study of younger and older adults", Am J Med 2004, Vol. 116, Issue 9, Page 634-9. Copyright © (2004), America Journal of Medicine. All Rights reserved.[18] Regression plot of difference in bone mineral density by 25(OH)D in younger (20 to 49 years, Fig. 1A) and older adults (50+ years, Fig. 1B). Symbols represent different ethnicities: circles are Caucasians, squares are Mexican Americans and triangles are African American individuals. The intercept was set to "0" for all race/ethnicity groups to focus on the difference in BMD by 25(OH)D levels, as oppose to differences in BMD by race/ethnicity. The reference range of the 25(OH)D assay (22.5-94 nmol/l) is marked as vertical lines. The reference range of the Diasorin assay has been provided by the company and was established using 98 samples from apparently healthy normal volunteers collected in the south-western United States (high latitude) in late autumn (www.fda.gov/cdrh/pdf3/k032844.pdf). Regression plots adjust for gender, age, body mass index, smoking, calcium intake, estrogen use, month and poverty income ratio. Weighting accounts for NHANES III sampling weights, stratification and clustering.

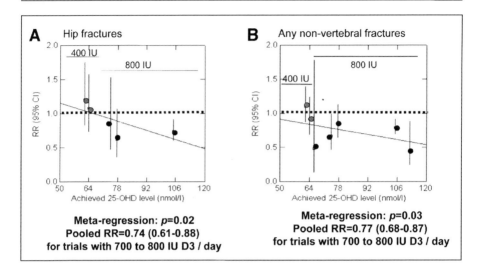

Figure 2A and B. Fracture efficacy by achieved 25(OH)D levels. Figures 2A and 2B are adapted from Bischoff-Ferrari HA et al. "Fracture Prevention with vitamin D supplementation: a meta-analysis of randomized controlled trials", JAMA 2005, Vol. 293, Issue 18, Pages 2257-64, Copyright © (2005), American Medical Association. All Rights reserved.[12] Dotted line represents relative risks (RRs) for the risk of any hip fracture among those who took vitamin D vs those on the control group. All trials identified for the primary analysis are included (from left to right: Lips et al[141] Meyer et al[142] Trivedi et al[143] Decalyos II,[144] Decalyos I[16]). Error bars represent 95% confidence intervals (CIs). Trendline is based on series of effect sizes (open squares). A meta regression, including 9294 individuals indicated a significant inverse relation between higher achieved 25(OH)D levels in the treatment group and hip fracture risk (Beta = −0.009; p = 0.02; meaning that the log RR of hip fracture is estimated to decrease by 0.009 per 1 nmol/l increase in 25(OH)D).
Figure 2B. Dotted line represents relative risks (RRs) for the risk of any nonvertebral fracture among Those who took vitamin D vs those on the control group. All trials identified for the primary analysis are included (from left to right: Lips et al[141] Meyer et al[142] Pfeifer et al[38] Trivedi et al[143] Decalyos II,[144] Decalyos I,[16] Dawson-Hughes et al[15]). Error bars represent 95% confidence intervals (CIs). Trend line is based on series of effect sizes (open squares). A meta regression, including 9820 individuals, indicated a significant inverse relation between higher achieved 25(OH)D levels in the treatment group and any nonvertebral fracture risk (Beta = −0.006; p = 0.03; meaning that the log RR of nonvertebral fracture is estimated to decrease by 0.006 per 1 nmol/l of 25(OH)D achieved in the treatment group). If the Record trial was added to the graph, it would be super-imposed to the trial of Lips et al on the far left (Record achieved 62 nmol/l 25(OH)D with 800 IU cholecalciferol per day in the treatment group and the RR of cholecalciferol preventing any low-trauma fracture in Record was 1.02, 95% CI [0.88,1.19][24]).
Diasorin equivalent values (Diasorin, Stillwater, Minnesota, USA[145]): Lips[41]: 54 nmol/l; Meyer[142]: as reported, Diasorin equivalent values not available[146]; Pfeifer[38]: as reported, Diasorin equivalent values not available; Decalyos II[144]: 63 nmol/l; Decalyos I[16]: 75 nmol/l; Trivedi[143]: 74 nmol/l; Dawson-Hughes[15]: 99 nmol/l).

the result of the meta-analysis (RR = 0.75; 95% CI [0.31, 1.78), however surrounded by a large confidence interval.

Figure 3 illustrates hip fracture efficacy by total vitamin D intake in the treatment group considering compliance and additional vitamin D intake (WHI women consumed a mean of 360 IU vitamin D throughout the trial).[19] The graph suggests that efficacy increases with higher predicted actual mean intake of vitamin D in the treatment group. Studies that were successful

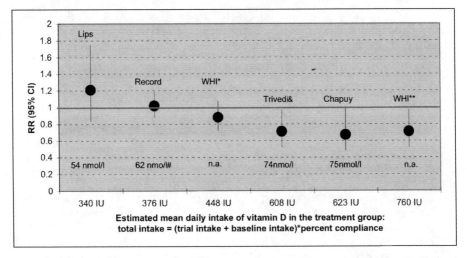

Figure 3. Fracture efficacy of Vitamin D by estimated total intake under consideration of compliance. Figure 3 is adapted from Bischoff-Ferrari HA "How to select the doses of vitamin D in the management of osteoporosis", Osteoporos Int 2007; 18(4):401-7. Copyright © (2007), Osteoporosis International. All Rights reserved.[147] Compliance in the different trials was reported as follows: Lips (400 IU per day) = 85%,[141] Record = 47%,[24] WHI* intent-to-treat analysis (400 IU per day plus additional reported mean vitamin D intake of 360 IU) = 59%,[19] Trivedi (100,000 IU every 4 months equals to 820 IU per day) = 76% (&includes hip plus forearm fractures),[143] Chapuy (800 IU per day) = 84%,[16] WHI**compliant women (400 IU per day plus additional reported mean vitamin D intake of 360 IU) = 100%.[19] In most studies being compliant was defined as taking 80% or more of the study medication. The x-axis gives the DiaSorin equivalent 25(OH)D levels in nmol/l achieved in the treatment arm of the trials. #For the Record trial a HPLC method has been used for 25(OH)D measurement with an unknown DiaSorin equivalent value. In the WHI trial, 25(OH)D levels have not been measured at follow-up in the study population (n.a. = not available).

in fracture reduction had an actual mean estimated intake of more than 600 IU per day and associated achieved mean 25(OH)D levels were close to 75 nmol/l. 25(OH)D levels are expressed in DiaSorin equivalent levels in Figure 3 as measurements of 25-OHD vary between assays[26] and the DiaSorin assay is widely used.

In summary, the data for bone health, based on BMD in younger and older adults, as well as prevention of hip and any nonvertebral fractures in older adults, suggest that serum 25(OH)D levels of at least 75 nmol/l are desirable.

25(OH)D and Lower Extremity Function

Background

The protective effect of vitamin D on fractures has been primarily attributed to the established benefit of vitamin D on calcium homeostasis and bone mineral density.[15,17,27-29] However, muscle weakness is also a prominent feature of the clinical syndrome of vitamin D deficiency[30,31] and may plausibly mediate fracture risk through an increased susceptibility to falls.[30,32-36]

A meta-analysis of RCTs published in 2004 addressed the effect of vitamin D on the risk of falling in older persons.[37] Based on 5 RCTs (n = 1237), vitamin D reduced the risk of falling by 22% (pooled corrected OR = 0.78; 95% CI [0.64, 0.92]) compared to calcium or placebo.[33,38-41] Subgroup analyses suggested that the reduction in risk was independent of the type of vitamin D, duration of therapy and gender. However, the results from one trial suggested that 400 IU of vitamin D may not be clinically effective in preventing falls in the elderly,[41] while two trials that used 800 IU of vitamin D per day plus calcium reduced the risk of falling.[33,38] For the two trials with 259 subjects using 800 IU of cholecalciferol, the corrected pooled OR was 0.65 (95% CI [0.40, 1.00]).[37] The importance of dose of vitamin D in regard to antifall efficacy was addressed within one double-blind RCT among 124 nursing home residents receiving 200, 400, 600 or 800 IU vitamin D compared to placebo over a 5 month period. Participants in the 800 IU group had a 72% lower adjusted-incidence rate ratio of falls than those taking placebo (rate ratio = 0.28; 95% confidence interval = 0.11-0.75) and their mean 25-hydroxyvitamin D level increased from 51 to 72 nmol/l.[42]

Since the 2004 meta-analysis, long-term antifall efficacy of cholecalciferol was shown in community-dwelling older women. The double-blind RCT compared 700 IU vitamin D plus 500 mg calcium to placebo over a 3-year intervention among 246 community-dwelling older men and women. Among women, treatment resulted in a 46% reduction in the odds of falling (odds ratio [OR], 0.54; 95% confidence interval [CI], 0.30-0.97).[43] Fall reduction was most pronounced in less active women (OR = 0.35; 95% CI, 0.15-0.81), while the effect in 199 community-dwelling older men was neutral (OR = 0.93; 95% CI, 0.50-1.72). Only, among compliant less active men, there was a suggestion of a benefit of treatment in regard to fall reduction (OR = 0.65; 95% CI, 0.18-2.29). 25(OH)D levels in this trial increased from 67 to 99 nmol/l (Diasorin adjusted levels).

A physiologic explanation for the beneficial effect of vitamin D on muscle strength is that 1,25-dihydroxyvitamin D (1,25(OH)$_2$D), the active vitamin D metabolite, binds to a vitamin D specific nuclear receptor in muscle tissue[44-46] leading to de novo protein synthesis,[30,34] muscle cell growth[34] and improved muscle function.[31,33,38,47] Higher serum 25(OH)D levels raise the substrate level for intracellular, tissue-specific 1-α-hydroxylases, thereby permitting intracellular levels of 1,25(OH)$_2$D to rise in muscle and other tissues.[48]

Optimal 25(OH)D Levels and Lower Extremity Function

A threshold for optimal 25(OH)D and lower extremity function has been addressed in two population-based surveys, one from the US (NHANES III including 4100 ambulatory older adults age 60 and older)[47] and one from the Netherlands (Longitudinal Study of Aging Amsterdam).[49] In the US survey, functional assessment included the 8-foot-walk test and sit-to-stand test.[50,51] Both tests depend on lower extremity strength and mirror functions needed in everyday life. In both tests, performance speed continued to increase throughout the reference range of 25(OH)D (22.5 to 94 nmol/l) with most of the improvement occurring in 25(OH)D levels going from 22.5 to approximately 50 nmol/l. Further improvement was seen in the range of 50-94 nmol, but the magnitude was less dramatic. For the 8-foot walk test, compared to the lowest quintile of 25(OH)D, the highest quintile showed an average improvement by 5.6% (test for trend: p < 0.001). For the sit-to-stand test, compared to the lowest quintile of 25(OH)D the highest quintile showed an average improvement by 3.9% (test for trend: p = 0.017)

Results were similar for subgroups of active and inactive individuals, men and women, three ethnic groups (Caucasians, African Americans and Mexican Americans) and persons with higher (>500 mg/day) and lower calcium intakes (≤500 mg/day).

This is supported by data from the Longitudinal Aging Study Amsterdam including 1351 Dutch men and women age 65 and older.[52] In that study, physical performance improved continuously from very low levels of serum 25(OH)D up to 75 nmol/l. Compared to individuals with 25(OH)D levels of 75 nmol/l and higher , individuals with serum levels below 25 nmol/l had a 2.54- fold cumulative odds (95% CI [1.63-3.97]) of scoring 1 point lower on the walking test (score range was 0-4), a 2.23-fold cummulitive odds (95% CI [1.45-3.41]) of scoring one point lower in the chair test and a 2.17-fold cumulative odds (95% CI [1.31-3.59]) of scoring one point lower on the tandem stand. For all tests there appeared to be a trend between better test performance and higher 25(OH)D levels.

Thus, data for lower extremity strength suggest that serum 25(OH)D levels of at least 50 nmol/l are desirable, but 75-100 nmol/l are best. Consistent with and likely closely linked to better function and lower fracture risk, the LASA data also showed a significant trend between baseline 25(OH)D levels and risk of nursing home admission over a 6 year follow-up. Compared to older individuals with adequate 25(OH)D levels of 75 nmol/l or higher, risk of nursing home admission was 3.48-fold higher (95% CI [1.39, 8.75) among individuals with 25(OH)D levels <25 nmol/l, 2.77-fold higher (95% CI [1.17-6.55]) individuals with 25(OH)D levels between 25-49 nmol/l and 1.92-fold higher (95% CI [0.79-4.66]) among individuals with 25(OH)D levels between 50-74 nmol/l (p-value for trend test = 0.002).

25(OH)D and Dental Health

Periodontal disease is a common chronic inflammatory disease in middle-aged and older persons characterized by the loss of periodontal attachment, including the periodontal ligaments and alveolar bone. Periodontal disease is the leading cause of tooth loss, particularly in older persons[53-56] and tooth loss is an important determinant of nutrient intake and quality of life.[57-59] Several epidemiological studies have reported positive associations between osteoporosis or low bone density and alveolar bone and tooth loss, indicating that poor bone quality may be a risk factor for periodontal disease.[60-66] Chronic marginal gingivitis, a chronic inflammation of the gingival tissues that is induced by bacterial dental plaque appears to be independent of underlying bone, but may in susceptible patients, eventually lead to the destruction of periodontal ligament and alveolar bone and may thus evolve into periodontal disease.

Vitamin D has been linked to both gingivitis and periodontal disease with an indication of a threshold of 75 nmol/l or above associated with best outcomes. Vitamin D may also reduce both gingivitis and periodontal disease through its antiinflammatory effect.[67,68] One epidemiologic study evaluated data from 77 503 gingival units (teeth) in 6700 never smokers aged 13 to 90 y from NHANES III. Compared with sites in subjects in the lowest 25(OH)D quintile (median: 32.4 nmol/L), sites in subjects in the highest 25(OH)D quintile (median: 99.6 nmol/L) were 20% (95% CI: 8%, 31%) less likely to bleed on gingival probing (p-value for trend test = 0.001).[69] The association appeared to be linear over the entire 25(OH)D range, was consistent across racial or ethnic groups and was similar among men and women. Furthermore, the association was independent of age, sex, income, BMI, intake of vitamin C, full crown coverage, calculus, frequency of dental visits, diabetes, use of oral contraceptives and hormone replacement therapy among women, number of missing teeth and diabetes.

Another epidemiologic study evaluated the association between 25(OH)D levels and alveolar attachment loss, a measure of periodontal disease, in NHANES III including 11,202 ambulatory subjects aged 20+ years.[70] The analysis revealed that 25(OH)D status was not significantly associated with attachment loss in younger men and women (20-50 years). However, in persons above 50 years of age, a significant association between 25(OH)D and attachment loss was observed in both genders independent of race/ethnicity (trend-test in men: p = 0.001; trend-test in women: p = 0.008). Figures 4 A and 4B display the quintiles of 25(OH)D levels in relation to degree of attachment loss. On average, the men aged 50 y who were in the lowest quintile of serum 25(OH)D3 concentration (<40 nmol/l) compared to those in the highest quintile (>85 nmol/l) lost 27% AL (95% CI: 12%, 42%). Similary women in the lowest quintile lost 23% (95% CI: 8%, 38%) compared to those women in the top quintile. Surprisingly, BMD of the total hip region was not associated with attachment loss and adjustment for this did not attenuate the association between 25(OH)D and attachment loss.

Today, one RCT tested the benefit of vitamin D (700 IU/day) plus calcium (500 mg/day) supplementation compared to placebo in regard to tooth loss. Treatment significantly reduced tooth loss in older individuals over a 3 year treatment period (OR = 0.4; 95% CI [0.2, 0.9]); while serum 25(OH)D levels increased from 71 nmol/l to 112 nmol/l.[71] Thus, available evidence suggests that for dental health serum 25(OH)D levels between 75-100 nmol/l are desirable.

25(OH)D and Cancer Incidence and Mortality

Serum 25(OH)D, after its conversion to 1,25-dihydroxyvitamin D, inhibits cell proliferation and induces cell differentiation and apoptosis in tumor cells[72] and thus may reduce cancer risk. It has

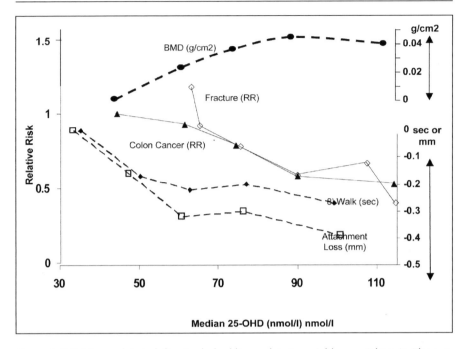

Figure 4. Solid lines relate to left axis, dashed lines relate to variables on right axis. The outcomes depicted as RRs are fracture risk (for more detail see Fig. 2) and colon cancer (data
from the Nurses Health Study[91]). For BMD, the example of older Caucasian was chosen (for
more detail see Fig. 1) and the unit is displayed in the upper part of the right side y-axis. For
lower extremity, we chose the 8-foot walk (8′walk) test results from NHANES III discussed
in this chapter[47] and the unit is seconds, as shown on the lower half of the right-side y-axis.
Attachment loss is based on data discussed in this chapter[70] and is given in mm units for
older men, as displayed on the lower half of the right side y-axis. Based on this summary of
all outcomes, the desirable serum 25(OH)D level to be achieved for optimal health is at least
about 75 nmol/l and best 90-100 nmol/l.

been suggested that for cancer prevention the conversion of 25(OH)D to 1,25-dihydroxyvitamin
D is primarily performed locally in various tissues, such as in colon cells by a local 1-alpha-hydrox-
ylase.[73] Importantly, this system critically depends on the substrate 25(OH)D.

A recent pooled analysis for breast cancer incidence and 25(OH)D levels among 1760 women
suggested a dose-response relationship.[74] Pooled odds ratios for breast cancer from lowest to highest
quintile for 25(OH)D were 1.00, 0.90, 0.70, 0.70 and 0.50 (p-value for trend test <0.001). The
medians of the pooled quintiles of serum 25(OH)D were 15, 45, 72.5, 92.5 and 120 nmol/l. Thus,
women with serum 25(OH)D levels of about 120 nmol/l had a 50% lower risk of developing breast
cancer compared to women with severe vitamin D deficiency with serum 25(OH)D levels below
15 nmol/l serum 25(OH)D of approximately 120 nmol/l had 50% lower risk of breast cancer.

Similarly, a recent pooled analysis for colorectal cancer incidence of five studies suggested a
dose-response between higher serum 25(OH)D and lower colorectal cancer risk.[75] Pooled odds
ratios for colorectal cancer from lowest to highest quintile of serum 25(OH)D, were 1.00, 0.82,
0.66, 0.59 and 0.46 (p-value for trend test <0.0001). The medians of the pooled quintiles of serum
25(OH)D were 15, 40, 55, 67.5 and 92.5 nmol/l. Thus, individuals with serum 25(OH)D levels of
about 93 nmol/l had a 54% lower risk of developing colorectal cancer compared to individuals with
severe vitamin D deficiency with serum 25(OH)D levels below 15 nmol/l serum 25(OH)D. Most
research in regard to cancer prevention with vitamin D has been performed for colorectal cancer

and all the studies of colorectal cancer that took into account supplementary vitamin D reported an inverse association.[76-82] In fact, after supplementation with vitamin D, circulating 25(OH)D levels are inversely associated with the size of the proliferative compartment in the colorectal mucosa in humans.[83] Mechanistically, colorectal cancer prevention with vitamin D is explained by several in vitro studies demonstrating the ability of 1,25-dihydroxyvitamin D or 25(OH)D to reduce proliferation and increase differentiation of colorectal cancer cells.[84-87]

Findings from WHI appear to contrast with the epidemiologic data for colorectal cancer.[88] However, two critical issues are dose and duration.[89] In the Nurses Health Study, a statistically significant reduction of colorectal cancer for higher vitamin D intake emerged only at doses above 550 IU per day in consistent users of greater than ten years (RR = 0.42, 95% CI, 0.19-0.91]).[90] In the WHI, median follow-up was only seven years. Furthermore, similar to the most recent findings on 25(OH)D levels and risk of colo-rectal cancer in the Nurses Health Study (Fig. 5),[91] there was a significant inverse trend between lower baseline serum 25(OH)D levels and an increased risk of colo-rectal cancer observed in the WHI participants (p-value = 0.02).

Incidence and mortality from all cause cancer among men in relation to estimated 25(OH)D levels was addressed recently.[92] Among 47,800 men of the Health Professionals Follow-Up Study an increment of 25 nmol/l in predicted 25(OH)D level was associated with a 17% reduction in total cancer incidence (multivariable relative risk [RR] = 0.83, 95% confidence interval [CI] = 0.74 to 0.92), a 29% reduction in total cancer mortality (RR = 0.71, 95% CI = 0.60 to 0.83) and a 45% reduction in digestive-system cancer mortality (RR = 0.55, 95% CI = 0.41 to 0.74). Thus, an incremental increase in 25(OH)D levels of 25 nmol/l could reduce total cancer incidence by 17% and digestive cancers by 45% among men.

Based on data for all cause cancer, breast cancer and colorectal cancer, estimated optimal serum 25(OH)D levels were at least 90 nmol/L. For the prevention of breast cancer serum 25(OH)D levels of 120 nmol/l may be desirable. Each incremental increase of serum 25(OH)D levels by 25 nmol/l appears to reduce total cancer risk by 17% and most pronounced digestive-system cancer risk by 45%. This conclusion is supported by a 2004 NIH (National Institute of Health) sponsored symposium where the role of vitamin D in cancer chemoprevention and treatment was discussed.[93-95]

Optimal 25(OH)D Levels for Blood Pressure Control

Central to cardiovascular health is blood pressure control. Ecologic studies have suggested an inverse association between latitude and blood pressure. In the INTERSALT study, which had 53 centers world-wide, a linear correlation between rise in blood pressure or the prevalence of hypertension and the latitudes north and south of the equator were observed.[96] Furthermore, observational studies found an inverse association between 1,25-dihydroxyvitamin D levels and blood pressure or plasma renin levels among both normotensive[97-100] and hypertensive[97,101,102] individuals. And the results from these observational studies are supported by one small RCT, in which vitamin D treatment reduced blood pressure in community-dwelling older women.[103] In the trial by Pfeifer and colleagues, within 2 months, treatment with vitamin D (800 IU/day) plus calcium (1200 mg/day) lead to a decrease in SBP by 13 mmHg (p = 0.02), a decrease in DBP by 6 mmHg (p = 0.10) and a decrease in heart rate by 4 beats/min (p = 0.02) compared to calcium alone (1200 mg/day). Similarly, in a randomized controlled trial by Krause and colleagues ultraviolet B light (UVB) significantly lowered SBP by 6 mmHg [−14;−1] and DBP by 6 mmHg [−12;−2] within six weeks if compared to ultraviolet A light (UVA).[104] 25-Hydroxyvitamin D levels increased in the UVB group from 58 to 151 nmol/l, while there was no increase in the UVA group.

Two possible mechanisms are suggested. *First,* several in vitro and animal studies suggest that vitamin D is a vasoactive agent and may play a protective role in the development of arterosclerosis: In vascular smooth muscle, several studies have documented the presence of the VDR[105,106] and in vitro studies found that 1,25-dihydroxyvitamin D antagonizes the mitogenic effect of epidermal growth factor on mesangial cell growth.[107,108]

Second, apart from establish renin regulators, such as renal perfusion pressure[109] and tubular sodium load,[110] recent studies suggest that vitamin D suppresses renin production.[111,112] Li and colleagues found that renin and angiotensin II expression was increased in mice lacking the vitamin D receptor (VDR (-I-) mice), whereas angiotensinogen expression was unaltered. As a consequence VDR (-I-) mice developed hypertension, since angiotensin II is a potent vasoconstrictor.[111]

Recent epidemiologic data provides evidence that the serum level of 25(OH)D that confers the maximum benefit in regard risk reduction of incident hypertension among men and women is at least 75 nmol/l (30 ng/ml).[113] Two large prospective cohort studies including 38,388 men from the Health Professionals' Follow-Up Study and 77,531 women from the Nurses' Health Study demonstrated that 25-hydroxyvitamin D levels are inversely associated with risk of incident hypertension.[113] Over a 4-year follow-up, men with serum 25-(OH)D levels of 75 nmol/l or higher had a 6.1-fold reduced risk of incident hypertension (95% confidence interval [CI]: 1.00 to 37.8) and women had a 2.7-fold reduced risk (95% CI: 1.05 to 6.79) if compared to vitamin D deficient individuals (25(OH)D levels <35 nmol/l).

Thus, available evidence suggests that for hypertension prevention serum 25(OH)D levels between 75-100 nmol/l are desirable.

Vitamin D Intake Needed to Achieve Optimal 25(OH)D Levels

Currently recommended intakes are 200 IU/d for young adults, 400 IU/d for those aged 51 to 70 years and 600 IU/d for those over age 70 years.[114]

The vitamin D intake needed to bring a large majority of adults to the desirable 90-100 nmol/l 25(OH)D range has not been defined precisely and depends to some extent on the starting level. Studies in older persons show that 25(OH)D levels could be increased by approximately 10 to 40 nmol/l to mean levels of about 60 nmol/l with 400 IU vitamin D/day,[41,115,116] by 31 nmol/l to mean levels of 79 nmol/l with 600 IU[117] or by 50-65 nmol/l to mean levels of 100 nmol/l with 800 IU of vitamin D per day.[15,16] Mean levels of 75 to 100 nmol/l are achieved with intakes of 700 to 1000 IU/d in groups of young and older adults.[118-120] In young men and women (age 41 ± 9 years SD) 4000 IU vitamin D per day (100 mcg/day) may increase 25(OH)D levels by 56 nmol/l to mean levels of 125 nmol/l.[121]

Adding Calcium to Vitamin D

As calcium absorption is improved with higher serum 25(OH)D levels,[122,123] future studies may need to evaluate whether current calcium intake recommendations with higher doses of vitamin D beyond 2000 IU per day are safe or require downward adjustment.[122] If dietary calcium is a threshold nutrient, as suggested by Dr. Heaney,[94] then that threshold for optimal calcium absorption may be at a lower calcium intake when vitamin D nutrition is higher.

Discussion

This chapter reviews optimal blood 25(OH)D levels for BMD and fracture risk reduction, lower extremity function, falls, risk of nursing home admission, dental health, cancer prevention and risk of incident hypertension. For all endpoints, the data suggested that the minimal target level of 25-OHD should be above 75 nmol/l (30 ng/ml) and optimally between 90 to 120 nmol/l (36 to 48 ng/ml). As such, reaching the optimal 25(OH)D range for bone health, which is the most widely acknowledged benefit of adequate vitamin D status, is expected to provide additional benefit for the investigated nonskeletal outcomes, which all have significant public health implications. Among older individuals, better lower extremity function, less falls and fractures, better dental health and a lower risk of hypertension directly define quality of life and independence at older age, which is reflected in a lower risk for nursing home admission among older individuals with adequate 25(OH)D from one prospective study. The target level of at least 75 nmol/l 25-OHD to achieve optimal health is supported by several experts.

Based on the 2005 fracture meta-analysis, achieved 25(OH)D levels of at least 74 nmol/l could prevent about one fourth of all hip and nonvertebral fractures in both ambulatory and institutionalized older persons.[12] Given the high cost of fracture treatment and the personal burden of disability after fractures, especially hip fractures, this finding has significant public health implications.[124,125] Furthermore, because the positive association between 25(OH)D levels and BMD in younger adults[18] (Fig. 1A) is consistent with the concept that higher levels of serum 25(OH)D may contribute to peak bone mass, maintaining high 25(OH)D levels in younger adulthood could further protect against fractures at older ages.[126]

For the prevention of cancer, higher achieved 25(OH)D levels between 90-120 nmol/l may be most desirable. With little at hand for the prevention of cancer, the suggested benefits of achieved 25(OH)D levels in the range between 90-120 nmol/l on breast cancer risk reduction (50%),[74] colorectal cancer risk reduction (54%)[75] and total cancer risk reduction (17%)[92] are very significant.

Based on a recent national US survey, only 31% of adult Caucasians between 20 and 49 years of age and less than 9% of older Caucasians and an even smaller fraction of the Mexican American and African American adults have serum 25(OH)D levels of 90 nmol/l or more.[18] Most vulnerable to low vitamin D levels are elderly,[21,127] individuals living in northern latitudes with prolonged winters,[10,128] obese individuals[129] and African Americans of all ages.[18,130,131] Other groups with dark skin pigmentation living in northern latitudes will also be at high risk of low vitamin D status. Thus a large majority of the population could benefit from vitamin D supplementation, a simple, highly affordable and well-tolerated strategy that could reduce osteoporosis and fractures and probably reduce falls associated with lower extremity weakness, poor dental health, colorectal cancer and hypertension in older adults.

Vitamin D intakes that may be required to achieve the optimal levels of 25(OH)D in most individuals are not established. Studies suggest that 700 to 1000 IU of vitamin D per day may bring 50% of younger and older adults up to 90-100 nmol/l.[118-120] Thus, to bring most adults to the desirable range of 90-100 nmol/l, vitamin D doses higher than 700-1000 IU would be needed. The current intake recommendation for older persons (600 IU per day) may bring most subjects to 50-60 nmol/l, but not to 90-100 nmol/l and for younger adults, the current recommendation of 200 IU per day is unlikely to be adequate.[18] According to studies in younger adults, intakes of as high as 4000 IU (100 mcg/day) to 10,000 IU (250 mcg/day) are safe[115,121,132] and 4000 IU may bring 88% of healthy young men and women to at least 75 nmol/l.[121] Heaney and colleagues, in a study of healthy men, estimated that 1000 IU cholecalciferol per day are needed during winter months in Nebraska to maintain a late summer starting level of 70 nmol/l, while baseline levels between 20-40 nmol/l may require a daily dose of 2200 IU vitamin D to reach and maintain 80 nmol/l.[94,115] A recent risk assessment on vitamin D based on relevant, well-designed human clinical trials of vitamin D documented the absence of toxicity in trials conducted in healthy adults that used vitamin D dose 10,000 IU vitamin D3.[132] The authors thus suggested an upward adjustment of the safe upper limit from currently 2000 IU to 10,000 IU per day.

If 75-100 nmol/l were the target range of a revised RDA (recommended daily allowance), the new RDA should meet the requirements of 97% of the population.[133] Based on a dose-response calculation proposed by Heaney and colleagues of about 1.0 nmol/(1 µg day) at the lower end of the distribution and 0.6 nmol/(1 µg day) at the upper end,[94] a daily oral dose of 2000 IU (50 mcg/day), the safe upper intake limit as defined by the National Academy of Science,[114] may shift the NHANES III distribution so that only about 10-15% of individuals were below 75 nmol/l. This may result in a 35 nmol/l shift in already replete individuals from between 75-140 nmol/l (NHANES III distribution) to 110-175 nmol/l, which are levels observed in healthy outdoor workers (i.e., farmers: 135 nmol/l[134] and lifeguards: 163 nmol/l[135]). Thus, 2000 IU may be a safe RDA even at the higher end of the normal 25(OH)D serum level distribution and for the lower end it may be conservative. As a first sign of toxicity, only serum 25(OH)D levels of above 220 nmol/l have been associated with hypercalcemia.[136,137]

Due to seasonal fluctuations of 25(OH)D levels,[10] some individuals may be in the target range during summer months. However, these levels will not sustain during the winter months even in sunny latitudes.[127,138] Thus winter supplementation with vitamin D is needed even after a sunny summer. Furthermore, several studies suggest that many older persons will not achieve optimal serum 25(OH)D levels during summer months suggesting that vitamin D supplementation should be independent of season in older persons.[127,139,140]

In summary, for bone health in younger adults and all outcomes in older adults, including antifracture efficacy, lower extremity strength, dental health, cancer prevention and hypertension prevention, serum 25(OH)D levels of at least 75 nmol/l should be the target. For cancer prevention, serum 25(OH)D levels between 90-120 nmol/l may be warranted. While several studies suggest that 50% of the population may achieve serum 25(OH)D levels of 75 nmol/l with a daily intake of about 1000 IU per day, limited data is available for intake estimates that would bring all adults up to this range. Given the low cost, safety and demonstrated benefit of higher 25(OH)D levels, vitamin D supplementation should become a public health priority to combat these common and costly chronic diseases. More studies are needed on the safety of higher doses of vitamin D applied to a population. Among healthy adults, 2000 IU per day may shift most individuals safely into the desired range. However, more data, especially among older individuals, are needed together with a reevaluation of calcium recommendations, which may need downward adjustment with higher vitamin D intakes.

Acknowledgement

This chapter is largely based on a recent review that was a shared effort between the following authors[1]: Dr. Heike A Bischoff-Ferrari, Dr. Edward Giovannucci (Dept. of Nutrition, Harvard School of Public Health, Boston, USA), Dr. Walter C. Willett (Dept. of Nutrition, Harvard School of Public Health, Boston, USA), Dr. Thomas Dietrich (Dept. of Health Policy and Health Services Research, Boston University Goldman School of Dental Medicine, Boston, USA) and Dr. Bess Dawson-Hughes (Jean Mayer USDA Human Nutrition Research Center on Aging, Tufts University, Boston, USA).

References

1. Bischoff-Ferrari HA, Giovannucci E, Willett WC et al. Estimation of optimal serum concentrations of 25-hydroxyvitamin D for multiple health outcomes. Am J Clin Nutr 2006; 84(1):18-28.
2. Freaney R, McBrinn Y, McKenna MJ. Secondary hyperparathyroidism in elderly people: combined effect of renal insufficiency and vitamin D deficiency. Am J Clin Nutr 1993; 58(2):187-91.
3. Dawson-Hughes B, Stern DT, Shipp CC et al. Effect of lowering dietary calcium intake on fractional whole body calcium retention. J Clin Endocrinol Metab 1988; 67(1):62-8.
4. Kitamura N, Shigeno C, Shiomi K et al. Episodic fluctuation in serum intact parathyroid hormone concentration in men. J Clin Endocrinol Metab 1990; 70(1):252-63.
5. Bischoff H, Stahelin HB, Vogt P et al. Immobility as a major cause of bone remodeling in residents of a long-stay geriatric ward. Calcif Tissue Int 1999; 64(6):485-9.
6. Lips P, Wiersinga A, van Ginkel FC et al. The effect of vitamin D supplementation on vitamin D status and parathyroid function in elderly subjects. J Clin Endocrinol Metab 1988; 67(4):644-50.
7. Malabanan A, Veronikis IE, Holick MF. Redefining vitamin D insufficiency. Lancet 1998; 351(9105):805-6.
8. Peacock M. Effects of calcium and vitamin D insufficiency on the skeleton. Osteoporos Int 1998; 8(Suppl 2):S45-51.
9. Chapuy MC, Preziosi P, Maamer M et al. Prevalence of vitamin D insufficiency in an adult normal population. Osteoporos Int 1997; 7(5):439-43.
10. Dawson-Hughes B, Harris SS, Dallal GE. Plasma calcidiol, season and serum parathyroid hormone concentrations in healthy elderly men and women. Am J Clin Nutr 1997; 65(1):67-71.
11. Krall EA, Sahyoun N, Tannenbaum S et al. Effect of vitamin D intake on seasonal variations in parathyroid hormone secretion in postmenopausal women. N Engl J Med 1989; 321(26):1777-83.
12. Bischoff-Ferrari HA, Willett WC, Wong JB et al. Fracture prevention with vitamin D supplementation: a meta-analysis of randomized controlled trials. JAMA 2005; 293(18):2257-64.
13. Raiten DJ, Picciano MF. Vitamin D and health in the 21st century: bone and beyond. Executive summary. Am J Clin Nutr 2004; 80(6 Suppl):1673S-7S.
14. Cummings SR, Nevitt MC, Browner WS et al. Risk factors for hip fracture in white women. Study of Osteoporotic Fractures Research Group. N Engl J Med 1995; 332(12):767-73.
15. Dawson-Hughes B, Harris SS, Krall EA et al. Effect of calcium and vitamin D supplementation on bone density in men and women 65 years of age or older. N Engl J Med 1997; 337(10):670-6.

16. Chapuy MC, Arlot ME, Duboeuf F et al. Vitamin D3 and calcium to prevent hip fractures in the elderly women. N Engl J Med 1992; 327(23):1637-42.
17. Ooms ME, Roos JC, Bezemer PD et al. Prevention of bone loss by vitamin D supplementation in elderly women: a randomized double-blind trial. J Clin Endocrinol Metab 1995; 80(4):1052-8.
18. Bischoff-Ferrari HA, Dietrich T, Orav EJ et al. Positive association between 25-hydroxy vitamin D levels and bone mineral density: a population-based study of younger and older adults. Am J Med 2004; 116(9):634-9.
19. Jackson RD, LaCroix AZ, Gass M et al. Calcium plus vitamin D supplementation and the risk of fractures. N Engl J Med 2006; 354(7):669-83.
20. Lips P, Duong T, Oleksik A et al. A global study of vitamin D status and parathyroid function in postmenopausal women with osteoporosis: baseline data from the multiple outcomes of raloxifene evaluation clinical trial. J Clin Endocrinol Metab 2001; 86(3):1212-21.
21. Theiler R, Stahelin HB, Tyndall A et al. Calcidiol, calcitriol and parathyroid hormone serum concentrations in institutionalized and ambulatory elderly in Switzerland. Int J Vitam Nutr Res 1999; 69(2):96-105.
22. Kinyamu HK, Gallagher JC, Balhorn KE et al. Serum vitamin D metabolites and calcium absorption in normal young and elderly free-living women and in women living in nursing homes. Am J Clin Nutr 1997; 65(3):790-7.
23. Holick MF, Shao Q, Liu WW et al. The vitamin D content of fortified milk and infant formula. N Engl J Med 1992; 326(18):1178-81.
24. Grant AM, Avenell A, Campbell MK et al. Oral vitamin D3 and calcium for secondary prevention of low-trauma fractures in elderly people (Randomised Evaluation of Calcium Or vitamin D, RECORD): a randomised placebo-controlled trial. Lancet 2005; 365(9471):1621-8.
25. Porthouse J, Cockayne S, King C et al. Randomised controlled trial of calcium and supplementation with cholecalciferol (vitamin D3) for prevention of fractures in primary care. Bmj 2005; 330(7498):1003.
26. Lips P, Chapuy MC, Dawson-Hughes B et al. An international comparison of serum 25-hydroxyvitamin D measurements. Osteoporos Int 1999; 9(5):394-7.
27. Gallagher JC, Kinyamu HK, Fowler SE et al. Calciotropic hormones and bone markers in the elderly. J Bone Miner Res 1998; 13(3):475-82.
28. Heaney RP, Barger-Lux MJ, Dowell MS et al. Calcium absorptive effects of vitamin D and its major metabolites. J Clin Endocrinol Metab 1997; 82(12):4111-6.
29. Lips P. Vitamin D deficiency and osteoporosis: the role of vitamin D deficiency and treatment with vitamin D and analogues in the prevention of osteoporosis-related fractures. Eur J Clin Invest 1996; 26:436-442.
30. Boland R. Role of vitamin D in skeletal muscle function. Endocrine Reviews 1986; 7:434-447.
31. Glerup H, Mikkelsen K, Poulsen L et al. Hypovitaminosis D myopathy without biochemical signs of osteomalacic bone involvement. Calcif Tissue Int 2000; 66(6):419-24.
32. Birge SJ, Haddad JG. 25-hydroxycholecalciferol stimulation of muscle metabolism. J Clin Invest 1975; 56(5):1100-7.
33. Bischoff HA, Stahelin HB, Dick W et al. Effects of vitamin D and calcium supplementation on falls: a randomized controlled trial. J Bone Miner Res 2003; 18(2):343-51.
34. Sorensen OH, Lund B, Saltin B et al. Myopathy in bone loss of ageing: improvement by treatment with 1 alpha-hydroxycholecalciferol and calcium. Clin Sci (Colch) 1979; 56(2):157-61.
35. Visser M, Deeg DJ, Lips P. Low vitamin D and high parathyroid hormone levels as determinants of loss of muscle strength and muscle mass (sarcopenia): the Longitudinal Aging Study Amsterdam. J Clin Endocrinol Metab 2003; 88(12):5766-72.
36. Sharkey JR, Giuliani C, Haines PS et al. Summary measure of dietary musculoskeletal nutrient (calcium, vitamin D, magnesium and phosphorus) intakes is associated with lower-extremity physical performance in homebound elderly men and women. Am J Clin Nutr 2003; 77(4):847-56.
37. Bischoff-Ferrari HA, Dawson-Hughes B, Willett CW et al. Effect of vitamin D on falls: a meta-analysis. JAMA 2004; 291(16):1999-2006.
38. Pfeifer M, Begerow B, Minne HW et al. Effects of a short-term vitamin D and calcium supplementation on body sway and secondary hyperparathyroidism in elderly women. J Bone Miner Res 2000; 15(6):1113-8.
39. Gallagher JC, Fowler SE, Detter JR et al. Combination treatment with estrogen and calcitriol in the prevention of age-related bone loss. J Clin Endocrinol Metab 2001; 86(8):3618-28.
40. Dukas L, Bischoff HA, Lindpaintner LS et al. Alfacalcidol Reduces the Number of Fallers in a Community-Dwelling Elderly Population with a Minimum Calcium Intake of More Than 500 Mg Daily. J Am Geriatr Soc 2004; 52(2):230-236.
41. Graafmans WC, Ooms ME, Hofstee HM et al. Falls in the elderly: a prospective study of risk factors and risk profiles. Am J Epidemiol 1996; 143(11):1129-36.

42. Broe KE, Chen TC, Weinberg J et al. A higher dose of vitamin d reduces the risk of falls in nursing home residents: a randomized, multiple-dose study. J Am Geriatr Soc 2007; 55(2):234-9.
43. Bischoff-Ferrari HA, Orav EJ, Dawson-Hughes B. Effect of cholecalciferol plus calcium on falling in ambulatory older men and women: a 3-year randomized controlled trial. Arch Intern Med 2006; 166(4):424-30.
44. Simpson RU, Thomas GA, Arnold AJ. Identification of 1,25-dihydroxyvitamin D3 receptors and activities in muscle. J Biol Chem 1985; 260(15):8882-91.
45. Bischoff HA, Borchers M, Gudat F et al. In situ detection of 1,25-dihydroxyvitamin D3 receptor in human skeletal muscle tissue. Histochem J 2001; 33(1):19-24.
46. Endo I, Inoue D, Mitsui T et al. Deletion of vitamin D receptor gene in mice results in abnormal skeletal muscle development with deregulated expression of myoregulatory transcription factors. Endocrinology 2003; 144(12):5138-44 Epub.
47. Bischoff-Ferrari HA, Dietrich T, Orav EJ et al. Higher 25-hydroxyvitamin D concentrations are associated with better lower-extremity function in both active and inactive persons aged ≥60 y. Am J Clin Nutr 2004; 80(3):752-8.
48. Zehnder D, Bland R, Williams MC et al. Extrarenal expression of 25-hydroxyvitamin d(3)-1 alpha-hydroxylase. J Clin Endocrinol Metab 2001; 86(2):888-94.
49. Wicherts IS, Schoor Van NM, Boeke AJP et al. Vitamin D deficiency and neuromuscular performance in the Longitudinal Ading Study Amsterdam (LASA). JBMR 2005; 20 Suppl 1, abstract 1134:S35.
50. Guralnik JM, Ferrucci L, Simonsick EM et al. Lower-extremity function in persons over the age of 70 years as a predictor of subsequent disability. N Engl J Med 1995; 332(9):556-61.
51. Seeman TE, Charpentier PA, Berkman LF et al. Predicting changes in physical performance in a high-functioning elderly cohort: MacArthur studies of successful aging. J Gerontol 1994; 49(3): M97-108.
52. Wicherts IS, van Schoor NM, Boeke AJ et al. Vitamin D status predicts physical performance and its decline in older persons. J Clin Endocrinol Metab 2007; 6:6.
53. Ong G. Periodontal reasons for tooth loss in an Asian population. J Clin Periodontol 1996; 23:307-309.
54. Phipps KR, Stevens VJ. Relative contribution of caries and periodontal disease in adult tooth loss for an HMO dental population. J Pub Health Dent 1995; 55:250-252.
55. Stabholz A, Babayof I, Mersel A et al. The reasons for tooth loss in geriatric patients attending two surgical clinics in Jerusalem, Israel. Gerodontology 1997; 14:83-88.
56. Warren JJ, Watkins CA, Cowen HJ et al. Tooth loss in the very old: 13-15-year incidence among elderly Iowans. Comm Dent Oral Epidemiol 2002; 30:29-37.
57. Ritchie CS, Joshipura K, Hung HC et al. Nutrition as a mediator in the relation between oral and systemic disease: associations between specific measures of adult oral health and nutrition outcomes. Crit Rev Oral Biol Med 2002; 13:291-300.
58. Marshall TA, Warren JJ, Hand JS et al. Oral health, nutrient intake and dietary quality in the very old. J Am Dent Assoc 2002; 133(10):1369-79.
59. Norlen P, Steen B, Birkhed D et al. On the relations between dietary habits, nutrients and oral health in women at the age of retirement. Acta Odontol Scand 1993; 51(5):277-84.
60. Payne JB, Reinhardt RA, Nummikoski PV et al. The association of cigarette smoking with alveolar bone loss in postmenopausal females. J Clin Periodontol 2000; 27(9):658-64.
61. Payne JB, Reinhardt RA, Nummikoski PV et al. Longitudinal alveolar bone loss in postmenopausal osteoporotic/osteopenic women. Osteoporos Int 1999; 10(1):34-40.
62. Tezal M, Wactawski-Wende J, Grossi SG et al. The relationship between bone mineral density and periodontitis in postmenopausal women. J Periodontol 2000; 71(9):1492-8.
63. Wactawski-Wende J, Grossi SG, Trevisan M et al. The role of osteopenia in oral bone loss and periodontal disease. J Periodontol 1996; 67(10 Suppl):1076-84.
64. Krall EA, Dawson-Hughes B, Papas A et al. Tooth loss and skeletal bone density in healthy postmenopausal women. Osteoporos Int 1994; 4(2):104-9.
65. Bando K, Nitta H, Matsubara M et al. Bone mineral density in periodontally healthy and edentulous postmenopausal women. Ann Periodontol 1998; 3(1):322-6.
66. Krall EA, Garcia RI, Dawson-Hughes B. Increased risk of tooth loss is related to bone loss at the whole body, hip and spine. Calcif Tissue Int 1996; 59(6):433-7.
67. Walters MR. Newly identified actions of the vitamin D endocrine system. Endocr Rev 1992; 13(4):719-64.
68. D'Ambrosio D, Cippitelli M, Cocciolo MG et al. Inhibition of IL-12 production by 1,25-dihydroxyvitamin D3. Involvement of NF-kappaB downregulation in transcriptional repression of the p40 gene. J Clin Invest 1998; 101(1):252-62.

69. Dietrich T, Nunn M, Dawson-Hughes B et al. Association between serum concentrations of 25-hydroxyvitamin D and gingival inflammation. Am J Clin Nutr 2005; 82(3):575-80.
70. Dietrich T, Joshipura KJ, Dawson-Hughes B et al. Association between serum concentrations of 25-hydroxyvitamin D3 and periodontal disease in the US population. Am J Clin Nutr 2004; 80(1):108-13.
71. Krall EA, Wehler C, Garcia RI et al. Calcium and vitamin D supplements reduce tooth loss in the elderly. Am J Med 2001; 111(6):452-6.
72. Chen TC, Persons K, Liu WW et al. The antiproliferative and differentiative activities of 1,25-dihydroxyvitamin D3 are potentiated by epidermal growth factor and attenuated by insulin in cultured human keratinocytes. J Invest Dermatol 1995; 104(1):113-7.
73. Bises G, Kallay E, Weiland T et al. 25-hydroxyvitamin D3-1alpha-hydroxylase expression in normal and malignant human colon. J Histochem Cytochem 2004; 52(7):985-9.
74. Garland CF, Gorham ED, Mohr SB et al. Vitamin D and prevention of breast cancer: Pooled analysis. J Steroid Biochem Mol Biol 2007; 103(3-5):708-11.
75. Gorham ED, Garland CF, Garland FC et al. Optimal vitamin D status for colorectal cancer prevention a quantitative meta analysis. Am J Prev Med 2007; 32(3):210-6.
76. Bostick RM, Potter JD, Sellers TA et al. Relation of calcium, vitamin D and dairy food intake to incidence of colon cancer in older women. American Journal of Epidemiology 1993; 137:1302-1317.
77. Kearney J, Giovannucci E, Rimm EB et al. Calcium, vitamin D and dairy foods and the occurrence of colon cancer in men. American Journal of Epidemiology 1996; 143:907-917.
78. Martinez ME, Giovannucci EL, Colditz GA et al. Calcium, vitamin D and the occurrence of colorectal cancer among women. Journal of the National Cancer Institute 1996; 88:1375-1382.
79. McCullough ML, Robertson AS, Rodriguez C et al. Calcium, vitamin D, dairy products and risk of colorectal cancer in the cancer prevention study II nutrition cohort (United States). Cancer Causes and Control 2003; 14:1-12.
80. Marcus PM, Newcomb PA. The association of calcium and vitamin D and colon and rectal cancer in Wisconsin women. International Journal of Epidemiology 1998; 27:788-793.
81. Zheng W, Anderson KE, Kushi LH et al. A prospective cohort study of intake of calcium, vitamin D and other micronutrients in relation to incidence of rectal cancer among postmenopausal women. Cancer Epidemiology, Biomarkers and Prevention 1998; 7:221-225.
82. Kampman E, Slattery ML, Caan B et al. Calcium, vitamin D, sunshine exposures, dairy products and colon cancer risk (United States). Cancer Causes and Control 2000; 11:459-466.
83. Holt PR, Arber N, Halmos B et al. Colonic epithelial cell proliferation decreases with increasing levels of serum 25-hydroxy vitamin D. Cancer Epidemiology, Biomarkers and Prevention 2002; 11:113-119.
84. Meggouh F, Lointier P, Saez S. Sex steroid and 1,25-dihydroxyvitamin D3 receptors in human colorectal adenocarcinoma and normal mucosa. Cancer Research 1991; 51(4):1227-1233.
85. Giuliano AR, Franceschi RT, Wood RJ. Characterization of the vitamin D receptor from the Caco-2 human colon carcinoma cell line: effect of cellular differentiation. Archives of Biochemistry and Biophysics 1991; 285(2):261-269.
86. Vandewalle B, Adenis A, Hornez L et al. 1,25-dihydroxyvitamin D3 receptors in normal and malignant human colorectal tissues. Cancer Letters 1994; 86(1):67-73.
87. Zhao X, Feldman D. Regulation of vitamin D receptor abundance and responsiveness during differentiation of HT-29 human colon cancer cells. Endocrinology 1993; 132(4):1808-1814.
88. Wactawski-Wende J, Kotchen JM, Anderson GL et al. Calcium plus vitamin D supplementation and the risk of colorectal cancer. N Engl J Med 2006; 354(7):684-96.
89. Giovannucci E. Calcium plus vitamin D and the risk of colorectal cancer. N Engl J Med 2006; 354(21):2287-8; author reply 2287-8.
90. Martinez ME, Giovannucci EL, Colditz GA et al. Calcium, vitamin D and the occurrence of colorectal cancer among women. J Natl Cancer Inst 1996; 88(19):1375-82.
91. Feskanich D, Ma J, Fuchs CS et al. Plasma vitamin d metabolites and risk of colorectal cancer in women. Cancer Epidemiol Biomarkers Prev 2004; 13(9):1502-8.
92. Giovannucci E, Liu Y, Rimm EB et al. Prospective study of predictors of vitamin D status and cancer incidence and mortality in men. J Natl Cancer Inst 2006; 98(7):451-9.
93. The Vitamin D Workshop 2004. J Steroid Biochem Mol Biol 2005; 97(1-2):1-2. Epub.
94. Heaney RP. The Vitamin D requirement in health and disease. J Steroid Biochem Mol Biol 2005; 15:15.
95. Bouillon R, Moody T, Sporn M et al. NIH deltanoids meeting on Vitamin D and cancer. Conclusion and strategic options. J Steroid Biochem Mol Biol 2005; 97(1-2):3-5. Epub .
96. Rostand SG. Ultraviolet light may contribute to geographic and racial blood pressure differences. Hypertension 1997; 30(2 Pt 1):150-6.
97. Resnick LM, Muller FB, Laragh JH. Calcium-regulating hormones in essential hypertension. Relation to plasma renin activity and sodium metabolism. Ann Intern Med 1986; 105(5):649-54.

98. Lind L, Wengle B, Wide L et al. Reduction of blood pressure during long-term treatment with active vitamin D (alphacalcidol) is dependent on plasma renin activity and calcium status. A double-blind, placebo-controlled study. Am J Hypertens 1989; 2(1):20-5.

99. Lind L, Hanni A, Lithell H et al. Vitamin D is related to blood pressure and other cardiovascular risk factors in middle-aged men. Am J Hypertens 1995; 8(9):894-901.

100. Kristal-Boneh E, Froom P, Harari G et al. Association of calcitriol and blood pressure in normotensive men. Hypertension 1997; 30(5):1289-94.

101. Burgess ED, Hawkins RG, Watanabe M. Interaction of 1,25-dihydroxyvitamin D and plasma renin activity in high renin essential hypertension. Am J Hypertens 1990; 3(12 Pt 1):903-5.

102. Imaoka M, Morimoto S, Kitano S et al. Calcium metabolism in elderly hypertensive patients: possible participation of exaggerated sodium, calcium and phosphate excretion. Clin Exp Pharmacol Physiol 1991; 18(9):631-41.

103. Pfeifer M, Begerow B, Minne HW et al. Effects of a short-term vitamin D(3) and calcium supplementation on blood pressure and parathyroid hormone levels in elderly women. J Clin Endocrinol Metab 2001; 86(4):1633-7.

104. Krause R, Buhring M, Hopfenmuller W et al. Ultraviolet B and blood pressure. Lancet 1998; 352(9129):709-10.

105. Koh E, Morimoto S, Fukuo K et al. 1,25-Dihydroxyvitamin D3 binds specifically to rat vascular smooth muscle cells and stimulates their proliferation in vitro. Life Sci 1988; 42(2):215-23.

106. Merke J, Hofmann W, Goldschmidt D et al. Demonstration of 1,25(OH)2 vitamin D3 receptors and actions in vascular smooth muscle cells in vitro. Calcif Tissue Int 1987; 41(2):112-4.

107. Hariharan S, Hong SY, Hsu A et al. Effect of 1,25-dihydroxyvitamin D3 on mesangial cell proliferation. J Lab Clin Med 1991; 117(5):423-9.

108. Mitsuhashi T, Morris RC Jr, Ives HE. 1,25-dihydroxyvitamin D3 modulates growth of vascular smooth muscle cells. J Clin Invest 1991; 87(6):1889-95.

109. Nobiling R, Munter K, Buhrle CP et al. Influence of pulsatile perfusion upon renin release from the isolated perfused rat kidney. Pflugers Arch 1990; 415(6):713-7.

110. Jelinek J, Hackenthal E, Hackenthal R. Role of the renin-angiotensin system in the adaptation to high salt intake in immature rats. J Dev Physiol 1990; 14(2):89-94.

111. Li YC, Kong J, Wei M et al. 1,25-Dihydroxyvitamin D(3) is a negative endocrine regulator of the renin-angiotensin system. J Clin Invest 2002; 110(2):229-38.

112. Li YC. Vitamin D regulation of the renin-angiotensin system. J Cell Biochem 2003; 88(2):327-31.

113. Forman JP, Giovannucci E, Holmes MD et al. Plasma 25-Hydroxyvitamin D Levels and Risk of Incident Hypertension. Hypertension 2007; 19:19.

114. Intakes SCotSEoDR. Dietary reference intakes: calcium, phosphorus, magnesium, vitamin D and fluoride. Washington, DC: National Academy Press, 1997.

115. Heaney RP, Davies KM, Chen TC et al. Human serum 25-hydroxycholecalciferol response to extended oral dosing with cholecalciferol. Am J Clin Nutr 2003; 77(1):204-10.

116. Chel VG, Ooms ME, Popp-Snijders C et al. Ultraviolet irradiation corrects vitamin D deficiency and suppresses secondary hyperparathyroidism in the elderly. J Bone Miner Res 1998; 13(8):1238-42.

117. Vieth R, Kimball S, Hu A et al. Randomized comparison of the effects of the vitamin D3 adequate intake versus 100 mcg (4000 IU) per day on biochemical responses and the wellbeing of patients. Nutr J 2004; 3:8.

118. Tangpricha V, Pearce EN, Chen TC et al. Vitamin D insufficiency among free-living healthy young adults. Am J Med 2002; 112:659-62.

119. Barger-Lux MJ, Heaney RP, Dowell S et al. Vitamin D and its major metabolites: serum levels after graded oral dosing in healthy men. Osteoporos Int 1998; 8(3):222-30.

120. Dawson-Hughes B. Impact of vitamin D and calcium on bone and mineral metabolism in older adults. In: Holick MF ed. Biologic Effects of Light 2001. Boston, MA: Kluwer Academic Publishers, 2002:175-83.

121. Vieth R, Chan PC, MacFarlane GD. Efficacy and safety of vitamin D3 intake exceeding the lowest observed adverse effect level. Am J Clin Nutr 2001; 73(2):288-94.

122. Heaney RP, Dowell MS, Hale CA et al. Calcium absorption varies within the reference range for serum 25-hydroxyvitamin D. J Am Coll Nutr 2003; 22(2):142-6.

123. Steingrimsdottir L, Gunnarsson O, Indridason OS et al. Relationship between serum parathyroid hormone levels, vitamin D sufficiency and calcium intake. JAMA 2005; 294(18):2336-41.

124. Ray NF, Chan JK, Thamer M et al. Medical expenditures for the treatment of osteoporotic fractures in the United States in 1995: report from the National Osteoporosis Foundation. J Bone Miner Res 1997; 12(1):24-35.

125. Melton LJ, 3rd, Gabriel SE et al. Cost-equivalence of different osteoporotic fractures. Osteoporos Int 2003; 14(5):383-8 Epub.

126. Tabensky A, Duan Y, Edmonds J et al. The contribution of reduced peak accrual of bone and age-related bone loss to osteoporosis at the spine and hip: insights from the daughters of women with vertebral or hip fractures. J Bone Miner Res 2001; 16(6):1101-7.
127. McKenna MJ. Differences in vitamin D status between countries in young adults and the elderly. Am J Med 1992; 93(1):69-77.
128. Webb AR, Kline L, Holick MF. Influence of season and latitude on the cutaneous synthesis of vitamin D3: exposure to winter sunlight in Boston and Edmonton will not promote vitamin D3 synthesis in human skin. J Clin Endocrinol Metab 1988; 67(2):373-8.
129. Parikh SJ, Edelman M, Uwaifo GI et al. The relationship between obesity and serum 1,25-dihydroxy vitamin D concentrations in healthy adults. J Clin Endocrinol Metab 2004; 89(3):1196-9.
130. Looker AC, Dawson-Hughes B, Calvo MS et al. Serum 25-hydroxyvitamin D status of adolescents and adults in two seasonal subpopulations from NHANES III. Bone 2002; 30(5):771-7.
131. Nesby-O'Dell S, Scanlon KS, Cogswell ME et al. Hypovitaminosis D prevalence and determinants among African American and white women of reproductive age: third National Health and Nutrition Examination Survey, 1988-1994. Am J Clin Nutr 2002; 76(1):187-92.
132. Hathcock JN, Shao A, Vieth R et al. Risk assessment for vitamin D. Am J Clin Nutr 2007; 85(1):6-18.
133. Yates AA. Process and development of dietary reference intakes: basis, need and application of recommended dietary allowances. Nutr Rev 1998; 56(4 Pt 2):S5-9.
134. Haddock L, Corcino J, Vazquez MD. 25(OH)D serum levels in the normal Puerto Rican population and in subjects with tropical sprue and paratyroid disease. Puerto Rico Health Sci J 1982; 1:85-91.
135. Haddad JG, Chyu KJ. Competitive protein-binding radioassay for 25-hydroxycholecalciferol. J Clin Endocrinol Metab 1971; 33(6):992-5.
136. Gertner JM, Domenech M. 25-Hydroxyvitamin D levels in patients treated with high-dosage ergo- and cholecalciferol. J Clin Pathol 1977; 30(2):144-50.
137. Vieth R. Vitamin D supplementation, 25-hydroxyvitamin D concentrations and safety. Am J Clin Nutr 1999; 69(5):842-56.
138. Grant WB, Holick MF. Benefits and requirements of vitamin D for optimal health: a review. Altern Med Rev 2005; 10(2):94-111.
139. Theiler R, Stahelin HB, Kranzlin M et al. Influence of physical mobility and season on 25-hydroxyvitamin D-parathyroid hormone interaction and bone remodelling in the elderly. Eur J Endocrinol 2000; 143(5):673-9.
140. Holick MF. Environmental factors that influence the cutaneous production of vitamin D. Am J Clin Nutr 1995; 61(suppl):638S-45S.
141. Lips P, Graafmans WC, Ooms ME et al. Vitamin D supplementation and fracture incidence in elderly persons. A randomized, placebo-controlled clinical trial. Ann Intern Med 1996; 124(4):400-6.
142. Meyer HE, Smedshaug GB, Kvaavik E et al. Can vitamin D supplementation reduce the risk of fracture in the elderly? A randomized controlled trial. J Bone Miner Res 2002; 17(4):709-15.
143. Trivedi DP, Doll R, Khaw KT. Effect of four monthly oral vitamin D3 (cholecalciferol) supplementation on fractures and mortality in men and women living in the community: randomised double blind controlled trial. Bmj 2003; 326(7387):469.
144. Chapuy MC, Pamphile R, Paris E et al. Combined calcium and vitamin D3 supplementation in elderly women: confirmation of reversal of secondary hyperparathyroidism and hip fracture risk: the Decalyos II study. Osteoporos Int 2002; 13(3):257-64.
145. Gunter EW, Lewis BL, Konkikowski SM. Laboratory Methods Used for the Third National Health and Nutrition Examination Survey (NHANES II), 1988-1994 (CD-ROM). Hyattsville, MD: Centers for Disease Control and Prevention [avaiable from National Information Service, Springfield, VA] 1996.
146. Falch JA, Oftebro H, Haug E. Early postmenopausal bone loss is not associated with a decrease in circulating levels of 25-hydroxyvitamin D, 1,25-dihydroxyvitamin D, or vitamin D-binding protein. J Clin Endocrinol Metab 1987; 64(4):836-41.
147. Bischoff-Ferrari HA. How to select the doses of vitamin D in the management of osteoporosis. Osteoporos Int 2007; 18(4):401-7.

CHAPTER 6

Ultraviolet Exposure Scenarios:
Risks of Erythema from Recommendations on Cutaneous Vitamin D Synthesis

Ann R. Webb* and Ola Engelsen

Abstract

Exposure to sunlight is a major source of vitamin D for most people yet public health advice focuses overwhelmingly on avoiding exposure of unprotected skin because of the risks of erythema and skin cancer. We have calculated the exposure required to gain a number of proposed oral-equivalent doses of vitamin D, as functions of latitude, season, skin type and skin area exposed, together with the associated risk of erythema, expressed in minimum erythema doses. The model results show that the current recommended daily intake of 400 IU is readily achievable through casual sun exposure in the midday lunch hour, with no risk of erythema, for all latitudes some of the year and for all the year at some (low) latitudes. At the higher proposed vitamin D dose of 1000 IU lunchtime sun exposure is still a viable route to the vitamin, but requires the commitment to expose greater areas of skin, or is effective for a shorter period of the year. The highest vitamin D requirement considered was 4000 IU per day. For much of the globe and much of the year, this is not achievable in a lunchtime hour and where it is possible large areas of skin must be exposed to prevent erythema. When the only variable considered was skin type, latitudinal and seasonal limits on adequate vitamin D production were more restrictive for skin type 5 than skin type 2.

Introduction

The ultraviolet (UV) region of the solar spectrum (280-400 nm) is responsible for a number of biological and chemical effects. For humans, the direct effects occur in organs that are exposed to sunlight i.e., the skin and eyes. Here we consider only the skin. In skin, the main competing responses to ultraviolet radiation are the synthesis of vitamin D (positive health benefit) and damage to cells and DNA manifested as erythema and an increased probability of skin cancer (negative health risk). Previous chapters have covered the synthesis and benefits of vitamin D and later chapters provide extensive details of current knowledge of skin cancer. Here we summarise only the points relevant to debate the relative risks and benefits of sun exposure.

Vitamin D has long been accepted as necessary for calcium metabolism and hence a healthy skeleton; more recently it has been linked with a protective effect against many life-threatening diseases, including a range of internal cancers and auto-immune diseases.[1,2] The so-called sunshine vitamin is also available through the diet, either in a very limited set of foods (mainly fatty fish, though some foods in some countries are fortified) or as supplements. As a dietary constituent, there are recommended guidelines for ingesting vitamin D. These are based only on bone health indicators and were aimed at eradicating the bone diseases of vitamin D deficiency: rickets and its adult form, osteomalacia. The guidelines range from zero dietary intake (assuming sunlight to

*Corresponding Author: Ann R. Webb, Centre for Atmospheric Sciences, School of Earth Atmospheric and Environmental Sciences, University of Manchester, Simon Building, Brunswick Street, Manchester, M13 9PL, U.K. Email: ann.webb@manchester.ac.uk

Sunlight, Vitamin D and Skin Cancer, edited by Jörg Reichrath. ©2008 Landes Bioscience and Springer Science+Business Media.

provide all necessary vitamin D) to 400-600 IU (international units) per day for those with extra growth requirements (pregnant and lactating women and children) or those "at risk" through potentially reduced capacity for cutaneous synthesis (the housebound and elderly).[3,4] The tolerable upper intake level for oral vitamin D is currently 2000 IU per day.[5] At higher doses long-term ingestion is deemed to have negative effects,[6] although this limit has been disputed.[7] Single therapeutic doses of up to 50,000 IU are given under medical supervision to cure bone disease, but this is a very different situation to unregulated home intake of supplements. With the suggestion that vitamin D benefits more than bone health have come calls for an increase in the recommended daily intake (RDI) of the vitamin. Recent intakes proposed to secure all the potential benefits of vitamin D range from 1000 IU[8] to 4000 IU per day.[7] Clearly the higher doses breach the current guidelines for oral intake and would be difficult to achieve since supplements of this strength are not widely available, but this does not take into account the role of sunlight in providing vitamin D.

In addition, there are differences in the effectiveness of different forms of vitamin D. Vitamin D_3 is formed in the skin, while vitamin D_2 (frequently used in food fortification and supplements) is the plant derived form of the vitamin. There is evidence that vitamin D_3, whether made cutaneously or ingested, is the more effective for increasing vitamin D status.[9-11]

Ultraviolet radiation, including that in sunlight, is a recognised carcinogen. Exposure to UV increases the risk of a cancer developing, although the details of the risk mechanism differ with the type of skin cancer. For the most life-threatening form, malignant melanoma, incidents of bad sunburn, especially in childhood, seem more important than the cumulative life time dose of UV that is implicated for squamous cell carcinoma, while basal cell carcinoma seems to combine elements of both sunburn and cumulative UV risks.[12-14] Current public health policy from e.g., UK, USA, Australia, World Health Organisation advises against sunlight exposure of unprotected skin, especially in the middle of the day (see websites for CRUK; EPA; Sunsmart; WHO)[15-18] when the advice is to stay indoors or cover up completely.

Existing recommendations to the public are contradictory: one assumes that UV exposure will, for a normal adult, provide necessary vitamin D, while the other advises minimising exposure to UV. This contradiction is exacerbated if calls to raise the recommended daily intake (or equivalent cutaneous synthesis) for vitamin D are considered, since achieving the higher suggested levels would involve ingesting twice the existing toxic limit for long-term intake of vitamin D, or increasing the minimum RDI-equivalent UV exposure by a factor of 10. Here we explore the possibilities of achieving current and suggested vitamin D status through sunlight exposure and assess the associated risks expressed in terms of erythema.

Differences between Vitamin D Synthesis and Erythema

Vitamin D synthesis and erythema both result from exposing unprotected skin to ultraviolet radiation, but there are significant differences between the two responses.

Action Spectra

A fundamental difference is that between the two action spectra. Vitamin D synthesis is very much a response to UVB radiation (280-315 nm), while erythema is elicited by both UVB and UVA (315-400 nm) radiation. The action spectra for the two responses are shown in Figure 1.

The biologically effective dose rate for each response is given by

$$\text{Biologically effective doserate} = \int E_\lambda \, A_\lambda \, d\lambda$$

Where E_λ is the incident radiation at a given wavelength, A_λ is the biological response at that wavelength and λ is wavelength. Since the solar spectrum is not a constant shape, especially in the UV, the ratio between erythema- and vitamin D- effective radiation is not a constant either.

Biological Endpoints

Erythema is damage to the skin and the endpoint of the damage is visible as a reddening and in extreme cases blistering, of the exposed skin. Vitamin D, by contrast, is synthesised in the skin but then enters the circulation and is hydroxylated in the liver to 25-hydroxyvitamin D (25OHD). It

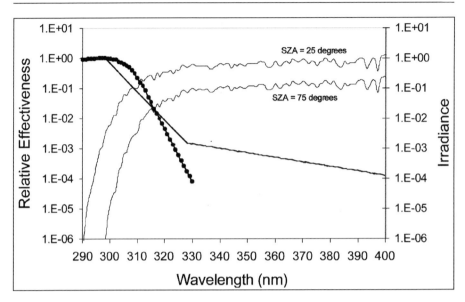

Figure 1. CIE erythema action spectrum[19] (bold line) and the action spectrum for the formation of previtamin D in human skin[20] (dots) with solar spectra measured at solar zenith angles of 25 and 75 degrees. The units of irradiance are $Wm^{-2}nm^{-1}$.

is the concentration of circulating 25OHD that is measured as an indicator of a person's vitamin D status since the hydroxylation to the active form in the kidney, 1,25 dihydroxyvitamin D (1,25), is tightly controlled by other factors. Vitamin D synthesised in all exposed skin contributes to the concentration of 25OHD in the blood, so increasing skin area exposed is one way to increase vitamin D status, rather than increasing exposure on a particular region of skin.

Other organs also have receptors for 25OHD and the cells can make their own 1,25 for internal use, hence the argument that once bone health requirements have been met, "left over" 25OHD can be used by the body for other health benefits. To gain these benefits the circulating 25OHD must be higher than the concentrations required simply to avoid rickets and the associated vitamin D intake/synthesis must increase correspondingly.[7]

Acute vs. Chronic Exposures

Erythema is experienced when UV exposure reaches or exceeds a personal minimum erythemal dose (MED) in a single exposure, or exposures close together. Two sub-erythemal doses gained a week apart are not additive for erythema, while the same two exposures either side of lunch on the same day could produce an erythemal response since there is inadequate time for repair processes to function.[21,22] All and any exposure will contribute to cumulative lifetime dose (and hence the risk of SCC), but avoiding erythema is a main goal in skin cancer prevention and risk-reduction for malignant melanoma.

The absolute UV dose that produces a slight reddening of the skin, i.e., an MED, is individual-dependent. It is broadly related to skin type[23] and skin colour, but neither is a very accurate predictor of MED.[24] The pigment melanin, which gives skin its brown colour, absorbs UV radiation and therefore prevents it from damaging DNA, or converting 7-dehydrocholesterol to previtamin D in the first step of vitamin D synthesis, but observation has shown that melanin is not the only determinant of MED.

The photochemical production of previtamin D, the first step in vitamin D synthesis requires sufficient UVB photons incident on the skin, but is then rapid. If the UVB requirement is met then previtamin D accumulation is limited by further photochemical reactions during any one (or several rapidly sequential) exposure(s). The previtamin D can be converted into several other biologically inert isomers and in sunlight the previtamin D in this isomer mixture never exceeds about 12%.[25] Prolonged exposure is therefore of no benefit once there is sufficient UVB to produce the initial previtamin D because the next stage of thermal isomerisation to vitamin D takes several hours and does not therefore remove the previtamin D from the mixture on photochemical time scales.

A generalised optimum exposure regime for acquiring and maintaining an adequate vitamin D status is therefore "little and often" e.g., a sub-erythemal dose of sufficiently UVB-rich radiation every day or two. The same regime is suitable for avoiding erythema and in this respect benefit gain and risk avoidance are served by the same behaviour. Indeed, regular sun exposure has also been shown to increase survival in cases of malignant melanoma, an effect that may be mediated by vitamin D.[26]

Implications for UV Exposure

Ambient Solar UV Radiation
The ambient solar UV radiation is most commonly expressed (measured or calculated) as the radiation incident on a flat, horizontal, unshaded plane. The human body is made of many surfaces, with orientations that change with the motion of the person relative to the position of the sun in the sky. Lacking any way to quantify the exposure of individuals relative to ambient, other than by personal dosimetry, the exposure of a flat horizontal plane will be taken as a default exposure that represents the local environment, while recognising that the exposure of any given body part will be a constantly changing fraction of this ambient UV.

The ambient UV depends first upon latitude, day of year and time, which factors combine to give the solar zenith angle (SZA, the angle between the local vertical and a line from the observer to the sun). The smaller the SZA (the higher the sun in the sky), the more intense is the solar radiation. This is due to two processes. When the direct solar beam strikes the surface at an oblique angle, the incident energy is spread over a larger surface area than when the radiation is normal to the surface, reducing the intensity by the cosine (SZA). In addition, as the SZA increases the pathlength of the radiation, that is the distance it travels from the Sun through the Earth's atmosphere, also increases thus increasing the scattering and absorption occurring along the path of the photons travelling towards the Earth and thus further reducing the radiation reaching the surface.

Superimposed on the very predictable cycle of SZA are the effects of components of the atmosphere, notably clouds, aerosols and ozone. These influences can change unpredictably on a range of time scales and modify the daily and annual cycles in incident radiation. Nonetheless, general experience and expectation is for maximum solar radiation in the summer time and in the middle of the day and minimum in winter and towards sunrise and sunset. Cloudless skies act as the default that allow maximum irradiance in the great majority of situations.

Solar Zenith Angle and the UV Spectrum
In addition to changes in incident solar energy, changes in SZA also change the shape of the solar spectrum, particularly in the UV region. This is a result of the changes in pathlength and hence the amount of atmospheric absorption and scattering. The absorption and scattering processes are wavelength dependent and this is particularly true of ozone absorption and Rayleigh scattering from air molecules. For clouds and aerosols this is less so. Ozone absorbs strongly at wavelengths less than 280 nm, so much so that no radiation at these wavelengths reaches the surface. Its absorptive properties then decrease rapidly through the UVB waveband and into the UVA, until there is no appreciable absorption for wavelengths greater than about 340 nm. The ozone absorption spectrum is mirrored in the rapidly increasing spectral irradiance in the UVB (see Fig. 1). As the distance the radiation has to travel through the stratospheric ozone layer increases, so does the absorption, attenuating the shortest wavelengths more than the longer UV wavelengths.

The scattering of solar radiation by air molecules is accurately described by Rayleigh scattering theory. The scattering is proportional to the inverse fourth power of the wavelength ($\alpha \lambda^{-4}$), which means that radiation at 300 nm is scattered about 3 times more than that at 400 nm. A major part of the ultraviolet radiation is back-scattered to space. At large SZA, most UV radiation is diffuse. Once more, increased pathlength leads to a disproportionate loss of the shorter UV wavelengths. Changes in stratospheric ozone will also alter the spectral shape, while cloud and aerosol effects are less wavelength dependent, but the dominant influence is SZA.

This spectral dependence on SZA means that for small SZA the proportion of UVB in the total UV waveband is greater than for large SZA. Since the action spectra for vitamin D synthesis (UVB) and erythema (UVB + UVA) differ, the ratio between their two biological doses changes as the solar zenith angle changes: there is more vitamin D effective radiation per dose of erythemally effective radiation at small SZA than at large SZA. Therefore the most efficient time to gain some UV exposure (maximising vitamin D synthesis for a fixed erythemal dose) is at small SZA. For a given location this is around noon on any day and in the summer months.[27,28]

Unprotected Skin Area

The area of skin exposed to UV radiation is extremely important in determining the resultant effect on vitamin D status since only exposed skin can synthesise vitamin D but circulating 25OHD is the resultant effect of vitamin D from any part of the body surface. Skin area does not determine the severity of erythema in any way, only the skin area that might suffer from reddening and the region of skin for which there has been an increase in cumulative lifetime dose. Thus the best way to increase vitamin D status while minimising the risk of erythema is to expose a large area of skin for a short period of time, rather than a small area of skin for a longer time.

Note that for either effect the skin exposed must be unprotected i.e., free of any covering, including sunscreen and other skincare products that may contain an element of sunscreen e.g., moisturisers and foundation creams. Face, neck and hands are the most frequently exposed skin areas (11.5%). At freezing temperatures, most people only expose the face (3.5%), except in extreme cold. In summer or during work-out, at least face, neck, arms, hands, legs (57.5%) are often exposed[29]

Realistic Exposure Times

A photobiological effect is the result of photons of suitable, effective wavelengths reaching target molecules in sufficient number that the resultant photochemical changes cause a noticeable biological reaction. In principle, even at very low irradiation rates, one can eventually acquire a sufficient dose to produce erythema, or a measurable change in circulating 25OHD. In practice the time might be so long that other processes (repair, or use of vitamin D) prevent a noticeable biological reaction and there is said to be no biological effect, even though the underlying photochemical reactions have occurred to a small degree.

For long durations of sun exposure a biological effect may become apparent, but would require a devotion to sunbathing that is unrealistic or impracticable, for example many hours exposure at high latitudes, where it may also be uncomfortably cold for prolonged exposure of bare skin. In considering the normal working adult we have taken one hour as the maximum period for a realistic daily exposure time, equating to a full lunch hour spent outdoors. Weekends and holiday periods provide the opportunity for more extensive exposure, but it has already been established that a regime of UV exposure "little and often" is most effective and beneficial.

Assessing the Erythema Risks of Exposures for Vitamin D Synthesis

To assess the risk of erythema associated with UV exposures sufficient to provide for our vitamin D requirements there are several variables that have to be determined: what are the vitamin D requirements? What skin type to consider? What skin area to expose? The UV radiation at the ground can then be modelled as a function of time and place, having defined some baseline atmospheric conditions, and applied to the conditions for vitamin D synthesis and erythema.

Throughout this study the FastRT UV simulation tool[30] was used to calculate UV irradiances on a flat, horizontal surface at sea level. The atmosphere was taken to be cloudless and the surface nonreflecting. The ozone layer thickness was fixed at 350 Dobson Units, a typical level. Aerosol was taken to be of rural type[31] with optical depth given by $\tau = \beta^* \lambda^{-\alpha}$ where the Ångström coefficient α

was set to 1.3 and the wavelengths (λ) are in micrometers. The Ångström coefficient β was related to 25 km visibility $R_m[km]$ using the parameterization of Iqbal (1983),[32] i.e.,

$$\beta = 0.55^{1.3}(3.912/R_m[km]\text{-}0.01162)[0.02472^*(R_m[km]\text{-}5) + 1.132].$$

In all other aspects, a US standard atmosphere[33] was assumed.

Vitamin D_3 effective doses were computed using the action spectrum for conversion of 7-DHC to previtamin D_3 in human skin[20] (CIE, 2006) (Fig. 1). The method used by Webb and Engelsen[28] (2006) for their standard vitamin D dose was applied for a range of conditions. A vitamin D dose, VD(X) was defined as corresponding to the UV equivalent of an oral dose of X IU vitamin D. Since radiation is incident on the skin and the response to either irradiation or oral dosing is measured in the blood, the dose VD(X) must be qualified by the conditions of skin exposure. The relation between the UV equivalent of an oral dose and skin area exposed was based on the work of Holick,[1,8] who equates exposure to ¼ of personal MED on ¼ skin area (hands, face and arms) to an oral dose of 1000 IU vitamin D. UV doses were then calculated under a reference condition, i.e., mid-latitude midday in spring (Boston, 21 March, 42.2° N, ozone = 350DU), after Webb and Engelsen (2006).[26] First to be calculated was the time required to acquire a ¼ MED around solar noon, using FastRT model[30] simulations. Then, using the same simulated solar spectra at the ground over the same time interval about noon, but weighting with the action spectrum for previtamin D_3 synthesis,[20] instead of the erythema action spectrum,[19] the vitamin D_3 effective dose acquired over the same time interval was calculated. This is the VD(1000) based on exposure of ¼ body surface area for a given MED.

Holick's formula has here been generalised by linear extrapolation:

$$VD(X, C, S) = 0.25^* \text{ MED}(S)^* 0.25/C^* X/1000$$

Where C is the fraction of the skin exposed to UV radiation and S is the skin type.

The calculations were performed for two MEDs equivalent to skin types 2 and 5.[23] The calculations were also repeated for different degrees of skin exposure, as shown in Table 1 which lists all the variables used in the calculations.

In the example above, a person exposing hands, face and arms would now make the equivalent of 1000 IU with 1 VD(1000) and would suffer a minimal erythema after 1 MED, which by definition is 4 times the VD exposure under the reference conditions (i.e., Boston, 21 March, 42.2° N, ozone = 350DU), but not necessarily for other conditions with a different shape to the solar spectrum at the ground.

Assumptions and Limitations

Calculations were all performed with an idealised atmosphere and receiving surface, neither of which would actually match reality in any but the rarest of cases.

Table 1. Variables of vitamin D dose, MED and skin area used in the model calculations

Variable	Value	Reference
X for VD(X)	400 IU	4
	1000 IU	8
	4000 IU	7
Skin type	2, MED = 250 J m⁻²	21
	5, MED = 600 J m⁻²	21
Skin area exposed	Face, neck and hands (11.5%)	29
	F,N,H and arms (25.5%)	29
	F,N,H, arms and legs (57.5%)	29

Nonetheless, the atmosphere represents a collection of standard conditions and a flat surface is unambiguous even if it only represents the tops of shoulders, head and feet for the upright human body. The angle of incidence for radiation at any body site changes continuously with motion of both the body and sun: for some sites, some of the time, incident radiation will be greater than on a horizontal surface, but in many cases irradiances will be lower than the case for a horizontal plane. To explore different atmospheric conditions, including ozone, cloud, aerosol, surface albedo and surface elevation the reader is directed to http://nadir.nilu.no/~olaeng/fastrt/VitD-ez_quart-MED.html where user selected inputs can be applied to the calculations. In the majority of real life cases we would expect the required exposure times to exceed those produced by the model.

Three recommendations for dietary intake of vitamin D have been used, representing the upper end of the current public health guidelines intended to prevent bone disease[3,4] and two suggestions for revised guidelines that, it is suggested, would confer all possible health benefits associated with vitamin D[7,8]. No account has been taken of any sections of the population such as the elderly or pregnant who may have different vitamin D requirements,[34,35] except insofar as they are intrinsically included in current guidelines based on bone health. Nor have confounding factors such as body fat[36] been considered.

The UV equivalence to an oral dose that is at the heart of these calculations is based on the assumption that the relation between body surface area exposed and change in circulating 25OHD is linear. We have used that assumption again in assessing exposures for different skin areas in table 1, but without clear proof that this linearity is anything more than sensible expectation. Additionally, the oral dose equivalence that we have used was not determined exactly, rather the whole-body exposure to 1 MED of UV was shown to produce a rise in 25OHD that fell between that produced by oral doses of 10,000 IU and 25,000 IU.[1] From this we followed Holick[8] in approximating 1 MED, full body to 16000 IU and thus ¼ MED and ¼ surface area to 1000 IU.

The action spectra used are, respectively, a mathematical fit to a collection of data, widely accepted through common use (erythema), or the only one available that is based on measurements in human skin (previtamin D synthesis). Alternatives to the latter are discussed by Webb and Engelsen (2006)[28] but no better candidate was identified. As with the base case atmosphere, these action spectra must be understood as representative, in this case of human skin, not necessarily exact for every person. Similarly, the MEDs used to quantify a skin type are average values from a wide range. MED and skin type are loosely related but each skin type can encompass a wide range of MED values and the ranges overlap.

In summary, the calculations shown here are for illustration. They should not be taken as precise recommendations for UV exposure since realistic situations will differ in many aspects from the limited range of conditions represented here. True exposure requirements may be either more or less than those shown depending on details of each location, the prevailing atmospheric conditions and personal characteristics. What the calculations do allow is a comparison between the various existing or suggested recommended daily intakes of vitamin D, expressed as a UV exposure equivalent and the associated risks of erythema in each case.

Results

A sample of the calculations for different vitamin D, skin type and skin area scenarios is used here for illustration. Note that the latitudinal and seasonal pattern seen in all plots is a function of the changing spectrum and intensity of the solar irradiance with latitude- and season- dependent solar zenith angle (represented, for example, by noontime SZA). If the solar spectrum remained the same all day then the permutations of dose, skin type and skin area would be simple scaling factors of a single example set e.g., 1000 IU, skin type 1, skin area 25%. .For example, a doubling of the desired dietary equivalent intake would require twice the exposure time. Likewise, exposing twice the skin area would half the required exposure time. A skin type requiring twice as much UV radiation to get burnt, would require twice the amount of exposure time with constant UV intensity.

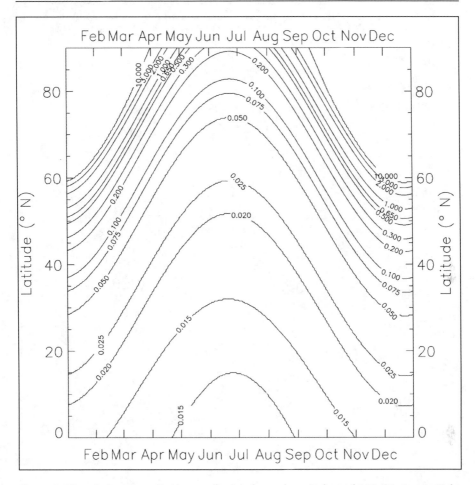

Figure 2. Time in hours required to synthesise the oral equivalent of 400 IU vitamin D for skin type 2 exposing hands, face, neck, arms and legs.

However, the spectrum changes with diurnal changes in SZA, with less irradiance and disproportionately less at shorter UVB wavelengths, as SZA increases (i.e., as the sun gets closer to the horizon). The calculations start at noon and move symmetrically away, taking account of the changing irradiance in doing so. Thus an exposure time of 30 minutes means 15 minutes before noon to 15 minutes after noon (during which time the SZA and spectrum will not change very much). An exposure of 6 hours means 3 hours before noon to 3 hours after noon, during which time the SZA and UV spectrum can change more significantly. Scaling for the variables will provide a reasonable approximation to the full calculation when exposure times are short and the scaling is small, so that both situations are encompassed by times close to noon when the spectrum does not change significantly. When times or scaling factors are large the changing solar spectrum introduces increasingly large errors to any attempt to directly scale results. However, as stated previously, we take an one hour exposure around noon to be the maximum feasible on a regular basis and then for a given latitude and month scaling can be applied.

Figure 2 shows the time required to achieve the oral equivalent of 400 IU vitamin D for skin type 2, exposing face, neck, hands and arms and legs (57.5% skin area). Even at 70⁰ latitude it is possible for a skin type 2 individual to synthesise the equivalent of 400 IU vitamin D in less than

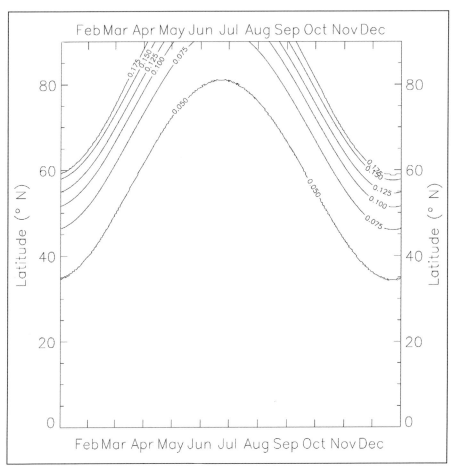

Figure 3. The fractional MED gained during the minimum exposure required for 400 IU vitamin D, skin type 2, skin area 57.5% (i.e., the situation in Fig. 2).

an hour for about 6 months of the year, by exposing all but the torso to sunlight. Whether this would be practical or desirable given the temperature is a further pragmatic consideration and the year round clear skies of the model do not occur. The associated MEDs can be seen in Figure 3. As skin area exposed decreases, exposure times increase and the viable vitamin D season shortens. Nonetheless, 400 IU vitamin D can be achieved without erythema by less than one hour exposure of hands, face and neck for several months even at 70° latitude, which we take as the limit of significant populations (400IU and 11.5% area exposed yield very similar results as 1000 IU and 25% area exposed[28] and is consequently not repeated here).

Figures 4 and 5 show the time required to achieve the oral equivalent of 4000 IU for skin types 2 and 5 with 11.5% skin area exposed. Figure 6 shows the associated MEDs acquired in the same time for skin type 2; the pattern is similar and the smallest MED (1.9 in the Tropics) is the same for skin type 5. Thus, to achieve 4000 IU without risk of sunburn is not possible unless large skin areas are exposed. Crude scaling of Figures 2-6 shows that 4000 IU can be achieved in this way in less than one hour and without incurring erythema at low latitudes.

As an example of mid-latitude exposures in all situations, Table 2 shows exposure times and number of MEDs acquired while achieving the stated UV dose for all permutations of variables

Table 2. Exposure time, in hours and associated MED (in parentheses) for Boston at the spring equinox for all permutations of variables

Vit. D >	400 IU		1000 IU		4000 IU	
Skin Type>	2	5	2	5	2	5
Area v						
F,N,H	0.15	0.35	0.36	0.89	1.49	3.95
(11.5%)	(0.21)	(0.21)	(0.54)	(0.54)	(2.16)	(2.16)
F,N,H,A	0.07	0.16	0.17	0.40	0.67	1.62
(25.5%)	(0.09)	(0.09)	(0.24)	(0.24)	(0.97)	(0.97)
F,N,H,A,L	0.03	0.07	0.07	0.18	0.29	0.70
(57.5%)	(0.04)	(0.04)	(0.10)	(0.10)	(0.43)	(0.43)

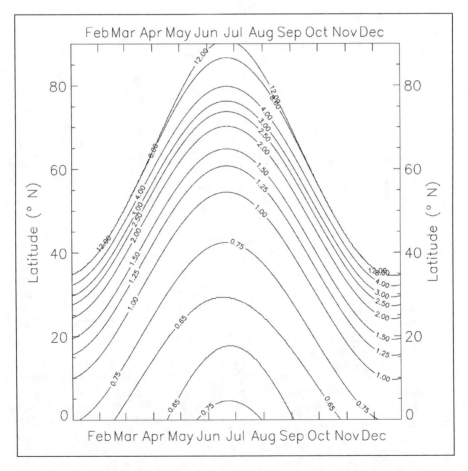

Figure 4. Time in hours required to synthesise the oral equivalent of 4000 IU vitamin D for skin type 2 exposing hands, face and neck.

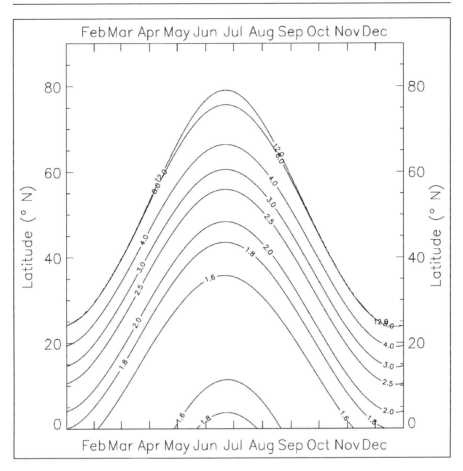

Figure 5. Time in hours required to synthesise the oral equivalent of 4000 IU vitamin D for skin type 5 exposing hands, face and neck.

for Boston (42° N) at the spring equinox, where the MEDs for 1000 IU, skin type 2, skin area 25% is 0.25 by definition (note skin area in the calculation is 25.5% so the MED is 0.24). At this time and location all exposure times except 4000 IU for skin type 5, 11.5% skin area, are within 1 hour either side of noon, so scaling is applicable. For other permutations, or alternative values of the variables readers may make their own calculations at http://nadir.nilu.no/~olaeng/fastrt/VitD-ez_quartMED.html

In summary, current recommendations for 400 IU vitamin D supply (cutaneous or oral) are achievable through sun exposure, without risk of erythema, for all or part of the year, albeit in contradiction to public health advice on sun exposure. Supplements are readily available for the locations and periods when cutaneous synthesis is not practically possible. At the intermediate recommendation of 1000 IU vitamin D sun exposure of less than one hour can still serve as a single source at low latitudes and at middle to high latitudes (results not shown here) for some or all of the year for those willing to expose sufficient skin area. As latitude (or skin pigment) increases the viable periods for sun-induced vitamin D become ever more constrained. Supplementation at these levels is possible if not easily available commercially and a combination of sunlight and supplementation makes this level of vitamin D intake achievable for most indigenous people—it is harder for migrant communities who have moved polewards and they would be more reliant on

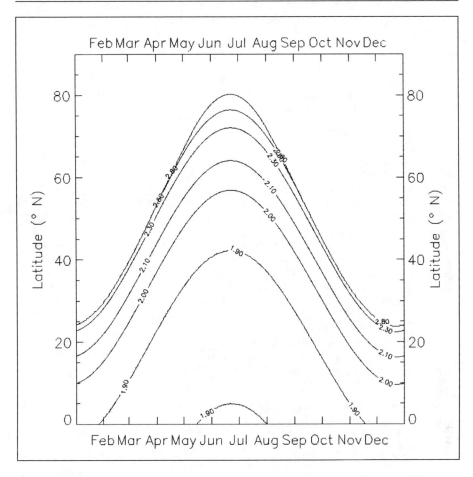

Figure 6. The The fractional MED gained during the minimum exposure required for 4000 IU vitamin D, skin type 2, skin area 11.5% (i.e., the situation in Fig. 4).

supplements. Achieving 4000 IU equivalent of vitamin D by sun exposure becomes problematical. Where it is theoretically possible to provide this vitamin D through skin synthesis e.g., for skin type 2 in the Tropics, the exposure time required also produces a significant erythemal dose: 1.9 MED for hand, face neck exposure and ~0.4 MED when arms and legs are also exposed. Skin type 5 can only acquire 4000 IU in less than an hour by exposing 25% or more skin area and incurring close to a full MED (at the smaller possible skin areas) even in the Tropics (results not shown here). It is not possible at this time to find over-the-counter vitamin supplements containing 4000 IU of vitamin D as this is twice the official tolerable limit.

Public Health and Personal Choice

One Size Does Not Fit All

It is clear from the illustrations above that there is no single, simple recommendation for sun exposure for vitamin D synthesis that will apply to all people and all locations. It is therefore a harder message to convey than the simple "Stay out of the sun" health policy that it contradicts. UV dose requirements, in absolute terms, will depend on skin pigmentation and age, as well as skin area exposed, while the time taken to achieve that dose will depend on location, season, time of day and weather conditions. The type of recommendation made by Holick[8] of ¼ MED on ¼ surface area for a 1000 IU equivalent dose is a practical way to account, at least approximately, for both personal characteristics and time-place-weather considerations. It does require some self-knowledge and a little understanding of influences on UV, or use of the UV index[28] as provided in weather forecasts. Surface areas and fractional MEDs can be changed to suit conditions or to provide the equivalent of other vitamin D requirements, within limits.

Understanding the Options

Sunlight exposure cannot be the complete answer to vitamin D supply as for large regions of the world it is not possible, or practical, to achieve significant cutaneous vitamin D synthesis for several months of the year. This problem is exacerbated for highly pigmented peoples living at high latitudes. It may be an adequate solution for a larger number of people if a short-term dip below optimum Vitamin D status is not detrimental to health, provided sufficient levels are maintained during the rest of the year, i.e., the observed seasonal cycle at mid-high latitudes is acceptable so long as the winter time low is not too deep or too long. This is an unknown factor.

Where sunlight cannot provide adequate vitamin D, whether because of latitude, weather, pigment, age, or because the selected requirements would in many cases incur erythema, oral intake (diet and supplements) is an alternative means to uphold vitamin D status. Food fortification is one means to increase the vitamin D content of modern diets, but this is variable from country to country and cannot be relied upon to reach those parts of the population most in need of extra vitamin D. A vitamin supplement containing a known dose of vitamin D is the most reliable method of ensuring a steady supply of the vitamin, but at the higher end of suggested vitamin intake no such supplement is available and the issue of health hazards from long-term use has still to be clarified. Vitamin supplements must be purchased and can also be costly in the long-run, while sunlight is free, if not always freely available.

References

1. Holick MF. Vitamin D: Importance in the prevention of cancers, type 1 diabetes, heart disease and osteoporosis. Am J Clin Nutr 2004a; 79:362-371.
2. Peterlik M, Cross HS. Vitamin D and calcium deficits predispose for multiple chronic diseases. Eur J Clin Invest 2005; 35:290-304.
3. Department of Health Nutrition and bone health: with particular reference to calcium and vitamin D. Report on Health and Social Subjects 49. London, HMSO, 1998.
4. Standing Committee on the Scientific Evaluation of Dietary Reference Intakes 1997 Dietary reference intakes: calcium, phosphorus, magnesium, vitamin D and fluoride. Washington, DC: National Academy Press.
5. Dietary Reference Intakes for Calcium, Magnesium, Phosphorus, Vitamin D and Fluoride. Food and Nutrition Board, Institute of Medicine. National Academy Press, Washington, DC, 1997.
6. Narang NK, Gupta RC, Jain MK et al. Role of vitamin D in pulmonary tuberculosis. J Assoc Physicians India 1984; 32:185-6.
7. Vieth R. Vitamin D supplementation, 25-hydroxyvitamin D concentrations and safety. Am J Clin Nutr 1999; 69:842-856.
8. Holick MF. The Vitamin D Advantage. iBooks, 2004, New York.
9. Trang MH, Cole DEC, Rubin LA et al. Evidence that vitamin D3 increases serum 25-hydroxyvitamin D more effectively than does vitamin D2. Am J Clin Nutr 1998; 68:854-858.
10. Armas LAG, Hollis BW, Heaney RP. Vitamin D2 is much less effective than vitamin D3 in humans. J Clin Endocrin Metabol 2004; 89:5387-5391.
11. Rapuri PB, Gallagher JC, Haynatzki G. Effect of vitamin D2 and D3 supplement use on serum 25OHD concentration in elderly women in summer and winter. Calcif Tissue Int 2004; 74:150-156.
12. Rosso S, Zanetti R, Pippione M et al. Parallel risk assessment of melanoma and basal cell carcinoma: skin characteristics and sun exposure. Melanoma Res 1998; 8(6):573-583.
13. Rosso S, Zanetti R, Martinez C et al. The multicentre south European study 'Helios'. II: Different sun exposure patterns in the aetiology of basal cell and squamous cell carcinomas of the skin. Br J Cancer 1996; 73(11):1447-54.
14. Zanetti R, Rosso S, Martinez C et al. Comparison of risk patterns in carcinoma and melanoma of the skin in men: a multi-centre case-case-control study. Br J Cancer 2006; 94(5):743-51.

15. http://info.cancerresearchuk.org/healthyliving/sunsmart/
16. http://www.epa.gov/radtown/sun-exposure.htm
17. http://www.cancersa.org.au/aspx/sunsmart.aspx
18. http://www.who.int/mediacentre/factsheets/fs261/en/
19. MacKinley AF, Diffey BL eds. A reference action spectrum for ultraviolet induced erythema in human skin. CIE J 1987; 6(1):17-22.
20. CIE 174 Action spectrum for the production of previtamin D3 in human skin. CIE publication 174. 2006, ISBN 3 901 906 50 9.
21. de Winter S, Vink AA, Roza L et al. Solar-simulated skin adaptation and its effect on subsequent UV-induced epidermal DNA damage. J Invest Dermatol 2001; 117(3):678-82.
22. Decraene D, Smaers K, Maes D et al. A low UVB dose, with the potential to trigger a protective p53-dependent gene program, increases the resilience of keratinocytes against future UVB insults. J Invest Dermatol 2005; 125(5):1026-31.
23. Fitzpatrick TB. The validity and practicality of sun-reactive skin types I through VI. Arch Dermatol 1988; 124(6):869-871.
24. Wiete Westerhof, Oscar Estevez-Uscanga, Joes Meens et al. The Relation Between Constitutional Skin Color and Photosensitivity Estimated from UV-Induced Erythema and Pigmentation Dose-Response Curves. J Invest Derm 1990; 94:812-816.
25. Webb AR, Kline L, Holick MF. Influence of season and latitude on the cutaneous synthesis of vitamin D3: Exposure to winter sunlight in Boston and Edmonton will not promote vitamin D3 synthesis in human skin. J Clin Endocrinol Metab 1988; 67:373-378.
26. Berwick M, Armstrong BK, Ben-Porat L et al. Sun Exposure and Mortality from Melanoma. J Nat Canc Inc 2005; 97:195-199.
27. Webb AR. Who, what, where and when- influences on cutaneous vitamin D synthesis. Prog Biophys Mol Biol 2006; (92):17-25.
28. Webb AR, Engelsen O. Calculated ultraviolet exposure levels for a healthy vitamin D status. Photchem Photobiol 2006; 82:122-128.
29. Lund CC, Browder NC. Estimation of areas of burns. Surgery, Gynecology and Obstretrics, 1944; 79:352-358.
30. Engelsen O, Kylling A. Fast simulation tool for ultraviolet radiation at the earth's surface. Opt Eng 2005; 44(4):041012.1-7.
31. Shettle EP. Models of aerosols, clouds, and precipitation for atmospheric propagation studies. AGARD Conf Proc 454, 1989; 15-32.
32. Iqbal M. An Introduction to Solar Radiation. 1983. Academic Press, San Diego.
33. Anderson GP, Clough SA, Kneizys FX et al. AFGL atmospheric constituent profiles (0-120 km). Tech. Rep. AFGL-TR-86-0110. Air Force Geophysics Laboratory, Hanscom Air Force Base, 1986, Massachusetts.
34. Arunabh S, Pollack S, Yeh J et al. Body fat content and 25-hydroxyvitamin D levels in healthy women. J Clin Endocrinol Metab 2003; 88(1):157-161.
35. Hollis BW, Wagner CL. Assessment of dietary vitamin D requirements during pregnancy and lactation. Am J Clin Nutr 2004; 79(5):717-726.
36. Vieth R, Ladak Y, Walfish PG. Age-related changes in the 25-hydroxyvitamin D versus parathyroid hormone relationship suggest a different reason why older adults require more vitamin D. J Clin Endocrinol Metab 2003; 88(1):185-191.

CHAPTER 7

At What Time Should One Go Out in the Sun?

Johan Moan,* Arne Dahlback and Alina Carmen Porojnicu

Abstract

To get an optimal vitamin D supplement from the sun at a minimal risk of getting cutaneous malignant melanoma (CMM), the best time of sun exposure is noon. Thus, common health recommendations given by authorities in many countries, that sun exposure should be avoided for three to five hours around noon and postponed to the afternoon, may be wrong and may even promote CMM. The reasons for this are (1) The action spectrum for CMM is likely to be centered at longer wavelengths (UVA, ultraviolet A, 320-400 nm) than that of vitamin D generation (UVB, ultraviolet B, 280-320 nm). (2) Scattering of solar radiation on clear days is caused by small scattering elements, Rayleigh dominated and increases with decreasing wavelengths. A larger fraction of UVA than of UVB comes directly and unscattered from the sun. (3) The human body can be more realistically represented by a vertical cylinder than by a horizontal, planar surface, as done in almost all calculations in the literature. With the cylinder model, high UVA fluence rates last about twice as long after noon as high UVB fluence rates do.

In view of this, short, nonerythemogenic exposures around noon should be recommended rather than longer nonerythemogenic exposures in the afternoon. This would give a maximal yield of vitamin D at a minimal CMM risk.

Introduction

In evaluations of positive and negative health effects of sun exposure, the human body is usually modeled as a horizontal, flat surface. Since ultraviolet B (UVB, 280-320 nm) is much more scattered in the atmosphere than ultraviolet A (UVA, 320-400 nm) is and has widely different health consequences, the choice of geometric representation for the human body is of fundamental importance. This holds for evaluations of latitudinal as well as of time effects, both being related to zenith angles of the sun. A vertical cylinder surface represents the human body much better than a horizontal planar surface. As we will demonstrate, the choice of geometry plays a major role for health evaluations of solar radiation and should be paid more attention to.

Methods

The radiative transfer model used in the calculations are described in another chapter in this book (Ultraviolet radiation and malignant melanoma). Whenever possible, the calculations were checked and evaluated by comparisons with measurements and found to agree well. In the present calculations a vertical cylinder was used as a model for the human body. When different wavelength regions are to be compared, these two models give widely different results as shown here.

*Corresponding Author: Johan Moan—Department of Radiation Biology, Institute for Cancer Research, Montebello, Oslo, Norway, and Department of Physics, University of Oslo, Oslo, Norway. Email: johan.moan@labmed.uio.no

Sunlight, Vitamin D and Skin Cancer, edited by Jörg Reichrath. ©2008 Landes Bioscience and Springer Science+Business Media.

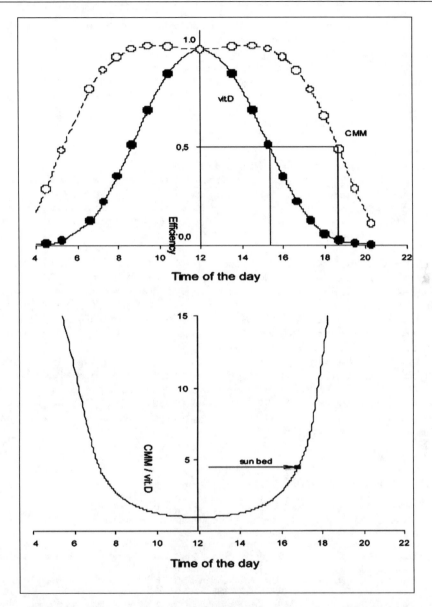

Figure 1. The time dependence on a midsummer day in Oslo (60° N) of vitamin D inducing- and melanoma generating fluence rates of solar radiation. For action spectra and other details, see the text. All curves are normalized to unity at noon.

There are at least five types of observation which indicate that UVA plays a major role in CMM induction by the sun and that melanin may be a cromophore for this: (1) CMM can be induced in the fish Xiphophorus by UVA;[1] (2) Albino black people who lack melanin, have very low incidence rates of CMM in spite of the fact that they have high incidence rates of non melanoma skin cancers;[2] (3) The latitude gradient of CMM is much smaller than those of non melanoma skin cancers, just as the latitude gradient of annual doses of UVA is smaller than that of annual doses of UVB;[3]

(4) Some of the mutations found in CMMs are not due to UVB induced pyrimidine dimers, but rather to UVA induced DNA damages;[4] (5) The action spectrum for light activation of melanin in Xiphophorus resembles that of CMM induction in the same fish.[5]

On this basis we have used the action spectrum for CMM induction in the fish Xiphophorus[1] in the calculations below. For vitamin D generation we have used the action spectrum of Galkin and Terenskaya,[6] which is supposedly more accurate in the wavelength region above 300 nm, which counts most heavily, than the spectrum measured in human skin.[7] For the present evaluations the two spectra lead to qualitatively similar conclusions.

Results and Discussion

As a representative example we carried out calculations for a midsummer day in Oslo, Norway, using cylinder geometry and the CMM and vitamin D action spectra. Typical ozone values for Oslo, midsummer were used. To check the validity of the calculations we also measured UVA and UVB fluence rates using a Robertson Berger meter with cosine diffusors. The UVA/UVB ratio of a commercial sun bed (Solarium Super Plus 100 W, Wolff System) was measured with the same instrument.

Figure 1 shows that after noon fluence rates of vitamin D generating radiation falls off much faster than those of CMM generating radiation do. The vitamin D generation rate is halved about 3 1/3 hours after noon, while the CMM induction rate is not halved before 6 1/2 hours after noon. The ratio of CMM to vitamin D generating fluence rate as a function of time is shown in the lower part of the figure.

Measurements of the UVB and UVA fluence rates of the commercial sun bed showed that its UVB rate was similar to that of solar radiation at noon and that the UVB to UVA ratio was similar to that of solar radiation 4 1/2 hours after noon.

We conclude that postponing moderate non erythemogenic sun exposures from noon to afternoon yields less vitamin D at a similar melanoma risk. The relative effects of a sun bed are similar to that of solar radiation 4-5 hours after noon. However, at that time longer sun exposures than sun bed exposures are needed to give the same vitamin D yield and CMM risk. In view of the present work, health authorities should consider to change their recommendations concerning "healthy and unhealthy" sun exposures.

Acknowledgements

The present work was supported by Sigval Bergesen D.Y. og hustru Nankis Foundation and by Helse Sør Medical Enterprise.

References

1. Setlow RB, Grist E, Thompson K et al. Wavelengths effective in induction of malignant melanoma. Proc Natl Acad Sci USA 1993; 90:6666-6670.
2. Diffey BL, Healy E, Thody AJ et al. Melanin, melanocytes and melanoma. Lancet 1995; 346:1713.
3. Moan J, Dahlback A, Setlow RB. Epidemiological support for an hypothesis for melanoma induction indicating a role for UVA radiation. Photochem Photobiol 1999; 70:243-247.
4. Hocker T, Tsao H. Ultraviolet radiation and melanoma: a systematic review and analysis of reported sequence variants. Hum Mutat 2007; 28:578-588.
5. Wood SR, Berwick M, Ley RD et al. UV causation of melanoma in Xiphophorus is dominated by melanin photosensitized oxidant production. Proc Natl Acad Sci USA 2006; 103:4111-4115.
6. Galkin ON, Terenetskaya IP. 'Vitamin D' biodosimeter: basic characteristics and potential applications. J Photochem Photobiol B 1999; 53:12-19.
7. MacLaughlin JA, Anderson RR, Holick MF. Spectral character of sunlight modulates photosynthesis of previtamin D3 and its photoisomers in human skin. Science 1982; 216:1001-1003.

CHAPTER 8

Epidemiology of Melanoma and Nonmelanoma Skin Cancer— The Role of Sunlight

Ulrike Leiter and Claus Garbe*

Abstract

Melanoma and nonmelanoma skin cancer (NMSC) are now the most common types of cancer in white populations. Both tumor entities show an increasing incidence rate worldwide but a stable or decreasing mortality rate.[1,2] The rising incidence rates of NMSC are probably caused by a combination of increased sun exposure or exposure to ultraviolet (UV) light, increased outdoor activities, changes in clothing style, increased longevity, ozone depletion, genetics and in some cases, immune suppression. A dose-dependent increase in the risk of squamous cell carcinoma (SCC) of the skin was found associated with exposure to Psoralen and UVA irradiation. An intensive UV exposure in childhood and adolescence was causative for the development of basal cell carcinoma (BCC) whereas for the aetiology of SCC a chronic UV exposure in the earlier decades was accused.

Cutaneous malignant melanoma is the most rapidly increasing cancer in white populations. The frequency of its occurrence is closely associated with the constitutive colour of the skin and depends on the geographical zone. The highest incidence rates have been reported from Queensland, Australia with 56 new cases per year per 100,000 for men and 43 for women. Mortality rates of melanoma show a stabilisation in the USA, Australia and also in European countries. The tumor thickness is the most important prognostic factor in primary melanoma. There is an ongoing trend towards thin melanoma since the last two decades. Epidemiological studies have confirmed the hypothesis that the majority of all melanoma cases are caused, at least in part, by excessive exposure to sunlight. In contrast to squamous cell carcinoma, melanoma risk seems not to be associated with cumulative, but intermittent exposure to sunlight. Therefore campaigns for prevention and early detection are necessary.

Introduction

Melanoma and nonmelanoma (basal and squamous cell carcinoma) skin cancer (NMSC) are now the most common types of cancer in white populations. Both tumor entities show an increasing incidence rate worldwide and also in Germany.[3-9] Nonmelanoma skin cancers (NMSCs) constitute more than one-third of all cancers in the US with an estimated incidence of over 600,000 cases per year. Of these 600,000 cases, approximately 500,000 are basal cell carcinomas (BCCs) and 100,000-150,000 are squamous cell carcinomas (SCCs).[3] The incidence of NMSC (BCC and SCC) is 18-20 times higher than that of malignant melanoma. However, incidence data of high epidemiological quality on NMSC are sparse because traditional cancer registries often exclude

*Corresponding Author: Claus Garbe—Division of Dermatoloncology, Department of Dermatology, University Medical Center, University of Tuebingen, Liebermeisterstr, 25, 72076 Tuebingen, Germany. Email: claus.garbe@med.uni-tuebingen.de

Sunlight, Vitamin D and Skin Cancer, edited by Jörg Reichrath. ©2008 Landes Bioscience and Springer Science+Business Media.

NMSC or are at least incomplete. Miller and Weinstock estimated the 1994 NMSC incidence to be higher, between 900,000 and 1,200,000.[10,11] The lifetime risks were estimated to be 28% to 33% for BCC and 7% to 11% for SCC (lifetime risk of developing NMSC for a child born in1994.)

The incidence of melanoma is much lower compared to NMSCs but has been rising in fair-skinned populations throughout the world for several decades.[12,13] The annual increase varies between populations but in general has been estimated to be between 3 and 7%, with mortality rates increasing less quickly. These estimates suggest a doubling of rates every 10-20 years. Cutaneous malignant melanoma is the most rapidly increasing cancer in white populations. The frequency of its occurrence is closely associated with the constitutive colour of the skin and depends on the geographical zone. Incidence among dark skinned ethnic groups is 1 per 100,000 per year or less, but is up to 50 per 100,000 per year among light-skinned Caucasians and higher in some areas of the world. The highest incidence rates have been reported from Queensland, Australia with 56 new cases per year per 100,000 for men and 43 for women.[14] The current estimated annual incidence of melanoma in the US among white populations, adjusted for the same standard population and for the same year (1987), is 14 and 11.33 In Northern Europe the incidence rates appear more moderate with less than 5 per 100,000.[2,3] The cumulative lifetime risk for melanoma is now in the order of 1:25 in Australia and it has been estimated to be around 1:75 in the US by the year 2000.[15] In Germany an estimation for MM incidence by the Robert Koch Institute indicates 6,225 new cases in Germany in 1998 (age-standardized incidence rate Europe about 7.0 per 100,000).[16] In Germany the incidence of melanoma is increasing continuously, no trend of a stabilisation or decrease could be observed. During 1976-2003 period, the incidence of CM approximately was tripled for males and females, reaching 10.3 and 13.3 per 100,000 per year, respectively.[17] An estimation for Great Britain reveals an ongoing increase of the incidence for another 30 years by which time the predicted age-standardized rate of melanoma may be around twice that presently observed.[18]

Mortality rates of melanoma show a stabilisation, no further increase could be reported.[19] This trend was found in different European countries.[2,20,21] The reason is benefits of intervention strategies, early detection of suspected lesions which lead to a constant decrease of tumor thickness at the time of diagnosis and a better prognosis.

Nonmelanoma Skin Cancer

Incidence of Nonmelanoma Skin Cancer

Nonmelanoma skin cancer (NMSC) is by far the most frequent cancer in white populations and numerous studies have shown that incidence rates of NMSC are increasing worldwide.[22-26] Incidence rates of NMSC vary vastly by geographical area with most extreme rates reported from Australia and New Zealand. In the United States, approximately 800,000 new cases of BCC and 200,000 new cases of SCC were diagnosed in 2000.[11,27] Nonmelanoma skin cancer generally occurs in persons older than 50 years and in this age group, its incidence is increasing rapidly.

In the white population in the USA, Canada and Australia a mean increase of NMSC of three to eight percent could be observed since 1960. Because the common basal cell and squamous cell cancers are not reportable to SEER, there are only few data counting for the incidence of basal cell carcinoma and squamous cell carcinoma.[28]

One study found nearly 50-fold differences in the incidence of basal cell carcinoma (BCC) and 100-fold differences in squamous cell carcinoma (SCC) between Caucasian populations in northern Europe and Australia.[26,29] Within Australia there is a marked North to South gradient with the most extreme incidence rates of NMSC recorded in Queensland.[26,30-32] A three year study recently conducted in Townsville found age-standardized incidence rates of BCC were 1,445 for men and 943 for women and of SCC were 805 for men and 424 for women.[26,32] This study also showed that within the three year study period 38.5% of the patients suffered from multiple NMSC.

In Europe, the incidence rate of NMSC was reported to be 129.3 in men and 90.8 in women (European standard), in northern Germany (Cancer Registry of Schlewig-Holstein) the crude incidence rate was 119.3/100,000 in men and 113.8/100,000 in women between 1998 and 2001.[2,33] The NMSC incidence rates in Germany corresponded well with data from Denmark (96 and 74 cases in 100,000 men and women, respectively).[34] In South Wales an NMSC incidence rate of 104 cases for men and 83 cases for women in 100,000 was observed.[1]

Basal Cell Carcinoma

Basal cell carcinoma demonstrates to be the most common malignant skin cancer worldwide, the incidence rate of basal cell carcinoma increased in the USA (New Mexico) have measurably increased in two time periods: 1977-1978 and 1998-1999 by 50% in males and 20% in females, whereas rates of squamous cell carcinoma roughly doubled in both males and females,[35] see Table 1. In Queensland, Australia yearly age standardized incidence rates (per 100,000 inhabitants) of basal cell carcinoma (BCC) were 2,058 for men, 1,194 for women in 1997. Compared to incidence rates, age-standardized rates of lesions of BCC were 2.1 times higher in men, 1.6 times higher in women.[32]

In Germany a crude incidence rate for basal cell carcinoma was given with 96.2 in men and 95.3 in women, standardized for the European Standard population with 80.8 for men and 63.3 for women (per 100,000 inhabitants), Table 1. Compared to Germany, the incidence rate standardized for the United States population and the world standard population was found to be up to 10 fold higher in the USA and up to 20 fold higher in Australia.

Squamous Cell Carcinoma

Squamous cell carcinoma is mostly associated with a higher age (mean age at diagnosis ca. 70 years), for squamous cell carcinoma an increase of age-adjusted incidence rates increased by 90% in males and by 109% in females from in the USA (New Mexico 1998/99, Men 356/100,000, Women 150/100,000), see Table 1. For SCC the percentage changed in SCC crude rates and increased with advancing age in males, the incidence rates were highest rates among those ages over 55 years.[35] In Australia the incidence rates accounted for 1,332 in men and 755 in women (1997, Queensland) per 100,000 inhabitants and year, age standardized for the United States population and world standard population, respectively, see Table 1. In Germany, the incidence rate for squamous cell carcinoma accounted for 30 per 100,000 inhabitants and year.[36]

Decrease of Mortality in Nonmelanoma Skin Cancer

Compared to the incidence the mortality of NMSC is quite low. A large American study showed an age adjusted NMSC mortality rate of 0.91 (per 100,000 persons per year), of which almost half (0.45) were due to genital carcinoma. Nonmelanoma skin cancer mortality increased

---

Table 1. Incidence rate of NMSC in New Mexico, USA, in Queensland, Australia and Germany, according to the Krebsregister Schleswig-Holstein

	New Mexico	USA	Queensland, Australia	Germany
	1977/1978	1998/1999	1997	2004
Basal cell carcinoma				
Men	619	920	2058	80.8
Women	399	486	1194	63.3
Squamous cell carcinoma				
Men	188	356	1332	18.2
Women	72	150	755	8.5

Incidence rates per 100,000 inhabitants and year, age standardized per the 2,000 United States population, for the World Standard Population and for the European Standard population.[32,35,36]

sharply with age. The mortality rate from nongenital NMSC in men was more than twice that in women, but for genital NMSC this ratio was reversed. Overall, nongenital squamous cell carcinoma and basal cell carcinoma death rates have declined and mortality due to genital carcinoma was about half of total NMSC deaths.[37] In Finland the mortality rate for BCC in 1991 through 1995 was 0.08 per 100,000 person-years in men and 0.05 in women and for NMSC, it was 0.38 in men and 0.23 in women. The mortality trend was decreasing for both cancer types.[23] The Rhode Island nongenital SCC mortality rate (adjusted to the US 1970 population) comparing two time periods (1979-1987 and 1988-2000) was estimated to decrease for men and women. Also, the BCC mortality rate for the current period is estimated at 0.05 compared with 0.10 for the earlier period. Hence, the BCC and nongenital SCC mortality rates appear to be declining over time in Rhode Island. Similar findings have been reported in Australia.[9-11,32,37-40]

An analysis of the mortality data 1968-1999 in western Germany revealed a continuous decrease of the mortality rates since the 70ties. This becomes even clearer if the age standardized mortality rates are considered. In men the age standardized mortality rate (world standard population) decreased from 0,56 in 1968 to 0,24 in 1999 (per 100,000 inhabitants and year), in women this rate decreased from 0.42 to 0.11.[9]

Clinical Epidemiology of NMSC

Nonmelanoma skin cancers (NMSCs) constitute more than one-third of all cancers in the US and the standardized ratio of BCC to SCC is roughly 4:1.2.[11,38,41]

Nonmelanoma skin cancer generally occurs in persons older than 50 years and in this age group, its incidence is increasing rapidly, patients with SCC were generally older at the time of diagnosis.[1,2,42] The anatomic pattern of increase in BCC and SCC incidence was consistent with an effect of greater sunlight exposure. Over 80% of NMSCs occur on areas of the body that are frequently exposed to sunlight, such as the head, neck and back of the hands. BCC is also most commonly found on the nose. Body site- and gender-specific incidence rates for skin cancer were estimated in an Australian study.[30] For NMSC the highest body site-specific incidence rates were found for lip, orbit, naso-labial and ear, nose, cheek and the dorsum of the hands. Studies of BCC and SCC occurrence are needed to identify possible behavioral and environmental factors and to assess possible changes in diagnostic practices that might account for the rise in incidence of these common malignancies.[1,2,42] The rising incidence rates of NMSC is probably due to a combination of increased sun exposure or exposure to ultraviolet (UV) light, increased outdoor activities, changes in clothing style, increased longevity and ozone depletion. Further etiological factors were genetics (Xeroderma pigmentosum), immune suppression and actinic keratoses, see Figures 1 and 2. A dose-dependent increase in the risk of SCC but not BCC of the skin associated with exposure to PUVA was reported by Stern et al.[43] This observation was concordant to the results of a large Canadian risk factor study, revealing that an intensive UV exposure in childhood and adolescence was causative fort the development of BCC whereas for the aetiology of SCC a chronic UV exposure in the earlier decades was accused.[42,44]

In organ transplant recipients a highly increased risk for nonmelanoma skin cancer was found in several studies. This cancer risk associated with transplantation is higher for sun-exposed than for nonsun-exposed epithelial tissues, even among populations living in regions with low insolation.[45,46] Infections with human papilloma virus HPV5 and HPV8 may represent an increased risk for SCC development in transplant recipients. The mechanisms by which these viruses may contribute to skin cancer development still remain unclear.

Sun Exposure and Nonmelanoma Skin Cancer

Sun exposure has long been regarded to be the major environmental risk factor for nonmelanoma skin cancer.[47-50] Lifelong cumulative sun exposure has been postulated to be a causal factor for SCC[48] while mixed effects of intermittent and cumulative sun exposure have been discussed as being causal for BCC.[47] A dose-response curve for sun exposure and basal cell carcinoma could be reported by several groups.[47] There is strong evidence to suggest that the role of ultraviolet (UV)

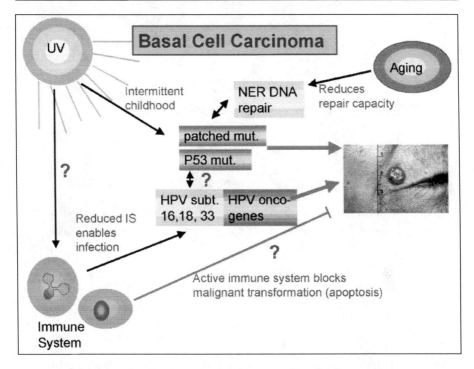

Figure 1. Hypothesized pathways to the development of basal cell carcinomas.

radiation in the development of skin cancer is multi-fold: (1) it causes mutations in cellular DNA that might ultimately lead to unrestrained growth and tumour formation, (2) it induces a state of relative cutaneous immune-suppression that might prevent tumour rejection and (3) might allow the persistent infection with Human Papilloma Viruses (HPV) as shown in immune-suppressed patients.[51] It could be demonstrated that mortality of NMSC could be prevented by reducing excessive exposure to UV light and prompt treatment of NMSC.[37]

Incidence rates of NMSC vary vastly by geographical area and latitude with most extreme rates reported from Australia and New Zealand.[26] Within Australia there is a marked North to South gradient with the most extreme incidence rates of NMSC recorded in Queensland.[26,30,32,52] Most UV-induced damage to the cellular DNA is repaired, however, mutations may occur as a result of base mispairing of the cellular DNA. The genes involved in the repair process are also potential UV targets. p53 is a nucleoprotein encoded by a tumour suppressor gene. Mutations of the tumour suppressor gene p53 are implicated in the genesis of a wide variety of human neoplasia including NMSC.[53] These mutations were reported to be present in 50% to 90% of SCCs[53] and approximately 55% of BCCs including very small lesions.[54] A second tumour suppressor gene, the gene for the patched (PTCH) protein in the epidermal growth-stimulating Hedgehog pathway, the human gene homolog of the Drosophila segment polarity gene patched, has also been shown to be mutated in more than 50% of sporadic BCCs, in patients with Gorlin-Goltz syndrome and with xeroderma pigmentosum.[55-58]

Furthermore, it has been reported that the observed point mutations both in the PTCH and the p53 genes were predominantly UV-specific transitions.[56,59] These results provide the first genetic evidence that UV radiation is the principal causal factor for NMSC. So far, mutations in the PTCH gene seem to be specific for BCC transformation, apart from SCCs in patients with a history of multiple BCCs.[59] On the other hand, in BCCs, UV-specific mutations of both p53 and the PTCH gene seem to frequently co-exist.[54,59,60]

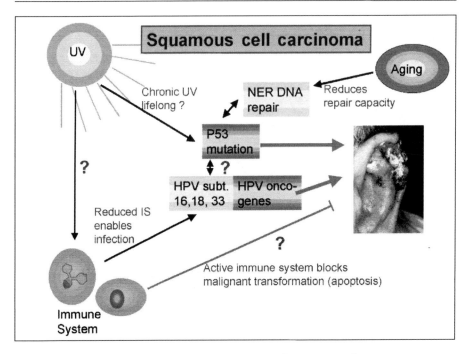

Figure 2. Hypothesized pathways to the development of squamous cell carcinomas.

The routine use of sunscreens on the skin by adults seems to be amenable to prevention of cutaneous squamous cell carcinoma, but not basal cell carcinoma.[61]

Melanoma

Increase of Melanoma Incidence in White Populations

The incidence of cutaneous melanoma (CM) increased most rapidly in the past decades until the late 1980s.[62-64] From the mid 1980s onwards, studies form Europe, Canada, the USA and Australia revealed that incidence rates were slowing down, stabilising or decreasing.[62-67] In the United States an increase of melanoma incidence was reported in men from 8 to 22/100,000 and in women from 7 to 15/100,000 in the time period from1975 to 2000, Figure 3. For 2003 54,200 new diagnoses and 7,600 deaths of melanoma were expected.[5,68]

The highest incidence rates were reported in Australia and New Zealand with 30 to 60 per 100,000 inhabitants/year.[14,67,69,70] In these countries, CM is one of the most frequent cancer types. The highest incidence rates were found in the northern equatorial parts of these countries as in Queensland (Australia) where incidence rates up to 60/100,000 inhabitants/year were found.

In Europe the highest increases of the incidence rates were found in Scandinavian Countries[7,71] but also in Central Europe and Southern Europe significant increases of melanoma incidences were found.[8,21,40,72] The lowest incidence rates were found in Mediterranean countries.[8,21,40,63,71,73] The reason for this North-South is a darker skin type (type III according to Fitzpatrick) in the Mediterranean population on one hand and different recreational activities, see Figure 4.

Stabilisation of Mortality Rates

Mortality from CMM has been increasing until the late 1980s in young and middle-aged populations from most European countries,[72,74] as well as from North America, Australia and New Zealand.[5] Mortality rates peaked in 1988-1990. Thereafter, trends have been less uniform, with mortality rates still rising in several European countries for middle aged adults, but with more favourable trends among women and some levelling off in rates for young adults, remaining roughly constant among men.[19] The favourable mortality trends have been related to changing patterns of sunshine exposure and sunburn in younger generations as well as to a better and earlier diagnosis of CMM[9,20,21,63,64,66,75-78] Additionally. A trend towards thinner and less invasive melanomas in both Central Europe and Queensland was observed in the last two decades.[4,79]

Clinical Epidemiology

Analyses for the clinical aspects of melanoma epidemiology are mainly based on data from the Central Malignant Melanoma Registry (CMMR),[80-82] which is presently one of the largest CM databases worldwide.[79] In 1983 the German Dermatological Society founded the Central Malignant Melanoma Registry (CMMR) a clinical-based melanoma registry in order to overcome the shortage of basic information on CM. Over the last two decades the CMMR developed into a large multi-centre project recording data retro- and prospectively from patients diagnosed with CM in 66 dermatological centres located in the former Federal Republic of Germany, 16 centres located in the former German Democratic Republic. Several dermatological centres provided their CM data bases dating back to the beginning seventies. Until 2005, 72,176 cases with CM were registered.

Compared to the 70ies where almost 2/3 of CM patients were women, equalization in both sexes was visible in the 90ies in Germany. Whereas in countries with a lower incidence as Great Britain still a higher ratio of women in melanoma patients con be found.[76] Countries with a high CM incidence as Australia show a more equivalence proportion or even a preponderance of men.[67,70,83]

Anatomic Site

The anatomic site varies according to gender. In men most of the tumors are localized on the trunk, in women the preferred site is lower extremity, see Table 2. In men 56% of CM are

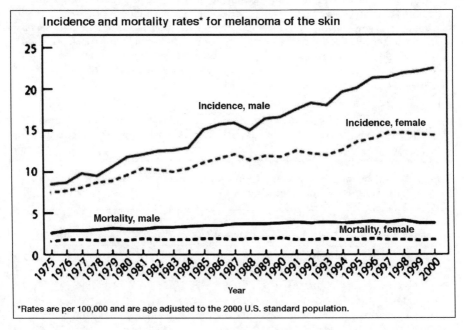

Figure 3. Incidence and mortality of melanoma in the USA according to SEER Cancer Statistics Review 1975-2000, JNCI 2003.

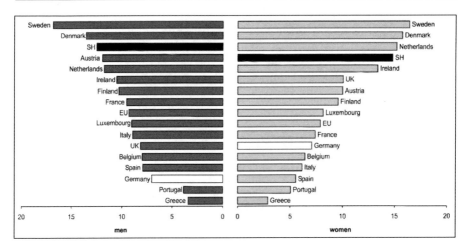

Figure 4. Melanoma incidence in Europe.[2]

localized at the trunk, thereof 38% at the back he followed by the lower leg in 16%. In women 42% of CM are localized at the lower extremity, of these 24% at the lower leg, followed by the trunk (26%). CM localized at the head and neck region and the upper extremity follow and are nearly equivalence in both sexes.[80,82,84]

This site distribution was found in most industrial nations with inhabitants of Caucasian origin as Europe, the USA and Australia.[8,31,62,66,85]

The site specific incidence of melanoma varies according to the age. The incidence of melanoma localized on the trunk and on the lower extremity decreases in higher ages, whereas a significant increase of melanoma localized in head and neck areas can be found in older patients.[86,87] Nearly 80% of melanoma in age groups of 80 and more years were found in head and neck areas.[86] Melanomas developing at different body sites are associated with distinct patterns of sun exposure. Melanomas of the head and neck are associated with chronic patterns of sun exposure whereas trunk melanomas are associated with intermittent patterns of sun exposure, supporting the hypothesis that melanomas may arise through divergent causal pathways.[87]

Histological Subtype

Superficial spreading melanoma is the most frequent histological subtype covering nearly 56% of all CM followed by the nodular melanoma (20% of all CM) and the lentigo maligna melanoma

Table 2. Anatomic sites of CM in the CMMR according to gender. The median age is given at the time point of diagnosis

Anatomic Site	Men %	Median Age	Women %	Median Age
Face	8.2%	66	10.1%	70
Scalp	5.1%	64	2.0%	61
Neck	2.2%	57	1.6%	56
Anterior trunk	16.3%	55	7.7%	45
Posterior trunk	39.3%	55	17.1%	48
Genital region	0.2%	59	0.8%	65
Upper extremity	12.2%	58	18.4%	59
Lower extremity	16.5%	52	42.3%	56

(9% of CM) and the acrolentiginous melanoma (4% of CM). A similar distribution is found in the analyses of incidence rates in the USA and Canada.[62,66]

Different age distributions are found for the respective histological subtypes. The peak for superficial spreading melanomas is found in patients of 55 to 59 years, for nodular melanomas in patients of 60 to 64 years, for acrolentiginous melanoma in patients of 65 to 69 years and in lentigo maligna melanoma in patients of 70 to 74 years.

Tumor Thickness

The tumor thickness is the most important prognostic factor in primary melanoma.[81] In this respect tumor thickness is the most important criterion for early diagnosis. In Germany there is an ongoing trend towards thin melanoma since the 1980ies.[4,79,81,84] The median tumor thickness decreased from 1.81 mm to 0.53 mm in the year 2000. The percentages of in situ and level II CM increased.[79] This trend is now alleviated and currently no distinct trend to a further decrease of tumor thickness is visible (Fig. 5).

The tumor thickness at the time point of primary diagnosis is also age dependent. Generally there's a significant decrease of melanoma with a tumor thickness of 1.0 mm or less in higher ages and is less than 50% at the age of 70. In contrast the fraction of thick melanoma increases significantly and reaches 20% at the age of 80 years in both genders.

An analysis of the prognosis 5,873 patients with primary CM of the clinical registry of the in consideration of tumor thickness was performed at the department of dermatology at the University of Tuebingen. In patients with a tumor thickness of 1.0 mm or less, 10 year survival rates were 96% and decreased to 85% in patients with a tumor thickness of >1.0 to 2.0 mm and to 70% in patients with a tumor thickness of 2.01-4.0 mm. Ten year survival rates were lowest (55%) in patients with a tumor thickness of more than 4 mm (Fig. 6). No changes could be observed over the recent decades.

Sun Exposure and Melanoma

To date, it is widely accepted that total risk of melanoma is determined through the interplay between genetic factors and exposure to sunlight.[88] 80% of melanoma develop in intermittently

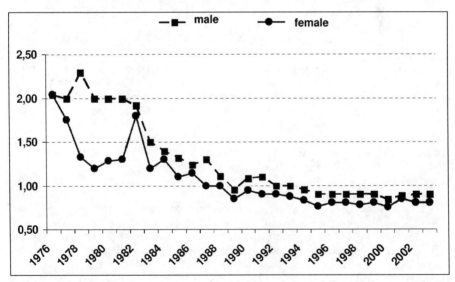

Figure 5. Time trends of median tumor thickness of in men and women between 1976 and 2005 recorded by the German CMMR. A significant decrease of tumor thickness can be found until the mid of 1990ies, afterwards tumor thickness stays nearly constant.

sun exposed regions. Intermittent sun exposure and sunburn history have been identified as risk factors for melanoma in epidemiologic studies.[89,90]

Melanocytic nevi have been identified as the most important risk factor for cutaneous melanoma. Sun exposure, sunburns and light pigmentation have been found to be associated with their development in childhood. In adulthood, sunburns and sun exposure is associated with the development of actinic lentigines.[90,91]

In a study of 1,812 German Kindergarten children high numbers of nevi in children were associated with the number of weeks on sunny holidays, outdoor activities at home, skin type, facial freckling, ethnicity and the number of nevi on the arms of parents. A strong association was found between nevus development in children and the number of parental moles, which most likely points to an inherited factor.[92] In Germany, moderate sun exposure such as outdoor activities during a German summer without sunburns seemed to be sufficient for induction of melanocytic nevi.[92-94]

The pathogenic effects of sun exposure could involve the genotoxic, mitogenic, or immunosuppressive responses to the damage induced in the skin by UV. Controversial is whether the UVB or the UVA component of solar radiation is more important in melanoma development.[95-97] To date it is not clear and further epidemiologic and basic science studies will be necessary to unravel the contribution that UVA or UVB might make in the production of BRAF mutations which were found to be present in about 60% of melanomas[98] and in 20%-80% of melanocytic nevi.[99-101] Among kindreds predisposed to multiple atypical melanocytic nevi and melanomas because of germ-line mutations in the *CDKN2A* gene encoding the tumor- suppressor proteins p16 and p19 or possibly other genes, retrospective analyses suggest that the incidence of melanoma has increased in recent generations, a phenomenon ascribed to the independent risk factor of increased sun exposure.[102,103]

There are particular genetic changes in melanomas in different sites, consistent differences related to ultraviolet exposure on sites that are chronically exposed (head and neck) or intermittently exposed (chest and back) and in acral and mucosal skin. For example, *CCND1* amplification occurs predominantly in acral regions, whereas activating mutations in *BRAF* occur most frequently in skin sites of intermittent sun exposure.[104-106]

Epidemiological studies have confirmed the hypothesis that the majority of all melanoma cases are caused, at least in part, by excessive exposure to sunlight.[5,12,13,15,70,107,108] For example, the greatest increases in incidence of melanomas have been seen in the regions of the body subjected to intermittent exposure, such as the torso in men and the lower legs in women. Indeed, it is likely that abrupt changes in sunlight exposure, is a causal factor in the increase in melanoma incidence observed in recent years. Epidemiological data have also suggested that a history of exposure to large doses of sunlight sufficient to cause sunburn in childhood is a particularly important melanoma risk factor.[109]

Latitude studies reveal a higher mean UV index to be significantly associated with an increase in melanoma incidence in non Hispanic whites in a large American study ($r = 0.85$, $P = .001$). Latitude also had a significant correlation with incidence in non Hispanic whites ($r = -0.85$, $P = .001$). A substantial portion of the variance in registry incidence in non Hispanic whites could be explained by the UV index ($R2 = 0.71$, $P = .001$). Melanoma incidence was shown to be associated with increased UV index and lower latitude in non Hispanic whites, but also in Hispanics and blacks.[110] Although, melanoma are uncommon in darker-skinned people; in the United States, the incidence among blacks is only 1/10 that among whites.[111]

The epidemiologic evidence implicating sun exposure in the causation of melanoma is supported by biologic evidence that damage caused by ultraviolet radiation, particularly damage to DNA, plays a central part in the pathogenesis of these tumors.[88,90,112-114] UV exposure in the childhood seems to be the main factor to induce mutations in the melanocytic system associated with an increased induction of melanocytic nevi and an increased risk for the development of melanoma.

Gilchrest et al described a potential explanation for the epidemiology of melanoma as compared with nonmelanoma skin cancer:[115] After exposure to ultraviolet radiation, the most severely dam-

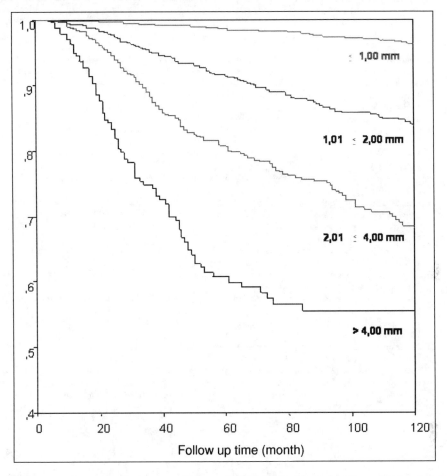

Figure 6. Ten year survival rates according to tumor thickness classes in primary CM in primary CM recorded by the German CMMR between 1976 and 2005. The current classification (AJCC2002) is mainly based on the tumor thickness.

aged keratinocytes undergo apoptosis, leaving the less damaged keratinocytes to up-regulate their DNA-repair capacity and to undergo nearly perfect repair. The skin tans, providing protective melanin to the surviving cells. Frequent subsequent exposure to ultraviolet radiation within the SOS-response period will then perpetuate the increases in repair capacity and melanin content, minimizing (but not eliminating) cumulative mutational damage. Intermittent high-dose exposures to ultraviolet radiation would have little effect on the development of basal-cell and squamous-cell carcinoma. Repeated low-dose exposure would be expected to cause multiple mutations in the retained cells of the basal compartment and hence to give rise to keratinocytic cancers. In melano-cytes, in contrast, a high dose of UV radiation will cause substantial damage but not apoptosis; the melanocytes will survive to mutate and divide. The appearance of freckles in children, is consistent with this speculation, because freckles are thought to represent clones of mutated melanocytes and their presence is associated with an increased risk of melanoma. Some mutations induced by ultraviolet radiation are thought to enable melanocytes to cross the epidermal basement membrane into the dermis, where subsequent proliferation gives rise to junctional nevi.

References

1. Holme SA, Malinovszky K, Roberts DL. Changing trends in nonmelanoma skin cancer in South Wales, 1988-98. Br J Dermatol 2000; 143:1224-9.
2. Katalinic A, Kunze U, Schafer T. Epidemiology of cutaneous melanoma and nonmelanoma skin cancer in Schleswig-Holstein, Germany: incidence, clinical subtypes, tumour stages and localization (epidemiology of skin cancer). Br J Dermatol 2003; 149:1200-6.
3. Diepgen TL, Mahler V. The epidemiology of skin cancer. Br J Dermatol 2002; 146 Suppl 61:1-6.
4. Garbe C, McLeod GR, Buettner PG. Time trends of cutaneous melanoma in Queensland, Australia and Central Europe. Cancer 2000; 89:1269-78.
5. Jemal A, Devesa SS, Hartge P et al. Recent trends in cutaneous melanoma incidence among whites in the United States. J Natl Cancer Inst 2001; 93:678-83.
6. Levi F, Te VC, Randimbison L et al. Trends in incidence of various morphologies of malignant melanoma in Vaud and Neuchatel, Switzerland. Melanoma Res 2005; 15:73-5.
7. Mansson-Brahme E, Johansson H, Larsson O et al. Trends in incidence of cutaneous malignant melanoma in a Swedish population 1976-1994. Acta Oncol 2002; 41:138-46.
8. Ocana-Riola R, Martinez-Garcia C, Serrano S et al. Population-based study of cutaneous malignant melanoma in the Granada province (Spain), 1985-1992. Eur J Epidemiol 2001; 17:169-74.
9. Stang A, Jockel KH. Declining mortality rates for nonmelanoma skin cancers in West Germany, 1968-99. Br J Dermatol 2004; 150:517-22.
10. Weinstock MA. Epidemiologic investigation of nonmelanoma skin cancer mortality: the Rhode Island Follow-Back Study. J Invest Dermatol 1994; 102:6S-9S.
11. Weinstock MA. Epidemiology of nonmelanoma skin cancer: clinical issues, definitions and classification. J Invest Dermatol 1994; 102:4S-5S.
12. Armstrong BK, Kricker A, English DR. Sun exposure and skin cancer. Australas J Dermatol 1997; 38 Suppl 1:S1-S6.
13. Armstrong BK, Kricker A. The epidemiology of UV induced skin cancer. J Photochem Photobiol B 2001; 63:8-18.
14. MacLennan R, Green AC, McLeod GR et al. Increasing incidence of cutaneous melanoma in Queensland, Australia. J Natl Cancer Inst 1992; 84:1427-32.
15. Rigel DS, Carucci JA. Malignant melanoma: prevention, early detection and treatment in the 21st century. CA Cancer J Clin 2000; 50:215-36.
16. Haberland J, Bertz J, Gorsch B et al. Krebsinzidenzschätzungen fur Deutschland mittels log-linearer Modelle. Gesundheitswesen 2001; 63:556-60.
17. Lasithiotakis KG, Leiter U, Gorkievicz R et al. The incidence and mortality of cutaneous melanoma in Southern Germany: trends by anatomic site and pathologic characteristics, 1976 to 2003. Cancer 2006; 107:1331-9.
18. Diffey BL. The future incidence of cutaneous melanoma within the UK. Br J Dermatol 2004; 151:868-72.
19. Stang A, Stang K, Stegmaier C et al. Skin melanoma in Saarland: incidence, survival and mortality 1970-1996. Eur J Cancer Prev 2001; 10:407-15.
20. Bosetti C, La Vecchia C, Naldi L et al. Mortality from cutaneous malignant melanoma in Europe. Has the epidemic levelled off? Melanoma Res 2004; 14:301-9.
21. Stracci F, Minelli L, D'Alo D et al. Incidence, mortality and survival trends of cutaneous melanoma in Umbria, Italy. 1978-82 and 1994-98. Tumori 2005; 91:6-8.
22. Gray DT, Suman VJ, Su WP et al. Trends in the population-based incidence of squamous cell carcinoma of the skin first diagnosed between 1984 and 1992. Arch Dermatol 1997; 133:735-40.
23. Hannuksela-Svahn A, Pukkala E, Karvonen J. Basal cell skin carcinoma and other nonmelanoma skin cancers in Finland from 1956 through 1995. Arch Dermatol 1999; 135:781-6.
24. Iversen T, Tretli S. Trends for invasive squamous cell neoplasia of the skin in Norway. Br J Cancer 1999; 81:528-31.
25. Karagas MR, Greenberg ER, Spencer SK et al. Increase in incidence rates of basal cell and squamous cell skin cancer in New Hampshire, USA. New Hampshire Skin Cancer Study Group. Int J Cancer 1999; 81:555-9.
26. Staples M, Marks R, Giles G. Trends in the incidence of nonmelanocytic skin cancer (NMSC) treated in Australia 1985-1995: are primary prevention programs starting to have an effect? Int J Cancer 1998; 78:144-8.
27. Weinstock MA. Issues in the epidemiology of melanoma. Hematol Oncol Clin North Am 1998; 12:681-98.
28. Elder DE. Skin cancer. Melanoma and other specific nonmelanoma skin cancers. Cancer 1995; 75:245-56.

29. Stern RS. The mysteries of geographic variability in nonmelanoma skin cancer incidence. Arch Dermatol 1999; 135:843-4.
30. Buettner PG, Raasch BA. Incidence rates of skin cancer in Townsville, Australia. Int J Cancer 1998; 78:587-93.
31. Green A, MacLennan R, Youl P et al. Site distribution of cutaneous melanoma in Queensland. Int J Cancer 1993; 53:232-6.
32. Raasch BA, Buettner PG. Multiple nonmelanoma skin cancer in an exposed Australian population. Int J Dermatol 2002; 41:652-8.
33. Krebsregister Schleswig-Holstein Instituts für Krebsepidemiologie. Krebs in Schleswig-Holstein 2004. Ref Type: Generic.
34. The Danish National Board of Health. Cancer Incidence in Denmark 1997. 2001. Ref Type: Generic.
35. Athas WF, Hunt WC, Key CR. Changes in nonmelanoma skin cancer incidence between 1977-1978 and 1998-1999 in Northcentral New Mexico. Cancer Epidemiol Biomarkers Prev 2003; 12:1105-8.
36. Katalinic A. [Population-based cancer registration in Germany. Essentials and perspectives]. Bundesgesundheitsblatt. Gesundheitsforschung Gesundheitsschutz 2004; 47:422-8.
37. Lewis KG, Weinstock MA. Nonmelanoma skin cancer mortality (1988-2000): the Rhode Island follow-back study. Arch Dermatol 2004; 140:837-42.
38. Schuz J, Schon D, Batzler W et al. Cancer registration in Germany: current status, perspectives and trends in cancer incidence 1973-93. J Epidemiol Biostat 2000; 5:99-107.
39. Stang A, Stegmaier C, Jockel KH. Nonmelanoma skin cancer in the Federal State of Saarland, Germany, 1995-1999. Br J Cancer 2003; 89:1205-8.
40. Vinceti M, Bergomi M, Borciani N et al. Rising melanoma incidence in an Italian community from 1986 to 1997. Melanoma Res 1999; 9:97-103.
41. Lehnert M, Eberle A, Hentschel S et al. [Malignant melanoma of the skin as evidenced by epidemiological cancer registries in Germany—incidence, clinical parameters, variations in recording]. Gesundheitswesen 2005; 67:729-35.
42. Gallagher RP, Hill GB, Bajdik CD et al. Sunlight exposure, pigmentation factors and risk of nonmelanocytic skin cancer. II. Squamous cell carcinoma. Arch Dermatol 1995; 131:164-9.
43. Stern RS. Risks of cancer associated with long-term exposure to PUVA in humans: current status—1991. Blood Cells 1992; 18:91-7.
44. Gallagher RP, Spinelli JJ, Lee TK. Tanning beds, sunlamps and risk of cutaneous malignant melanoma. Cancer Epidemiol Biomarkers Prev 2005; 14:562-6.
45. Ulrich C, Schmook T, Nindl I et al. Cutaneous precancers in organ transplant recipients: an old enemy in a new surrounding. Br J Dermatol 2003; 149 Suppl 66:40-2.
46. Ulrich C, Schmook T, Sachse MM et al. Comparative epidemiology and pathogenic factors for nonmelanoma skin cancer in organ transplant patients. Dermatol Surg 2004; 30:622-7.
47. English DR, Armstrong BK, Kricker A et al. Case-control study of sun exposure and squamous cell carcinoma of the skin. Int J Cancer 1998; 77:347-53.
48. Kricker A, Armstrong BK, English DR. Sun exposure and nonmelanocytic skin cancer. Cancer Causes Control 1994; 5:367-92.
49. Kricker A, Armstrong BK, McMichael AJ. Skin cancer and ultraviolet. Nature 1994; 368:594.
50. Kricker A, Armstrong BK, English DR et al. Does intermittent sun exposure cause basal cell carcinoma? a case-control study in Western Australia. Int J Cancer 1995; 60:489-94.
51. de Villiers EM. Human papillomavirus infections in skin cancers. Biomed Pharmacother 1998; 52:26-33.
52. Green A, Marks R. Squamous cell carcinoma of the skin (nonmetastatic). Clin Evid 2005; 2086-90.
53. Ziegler A, Leffell DJ, Kunala S et al. Mutation hotspots due to sunlight in the p53 gene of nonmelanoma skin cancers. Proc Natl Acad Sci USA 1993; 90:4216-20.
54. Zhang H, Ping XL, Lee PK et al. Role of PTCH and p53 genes in early-onset basal cell carcinoma. Am J Pathol 2001; 158:381-5.
55. Athar M, Tang X, Lee JL et al. Hedgehog signalling in skin development and cancer. Exp Dermatol 2006; 15:667-77.
56. Daya-Grosjean L, Sarasin A. UV-specific mutations of the human patched gene in basal cell carcinomas from normal individuals and xeroderma pigmentosum patients. Mutat Res 2000; 450:193-9.
57. Levanat S, Mubrin MK, Crnic I et al. Variable expression of Gorlin syndrome may reflect complexity of the signalling pathway. Pflugers Arch 2000; 439:R31-R33.
58. Situm M, Levanat S, Crnic I et al. Involvement of patched (PTCH) gene in Gorlin syndrome and related disorders: three family cases. Croat Med J 1999; 40:533-8.
59. Ping XL, Ratner D, Zhang H et al. PTCH mutations in squamous cell carcinoma of the skin. J Invest Dermatol 2001; 116:614-6.

60. Ling G, Ahmadian A, Persson A et al. PATCHED and p53 gene alterations in sporadic and hereditary basal cell cancer. Oncogene 2001; 20:7770-8.
61. Green A, Williams G, Neale R et al. Daily sunscreen application and betacarotene supplementation in prevention of basal-cell and squamous-cell carcinomas of the skin: a randomised controlled trial. Lancet 1999; 354:723-9.
62. Bulliard JL, Cox B, Semenciw R. Trends by anatomic site in the incidence of cutaneous malignant melanoma in Canada, 1969-93. Cancer Causes Control 1999; 10:407-16.
63. de Vries E, Bray FI, Coebergh JW et al. Changing epidemiology of malignant cutaneous melanoma in Europe 1953-1997: rising trends in incidence and mortality but recent stabilizations in western Europe and decreases in Scandinavia. Int J Cancer 2003; 107:119-26.
64. Geller AC, Miller DR, Annas GD et al. Melanoma incidence and mortality among US whites, 1969-1999. JAMA 2002; 288:1719-20.
65. Dennis LK. Melanoma incidence by body site: effects of birth-cohort adjustment. Arch Dermatol 1999; 135:1553-4.
66. Hall HI, Miller DR, Rogers JD et al. Update on the incidence and mortality from melanoma in the United States. J Am Acad Dermatol 1999; 40:35-42.
67. Marrett LD, Nguyen HL, Armstrong BK. Trends in the incidence of cutaneous malignant melanoma in New South Wales, 1983-1996. Int J Cancer 2001; 92:457-62.
68. Anonymus. Stat bite: Incidence of and mortality from melanoma of the skin, 1975-2000. J Natl Cancer Inst 2003; 95:933.
69. Jones WO, Harman CR, Ng AK et al. Incidence of malignant melanoma in Auckland, New Zealand: highest rates in the world. World J Surg 1999; 23:732-5.
70. Marks R. Epidemiology of melanoma. Clin Exp Dermatol 2000; 25:459-63.
71. Osterlind A, Hou-Jensen K, Moller JO. Incidence of cutaneous malignant melanoma in Denmark 1978-1982. Anatomic site distribution, histologic types and comparison with nonmelanoma skin cancer. Br J Cancer 1988; 58:385-91.
72. Balzi D, Carli P, Giannotti B et al. Cutaneous melanoma in the Florentine area, Italy: incidence, survival and mortality between 1985 and 1994. Eur J Cancer Prev 2003; 12:43-8.
73. de Vries E, Bray FI, Eggermont AM et al. Monitoring stage-specific trends in melanoma incidence across Europe reveals the need for more complete information on diagnostic characteristics. Eur J Cancer Prev 2004; 13:387-95.
74. Stang A, Jockel KH. Changing patterns of skin melanoma mortality in West Germany from 1968 through 1999. Ann Epidemiol 2003; 13:436-42.
75. de Vries E, Schouten LJ, Visser O et al. Rising trends in the incidence of and mortality from cutaneous melanoma in the Netherlands: a Northwest to Southeast gradient? Eur J Cancer 2003; 39:1439-46.
76. MacKie RM, Bray CA, Hole DJ et al. Incidence of and survival from malignant melanoma in Scotland: an epidemiological study. Lancet 2002; 360:587-91.
77. Berwick M, Armstrong BK, Ben Porat L et al. Sun exposure and mortality from melanoma. J Natl Cancer Inst 2005; 97:195-9.
78. Berwick M, Halpern A. Melanoma epidemiology. Curr Opin Oncol 1997; 9:178-82.
79. Buettner PG, Leiter U, Eigentler TK et al. Development of prognostic factors and survival in cutaneous melanoma over 25 years: An analysis of the Central Malignant Melanoma Registry of the German Dermatological Society. Cancer 2005; 103:616-24.
80. Garbe C, Orfanos CE. Epidemiology of malignant melanoma in central Europe: risk factors and prognostic predictors. Results of the Central Malignant Melanoma Registry of the German Dermatological Society. Pigment Cell Res 1992; Suppl 2:285-94.
81. Garbe C, Weiss J, Kruger S et al. The German melanoma registry and environmental risk factors implied. Recent Results Cancer Res 1993; 128:69-89.
82. Garbe C, Buttner P, Bertz J et al. Primary cutaneous melanoma. Prognostic classification of anatomic location. Cancer 1995; 75:2492-8.
83. Marks R. The changing incidence and mortality of melanoma in Australia. Recent Results Cancer Res 2002; 160:113-21.
84. Garbe C, Wiebelt H, Orfanos CE. Change of epidemiological characteristics of malignant melanoma during the years 1962-1972 and 1983-1986 in the Federal Republic of Germany. Dermatologica 1989; 178:131-5.
85. Carli P, Borgognoni L, Biggeri A et al. Incidence of cutaneous melanoma in the centre of Italy: anatomic site distribution, histologic types and thickness of tumour invasion in a registry-based study. Melanoma Res 1994; 4:385-90.
86. Hoersch B, Leiter U, Garbe C. Is head and neck melanoma a distinct entity? A clinical registry-based comparative study in 5,702 patients with melanoma. Br J Dermatol 2006; 155:771-7.

87. Whiteman DC, Stickley M, Watt P et al. Anatomic site, sun exposure and risk of cutaneous melanoma. J Clin Oncol 2006; 24:3172-7.
88. Jhappan C, Noonan FP, Merlino G. Ultraviolet radiation and cutaneous malignant melanoma. Oncogene 2003; 22:3099-112.
89. Gandini S, Sera F, Cattaruzza MS, et al. Meta-analysis of risk factors for cutaneous melanoma: II. Sun exposure. Eur J Cancer 2005; 41:45-60.
90. Elwood JM, Jopson J. Melanoma and sun exposure: an overview of published studies. Int J Cancer 1997; 73:198-203.
91. Garbe C, Buttner P, Weiss J et al. Associated factors in the prevalence of more than 50 common melanocytic nevi, atypical melanocytic nevi and actinic lentigines: multicenter case-control study of the Central Malignant Melanoma Registry of the German Dermatological Society. J Invest Dermatol 1994; 102:700-5.
92. Wiecker TS, Luther H, Buettner P et al. Moderate sun exposure and nevus counts in parents are associated with development of melanocytic nevi in childhood: a risk factor study in 1,812 kindergarten children. Cancer 2003; 97:628-38.
93. Bauer J, Buttner P, Wiecker TS et al. Interventional study in 1,232 young German children to prevent the development of melanocytic nevi failed to change sun exposure and sun protective behavior. Int J Cancer 2005.
94. Bauer J, Buttner P, Wiecker TS et al. Effect of sunscreen and clothing on the number of melanocytic nevi in 1,812 German children attending day care. Am J Epidemiol 2005; 161:620-7.
95. De Fabo EC, Noonan FP, Fears T et al. Ultraviolet B but not ultraviolet A radiation initiates melanoma. Cancer Res 2004; 64:6372-6.
96. Wang SQ, Setlow R, Berwick M et al. Ultraviolet A and melanoma: a review. J Am Acad Dermatol 2001; 44:837-46.
97. Thomas NE, Berwick M, Cordeiro-Stone M. Could BRAF mutations in melanocytic lesions arise from DNA damage induced by ultraviolet radiation? J.Invest Dermatol 2006; 126:1693-6.
98. Dong J, Phelps RG, Qiao R et al. BRAF oncogenic mutations correlate with progression rather than initiation of human melanoma. Cancer Res 2003; 63:3883-5.
99. Kumar R, Angelini S, Snellman E et al. BRAF mutations are common somatic events in melanocytic nevi. J Invest Dermatol 2004; 122:342-8.
100. Pollock PM, Harper UL, Hansen KS et al. High frequency of BRAF mutations in nevi. Nat Genet 2003; 33:19-20.
101. Yazdi AS, Palmedo G, Flaig MJ et al. Mutations of the BRAF gene in benign and malignant melanocytic lesions. J Invest Dermatol 2003; 121:1160-2.
102. Battistutta D, Palmer J, Walters M et al. Incidence of familial melanoma and MLM2 gene. Lancet 1994; 344:1607-8.
103. Monzon J, Liu L, Brill H et al. CDKN2A mutations in multiple primary melanomas. N Engl J Med 1998; 338:879-87.
104. Maldonado JL, Fridlyand J, Patel H et al. Determinants of BRAF mutations in primary melanomas. J Natl Cancer Inst 2003; 95:1878-90.
105. Miller AJ, Mihm MC Jr. Melanoma. N Engl J Med 2006; 355:51-65.
106. Sauter ER, Yeo UC, von Stemm A et al. Cyclin D1 is a candidate oncogene in cutaneous melanoma. Cancer Res 2002; 62:3200-6.
107. Armstrong BK, Kricker A. Epidemiology of sun exposure and skin cancer. Cancer Surv 1996; 26:133-53.
108. MacKie RM. Incidence, risk factors and prevention of melanoma. Eur J Cancer 1998; 34 Suppl 3 S3-S6.
109. Autier P, Dore JF. Influence of sun exposures during childhood and during adulthood on melanoma risk. EPIMEL and EORTC Melanoma Cooperative Group. European Organisation for Research and Treatment of Cancer. Int J Cancer 1998; 77:533-7.
110. Eide MJ, Weinstock MA. Association of UV index, latitude and melanoma incidence in nonwhite populations—US Surveillance, Epidemiology and End Results (SEER) Program, 1992 to 2001. Arch Dermatol 2005; 141:477-81.
111. Parkin DM, Pisani P, Ferlay J. Estimates of the worldwide incidence of 25 major cancers in 1990. Int J Cancer 1999; 80:827-41.
112. Hu S, Ma F, Collado-Mesa F, et al. UV radiation, latitude and melanoma in US Hispanics and blacks. Arch.Dermatol 2004; 140:819-24.
113. Holman CD, Armstrong BK, Heenan PJ. A theory of the etiology and pathogenesis of human cutaneous malignant melanoma. J Natl Cancer Inst 1983; 71:651-6.
114. Whiteman DC, Whiteman CA, Green AC. Childhood sun exposure as a risk factor for melanoma: a systematic review of epidemiologic studies. Cancer Causes Control 2001; 12:69-82.
115. Gilchrest BA, Eller MS, Geller AC et al. The pathogenesis of melanoma induced by ultraviolet radiation. N Engl J Med 1999; 340:1341-8.

CHAPTER 9

Ultraviolet Radiation and Malignant Melanoma

Johan Moan,* Alina Carmen Porojnicu and Arne Dahlback

Abstract

Essential features of the epidemiology and photobiology of cutaneous malignant melanoma (CMM) in Norway were studied in comparison with data from countries at lower latitudes. Arguments for and against a relationship between ultraviolet radiation (UV) from sun and sun beds are discussed. Our data indicate that UV is a carcinogen for CMM and that intermittent exposures are notably melanomagenic. This hypothesis was supported both by latitude gradients, by time trends and by changing patterns of tumor density on different body localizations. However, even though UV radiation generates CMM, it may also have a protective action and/or an action that improves prognosis. The same may be true for a number of internal cancers.

There appears to be no, or even an inverse latitude gradient for CMM arising on non-UV exposed body localizations (uveal melanoma). Furthermore, CMM prognosis was gradually improved over all years of increasing incidence (up to 1990), but during the last 10 to 15 years, incidence rates decreased and prognosis was not further improved.

While CMM incidence rates are twice as high in South Norway as in North Norway, the ratios of death rates to incidence rates are higher in the North, where the annual UV fluences are lower. Death- and incidence rates in Australia and New Zealand fully support this.

Comparisons of skin cancer data from Norway and Australia/New Zealand indicate that squamous cell carcinoma and basal cell carcinoma are mainly related to annual solar UVB fluences, while UVA fluences play a larger role for CMM.

Introduction

Ultraviolet radiation (UV) from the sun is an important risk factor for skin cancer.[1-3] For squamous call carcinoma (SCC) and basal cell carcinoma (BCC) there is a clear relationship with UV, although for BCC the dose-response relationship has not been firmly established in all investigations.[2] For cutaneous malignant melanoma (CMM) the relationship has been debated for decades,[2-12] although most investigators tend to conclude that UV is CMM-generating in humans.

As it will be discussed in this chapter, there are arguments both for and against a relationship. A complicating factor is that the exposure pattern (continuous occupational exposure versus episodes of intense exposure, often termed intermittent exposure) seems to be of importance for CMM.

Scandinavia is located at high latitudes (>54°N). Therefore, the annual UVB (280-320 nm) exposures are limited and are of the order of 25% of the Equatorial UVB exposures.[10] In spite of this, CMM is a significant health problem in Scandinavia, in fact much more important than one might expect in view of the high latitudes, with Norway presenting surprisingly high incidence

*Corresponding Author: Johan Moan—Department of Radiation Biology, Institute for Cancer Research, Ullernchausseen 70, Montebello, 0310, and Department of Physics, University of Oslo, Oslo, Norway. Email: johan.moan@labmed.uio.no

Sunlight, Vitamin D and Skin Cancer, edited by Jörg Reichrath. ©2008 Landes Bioscience and Springer Science+Business Media.

rates. In 2002, the estimated age adjusted incidence rate of CMM for women in Norway was 15,7 as compared with 11,3 in France, 5,5 in Spain, 6,2 in Italy and 9 in Germany.[13]

While BCC and SCC, like most other cancers, are diseases of old people, with risks increasing sharply with age almost in an exponential manner, CMM is most frequent among middle aged people. The localization pattern on the body is also different for the three skin cancer forms, and this pattern is changing with time.

The fact that the incidence rates of CMM have increased over many decades has been a serious concern for health authorities. Therefore, large campaigns against sun- and sun bed exposure and for sunscreen use have been launched. An emerging, complicating factor associated with such campaigns is that the health benefits of vitamin D have become evident during the last decade. Not only solar radiation, but also radiation from sun beds produces vitamin D,[14] while sunscreens, applied as recommended, eliminate the production.[15]

In this chapter we will summarize the epidemiology of CMM in Norway, compare it with data from other countries and try to elucidate some of the puzzles mentioned above. We will start with a list of the arguments against and for a melanoma-generating effect of solar radiation and attempt to perform an evaluation of the arguments.

Does UV Radiation Induce CMM?

Arguments against a Relationship[8,11,16-18]

1. CMM is more frequent among people with occupation giving low accumulated UV exposure, so called white collar workers, than among people with large accumulated UV exposures (farmers, fishermen, etc).
2. The localization pattern of CMM on the body is different from that of SCC.
3. CMM appears to be uncommon among albino Africans; opposite to what is found for BCC and SCC.
4. The incidence rate of CMM in sunny Australia is only about two times higher than in the high-latitude country Norway, while the incidence rates of BCC and SCC are 20 to 40 times higher.
5. In Europe, CMM is more frequent in the north than in the south. The whole area is mainly populated by Caucasians.
6. Not all case-control epidemiological studies show an increase of CMM incidence with increasing UV exposure.
7. Some sunscreen investigations indicate no CMM protective effect of UVB absorbing sunscreens.
8. Some sun bed investigations indicate a protective rather than a generating effect of artificial UV sources.
9. Around CMM lesions little solar elastosis is found. Solar elastosis is related to cumulative UV exposure.
10. Sun and artificial sources of UVB are efficient generators of vitamin D. Vitamin D reduces carcinogenesis and tumor progression.
11. CMM may be a disease related to affluence, since the incidence rates appear to increase with increasing GDP (gross domestic product).

Arguments for a Relationship[2,4,6-11,16-20]

1. In populations with strictly similar skin type there is a clear latitudinal gradient for CMM, although it is smaller than that for BCC and SCC.
2. The risk of getting CMM decreases with increasing pigmentation.
3. Migration to more sunny countries increases the CMM risk.
4. UV induces pigmented nevi, and CMMs often arise in the borders of such nevi.
5. Sunburn episodes appear to increase the CMM risk, although conflicting results have been reported.

6. CMM patients often have low DNA repair capacity and low minimum erythema doses (MEDs).
7. Lentigo maligna melanoma is clearly related to UV exposure.
8. Patients with Xeroderma Pigmentosum (related to abnormal DNA repair) have at least 1000 times increased CMM risks compared with control persons.
9. Some CMMs contain UV fingerprint mutations.
10. CMM-resembling tumors can be induced in some animals by UV (examples: Angora goats, Sinclair swine, Monodelphis Domestica (an opossum), white horses and Xiphophorus (a small swordfish).
11. Patients with CMM have increased risk of BCC.
12. Some investigations indicate increased risk of getting CMM for persons frequently using sun beds.

Materials and Methods

The epidemiological data presented for Norway are extracted from the database of the Norwegian Cancer Registry. Rates are given per 100 000 and adjusted to the world (W) standard population. Data from other sources are also used, as referred to in the text. The two largest cities, Oslo and Bergen, are excluded from the study, to reduce the errors that may arise from different sun-exposure habits of urban and rural populations, although this does not seem to be of major importance for skin cancer incidence in Norway.[2]

The global solar UV (i.e., direct + diffuse radiation on a horizontal surface) was calculated with a radiative transfer model.[21,22] The daily ozone values measured by the TOMS instruments the Nimbus-7 and Earth Probe satellites were used as inputs to the model. The daily cloud cover for each site used in the calculations was derived from measured reflectivities from an ozone-insensitive channel in the same satellite instruments. Notably, costal regions (Regions 11-15, Fig. 1) are cloudier than inland regions (Region 1, 2, 4-6, Fig. 1). The effect of snow cover in different regions was estimated by comparing the calculations with UV measurements from the Norwegian UV monitoring network. The calculated annual UV fluences given in this chapter are based on available satellite measurements in the period 1980-2000.

The fluences of carcinogenic UV from the sun were determined, assuming that the action spectrum of CMM is similar to the CIE reference spectrum for human erythema.[23] Similar results, although with slightly different latitude slopes of the incidence curves, would have been obtained if the fish melanoma spectrum[24] had been used.

Annual fluences are given, although summer values (May-August) are probably dominant with respect to real fluences obtained by the population. However, as earlier shown by comparisons with SCC incidence rates, the annual fluences are good approximations for the skin cancer generating fluences received by the population.[25] Average summer temperatures may be relevant for CMM induction, but are similar for all regions.[26]

Results and Discussion

Latitude Gradients

Latitude gradients are conveniently described by the so called biological amplification factor, A_b, which is defined by the equation $A_b = (dR/R)/(dD/D)$, where R is the age adjusted incidence rate and D is the annual exposure to carcinogenic solar radiation. D is often calculated by using the CIE reference spectrum for erythema[23] and so is done in the present chapter. Using a planar, horizontal surface in the exposure calculations, D increases by 50% per 10° latitude decrease in Norway.[10] The Norwegian skin cancer data are well described by the equation $\ln R = A_b \ln D + const$,[2,10,27] corresponding to the equation of definition for A_b above.

For SCC and BCC values of A_b between 1.5 and 2.5 are found, slightly smaller than those for CMM.[2,10,27] For BCC and SCC the Norwegian and Australian data agree quite well and A_b values of 2.3-2.5 are obtained when the two data sets are combined.[2] A_b values of 1.5 and 2 correspond to 75% and 100%, respectively, increase in skin cancer incidence rates per 10° decrease in latitude. Thus, the risks of SCC and BCC are roughly twice as large in South Norway (60° N) as in North Norway (70° N).

In our analysis Norway is divided in 20 counties (Fig. 1). Earlier we have found biological amplification factors of about 3 for CMM in Norway.[2] There were no significant differences between urban and rural areas, neither between different body localizations.[2] Furthermore, the factor remained constant over the time period from 1966 to 1986.[2] As shown in figure 2A and 2B, the relationship between age adjusted incidence rates of CMM (averaged for the period 1960 to 2001) and CIE weighted exposure is also well described by the same equation as given above for BCC and SCC and as earlier found for CMM,[2] but the biological amplification factor is slightly smaller, about 2.4 for both men and women (Fig. 2). The death rates follow the same equation, but with slightly smaller slopes i.e., A_b values. This is demonstrated by the ratios of death rates (DR) to incidence rates (R) in the lower part of figure 2. For men the slope of this curve is $(-8.6 \pm 8.3)10^{-4}$ and for women the slope is $(-3 \pm 1)10^{-3}$. Thus, the prognosis is improving with increasing annual UV exposure. The Norwegian data for the latitude dependency of DR/R agree with the combined data from Scandinavia, New Zealand and Australia (see table 1 in Ref. 28). The death to incidence ratios for CMM are, according to 2002 estimates, about 0.09 (women) and 0.14 (men) for New Zealand and Australia. The corresponding ratios for Northern Europe are significantly larger: 0.16 and 0.26, respectively. The incidence rates are much higher in Australia and New Zealand than in Northern Europe: 29.4 (women), 37.7 (men) versus 10 (women), 8.4 (men) in Europe. These data are in full agreement with our data. No difference in CMM diagnosis, nor in therapy, is expected

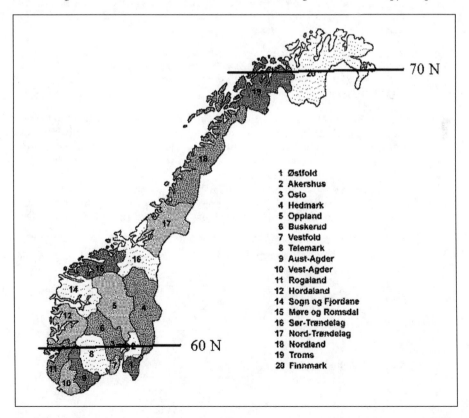

Figure 1. A map of Norway showing the different counties, given the numbers used in this chapter.

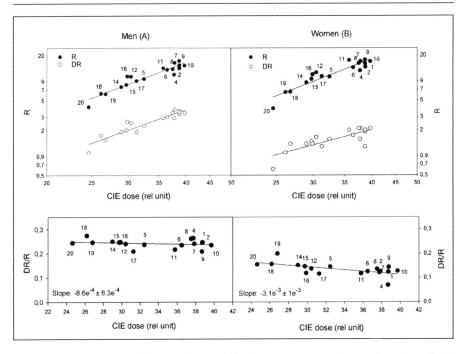

Figure 2. Incidence rates (filled circles) and death rates (open circles) as functions of CIE weighted annual UV doses for CMM in men (A) and women (B) in Norway. Age adjusted rates for the period 1960 to 2004 are given. The ratio of death rates to the incidence rates are shown in the lower panels.

to be found in the different regions of Norway and our data seem to indicate that prognosis of CMM is really improving with increasing sun exposure, in agreement with the work of Berwick et al[29] and with the recent immunological work by Sigmundsdottir et al.[30] Their findings indicate that small UV doses may improve the potency of the immune system of the skin, possibly through generation of vitamin D from 7-dehydrocholesterol.

The dependency of ocular melanoma on latitude in USA[31] can be interpreted in a similar way: stimulation of the immune system by UV radiation via vitamin D synthesis may explain why uveal melanoma decreases in rate with increasing UV exposure, opposite to what is found for CMM.

Table 1. Age adjusted incidence rates (W) by skin cancer type in Norway and Australia

Age Standardized Rates Per 100,000 (W)	1990-1994	1995-1999	2000-2004
Basal cell carcinoma			
Norway	18.5	30.7	33.3
Australia[33]	726	788	884
Squamous cell carcinoma			
Norway	9.1	10.75	11.85
Australia[33]	250	321	387
Cutaneous malignant melanoma			
Norway	15.4	15.3	15.5
Australia[32,13]	29.7	38.1	44.3

When the CMM rates in Australia and New Zealand are brought into consideration together with the Scandinavian data, the value of A_b becomes smaller, about 1 (Fig. 3B). However, using recent data for SCC and BCC in Australia[13,32,33] and in Norway we find that SCC and BCC are about factors of 35 and 25, respectively, more frequent in Australia than in Norway per 100,000 persons (Table 1), while CMM is only a factor of about 2 more frequent (Fig. 3). As earlier proposed,[27] this may have two explanations: 1) Scandinavians may follow a more melanomagenic sun exposure pattern i.e. a more intermittent pattern than Australians. 2) UVA from the sun may play a larger role for CMM induction than for BCC and SCC induction, in agreement with Setlow's action spectrum for melanoma in Xiphophorus, as earlier discussed.[27]

In some investigations latitude gradients opposite to those shown in the present work, are found.[34,35] In USA most states that are in the two highest CMM death rate quartiles are not found at the lowest latitudes. Furthermore, the north-south incidence gradient has been decreasing since the 1950ies, so that within some years no gradient is expected.[36] Furthermore, in southern Europe the CMM incidence rates are much smaller than in Scandinavia.[26] This may have at least two reasons: 1) Southern Europeans generally have darker skin and darker hair than blond or red-haired Scandinavians and Celts. 2) We have shown that CMM incidence rates of different countries seem to increase with GDP/capita (gross domestic product, a measure of economic standard).[26] This may influence on the sun exposure pattern, since one may assume that rich people can afford more vacations and weekend tours associated with strong intermittent exposures. Several CMM epidemiologists have stated that CMM is more of a "white collar" than a "blue collar" disease.

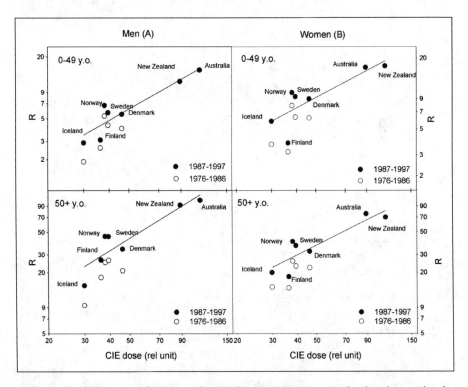

Figure 3. Incidence rates of CMM in the Nordic countries, New Zealand and Australia, for two time periods (1976-1986, filled circles and 1987-1997, open circles) for men (A) and women (B) as functions of CIE weighted annual UV doses. Two age groups are included: 0-49 and 50+ years.

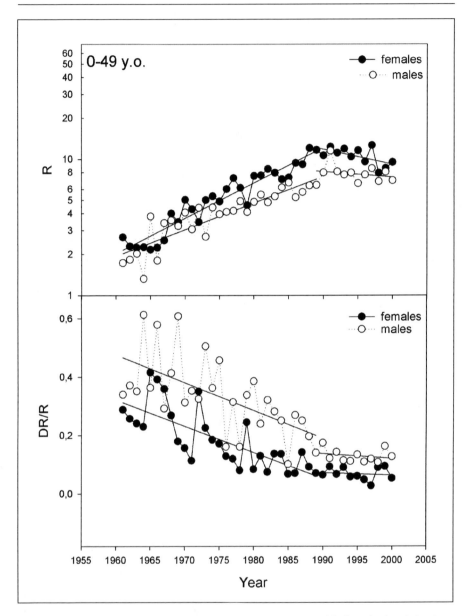

Figure 4. Incidence rates of CMM (men open circles, women filled circles) and death to incidence ratios (DR/R) in Norway as functions of the time of diagnosis. The data are for the period 1960 to 2004.

Recently, and as mentioned, the latitude dependencies of CMM and ocular melanoma in some states in USA were studied.[31] Latitude gradients, similar to those reported in the present work, were found for CMM and for external, ocular melanomas (eyelid and conjunctivae melanomas). For uveal melanomas (internal ocular melanomas) an opposite gradient was found: increasing incidence with increasing latitude. In agreement with our suggestions, it was concluded that solar radiation has both a protective and a generating effect with respect to melanomas. Obviously,

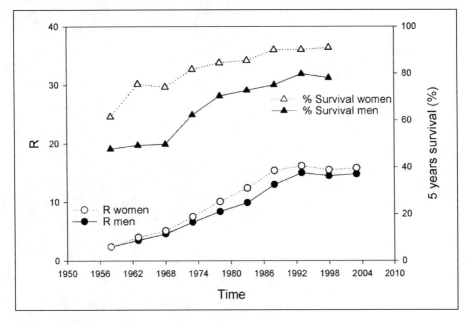

Figure 5. Incidence rates of CMM in Norway and five years survival percentage as functions of time. Men filled circles, women opened circles.

total exposures as well as exposure patterns are crucial for the balance between the two effects: High, intermittent exposures will mainly act generating, while low, regular exposures will act more protective. Time trends of uveal melanomas seem to be opposite of those of CMM: While the incidence rates of CMM increased in many countries upto around 1990 (see below), those of uveal melanomas tended to decrease.[37-39]

Time Trends

For several decades the incidence rates of all three skin cancer forms were increasing in Norway, as in most other Western countries.[2,26] However, during the last decade the increase of the rates of CMM has stopped, and for the youngest persons, even a decreasing trend is seen (Fig. 4). Similar trends have been reported from other countries.[40,41] The prognosis of CMM improved over all the years of increasing incidence, as indicated by the decreasing DR/R ratio (Fig. 4, lower part). However, after 1990, when the rates changed from an increasing to a decreasing trend, the improvement of prognosis appears to have stopped, although our data do not allow any firm conclusion yet (Fig. 4). Another way to study prognosis is to determine the five-year survival percentage (Fig. 5). From 1960 to about 1990 the percentage of CMM patients surviving five years after diagnosis increased from below 50% to about 75% for men and from about 65% to about 90% for women, while after 1990 no significant change has taken place, neither for men, nor for women (Fig. 5). Again a relationship with the flattening incidence curves (Figs. 4 and 5) seems possible. In agreement with these observations is the finding that the ratio of the number of old (≥ 50 years) to that of young (< 50 years) patients has been increasing, notably for men in the southern regions of the country.[26]

Upto 1990 the time trends of CMM incidence rates are similar in all Nordic countries, in all regions of Norway and for all age cohorts above 35 years.[2]

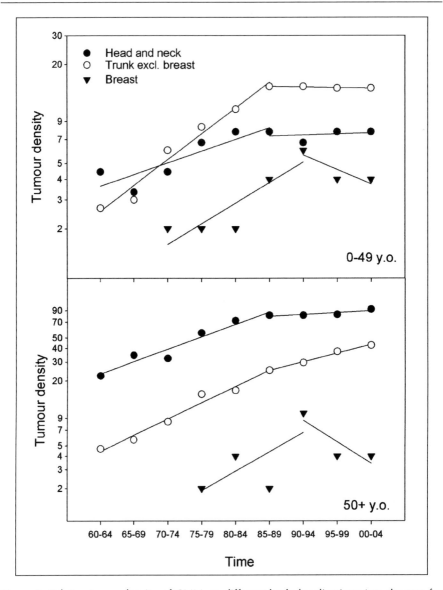

Figure 6. Relative tumor density of CMM on different body localizations (see the text for definition) among women in two age groups (0-49 and 50+ years) in Norway as a function of time.

Body Localization

Relative tumor density (RTD) is here defined as the age adjusted incidence rate of CMM on a given body localization (head and neck, trunk, breast etc) divided by the fraction of the total body area occupied by the given localization. Thus, the higher the RTD is, the more CMMs arise per cm.[2] The values of the fraction of the skin at different sites are taken from Lund and Browder and are 0.09 for head and neck, 0.3 for trunk and 0.05 for breasts.[42]

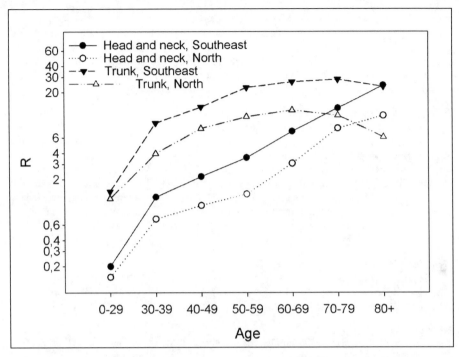

Figure 7. Age specific incidence rates of CMM among women in Norway. Data for the period 1992-2001. Body localizations: head and neck (circles) trunk (triangles), filled symbols: south-east Norway (counties 1, 2, 6-11), open symbols: north Norway (counties 18-20).

Figure 6 shows that for women older than 50 years the RTD is, as expected in view of solar exposure, larger on head and neck than on trunk, excluding breast and larger on trunk than on breast. However, surprisingly, for women younger than 50 years the RTD is larger on trunk than on head and neck, notably after 1960. For younger women the RTD on breast is higher than for older women. This gives valuable information about the impact of the changing pattern of sun exposure. The fact that the RTD on trunk, excluding breast, is larger than that on head and neck, which certainly are much more heavily UV exposed, is a strong indication that intermittent UV exposure is a carcinogen for melanoma, while regular exposure is a much weaker one. Practically no CMMs arose on the breasts of Norwegian women before the advent of the topless fashion at about 1970. This is a strong argument for the melanomagenic power of solar exposure. As indicated by the curves for the breasts (Fig. 6), the topless fashion may have culminated some time before 1994. These data are in agreement with our earlier findings.[2,26]

The incidence rates of CMM on head and neck and that on trunk have different age dependencies (Fig. 7). While the age specific rate of CMM on head and neck increases uniformly with age (as do those for SCC, BCC and practically all internal cancers), that for CMM on the trunk has a maximum at an age of 50-70 years. This is true for the north as well for the south part of Norway and agrees with earlier findings.[2] We conclude that the risk of CMM on head and neck, areas regularly sun exposed, increases with age, while that on trunk has a maximum between 50 and 70 years when the population as a whole is considered, i.e., at a slightly higher age than found for the period 1976 to 1985.[2] This is certainly related to changing habits of clothing and sun exposure. People who are now 70-80 years did not follow an intermittent exposure pattern when they were young to the same extent as young people do now.

Seasonal Variation of Incidence and Prognosis

As earlier shown, there is a peak of diagnosed cases of CMM in June and minima in July and December.[26] This is probably related to summer- and Christmas vacations. Furthermore, for the youngest patients (< 29 years), the prognosis is best for summer diagnosis,[26] just as earlier found for several internal cancers.[25,43-45] We have proposed that the optimal survival after summer and autumn diagnosis is due to the optimal vitamin D level at these seasons.

Effects of Sun Beds and Sunscreens

A slight increase of CMM incidence rates was found for sun bed users in Norway.[46] However, other investigations have observed decreasing rates as well as increasing rates.[47-50] We have recently found that two weekly, moderate (10-15 minutes, completely non-erythemogenic) sun bed exposures for 5 weeks almost doubled the serum calcidiol (25 hydroxyvitamin D, serum marker of the vitamin D status) level, from winter values to summer values, and that the recommended vitamin D intake of 200 IU per day was not enough to maintain that level,[51] (manuscript in preparation). Furthermore, we have found that recommended application of a sunscreen with a moderate or high UVB protection factor almost eliminates the vitamin D synthesis, by sun as well as by sun beds,[52] (manuscript submitted).

Acknowledgement

The present work was supported by Sigval Bergesen DY og hustru Nankis Foundation and by Helse Sør Medical Enterprise. The TOMS data were provided by NASA/GSFC. We thank Steinar Hansen at Norwegian Cancer Registry for technical assistance in obtaining CMM data.

References

1. Armstrong BK, Kricker A, English DR. Sun exposure and skin cancer. Australas J Dermatol 1997; 38 Suppl 1:S1-S6.
2. Moan J, Dahlback A. Ultraviolet radiation and skin cancer: epidemiological data from Scandinavia. In: Young AR, Bjørn LO, Moan J, Nultsch W, eds. Environmental UV Photobiology. New York/London: Plenum Press; 1993:255-93.
3. Whiteman DC, Green AC. Melanoma and sun exposure: where are we now? Int J Dermatol 1999; 38:481-489.
4. Elwood JM, Whitehead SM, Gallagher RP. Epidemiology of human malignant skin tumours with special reference to natural and artificial ultraviolet radiation exposure. In: Conti CJ, Slaga TJ, Klein-Szanto AJP, eds. Skin tumors: experimental and clinical aspects. New York: Raven Press; 1989:55-84.
5. Elwood JM. Melanoma and sun exposure: contrasts between intermittent and chronic exposure. World J Surg 1992; 16:157-165.
6. Green A, Williams G. Ultraviolet radiation and skin cancer: epidemiological data from Australia. In: Young AR, Bjørn LO, Moan J, Nultsch W, eds. Environmental UV photobiology. New York/London: Plenum Press: 1993, 233-54.
7. Holman CD, Armstrong BK, Heenan PJ. Relationship of cutaneous malignant melanoma to individual sunlight-exposure habits. J Natl Cancer Inst 1986; 76:403-414.
8. Koh HK, Kligler BE, Lew RA. Sunlight and cutaneous malignant melanoma: evidence for and against causation. Photochem Photobiol 1990; 51:765-779.
9. Magnus K. Habits of sun exposure and risk of malignant melanoma: an analysis of incidence rates in Norway 1955-1977 by cohort, sex, age and primary tumor site. Cancer 1981; 48:2329-2335.
10. Moan J, Dahlback A. Predictions of health consequences of a changing UV-fluence. In: Dubertret L, Santus R, Morliere P, eds. Ozone, sun, cancer. Paris: Les Editions Inserm, 1995:87-100.
11. Weinstock MA. Ultraviolet radiation and skin cancer: epidemiological data from the United States and Canada. In: Young AR, Bjørn LO, Moan J, Nultsch W, eds. Environmental UV photobiology. New York/London: Plenum Press, 1993:295-344.
12. Miller AJ, Mihm MC, Jr. Melanoma. N Engl J Med 2006; 355:51-65.
13. AICR. Globocan 2002 database. Available online at http://www-dep.iarc.fr/ (Accessed on February 2007).
14. Tangpricha V, Turner A, Spina C et al. Tanning is associated with optimal vitamin D status (serum 25-hydroxyvitamin D concentration) and higher bone mineral density. Am J Clin Nutr 2004; 80:1645-1649.
15. Matsuoka LY, Ide L, Wortsman J et al. Sunscreens suppress cutaneous vitamin D3 synthesis. J Clin Endocrinol Metab 1987; 64:1165-1168.
16. Christophers AJ. Melanoma is not caused by sunlight. Mutat Res 1998; 422:113-117.

17. Rampen FH, Fleuren E. Melanoma of the skin is not caused by ultraviolet radiation but by a chemical xenobiotic. Med Hypotheses 1987; 22:341-346.
18. Rockley PF, Trieff N, Wagner RF et al. Nonsunlight risk factors for malignant melanoma. Part I: Chemical agents, physical conditions and occupation. Int J Dermatol 1994; 33:398-406.
19. Beitner H, Ringborg U, Wennersten G et al. Further evidence for increased light sensitivity in patients with malignant melanoma. Br J Dermatol 1981; 104:289-294.
20. Maestro R, Boiocchi M. Sunlight and melanoma: an answer from MTS1 (p16). Science 1995; 267:15-16.
21. Dahlback A, Stamnes K. A new spherical model for computing the radiation field available for photolysis and heating rate at twilight. Planet Space Sci 1991; 671-683.
22. Stamnes K, Tsay SC, Wiscombe W et al. Numerically stable algorithm for discrete-ordinate-method for radiative transfer in multiple scattering and emitting layered media. Appl Opt 1988; 2502-2509.
23. McKinlay AF, Diffey AL. A reference action spectrum for ultraviolet induced erythema in human skin. CIE J 1987; 6:17-22.
24. Setlow RB, Grist E, Thompson K et al. Wavelengths effective in induction of malignant melanoma. Proc Natl Acad Sci USA 1993; 90:6666-6670.
25. Porojnicu AC, Robsahm TE, Dahlback A et al. Seasonal and geographical variations in lung cancer prognosis in Norway. Does vitamin D from the sun play a role? Lung Cancer 2005 DOI: 10.1016/j lungcan 2006.11.013.
26. Moan J, Porojnicu AC, Dahlback A. Epidemiology of cutaneous malignant melanoma. In: Ringborg U, Brandberg Y, Breitbart EW, Greinert R, eds. Skin cancer prevention. New York: Informa Healthcare; 2006:179-201.
27. Moan J, Dahlback A, Setlow RB. Epidemiological support for an hypothesis for melanoma induction indicating a role for UVA radiation. Photochem Photobiol 1999; 70:243-247.
28. Diffey B. Do we need a revised public health policy on sun exposure? Br J Dermatol 2006; 154:1046-1051.
29. Berwick M, Armstrong BK, Ben Porat L et al. Sun exposure and mortality from melanoma. J Natl Cancer Inst 2005; 97:195-199.
30. Sigmundsdottir H, Pan J, Debes GF et al. DCs metabolize sunlight-induced vitamin D3 to 'program' T cell attraction to the epidermal chemokine CCL27. Nat Immunol 2007. DOI: 10.1038/ni 1433.
31. Yu GP, Hu DN, McCormick SA. Latitude and Incidence of Ocular Melanoma. Photochem Photobiol 2006.
32. Lens MB, Dawes M. Global perspectives of contemporary epidemiological trends of cutaneous malignant melanoma. Br J Dermatol 2004; 150:179-185.
33. Staples MP, Elwood M, Burton RC et al. Nonmelanoma skin cancer in Australia: the 2002 national survey and trends since 1985. Med J Aust 2006; 184:6-10.
34. Tucker MA, Goldstein AM. Melanoma etiology: where are we? Oncogene 2003; 22:3042-3052.
35. Gandini S, Sera F, Cattaruzza MS et al. Meta-analysis of risk factors for cutaneous melanoma: II. Sun exposure. Eur J Cancer 2005; 41:45-60.
36. Lee JA. Declining effect of latitude on melanoma mortality rates in the United States. A preliminary study. Am J Epidemiol 1997; 146:413-417.
37. Stang A, Parkin DM, Ferlay J et al. International uveal melanoma incidence trends in view of a decreasing proportion of morphological verification. Int J Cancer 2005; 114:114-123.
38. Stang A, Schmidt-Pokrzywniak A, Lehnert M et al. Population-based incidence estimates of uveal melanoma in Germany. Supplementing cancer registry data by case-control data. Eur J Cancer Prev 2006; 15:165-170.
39. Bergman L, Seregard S, Nilsson B et al. Incidence of uveal melanoma in Sweden from 1960 to 1998. Invest Ophthalmol Vis Sci 2002; 43:2579-2583.
40. de VE, Bray FI, Coebergh JW et al. Changing epidemiology of malignant cutaneous melanoma in Europe 1953-1997: rising trends in incidence and mortality but recent stabilizations in western Europe and decreases in Scandinavia. Int J Cancer 2003; 20;107:119-126.
41. De Vries E, Tyczynski JE, Parkin DM. Cutaneous malignant melanoma in Europe. ENCR Cancer fact sheets 4. 2003; France, European network of cancer registries.
42. Lund CC, Browder NC. The estimation of area of burns. Surg Gynecol Obstet 1944; 79:352-361.
43. Robsahm TE, Tretli S, Dahlback A et al. Vitamin D3 from sunlight may improve the prognosis of breast-, colon- and prostate cancer (Norway). Cancer Causes Control 2004; 15:149-158.
44. Moan J, Porojnicu AC, Robsahm TE et al. Solar radiation, vitamin D and survival rate of colon cancer in Norway. J Photochem Photobiol B 2005; 78:189-193.
45. Lim HS, Roychoudhuri R, Peto J et al. Cancer survival is dependent on season of diagnosis and sunlight exposure. Int J Cancer 2006; 119:1530-1536.

46. Veierod MB, Weiderpass E, Thorn M et al. A prospective study of pigmentation, sun exposure and risk of cutaneous malignant melanoma in women. J Natl Cancer Inst 2003; 95:1530-1538.
47. Levine JA, Sorace M, Spencer J et al. The indoor UV tanning industry: a review of skin cancer risk, health benefit claims and regulation. J Am Acad Dermatol 2005; 53:1038-1044.
48. Abdulla FR, Feldman SR, Williford PM et al. Tanning and skin cancer. Pediatr Dermatol 2005; 22:501-512.
49. Ivry GB, Ogle CA, Shim EK. Role of sun exposure in melanoma. Dermatol Surg 2006; 32:481-492.
50. The association of use of sunbeds with cutaneous malignant melanoma and other skin cancers: A systematic review. Int J Cancer 2007; 120:1116-1122.
51. Moan J, Lagunova Z, Porojnicu AC. Vitamin D, photobiology and relevance for cancer. Sunlight, Vitamin D and Health, 2006:33-40. Proceedings of the meeting Sunlight, Vitamin D and Health House of Commons London.
52. Pagh Nielsen K, Porojnicu AC, Lagunova Z et al. Solarier og sol produserer D-vitamin, mens solkremer med høy beskyttelsesfaktor reduserer produksjonen kraftig. Submitted, 2006.

CHAPTER 10

Solar UV Exposure and Mortality from Skin Tumors

Marianne Berwick,* Anne Lachiewicz, Claire Pestak and Nancy Thomas

Abstract

Solar ultraviolet radiation (UVR) exposure is clearly associated with increased mortality from nonmelanoma skin cancer—usually squamous cell carcinoma. However, the association with cutaneous melanoma is unclear from the evidence in ecologic studies and the few analytic studies show that high levels of intermittent UV exposure prior to diagnosis are somehow associated with improved survival from melanoma. Understanding this conundrum is critical to present coherent public health messages and to improve the mortality rates from melanoma.

Introduction

Solar UV Exposure. Solar ultraviolet radiation (UVR) exposure can be measured in a multitude of ways, but there is no "gold standard" applicable to epidemiologic studies of incidence and mortality at the moment. This problem leads to the lack of consistent observations regarding mortality from skin cancer that currently exist in the literature. Solar UVR exposure consists of two broad types of wavelengths—UVB (280-320 nm) and UVA (320-400 nm). UVB at ground level is reduced by its passage through the thin stratospheric ozone shield around the earth at 10-16 km above the earth's surface and by factors in the atmosphere, such as cloud cover, pollution and water vapor. UVA is not substantially modified by stratospheric or atmospheric conditions and accounts for approximately 90% of UVR reaching the earth's surface. Another measure utilized is erythemal UV irradiance, a measure of spectral irradiance between 250 and 400 nm weighted for ultraviolet by erythema-inducing capacity in human skin.

Measurement. Multiple studies use an "ecological" approach to assessing the role of sunlight and mortality from cancer, particularly melanoma. However, both latitude and satellite measures can only measure potential exposure at the site and do not take into account a particular individual's characteristics or behavior. Using latitude alone also ignores the complexity of other geographic factors that modify solar UV exposure, such as altitude and cloud cover. On the other hand, latitude is a static variable and is readily available for ecological analyses.

Ground level meter readings. Robertson-Berger meters have been placed at ground level at various weather stations throughout the world and give readings for the erythemal action spectrum. Unfortunately, these are not often calibrated and so the readings are somewhat suspect.

Satellite measures and mathematical algorithms. Several algorithms using satellite measures have been used and are generally considered more accurate than the Robertson-Berger meter readings. Satellite measures and mathematical algorithms have advantages over latitude in that they also can take into account variations in the Earth-Sun distance, cloud cover, ozone column and surface elevation.

*Corresponding Author: Marianne Berwick—Department of Internal Medicine and the University of New Mexico Cancer Center, Albuquerque, NM 87131-0001, U.S.A. Email: mberwick@salud.unm.edu

Sunlight, Vitamin D and Skin Cancer, edited by Jörg Reichrath. ©2008 Landes Bioscience and Springer Science+Business Media.

Self-reported outdoor activities. Occupationally associated ultraviolet exposure is generally determined by a combination of an individual's self-reported occupation—either as a history or as that occupation engaged in for the longest period. This information is then often converted by an occupational hygienist into an exposure matrix and a summary variable of exposure is generated. Recreational ultraviolet radiation exposure is also determined from numerous self-reported activities, time outdoors and combinations thereof.

Combination of satellite measures and self-reported outdoor activities. Perhaps the most rigorous estimation has been published by Kricker et al[1] where a number of types of exposures are presented in relation to risk of melanoma, including: potential lifetime and early life ambient erythemal UV exposure estimated using lifetime residential history and a satellite-based model and history of sunburns, holiday hours in sunnier climates and hours in outdoor beach and waterside recreational activities. Less rigorous algorithms often use latitude of current residence combined with beach activities, or another similar combination.

Observed Relationships for Nonmelanoma Skin Cancer

The relationships for solar exposure and mortality in nonmelanoma skin cancer—squamous cell carcinoma and basal cell carcinoma—seem to be more straightforward than for melanoma skin cancer. That said, it should be pointed out that most deaths from nonmelanoma skin cancer are from squamous cell carcinoma; few individuals die of basal cell carcinoma. Possibly because there is a somewhat linear relationship between solar ultraviolet light exposure and squamous cell carcinoma, there is a consistent association between any of the measures of solar ultraviolet radiation and mortality from squamous cell carcinoma. However, this relationship is not so clear for melanoma skin cancer.

An analysis of solar ultraviolet radiation and nonmelanoma skin cancer comes from a death certificate based study[2] in which usual occupation derived from death certificates was the surrogate for occupational sunlight exposure and 24 states were categorized as low, medium or high residential exposure using data from the United States Weather Bureau. Analyses were controlled for age, sex, race, physical activity and socioeconomic status. These data show for Caucasians that living in a state with "high" ultraviolet radiation increased mortality from nonmelanoma skin cancer significantly (Odds Ratio [OR] 1.23, 95% Confidence Interval [CI] 1.14-1.33) and that having an outdoor occupation also increased the mortality from nonmelanoma skin cancer significantly (OR 1.30, 95% CI 1.14-1.47). This study illustrates the problems with ecological analyses, even though it was based on individual death certificates. There is always the potential misclassification of underlying cause of death, occupation and residential exposure. Lifetime residential history, individual behaviors and accurate measures of ground level ultraviolet radiation are unavailable in such a study.

A more sophisticated analysis of cancer mortality and latitude was conducted by Grant[3] using Spanish data. He concluded that data on the latitudinal gradient for melanoma and nonmelanoma skin cancer distinctly differentiates the two cancers and that nonmelanoma skin cancer mortality is a good proxy for chronic solar exposure, whereas melanoma is due to intermittent sun exposure and thus an analysis based on latitude alone will not capture this type of exposure. Further, in Spain at least, latitude seems to correlate more strongly with smoking than with sun exposure in the association with nonmelanoma skin cancer. In Spain, melanoma mortality was inversely but not significantly associated with latitude. An important and highly salient point made by Grant, using the 2002 International Agency for Cancer Research Globocan data, is that melanoma mortality rates increase with increasing latitude from those living in their ancestral homelands, but rates decrease with increasing latitude for pale-skinned populations who have migrated to countries such as Australia, New Zealand, Israel and the United States.

Interest has focused on nonmelanoma skin cancer among subgroups such as blacks. Pennello et al[4] compared non melanoma skin cancer rates among whites and blacks using Robertson-Berger meter readings as the exposure variable. Although there is a trend for mortality among whites by UVB tertile, there is no clear trend for blacks. White males move from 0.83 deaths per 100,000 in the lowest tertile to 1.19 in the highest and, similarly, white females move from 0.39 in the lowest tertile to 0.49 in the highest. However, although black males do move from 0.58 deaths per 100,000 in the lowest tertile to 0.68 in the highest, the trend is not linear. The trend is even flatter for black females moving from 0.37 in the lowest tertile to 0.39 in the highest.

Observed Relationships for Cutaneous Melanoma

Ecologic Studies

As stated above, ecologic studies are subject to many unknown biases. However, they can also provide insights into scientific problems and so have some utility. In the area of melanoma mortality there are few large studies that have been conducted, so the large data bases maintained by the U.S. SEER program and the WHO data base can be helpful to evaluate trends over time and by latitude. Lemish et al[5] observed that survival from melanoma increased with increasing melanoma incidence among several populations and suggested that high levels of ambient sun exposure might induce a more biologically benign type of melanoma. Recent data evaluating a very large number of populations support this association between the positive temporal and geographic association with incidence and survival.[6]

Conflicting analyses, however, occur (Table 1). For example, two studies have found no association between latitude or other measures of UV exposure and mortality from melanoma in the US,[7,8] and Bulliard et al[9] reported a positive association between increasing latitude (decreasing UV) and increasing melanoma rates in New Zealand. The mean percentage increase in mortality rates per degree of latitude ranged from 0.27% to 4.01%. On the other hand, two other studies have found a positive (or inverse) association[10,11] between melanoma mortality and latitude. An important difference among these studies, however, is that Lachiewicz (in preparation) evaluated individual tumor characteristics whereas Boscoe and Schymura only evaluated latitude and mortality without adjustment for critical covariates that can be obtained from the SEER registries, as their analysis evaluated multiple cancers. Clearly, the more refined and specific data analysis is likely to be more informative. Finally, WHO data, Garland et al[12] found a strong negative association between melanoma mortality and UVA as well as UVB in 45 countries.

A different measure of previous sun exposure derived for ecologic study is season of diagnosis. Seasonality of mortality has been shown to be associated with melanoma mortality in one study. Boniol et al[13] found that in Australia those diagnosed in the summer had a significantly reduced risk of dying from melanoma compared to those diagnosed in the winter (HR = 0.72, 95% CI = 0.65-0.81). In contrast, a report from Spain[14] showed a significant association between diagnosis in July and August and mortality from melanoma.

Occupation is sometimes used as a surrogate for solar exposure. Gass et al[15] reported that in Switzerland, occupation outdoors was slightly protective for mortality from melanoma, whereas indoor workers had an increased risk, consistent with meta-analyses of incidence.[16-18]

It is clear that despite the complexity and inherent bias in ecologic studies that the preponderance of the evidence upholds Lee's[19,20] projections—that the upward gradient noted by Elwood[11] in 1974 has been decreasing since 1950 and that rates of mortality in the contiguous US would be unaffected by latitude by the early 21st Century. A study by Fears et al[21] suggests that ecological data assigning UV exposure to an individual based on the place of diagnosis (or by inference death) is more likely to be measuring current rather than lifetime UV exposure. He found that among melanoma patients studied at sites in Philadelphia and San Francisco only 13% had spent their life there. Most participants had spent only about half their life at the place of diagnosis.

No particular associations between measures of UV and melanoma mortality were noted by Page[22] when evaluating deaths from melanoma among WWII veterans of the Pacific and the European theatres, or by Larsen[23] in evaluating associations among histology, survival and solar elastosis—a marker of sun damage and a large study of mortality among children and UV levels found no association with UV irradiance and the hazard of dying from melanoma.

Table 1. Association between time and location and incidence and survival of cutaneous melanoma

Author Year	Country or Population	Time Period	Number Followed	Mortality Rate	Comments
Boniol M 2006	Australia	1989-1998	10,869 F 14,976 M	2,710 (10.5%)	Fatality for melanoma lower for that diagnosed in summer than winter 0.72 (0.65-81) Sun exposure @ time of diagnosis led to lower fatalities.
Boscoe FP 2006	United States	1993-2002	3 million	Mortality 0.7 M 0.83 F	Paper relates UV exposure and cancer incidence on a population basis. UV exposure was positively associated with melanoma mortality.
Garland CF 2003	World	1990	45 countries	Range	Melanoma mortality rates decreased with increasing UVB in men (r = −0.48) and women (r = −0.57) and increasing UVA in both. However, mortality rates were positively associated with the increasing ratio in UVA/UVB. Controlling for skin pigmentation left only UVA associated with male mortality.
Page WF 2000	WWII veterans of Pacific & European theatres	50 year follow up	9237 male	18 deaths	Prisoner of war (POW) status is associated with high levels of melanoma mortality although station in the Pacific was not different from Europe.
Gass R 2005	Switzerland males	Mortality rates of 1979/83 and 1997/2001		Mortality rates diminished by 66% (p < 0.02)	Analysis of mortality by occupational groups shows indoor workers males have increased risk. Outdoor workers with chronic sunlight exposure are slightly protected.
Jemal A 2000	US White population	1950-1959 1990-1995		0.08-0.01 F 0.11-0.12 M	Mortality not significantly associated with latitude.
Bulliard A 2000	New Zealand	1968-1993	3,150 deaths	4.55—males 2.95—females	Incidence gradient steeper for males than females and greater for incidence than mortality.

continued on next page

Table 1. *Continued*

Author Year	Country or Population	Time Period	Number Followed	Mortality Rate	Comments
Lee JA 1997	US whites	1950-1992		2.2-5.0 for males; 0.8-2.3 for females	Upward gradient of mortality from north to south has been decreasing since 1950. Rates of mortality in contiguous US expected to be unaffected by latitude by early 21st century.
Lee JA 1993	US whites				Decline from old age to youth in the influence of latitude on mortality for both men and women.
Suarez-Varlea MM 1990	Spain	1975-1983			Statistically significant relation observed between mortality and solar radiation during July and August.
Larsen TE 1979	Scandinavia	Series	399		No association among 3 major histologic subtypes, solar elastosis and survival.
Elwood JM 1974	US & Canada	1950-1967			The rates of mortality rate w/ latitude are similar in each sex, greater in males than females. Strong negative assoc w/ latitude, similar degree of correlation w/ mortality rates.
Dark-skinned populations:					
Pennello G 2000	US Blacks	1970-1994			Age-adjusted risk of mortality for 50% increase in UVB radiation significantly above 1 for malignant melanoma for M. for both M & F relative risk of incidence was not significantly elevated 1973-94.

So, in summary, the ecologic studies are mixed in their results, but the weight of the evidence no longer supports a strong positive association between latitude or UV exposure, regardless of how measured and mortality from melanoma.

Analytic Studies

Unfortunately, few analytic studies have interviewed patients for sun exposure and residential histories and then followed subjects for mortality.

In the most recent study, Berwick et al[24] reported an inverse association between measures of solar exposure and melanoma mortality among a population of 528 subjects who had been interviewed within 3 months of diagnosis and then followed for a mean of 5 years for mortality. Variables associated with sun exposure over a lifetime were inversely and significantly associated with mortality from melanoma in univariate analyses: A history of ever having been severely sunburned (Hazard ratio [HR] 0.5, 95% Confidence Interval [CI] 0.3-0.9, P = 0.02), a history of high levels of intermittent sun exposure (HR 0.6, 95% CI 0.3-1.0, P =0.04) and the presence of any solar elastosis in the matrix surrounding the lesional biopsy (HR 0.5, 95% CI 0.5-0.9, P = 0.02). This study was unique in that individual level characteristics of surveillance were carefully and thoroughly collected: skin self-examination practices, physician skin examination and skin examination by a partner, as well as "awareness" of skin. A self-reported awareness of skin for cosmetic or medical reasons resulted in a reduced risk of dying from melanoma (HR 0.4,95% CI = 0.2-0.7, P < 0.001).

In multivariate analyses, controlling for clinical characteristics known to be important prognostic factors, solar elastosis remained an important predictor for reduced mortality (HR 0.4, 95% CI 0.2-0.8, P = 0.009). The authors suggested that this provocative finding might be related to this beneficial effect of sun exposure in relationship to survival with melanoma could be mediated by vitamin D. Alternative hypotheses were also offered: that previous sun exposure might induce more indolent melanomas through increased melanization and DNA repair capacity.

Interestingly, Heenan et al[25] published a somewhat similar analysis among 486 subjects diagnosed with melanoma in 1980/1981. In their univariate analyses, they found that solar elastosis was of borderline significance (P for trend = 0.07) and inversely associated with death from melanoma: Mild solar elastosis resulted in a rate ratio of 0.64 (95% CI = 0.30-1.37) and severe solar elastosis a rate ratio of 0.46 (95% CI = 0.19-1.12) and because of the borderline significance, this variable was not included in multivariate analyses. This study is the only other study evaluating melanoma mortality and solar elastosis in the literature and, interestingly, had very similar findings to the Berwick paper.

Zanetti et al[26] have also suggested that intense sun exposure prior to the diagnosis of melanoma is associated with an improved survival. They found that intermittent sun exposure (time spent over a lifetime at the beach) was inversely associated with risk of death from melanoma (HR = 0.41 95% CI = 0.17 to 0.98).

In summary, there are few analytic studies evaluating mortality in relationship to solar exposure prior to diagnosis. The three found show an inverse association that is worthy of additional investigation. Analytic studies are generally considered to be more valid than ecologic studies and could come up with different interpretations of data because they may suffer less from misclassification of solar UV and the measures of individual sun exposure are more precise than those estimated by latitude.

Potential Mechanisms

If UV exposure prior to a diagnosis of melanoma is protective, then there are multiple hypotheses as to how that could happen. Sun exposure prior to the diagnosis of melanoma, i.e., lifetime exposure, may lead to the development of less aggressive melanomas[5] and potentially increases DNA repair[27] and possibly the higher levels of serum Vitamin D stimulated by the UVB exposure delay tumor onset. In addition, sun exposure after diagnosis—or near the time of diagnosis—may increase serum levels of Vitamin D that may limit tumor progression. To know how UV is associated with incidence and mortality we need to rely on a more clear understanding of the biology of melanoma progression. Thus, none of the ecological studies are necessarily in conflict with the Berwick study finding that solar elastosis may be an independent indicator of better survival—if in fact the temporal relationship of sun exposure to melanoma differs by incidence and mortality. Unfortunately, this is an area where we have little hard evidence.

Vitamin D 25-hydroxy vitamin D_3 has antiproliferative and proapoptotic effects.[28,29] UVB induces serum vitamin D yet it also plays an important role in the development of melanoma. Possibly the circulating vitamin D levels are insufficient to reduce the risk of developing melanoma, particularly as melanocytes may have been programmed toward the development of melanoma quite early on. However, perhaps sun exposure does increase the protective reaction[30] of tanning and enhanced DNA repair capacity, in combination with the antiproliferative and proapoptotic effects of vitamin D, so that in combination, these factors are able to keep the invasive lesion "in check". Evidence for the vitamin D theory suggests vitamin D limits tumor progression—perhaps people with melanoma stay out of the sun during and following melanoma diagnosis, thus they do not receive the survival benefit (this would correspond to Boscoe's study examining current environment risk factors, all ecological). Since migration is so frequent, we would expect ecological data (like assigning UV to SEER sites) to measure current sun exposure as well. Garland's study, on the other hand, although ecological as well, might be capturing lifetime exposure as well as current exposure if people are less likely to migrate between countries than within countries. Additionally, countries with higher incidence of melanoma, like Australia, have relatively better survival potentially due to increased incidence of less aggressive melanomas.

Thus, none of the ecological studies are necessarily in conflict with the Berwick study finding that solar elastosis may be an independent indicator of better survival, if in fact they are measuring two different temporal aspects of sun exposure.

Conclusions

Clearly, there is much more to understand about the specific wavelengths involved in the development and progression of cutaneous melanoma and clearly sun exposure is a classic "two-edged sword". Data to date are only provocative and not convincing. If we assume that most ecological studies are measuring current UV exposure rather than lifetime exposure, the null or positive associations between melanoma mortality and UV exposure could be due to (1) a tendency for melanoma patients to tend to avoid sun exposure following diagnosis so they are not getting the benefit from Vitamin D, (2) a lack of variability in Vitamin D levels among melanoma patients (e.g., light pigmentation or sun avoidance) to detect any association with vitamin D levels, or (3) the fact that melanoma is a cancer, like renal cell carcinoma, more responsive to immune system response than other cancers; thus the rationale for interferon therapy and the occurrence of vitiligo among melanoma patients. It is possible that the effect of a UV-induced decrease in cellular immunity negates any benefit from Vitamin D antiproliferative and proapoptotic effects.

Much more work needs to be carried out to elucidate the effects of solar UV on melanoma development and progression before any conclusions can be drawn. Unfortunately, these data indicate that our public health messages—which are already confusing ("wear sunscreen all the time and stay out of the sun"—versus "some sun is good for you")—are not biologically driven and in order to stem the rising incidence of melanoma, it is critically important to understand better the basic biology of the disease.

References
1. Kricker A, Armstrong BK, Goumas C et al. Ambient UV, personal sun exposure and risk of multiple primary melanomas. Cancer Causes Control 2007; 18(3):295-304.
2. Freedman DM, Dosemeci M, McGlynn K. Sunlight and mortality from breast, ovarian, colon, prostate and nonmelanoma skin cancer: a composite death certificate based case-control study. Occup Environ Med 2002; 59(4):257-62.
3. Grant WB. An ecologic study of cancer mortality in Spain with respect to indices of solar UVB irradiance and smoking. International Journal of Epidemiology 120(5):1123-1128.

4. Pennello, Gene. Devesa Susan, Gail et al. Association of Surface Ultraviolet B Radiation Levels with Melanoma and Nonmelanoma skin Cancer in United States Blacks. Cancer Epidemiology, Biomarkers and Prevention 2000; 9:291-197.
5. Lemish WM, Heenan PJ, Holman CD et al. Survival from pre-invasive and invasive malignant melanoma in Western Australia. Cancer 1983; 52:580-5.
6. Armstrong BK. Ch 6. Epidemiology of melanoma and current trends. In Textbook of Melanoma, London; Martin Dunitz 2006; 65-80.
7. Lachiewicz AM, Berwick M, Wiggins CL et al. N Survival Differences between Scalp/Neck Melanoma and Melanoma of Other Sites in the Surveillance, Epidemiology and End Results (SEER) Program (In preparation).
8. Jemal A, Sevesa S, Fears T et al. Cancer surveillance series: changing patterns of cutaneous malignant melanoma mortality rates among whites in the United States. Journal of the National Cancer Institute 2000; 92:811-818.
9. Bulliard JL. Site-Specific risk of cutaneous malignant melanoma and pattern of sun exposure in New Zealand. Int J Cancer 2000; 85:627-632.
10. Boscoe FP, Schymura MJ. Solar ultraviolet-B exposure and cancer incidence and mortality in the United States, 1993-2002. BMC Cancer 2006; 6:264.
11. Elwood JM, Lee JA, Walter SD et al. Relationship of melanoma and other skin cancer mortality to latitude and ultraviolet radiation in the United States and Canada. Int J Epidemiol 1974; 3:325-32.
12. Garland CF, Garland FC, Gorham ED. Epidemiologic evidence for different roles of Ultraviolet A and B Radiation in melanoma mortality rates. Annals of Epidemiology 2003; 13:395-404.
13. Boniol M, Armstrong BK, Doré JF. Variation in incidence and fatality of melanoma by season of diagnosis in New South Wales, Australia. Cancer Epidemiol Biomarkers Prev 2006; 15:524-6.
14. Morales Suarez-Varela M, Llopis-Gonzalez A, Lacasana-Navarro M et al. Trends in malignant skin melanoma and other skin cancers in Spain, 1975-1983 and their relation to solar radiation intensity. Journal Environmental Pathology, Toxicology, Oncology 1990; 10:245-253.
15. Gass R, Bopp M. Mortality from malignant melanoma: epidemiological trends in Switzerland. Schweiz Rundsch Med Prax 2005; 94:1295-300.
16. Nelemans PJ, Rampen FH, Ruiter DJ et al. An addition to the controversy on sunlight exposure and melanoma risk: a meta-analytical approach. J Clin Epidemiol 1995; 48:1331-42.
17. Elwood JM, Jopson J. Melanoma and sun exposure: an overview of published studies. Int J Cancer 1997; 73:198-203.
18. Gandini S, Sera F, Cattaruzza MS et al. Meta-analysis of risk factors for cutaneous melanoma: II. Sun exposure. Eur J Cancer 2005; 41(1):45-60.
19. Lee JA. Declining effect of latitude on melanoma mortality rates in the United States. A preliminary study. Am J Epidemiol 1997; 146:413-7.
20. Lee JA, Scotto J. Melanoma: linked temporal and latitude changes in the United States. Cancer Causes Control 1993; 4:413-8.
21. Fears et al.
22. Page W, Whiteman D, Murphy M. A comparison of melanoma mortality among WWII veterans of the Pacific and European theatres. Ann Epidemiol 2000; 10:192-195.
23. Larsen TE, Grude TH. A retrospective histological study of 669 cases of primary cutaneous malignant melanoma in clinical stage I. 6. The relation of dermal solar elastosis to sex, age and survival of the patient and to localization, histological type and level of invasion of the tumour. Acta Pathol Microbiol Scand 1979; 87A:361-366.
24. Berwick M, Armstrong BK, Ben-Porat L et al. Sun exposure and mortality from melanoma. Journal of the National Cancer Institute 2005; 97:195-198.
25. Heenan PJ, English DR, Holman CD et al. Survival among patients with clinical stage I cutaneous malignant melanoma diagnosed in Western Australia in 1975/76 and 1980/81. Cancer 1991; 65:2079-87.
26. Zanetti R, Rosso S and the Helios Study. Sun exposure habits in an Italian population and survival from melanoma (In preparation).
27. Gilchrest BA, Eller MS, Geller AC et al. The pathogenesis of melanoma induced by ultraviolet radiation. New England J Med 1999; 340(17)1341-1348.
28. Vandwalle B, Wattez N, Lefebvre J. Effects of vitamin D3 derivatives on growth, differentiation and apoptosis in tumoral colonic HT 29 cells: possible implication of intracellular calcium. Cancer Lett 1995; 97:99-106.
29. Bernardi R, Jonson CS, Modzeleski RA et al. Antiproliferative effects of 1-alpha, 25-hydroxyvitamin D(3) and vitamin D analogs on tumor-derived endothelial cells. Endocrinology 2002; 143:2508-14.
30. Cui R, Widlund HR, Feige E et al. Central Role of p53 in the suntan response and pathologic hyper-pigmentation. Cell 2007; 128(5):853-864.

CHAPTER 11

Health Initiatives for the Prevention of Skin Cancer

Rüdiger Greinert,* Eckhard W. Breitbart, Peter Mohr and Beate Volkmer

Introduction

Skin cancer represents the most common type of cancer in the white population worldwide and the incidence has dramatically increased during the last decades. UV radiation is the most important risk factor responsible for this development. Socio-economical and cultural changes in behaviour of large groups of the society led to an increase in UV-exposure due to life-style trends which go along with more leisure time and holidays spent in the sun and (in the last decades) with frequent exposure to artificial UV in sunbeds.

While at the end of the 19th century a pail taint was still associated with persons forming part of the "upper social class", who don't had to work outdoors or on the fields, the 20th century started with changing attitudes to sun exposure. A tan became a new status symbol because only the wealthy could afford holidays in foreign countries seeking sporting activities at the sea or in the mountains. Already in 1910 the *Lancet* reported: "Rightly or wrongly, the face browned by the sun is regarded as an index of health".[1]

This and comparable estimates were adopted by a majority in the white population worlwide and was supported and expanded by the industry and different trendsetters in fashion and lifestyle which "advertised" a tan to by associated not only with being healthy but also trendy, sexy and successful. This led (especially after World War II) to a tremendous increase in outdoor activities and in tourism to sunny places and countries where people exposed themself to UV-radiation of the sun, unadapted, unwise and without any caution and protection. During the last decades this behaviour was further uncouraged through the wellness-movement which, additionally introduced exposure to artificial UV in sunbeds, which is also known to increase the risk of skin cancer.[2]

Individual behaviour under certain conditions of UV-exposure has, therefore, to be considered as the main "risk factor" responsible for the drastic, worldwide increase in skin cancer incidence which has been monitored during the last decades.[3-5] Environmental changes, however, like the depletion of stratospheric ozone, due to man-made chlorofluorocarbons (CFCs) released into the atmosphere and which increase the amount of UVB radiation reaching Earth's surface,[6-8] played an important role and will gain further significance if climate changes are not stopped and hopefully reversed in the future.[9]

Already at the end of the 19th century early reports about the the association between sun exposure and skin cancer appeared in dermatological publications. They attracted only little attention in the public community. During the next decades, however, knowledge about the hazardous effects of excessive sun exposure as well as about the etiology of skin cancer increased, mainly because of epidemiological analysis of the skin cancer problem in Australia, where the incidence is particularly high because of geographical, environmental and ethnical reasons.[10]

*Corresponding Author: Rüdiger Greinert—Center of Dermatology, Elbenkliniken Stade/ Buxtehude, D-21614 Buxtehude, Germany. Email: grein25@gmx.de

Sunlight, Vitamin D and Skin Cancer, edited by Jörg Reichrath. ©2008 Landes Bioscience and Springer Science+Business Media.

Therefore it is understandable that primary and secondary prevention of skin cancer originated in Australia and that new health initiatives have been developed on the basis of Australian experience during the last 10-30 years.

Prevention of Skin Cancer

Development of skin cancer can be influenced at three temporally different levels of prevention. Primary and secondary prevention as well as tertiary prevention (which already includes therapy and rehabilitation). This is schematically shown in Figure 1.

Skin cancer is a type of cancer which is highly preventable because the main risk factor, UV-radiation, is know and excessive UV-exposure can be reduced to a great extend by using simple strategies which can be educated by means of primary prevention. Even if first signs of skin cancer already appear, early detection, as a strategy of secondary prevention, goes along with nearly 100% curability. This holds for basal cell carcinoma (BCC), squamous cell carcinoma (SCC) but also for malignant melanoma (MM) of the skin. In this contribution we will focus on primary prevention.

Primary Prevention of Skin Cancer

Initiatives in primary prevention of skin cancer should inform and enlighten the public as well as representatives in public health and politcs about possible health benefits and health risks of natural and artificial UV-exposure in the sense of avoidance of causality through changes in risk-awareness. It is the aim, on the short and long tem, that primary prevention will change social behaviour of the public in direction of save an more conscious use of UV-radiation.

The prominent role of UV-radiation in the etiology of skin cancer renders this type of cancer most suitable for primary prevention, because the main risk factor can easily be avoided by sticking to simple rules for the behaviour in the sun or under artificial UV (e.g., sunbeds).

Programmes to limit excessive sun-exposure started in the early 1980s in Australia with the "Slip (on a shirt), Slop (on some sunscreen), Slap (on a hat)" initiative. The programme and the subsequent SunSmart[11] campaign has highly influencend other countries to develop their own intervention programmes. Several international consensus meetings profited from Australian experiences and formulated common aims in the primary prevention of skin cancer:

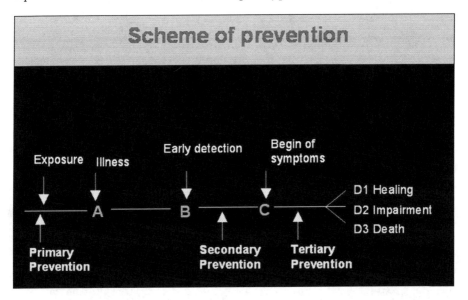

Figure 1. Different types of prevention at different time points of development of illness.

- Consensus meeting "Educational needs for primary and secondary prevention of melanoma in Europe", 1991, by the EORTC Melanoma Group[12]
- Consensus Conference "Early Melanoma", 1992, by the National Institut of Health (NIH), USA[13]
- Consensus meeting "How to decrease morbidity and mortality of skin cancer, 1994, by the Commission of Early Detection and Prevention of Skin Cancer of the working group of dermatological prevention (ADP e.V) in Germany.[13,14]

The United Nations (UN) also became aware of the worldwide problem of increase in skin cancer incidence and recommended 1992 at the United Nations Conference of Environment and Development under Agenda 21: "to undertake as a matter of urgency, research on the effects on human health of increasing ultraviolet radiation reaching Earth's surface as a consequence of depletion of the stratospheric ozone layer"; and furthermore "on the basis of the outcome of this research, to consider taking appropriate remedial measures to migrate the above mentioned effects on human beings".

In response to this, WHO established the Global UV Project, INTERSUN,[15] in collaboration with the United Nations Environment Programme (UNEP), the World Meteorological Organization (WMO), the International Agency for the Research on Cancer (IARC) and the International Commission for Non-Ionizing Radiation Protection (ICNIRP). In accordance with this project several institutions and organizations developed (country-) specific prevention strategies throuhout the world to reduce the burden of disease resulting from the exposure to UV-radiation. Just to mention a few, there have been huge, ongoing campains of primary prevention of skin cancer in the USA by the Skin Cancer Foundation (http://www.skincancer.org), in the UK by the Health Protection Agency (HPA, formerly NRPB: http://www.hpa.org.uk), in France by Association Securite Solaire (http://www.vivreaveclesoleil.info) or in Germany by the German Cancer Aid (Deutsche Krebshilfe: http://www.krebshilfe.de) in collaboration with the Association of Dermatological Prevention (Arbeitsgemeinschaft Dermatologische Prävention, ADP: http://www.unserehaut.de). These and other programmes tried to reach the public as a whole or certain target groups. Especially children at school have been in focus of certain intervention programmes, which have been described and partly evaluated.[16-18] These studies show that interventions in schools involving childrens of different grade classes are suitable to change knowledge about harmful effects of UV-radiation and how to protect against them. New studies from the USA demonstrate that, e.g., intentions to play in the shade increase significantly in children of primary and scondary schools (grade K-8) during the SunWise School Programme. Modest changes in the intention to use sunscreens were described as well as a significant decrease in attitudes regarding the healthness of a tan.[19] However, studies already starting with interventions at kindergarten level also show that sun protection education has to be provided continously over several school years in order to produce changes in sun safety behaviour.[20] This result holds also for other target or age groups which shall be reached by cetain intervention programmes for skin cancer prevention (see below).

Initiatives for the prevention of skin cancer throughout the world more or less use the same kind of messages, although there is still a need for harmonization.[21] The main fields which should be affected by these messages in primary prevention have been summarized by WHO when the INTERSUN Programme was relaunched.[22] They include:[10]

- development and use of an internationally recognized UV Index (UVI) to fascilitate sun protection messages related to daily UV-intensity
- special programmes for schools to teach children and teachers about sun protection
- guidance for tour operators providing services to customers travelling to sunny places
- recommendations to limit sunbed use
- guidance on decreasing occupational UVR exposure for outdoor workers (http://www.who.int.uv.en)

These activities should encourage people to enjoy the sun safely and protect themselves against UV-radiation to avoid excessive exposure, especially in childhood, because it is well established meanwhile that childhood UV-exposure is a main risk factor for skin cancer as an adult.

Focussing on primary prevention in childhood and adolescence is supported by many organizations, institutions and partly by governments. For example in 2001, the European Society of Skin Cancer Prevention, EUROSKIN, organized an international conference "Children under the Sun" in Orvieto, Italy, which included a WHO workshop "Children's Sun Protection education". It has been recommended after this conference that:

"Health authorities and relevant international responsible bodies, such as the EC should be reminded of the importance of addressing the UVR health messages to the parents, teachers and other carers of children using key interventions and of the importance of providing support for resources to achieve this".[23]

In order to achieve these goals, the Association of Dermatological Prevention (ADP) introduced a "Periods-of-Life-Programme" (POLP) during the EUROSKIN conference "Children under the Sun". POLP defines certain target groups for age-specific education levels in the population. This target grouping starts with parents of unborns (lasting from fertilization to birth), followed by babies (up to 12 month), children (1-6 years of age), youth (12-17 years of age), adults (≥18 years of age) and parents (see Fig. 2). As can be seen from Figure 2, the target group of children can be subdivided in three further groups: children at the age of 1-3 years, kindergarten children (3-6 years of age), children at the age after (ground-) school entry (6-11 years of age).

For all target groups certain caretakers in the health and education system have been identified and special information and eduction material has been developed and was distributed to them. This was done in order to integrate their help as important members of supporting target groups.

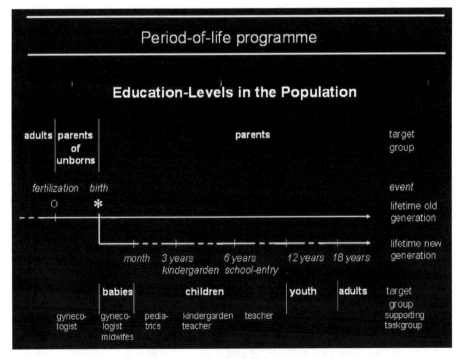

Figure 2. Schematic representation of the Periods-of Life-Proramme (for further explanation, see text.).

These include gynecologists, midwifes, pediatrics, kindergarten teachers, teachers at schools and (always) parents (see Fig. 2).

In 2002 the ADP started POLP in Germany with the target group of babies and their parents. This was followed in 2003 by an intervention campaign targeting kindergarten children. In 2004 children entering (ground-) school represented the next target group. This campaign closely followed WHO's "Sun Protection programmes in schools" (download: http://www.who.int/phe/uv). Materials have been developed and distributed to more than 16,000 ground schools in Germany, containing information and materials for pupils as well as for their teachers. These education materials were cpmplemented by a special CD of a German song writer who composed a number of "sun-songs", which were easily learned, adopted and often song by pupils at school. The 2005 campaign tries to reach the group of teens (12-17 years of age). For this age group prizes were awarded for best video-clips produced by groups at school, transporting sun-protection- and sun-behaviour-messages like "seek shade", "use textile protection", "use sun screens", etc.

All interventions in context of a POLP since 2002 have been accompanied by huge efforts in public relations, including press conferences, spots for TV and in cinemas, as well as by nation-wide bill-posting of so called "eye-openers" to awake interest in the public. Some examples are shown in Figs. 3 and 4. All efforts have been financially supported by the German Cancer Aid (Deutsche Krebshilfe e.V.).

Further Developments

In a recent systematic review Saraiya et al suggested a classification of interventions into four broad groups:

- individual-directed strategie
- environmental and policy interventions

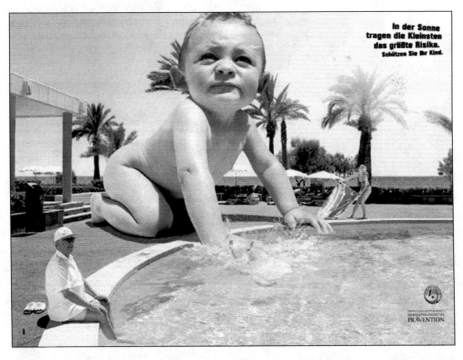

Figure 3. Example of a poster ("eye-opener") used in the German POLP (target group: babies and their parents). The German text in the upper right corner translates to: "In the sun babies carry the highest risk. Save your child".

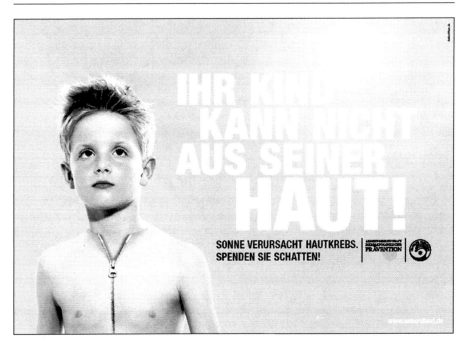

Figure 4. Example of a poster ("eye-opener") used in the German POLP (target group: ground school children). The German text in the poster translates to: "Your child is not able to escape it's skin! Sun causes skin cancer. Please donate shade".

- media campaigns
- multicomponent programs and comprehensive community-wide interventions

and subdivided individual-directed strategies further according to settings, i.e., childcare, primary school, secondary school, collage, recreational and tourism sites, occupational and healthcare settings.[24] The authors concluded that education and policy approaches to increase sun-protection behaviours were only effective when implemented in primary schools and in recreational and tourism settings. However, they found insufficient evidence for effectiveness of educational and policy approaches in other settings like childcare centers, secondary schools, colleges and occupational settings. Prevention activities also showed little effectiveness when targeting healthcare settings and providers, media campaigns alone, interventions oriented to parents and community-wide multicomponent interventions.

Although specific intervention activities in primary prevention of skin cancer have been reported to be successful by others, Brändström points out[25] that the comprehensive review by Saraiya and coworkers[24] highlights the need for more well-evaluated studies of skin cancer preventive interventions. Brandström concludes that "one way to use theories of individual health behaviour in prevention is to use them to identify individuals or groups with specific needs for information or preventive interventions. A successful assessment of groups with differing needs for interventions enables tailoring or targeting of preventive strategies towards these groups. Assessing and targeting people with different sun-exposure profiles is one way to match different needs with appropriate intervention".[25]

POLP (see above) is a practical approach to primary prevention of skin cancer which identifies individuals or groups with specific needs for information and targets them to specific prevention strategies. On a more theoretical basis it becomes evident that skin cancer prevention tries to reach individuals and/or groups with different sun- and/or artificial UV-behaviour (e.g., in the case of indoor tanning). The categorization of this behaviour defines UV-exposure profiles with different motivations for being exposed or protected from UV-radiation and thus different preventive strategies are needed to change the behaviour.[25] These profiles can be described by the tanning- (exposure-) behaviours of individuals. The profiles depend on different times, situations and places and are not mutually exclusive for a certain individual. Nevertheless, they can be used to specify and develop specific preventive interventions. Characterization and typical behaviour patterns of profiles can be found in the recent excellent review by Brändström.[25] Briefely, these profiles can summarized as follows:

- *Compulsive sunbathers (intentional tanning)*
  Example: Travelers to sunny vacation resorts, who like to subathe, see no or few risks, do not want to change their behaviour and do not seek information.
- *Professional tanners (intentional tanning)*
  Example: Travelers to sunny vacation resorts and/or sunbed users, who like to sunbathe, see some risk with tanning, do not want to stop sunbathing (exposing themselves to artificial UV-radiation) and seek information.
- *Incidental tanners*
  Example: People who spend time on outdoor activities (e.g., gardening, sailing, golfing, etc.), who do not necessarily like to sunbathe, see some risk with tanning, do not want to change and do not seek information.
- *Inevitable sun-exposed*
  Example: people like outdoor workers, who might like to sunbathe, might be unconscious of risks and do not seek information.
- *Unprotected children*:
  Example: Young children on shade-less beach, who do not like to sunbathe, who are unconscious of risks and do not seek information.

Althought this list of profiles already covers a broad range of UV-exposure behaviours it has, surely, to be completed by at least one further profile which characterizes

- *Professional sunbed users*:
  Example: People who frequently use sunbeds, who like to get a tan for cosmetic reasons, who see some risk with tanning, do not want to stop tanning and might seek information.

This profile describes the quickly growing number of individuals (especially young women and adolsescents) which has to be treated by specific preventive interventions which provide information about the health risks of exposure to arificial UV-radiation in sunbeds, which is known to increase skin cancer risks remarkably.[2]

A number of specific preventive strategies for the different profiles have been suggested.[25] These have been used already in a number of intervention campaigns and it is interesting to note that unconventional strategies are effective. The group of professional tanners, e.g., seems to react more sensible on messages emphasizing the negative consequences of sun exposuere for appearance (early skin aging) than on messages concerning negative health effects.[26-28]

This also might be a good strategy for the special case of professional sunbed users for whom intervention campaigns, however, should provide further information which clearly shows that there are no health benefits of artificial UV exposure at all and that sunbed use is not recommended by international health organizations (WHO, ICNIRP, EUROSKIN) because of the known increase in the risk of skin cancer development after frequent sunbed use.[2] If, nevertheless indoor tanning is used, this should only be done in sunbed studios which are regulated according to national or international guidelines which try to enable UV-exposure at putative reduced risk (e.g., by limiting the maximum irrdiance to 0.3 w/m,^{2} mandatory for Europe for new irradiation devices on the market from July 2007 on)

(http://ec.europa.eu/health/ph_risk/committees/04_sccp/docs/sccp_o_031b.pdf).

In many cases it's to early already to decide if certain campaigns have been successful. However, profile categorization should help to tailor and target preventive messages more effectively and to better evaluate the outcome of intervention programmes.

Balanced Messages (Concerning Vitamin D)

Because of the knonw risk factor (UV-radiation) skin cancer represents an ideal target cancer for primary prevention, because UV-radiation can easily be avoided by sticking to simple rules for the behaviour in the sun or under artificial UV (e.g., sunbeds).

However, because UV-exposure can not and should not be avoided totally, recommendations and information for the public should be as clear and as weighted as possible. Advices to avoid UV-exposure at a certain age or for a certain group (profile) should not introduce any deficits in possible benefitial health effects of UV-radiation. Nevertheless, WHO is adresssing the issue wether current sun protection messages in primary prevention might be to strong and if they are balanced, especially in connection with UV(B) (280-315 nm)—induced vitamin D photosynthesis and the role of this vitamine in individual's health. WHO concentrates on questions like:[10]

- What is the balance between healthy sun exposure that provides the body's requirements for vitamin D and excessive exposure that leads to skin cancer later in life?
- Is it possible to recommend dietary supplements in countries that lack sufficient sunshine (i.e., high lattitude countries in winter) to account for the loss of natural vitamin D production?
- Are there UVR-mediated beneficial effects on health, other than those stemming from the production of vitamin D?

These and other questions have already been discussed on an "International Worshop on UV exposure Guidance", 2005 in Munic, Germany, which was organized by ICNIRP, hosted by the German Radiation Protection Offices (BfS) and cosponsored by the German Federal Environmental Ministry (BMU), WHO and *EUROSKIN*. It was the principal aim of this workshop to review current knowledge and undertake a scientific based evaluation of sun exposure which counterbalances health risks and benefits of UV-radiation.

The vitamin D issue was particularly considered, because it is known, that UV(B) induced vitamin D, which is produced in exposed skin, regulates calcium levels in the blood and is needed for bone musculoskeletal health. Furthermore, only recently a number of ecological, observational and experimental studies seem to support the view of beneficial effects of sun exposure by revealing a link between a number of cancers, e.g., breast, prostate and colon cancers and low vitamin D levels.[29-34] There are also reports which indicate that vitamin D lowers the risk of autoimmune diseases, e.g., multiple sclerosis, diabetes type I and II as well as rheumatoid arthritis.[35-39] However, evidence of these findings has been assessed as not yet convincing.[10] This might be explained by the fact, that there exists still an expert's controversy about how much vitamin D a healthy person actually needs and, if vitamin D deficiency is really a problem for large parts of the white population, although there is some evidence that even in sunny countries and in lightly pigmented populations, vitamin D insufficiency is not uncommon.[10,40,41]

The range of concentration of vitamin D in the blood (which means the concentration of 25-hydroxyvitamin D, [25(OH)D]) that is considered "normal" varies, depending on the literature which is taken to be relevant.[42-45] Sometimes 50 nmol/l 25(OH)D seem to be currently accepted as a lower limit of sufficiency,[10] although recent results seem to indicate that at least 80 nmol/l are required to prevent physiological changes associated with vitamin D insufficiency.[42,46] Holick states[45] that it has been suggested that the body uses between 3000—5000 IU[47] of vitamin D per day to satisfy physiological needs, which will not be achieved by vitamin D supplementation, which is not widely practiced and might not be sufficient, because most supplements only contain 400 IU of vitamin D. There seems to be, however, kind of an agreement between experts, that a daily intake of 1000 IU of vitamin D, in the absence of sun exposure (!), is sufficient to maintain a healthy blood level of 25(OH)D of between 75—125 nmol/l (20—50 ng/ml).[48] On the other hand, the Institute of Medicine for the National Acadamy of Science (USA) suggested in 1997 that an adequate intake of vitamin D of children and adults up to the age of 50 years of 200 IU (5 µg) is sufficient, because this age group recieves adequate amounts of sunlight. For adults 50 to 70 years and older than 70 years 400 and 600 IU daily have been recommended.[49] Nevertheless, scientifical and epidemiological knowledge about sufficient levels of vitamin D for healthy individuals still seems to be insuffient and a urgent need for evidence based recommendation exists.[50]

Wether UV-induced vitamin D production is connected to a decrease in the incidence of certain forms of cancer or has a protective effect for other diseases still has to be elucidated in more detail. Surely, this issue has to be considered in terms of balanced messages used in preventive intervention programmes which try to reduce the risks of skin cancer development, because 95% of human body's requirement of vitamin D comes from exposure to UV(B)-radiation of the sun. For a healthy person this can easily achieved by a reasonable, intelligent and save use of the sun. It has been recommended that exposure of hand, arms and face two or three times the week to approximately one quarter or on third of an minimal erythemal dose (MED) of UV-radiation from the sun is more than adequate to satisfy a skintype II body's requirement. Holick and co-workers have estimated, that if only 6% of the body surface is exposed to one MED (about 250 J/m^2), approximately 600 to 1000 IU vitamin D are produced.[51] Whole body exposure of young adults to one MED is sufficient to produce an amount of vitamin D equivalent of taking between 10,000 to 25,000 IU.[45,51,52]

Having these numbers in mind it can easily be calculated, that moderate, sub-erythemal esposure to the sun's UV-radiation is sufficient to produce enough vitamin D for a healthy person. For example, at an UV-Index (UVI) of 6 (which is typical for a month at noon time in summer at a lattitude of 50-52° N, e.g., in the UK or Germany) an equivalent of 200 IU vitamin D is produced in about only 8 min, if only 6% of the body (hands, arms, face) are UV-exposed. Even at a very low UVI = 1, which, still can be reached even in wintertimes, or in summer before 11:00 am or after 3:00 pm, the comparable time will be about 50 min. Exposure of larger parts of the body will even reduce these times to clearly sub-erythemal doses to produce the same amounts of vitamin D. Knowing that one unit of the UVI corresponds to 0.42 MED/h, exposure times for other vitamin D requirements (e.g., for older peolple) and for different UVI-values can be calculated, showing that a moderate, suberythemal exposure to the sun is more than sufficient to satisfy the health requirements of the human body.

There is no need for an excessive natural UV-exposure (from the sun) or an additional exposure to artificial UV (e.g., in sunbeds). On the contrary, excess UV-exposure will degrade vitamin D into inert photoproducts.[53,54] Even if there exists a treshold level of UV(B) radiation required to induce vitamin D production,[55] which is not generally reached during the winters in areas above a lattitude of 40°, adequate stores of vitamin D can be built up during spring, summer and autumn, or vitamin D supplementation (e.g., by vitamin D fortificated milk or other food products) should be used.[10] Furthermore, as WHO states, the use of sunbeds remains unsafe because of its link to an increased skin cancer risk.[2,10] Sunbeds emit mostly UVA rather than vitamin D inducing UVB, thus increasing the risk of skin damage without a concomitant increase in beneficial vitamin D production.[56] This judgement is in full agreement with conclusions which have been drawn from the "International Workshop on UV exposure Guidance", 2005 in Munich, Germany. There was general agreement[57] that:

- Sun exposure is responsible for a substantial burden of skin and eye disease and may play a role in reactivating some viral diseases.
- A lack of vitamin D is a serious health problem.
- There is still much to be learned about the quantitative relationship between 25(OH)D health and much more research is necessary to address this issue.
- More research is needed on investigating optimal levels of vitamin D for different groups within the general population and on deriving "upper safe limits" on vitamin D uptake.
- Little is know about the effects of UVR exposure on vaccination efficacy and infectious deseases and research is needed in this area.
- The use of sunbeds is not recommended for vitamin D enhancement.
- Sun protection messages need to be aimed at the ididividuals or groups risk and the factors affecting that risk such as location and time of the year and that the solar UV Index should be actively promoted as part of protection programmes.

- Moderation of sun exposure is an important goal and a key message is to ensure that people protect themselves when the Solar UV Index is greater than 3.

Conclusion

If open questions in the above list are answered and given recommendations are implemented into health initiatives for the prevention of skin cancer, they will be able to provide the public with balanced messages which support the reduction of health risks of excessive UV-exposure. On a long term this should increase the awareness of adverse health effects of natural and artificial UV-exposure and produce changes in sun-related behaviour. First results from Australia and New Zealand show that educational interventions are moderately effective in improving at least short-term knowledge and behavioural intentions to be protected in the sun.[58,59] Furthermore, recent results from Australia and Switzerland already show a decrease in incidence of nonmelanoma skin cancers for people younger than 50 years, despite an increase in the overall age-standardized incidence.[60,61] It is also interesting to note that, although the incidence of malignant melanoma still sharply increases in Southern and Eastern Europe,[62] in Canada, Northern Europe, Australia and New Zealand a trend for a plateau in the incidence of cutaneous malignant melanoma becomes appearant.[10,62-65] These changes probably reflect the effectiveness of sun-avoidance programmes over the last 50 years.[10] This also shows that the main messages of primary prevention:

- enjoy the sun but save your skin
- use textile sun protection
- don't stay unprotected in the sun between 11:00 am and 3:00 pm (seek shade)
- use sunscreens properly
- wear a hat in the sun
- wear sun glasses
- during your holidays at sunny places, behave like the local residents
- take care for your kids in the sun (be an example in sun protection)
- don't use sunbeds

which have been used over the years in many campaigns throughout the world seem to be effective in reducing the risk of skin cancer. There are no convincing indications until now, that these messages have produced any adverse health effects, e.g., problems in the vitamin D physiology, because amounts of UV needed are small. However, if vitamin D insufficiency for certain age or risk groups turns out to be a problem, this can be counteracted by proper diet and/or special advice for sun behaviour without excessive UV-exposure. There is surely no "one message fits all" approach,[10] but balanced information in health initiatives for the prevention of skin cancer, which use evidence-based modern strategies, will further be needed in the future to reduce the incidence, morbidity and mortality of the most frequent cancer worldwide.

References
1. The sun-burnt face. Lancet 1910; 2:132-135.
2. The association of use of sunbeds with cutaneous malignant melanoma and other skin cancers: A systematic review. Int J Cancer 2007; 120:1116-1122.
3. Albert MR, Ostheimer KG. The evolution of current medical and popular attitudes toward ultraviolet light exposure: part 1. J Am Acad Dermatol 2002; 47:930-937.
4. Albert MR, Ostheimer KG. The evolution of current medical and popular attitudes toward ultraviolet light exposure: part 3. J Am Acad Dermatol 2003; 49:1096-1106.
5. Albert MR, Ostheimer KG. The evolution of current medical and popular attitudes toward ultraviolet light exposure: part 2. J Am Acad Dermatol 2003; 48:909-918.
6. de Gruijl FR, Longstreth J, Norval M et al. Health effects from stratospheric ozone depletion and interactions with climate change. Photochem Photobiol Sci 2003; 2:16-28.
7. Andrady A, Aucamp PJ, Bais AF et al. Environmental effects of ozone depletion and its interactions with climate change: progress report, 2004. Photochem Photobiol Sci 2005; 4:177-184.
8. Andrady AL, Aucamp PJ, Bais AF et al. Environmental effects of ozone depletion: 2006 assessment: interactions of ozone depletion and climate change. Executive summary. Photochem Photobiol Sci 2007; 6:212-217.
9. Norval M, Cullen AP, de Gruijl FR et al. The effects on human health from stratospheric ozone depletion and its interactions with climate change. Photochem Photobiol Sci 2007; 6:232-251.

10. Lucas RM, Repacholi MH, McMichael AJ. Is the current public health message on UV exposure correct? Bull World Health Organ 2006; 84:485-491.
11. The Cancer Concil of Victoria. SunSmart overview: Our history. 2007. http://www.sunsmart.com.au. Ref Type: Internet Communication.
12. MacKie RM, Osterlind A, Ruiter D et al. Report on consensus meeting of the EORTC Melanoma Group on educational needs for primary and secondary prevention of melanoma in Europe. Results of a workshop held under the auspices of the EEC Europe against cancer programme in Innsbruck. Eur J Cancer 1991; 27:1317-1323.
13. NIH. Consensus Developmental Conference: Diagnosis and treatment of early melanoma. 1992; 10:1-25. Cosensus Statement. Ref Type: Conference Proceeding.
14. How to decrease morbidity and mortality of skin cancer: primary prevention of skin cancer/screening of skin cancer. Report of a workshop held under the auspices of the society of dermatological prevention (ADP e.V.), Commission of early detection and prevention of skin cancer 1994. Hamburg, Germany. Eur J Cancer Prev 1996; 5:297-299.
15. WHO. INTERSUN. The global UV project: a guide and compendium. Geneva 2003.
16. Girgis A, Sanson-Fisher RW, Tripodi DA et al. Evaluation of interventions to improve solar protection in primary schools. Health Educ Q 1993; 20:275-287.
17. Hughes BR, Altman DG, Newton JA. Melanoma and skin cancer: evaluation of a health education programme for secondary schools. Br J Dermatol 1993; 128:412-417.
18. Kölmel FKCURMBEW. Sonne, Kind und Melanome. Kinderarzt 1993; 4:470-481.
19. Geller AC, Rutsch L, Kenausis K et al. Can an hour or two of sun protection education keep the sunburn away? Evaluation of the Environmental Protection Agency's Sunwise School Program. Environ Health 2003; 2:13.
20. Buller DB, Buller MK, Beach B et al. Sunny days, healthy ways: evaluation of a skin cancer prevention curriculum for elementary school-aged children. J Am Acad Dermatol 1996; 35:911-922.
21. Greinert R, McKinlay A, Breitbart EW. The European Society of Skin Cancer Prevention—EUROSKIN: towards the promotion and harmonization of skin cancer prevention in Europe. Recommendations. Eur J Cancer Prev 2001; 10:157-162.
22. Repacholi MH. Global Solar UV Index. Radiat Prot Dosimetry 2000; 91:307-311.
23. McKinlay A, Breitbart EW. Ringborg U et al. 'Children under the Sun'—UV radiation and children's skin. WHO Workshop—Children's sun protection education. Eur J Cancer Prev 2002; 11:397-405.
24. Saraiya M, Glanz K, Briss PA et al. Interventions to prevent skin cancer by reducing exposure to ultraviolet radiation: a systematic review. Am J Prev Med 2004; 27:422-466.
25. Brändström R. Skin Cancer Prevention. In: Ringborg U, Brandberg Y, Breitbart EW, Greinert R. eds, pp. 315-337 (informa Helathcare, New York, London, 2007).
26. Mahler HI, Kulik JA, Gibbons FX et al. Effects of appearance-based interventions on sun protection intentions and self-reported behaviors. Health Psychol 2003; 22:199-209.
27. Mahler HI, Kulik JA, Harrell J et al. Effects of UV photographs, photoaging information and use of sunless tanning lotion on sun protection behaviors. Arch Dermatol 2005; 141:373-380.
28. Mahler HI, Kulik JA, Gerrard M et al. Long-term effects of appearance-based interventions on sun protection behaviors. Health Psychol 2007; 26:350-360.
29. Giovannucci E. The epidemiology of vitamin D and colorectal cancer: recent findings. Curr Opin Gastroenterol 2006; 22:24-29.
30. Bodiwala D, Luscombe CJ, French ME et al. Associations between prostate cancer susceptibility and parameters of exposure to ultraviolet radiation. Cancer Lett 2003; 200:141-148.
31. Grant WB. An ecologic study of dietary and solar ultraviolet-B links to breast carcinoma mortality rates. Cancer 2002; 94:272-281.
32. Grant WB. Ecologic studies of solar UV-B radiation and cancer mortality rates. Recent Results Cancer Res 2003; 164:371-377.
33. Grant WB. Epidemiology of disease risks in relation to vitamin D insufficiency. Prog Biophys Mol Biol 2006; 92:65-79.
34. Welsh J. Vitamin D and breast cancer: insights from animal models. Am J Clin Nutr 2004; 80:1721S-1724S.
35. Munger KL, Levin LI, Hollis BW et al. Serum 25-hydroxyvitamin D levels and risk of multiple sclerosis. JAMA 2006; 296:2832-2838.
36. Staples JA, Ponsonby AL, Lim LL et al. Ecologic analysis of some immune-related disorders, including type 1 diabetes, in Australia: latitude, regional ultraviolet radiation and disease prevalence. Environ Health Perspect 2003; 111:518-523.
37. Hypponen E, Laara E, Reunanen A et al. Intake of vitamin D and risk of type 1 diabetes: a birth-cohort study. Lancet 2001; 358:1500-1503.

38. Chiu KC, Chu A, Go VL et al. Hypovitaminosis D is associated with insulin resistance and beta cell dysfunction. Am J Clin Nutr 2004; 79:820-825.
39. Merlino LA, Curtis J, Mikuls TR et al. Vitamin D intake is inversely associated with rheumatoid arthritis: results from the Iowa Women's Health Study. Arthritis Rheum 2004; 50:72-77.
40. McGrath JJ, Kimlin MG, Saha S et al. Vitamin D insufficiency in south-east Queensland. Med J Aust 2001; 174:150-151.
41. Hanley DA, Davison KS. Vitamin D insufficiency in North America. J Nutr 2005; 135:332-337.
42. Lamberg-Allardt C. Vitamin D in foods and as supplements. Prog Biophys Mol Biol 2006; 92:33-38.
43. Reichrath J. The challenge resulting from positive and negative effects of sunlight: how much solar UV exposure is appropriate to balance between risks of vitamin D deficiency and skin cancer? Prog Biophys Mol Biol 2006; 92:9-16.
44. Vieth R. What is the optimal vitamin D status for health? Prog Biophys Mol Biol 2006; 92:26-32.
45. Holick MF. Vitamin D: its role in cancer prevention and treatment. Prog Biophys Mol Biol 2006; 92:49-59.
46. Lamberg-Allardt CJ, Outila TA, Karkkainen MU et al. Vitamin D deficiency and bone health in healthy adults in Finland: could this be a concern in other parts of Europe? J Bone Miner Res 2001; 16:2066-2073.
47. Barger-Lux MJ, Heaney RP, Dowell S et al. Vitamin D and its major metabolites: serum levels after graded oral dosing in healthy men. Osteoporos Int 1998; 8:222-230.
48. Tangpricha V, Koutkia P, Rieke SM et al. Fortification of orange juice with vitamin D: a novel approach for enhancing vitamin D nutritional health. Am J Clin Nutr 2003; 77:1478-1483.
49. Institute of Medicine. Dietary Reference Intakes for Calcium, Phosphorus, Magnesium, Vitamin D and Fluoride, pp. 250-287 (National Academic Press, 1997).
50. Vieth R, Bischoff-Ferrari H, Boucher BJ et al. The urgent need to recommend an intake of vitamin D that is effective. Am J Clin Nutr 2007; 85:649-650.
51. Holick MF. A perspective on the benefitial effects of moderate exposure to sunlight: bone health, cancer prevention, mental health and well being. In: Giacomoni, PU, ed. Sun protection in men. Amsterdam, London, New York: Elsevier, 2001:11-37.
52. Hollis BW. Circulating 25-hydroxyvitamin D levels indicative of vitamin D sufficiency: implications for establishing a new effective dietary intake recommendation for vitamin D. J Nutr 2005; 135:317-322.
53. MacLaughlin JA, Anderson RR, Holick MF. Spectral character of sunlight modulates photosynthesis of previtamin D3 and its photoisomers in human skin. Science 1982; 216:1001-1003.
54. Webb AR. Who, what, where and when-influences on cutaneous vitamin D synthesis. Prog Biophys Mol Biol 2006; 92:17-25.
55. Matsuoka LY, Wortsman J, Haddad JG et al. In vivo threshold for cutaneous synthesis of vitamin D3. J Lab Clin Med 1989; 114:301-305.
56. WHO. Sunbeds, tanning and UV exposure (Fact sheet). 2005; 287.
    Ref Type: Report.
57. McKinlay A. Workshop round-up session rapporteur's report. Prog Biophys Mol Biol 2006; 92:179-184.
58. Schofield PE, Freeman JL, Dixon HG et al. Trends in sun protection behaviour among Australian young adults. Aust N Z J Public Health 2001; 25:62-65.
59. Hill D. Sun Protection behaviour—determinants and trends. Cancer Forum 1996; 20:204-211.
60. Staples M, Marks R, Giles G. Trends in the incidence of nonmelanocytic skin cancer (NMSC) treated in Australia 1985-1995: are primary prevention programs starting to have an effect? Int J Cancer 1998; 78:144-148.
61. Levi F, Te VC, Randimbison L et al. Trends in skin cancer incidence in Vaud: an update, 1976-1998. Eur J Cancer Prev 2001; 10:371-373.
62. de Vries E, Bray FI, Coebergh JW et al. Changing epidemiology of malignant cutaneous melanoma in Europe 1953-1997: rising trends in incidence and mortality but recent stabilizations in western Europe and decreases in Scandinavia. Int J Cancer 2003; 107:119-126.
63. Bulliard JL, Cox B, Semenciw R. Trends by anatomic site in the incidence of cutaneous malignant melanoma in Canada, 1969-93. Cancer Causes Control 1999; 10:407-416.
64. Marrett LD, Nguyen HL, Armstrong BK. Trends in the incidence of cutaneous malignant melanoma in New South Wales, 1983-1996. Int J Cancer 2001; 92:457-462.
65. Martin RC, Robinson E. Cutaneous melanoma in Caucasian New Zealanders: 1995-1999. ANZ J Surg 2004; 74:233-237.

CHAPTER 12

Sunscreens

Guido Bens*

Ultraviolet Radiation

Naturally occurring ultraviolet radiation (UVR) from the sun has been divided into two broad band regions: low-energy UVA (with wavelengths of 320 to 400 nm) and high-energy UVB (280-320 nm). Relative effectiveness of different wavelengths in producing a biologic reaction is called action spectrum for this particular reaction. The most obvious acute reaction of white skin to UVR is erythema which is commonly addressed to as "sunburn". The action spectrum of solar erythema lies mainly in the UVB band region, with a peak at 295 nm and rapid decline towards the UVA region (Fig. 1): 295 nm UVB radiation (UVBR) is about 1000 times more erythemogenic than short-wave UVAR. Under normal conditions, middle and long-wave UVAR do not induce sunburn. UVAR has therefore been further broken down into two bands UVA1 (340-400 nm) and UVA2 (320-340 nm) because of the increased erythemogenic activity of UVA2 compared to UVA1.

Solar radiation is significantly modified by the earth's atmosphere with ozone in the stratosphere being the major photoprotective agent that absorbs all high-energy cosmic radiation, UVCR (200-280 nm) and short-wave UVBR up to 290 nm. Clouds, pollutants and fog furthermore decrease UVR by scattering and absorption. However, UVAR and visible light (400-700 nm) are much less affected by the way through the atmosphere. Less than 5% of the sunlight that reaches the earth's surface is UVR, with a ratio of UVA to UVB of about 20:1, depending on geographical latitude, altitude, season of the year, time of day and meteorological conditions.[1] UVAR but not UVBR traverses window glass and is therefore present also indoor. UV exposure does not only occur by direct sunshine on the skin, but also by light reflection, e.g., by snow, glass, sand and light-colored metals, with once more wavelengths in the UVA band being more reflected than UVBR. About 50% of effective UVA exposure has been estimated to occur in the shade.[2] The predominance of UVA in the solar energy in our environment permits UVA to play a far more important role in contributing to the harmful effects of sun exposure than previously suspected.

Effects of Ultraviolet Radiation in Human Skin

UVA penetrates far deeper into the skin than UVB does (Fig. 2): The major part (70%) of UVB is absorbed or scattered by the stratum corneum. Twenty percent of UVB reaches living cells in the epidermal spinous layer and 10% superficial dermis. UVAR and visible light are less filtered by stratum corneum, but after absorption by melanin, 30% of UVA hits basal cells of epidermis and still 20% reaches reticular dermis. One percent of UVA1 penetrates up to the limits of subcutis.[3] The skin penetration of visible light is even more important, but little is known about its biologic effects in human skin.

Positive and harmful effects of UVR in the skin are tightly woven as they contribute to the natural mechanisms of photoprotection. UVR that is not scattered by the superficial horny layer is absorbed by endogenous chromophores. Photochemical reactions of these absorbing biomolecules

*Guido Bens—Clermont-Ferrand University Hospital, Department of Dermatology Hôtel-Dieu, Boulevard Léon Malfreyt, 63058 Clermont-Ferrand cedex 1, France.
Email: gbens@chu-clermontferrand.fr

Sunlight, Vitamin D and Skin Cancer, edited by Jörg Reichrath. ©2008 Landes Bioscience and Springer Science+Business Media.

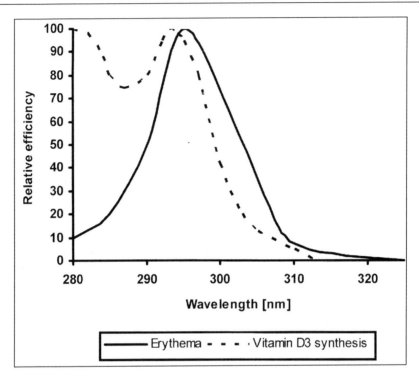

Figure 1. Action spectrum of natural terrestric UVR for solar erythema and vitamin D3 synthesis. (adapted from ref. 3).

result in alterations of skin biology that lead to the immediate or delayed UV effects represented in Figure 3.

Epidermal chromophores with absorption spectra within the UVB range are urocanic acid, melanin, aromatic amino acids such as tryptophane and tyrosine in epidermal proteins and nuclear DNA.[4] Urocanic acid is most expressed in the superficial layers of epidermis. It absorbs UVB by a trans to cis isomerization. Its synthesis from histidine liberated by filaggrin breakdown is triggered by UVBR.[3] Another major target for UVB and UVA2 are nucleotides. Absorption of UVR by pyrimidine and purine bases results in DNA photoproduct formation, mainly pyrimidine dimers, but also pyrimidine (6-4) pyrimidone photoproducts. These DNA photoproducts are continuously excised by DNA repair enzymes. If repair fails, they can lead to p53-mediated apoptosis or, after replication, to DNA mutations.[1] C→T and CC→TT mutations are considered as a nuclear fingerprint of UVB-induced photodamage. UVB-generated thymine dimers induce p53 which is a pro-apoptotic protein that helps to eliminate cells in which DNA is too heavily damaged to be repaired.[5] UVB triggers in the skin the production of cholecalciferol (vitamin D3) from 7-dehydrocholesterol (DHC). The action spectrum for this synthesis is nearly identical to the one for solar erythema (Fig. 1). UVA alone does not permit cutaneous vitamin D3 synthesis.[6] UVB exposure stimulates mitotic activity in epidermis and, to a lesser extent, also in papillary dermis that persists from days to weeks. This results in acanthosis and hyperkeratosis with an approximate two-fold thickening of these skin layers that is best characterized by the German term *"Lichtschwiele"* ("light-induced callosity"). This phenomenon provides supplementary UV protection to the underlying living cells. UVA does not induce such epidermal thickening.

While UVB effects in the skin occur by direct UVB photon absorption by the target molecules, UVA effects are mostly mediated by the formation of radicals:[1] Absorption of UVAR

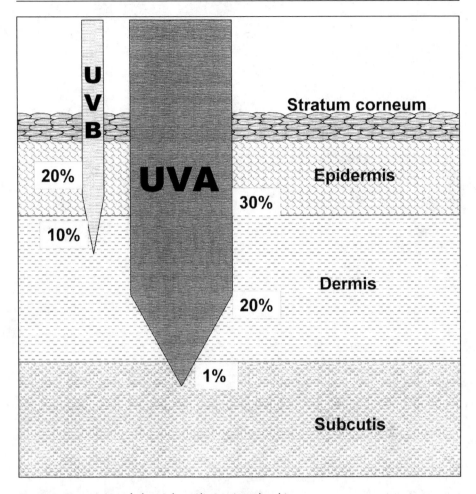

Figure 2. Penetration of ultraviolet radiation into the skin.

by appropriate chromophores such as urocanic acid, NADH, flavins and unsaturated lipids promotes these molecules into an excited state. Dissipation of this energy occurs either by internal conversion which may generate an organic radical, or, more frequently, by reaction with tissular oxygen or oxygen-containing molecules which leads to formation of so-called reactive oxygen species (ROS).[7] ROS are unstable and extremely chemically reactive molecules that can cause lipid peroxidation in plasma, nuclear and mitochondrial membranes. They can damage cellular proteins and cause DNA strand breaks and oxidation of nucleic acids.[8] The corresponding characteristic DNA fingerprint is 8-hydroxyguanine which generates G:C→ T:A mutations by error pairing of 8-hydroxyguanine with adenine instead of cytosine during following replication. These mutations generated by oxidative stress do not induce p53 and escape therefore more easily to apoptotic control than UVB-induced mutations.[9] Melanocytes seem to be more sensitive to UVA-induced DNA damage than keratinocytes.[10] Pyrimidine dimers are not only formed by direct UVBR but also by oxidative stress after UVA irradiation. DNA repair of pyrimidine dimers induced by UVAR is less effective than excision repair of UVB-induced DNA damage.[11]

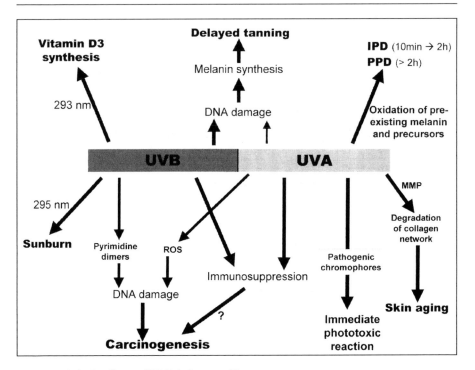

Figure 3. Biologic effects of UVR in human skin.

In response to damage to DNA and to other chromophores by UVB and UVA, cytokines and inflammatory mediators are released into the skin following UVR.[12] This is responsible for sunburn as acute clinical effect of overexposure to sunlight.

DNA damage by UVB or UVA2 triggers a tanning response in human skin.[12] Nucleotide fragments removed from the DNA after repair activate melanocyte tyrosinase, the key enzyme in melanogenesis.[13,14] UVBR seems to be most effective in stimulating de novo melanogenesis from pre-existing melanin monomers and precursors. Melanocyte dendrites elongate and branch, melanosome numbers and sizes increase and their transfer from melanocytes to keratinocytes is enhanced. This results in delayed tanning that becomes visible within 3 days after UV exposure.[12] In white skin, melanosomes are diffusely distributed within keratinocyte cytoplasm but they aggregate above the nucleus to form a kind of cap. Melanin is a large opaque molecule absorbing throughout the UV and visible light band. It is photostable, i.e., it converts the absorbed energy into heat rather than into chemical energy.[1] Both constitutive and induced melanin pigmentation protect against UV-induced DNA damage. UVA-induced tan seems to be less protective than the one induced by UVB.[15] This may be explained by the more basal localization of UVA2-induced pigmentation and the lack of epidermal thickening after UVAR. UVA2, UVA1 and short-wave visible light also induce another kind of pigment reaction after exposure: In little doses, these wavelengths generate a greyish skin color within 15 minutes after exposure that is called immediate pigment darkening (IPD).[12] It progressively declines and disappears within 2 hours. Higher UVA doses induce a longer-standing pigmentation of more brownish color called persistent pigment darkening (PPD) that persists after 2 hours. IPD and PPD do not represent de novo melanin synthesis, but they are a product of photo-oxidation of pre-existing melanin and precursors in presence of oxygen. Neither IPD nor PPD provide protection against UV-induced skin damage. They do not prevent sunburn.

Oxidative stress by UVAR can be massively enhanced by the presence of pathogenic chromophores in the skin that generate after UV irradiation far greater amounts of ROS than do cutaneous chromophores under normal conditions. The resulting acute cutaneous inflammation is addressed to as phototoxic reaction. Examples of phototoxic agents are furocoumarins contained in plants causing phytophotodermatitis after UVA irradiation or phototoxic drugs, e.g., cyclins.

Penetrating up to the dermis, UVAR is responsible for photoaging changes: The action spectrum for these degrading mechanisms lies mainly in the UVA1 band. UVB alone does not induce photoaging. UVA induces a series of matrix metalloproteinases that degrade the dermal collagen framework.[7] The presence of collagen detritus inhibits dermal procollagen synthesis and thereby aggravates the degenerative process.[16] UVA-induced oxidative stress also increases elastin messenger RNA levels in dermal fibroblasts which explains the elastotic changes that are characteristic of photoaged skin.[17]

Both UVA and UVB have immunosuppressive potential even at suberythemal doses:[18] After UV irradiation Langerhans cells in the skin are diminished in number and their morphology and function are altered. This effect is used for therapeutic purposes in dermatologic phototherapy. UVA suppresses delayed-type contact hypersensitivity.[19] Nghiem et al showed in a mouse model that even established systemic immune response is impaired by short-wave UVA.[20] It remains unclear, however, if UVA2 effectively suppresses anti-microbial immune response in humans.

The 20-fold increased risk of skin cancer in therapeutically immunosuppressed organ transplant patients suggests a role of the immune system in preventing those skin tumors. Photo-induced immunosuppression is therefore thought to contribute to the carcinogenic effect of UVR. The mutagenic action of UVR is physiologically controlled by several mechanisms: DNA repair enzymes in first line, pro-apoptotic regulation, e.g., by p53 in second line and cellular immune defense in third line. UVR can affect each one of these three defense lines: UVAR has been shown to inhibit DNA repair enzymes.[9,11] When mutations concern the p53 gene, apoptosis control is impaired and actinic keratoses, squamous and basal cell carcinomas may arise.[21] When UV-induced DNA mutations hit the patched gene, this can contribute to the carcinogenesis of basal cell carcinoma.[22] Finally the UVR-induced cutaneous immunosuppression probably concerns in the same way local anti-tumor immunity, although this has not been demonstrated in human skin so far.

Topical Photoprotection Agents

The numerous deleterious effects of UVR make protective measures necessary. Total avoidance and protective clothing are without any doubt the most effective methods but they are not practicable for daily consequent protection. Moreover, modern lifestyle going along with a great popularity of sunbathing encourages acute intermittent sun exposure. For this reason topically applied sunscreens are since 40 years the most used photoprotective means.

Suncare products are available as oils, creams, lotions, sprays, gels and sticks. They are composed of different UV filter agents and, depending on their galenic presentation, of moisturizers, conservatives and often alternative photoprotectants such as antioxidants. UV protection increases with filter concentration in sunscreens, but toxicity and poor cosmetic acceptance limit UV filter concentration for in vivo use in human beings. Classic recommendation for sunscreen use is to apply 15 to 30 minutes before sun exposure and to repeat application every two hours. The product has to be reapplied earlier after activity that may wash or rub off the sunscreen, i.e., after swimming, sweating or towel drying. "Water-resistant" suncare products are defined as protecting skin for 40 minutes of bathing whereas "waterproof" (or "very water-resistant" in the EU) sunscreens protect for 80 minutes.[23] The term "remanence" describes a sunscreen's resistance to external elimination by water, sweat or rubbing. Tightly related to remanence is a product's "substantivity" that characterizes the capacity of a filter substance to fix to structures in the upper epidermis which ensures a long lasting action.

The ideal sun protection agent should provide high protection that is equally effective against UVA and UVB. Moreover, it should be waterproof, sweat-proof, photostable, cosmetically acceptable and nontoxic.

Regulations and Marketing

Sunscreen marketing is submitted to national legislation. These regulations are harmonized among the member states of the European Union where UV filters are listed as cosmetics by the European Cosmetic Toiletry and Perfumery Association (COLIPA). In the United States, in contrast, sunscreens are considered as over-the-counter drugs that are subject to Food and Drug Administration (FDA) regulation. They must therefore undergo considerable safety and allergy testing in clinical trials that is responsible for high costs to the manufacturers and important delay before marketing as compared to the EU where new filter products can enter the market more rapidly. Strict FDA regulations—and bureaucracy—have conducted to a kind of regrettable underdevelopment of the US suncare market. For this reason, although it was in the United States where the first commercial UV filter preparation was available in the 1920s, 80 years later French, German and Swiss manufacturers are global market leaders in this domain.

The following discussion of filter substances that are listed in Table 1 is adapted to the positive list of the European Cosmetics Directive. I regard this filter selection as more representative of today's possibilities in the UV filter domain than the substances listed in the US FDA sunscreen monograph. The UV filters in the European list are commercially available in most countries outside the US.

Measuring Photoprotection

The sun protection factor (SPF) of sunscreens expresses their capacity of protection from erythema after UV exposure. SPF therefore essentially translates protection from UVBR.

For SPF testing, erythema is induced by a xenon lamp solar simulator. The smallest dose causing a minimally perceptible erythema with well-defined borders at 24 hours after one single irradiation is called minimal erythema dose (MED). Basic MED mainly depends on the individual's natural photoprotective potential provided by constitutive and adaptive pigmentation and skin thickening, but also on variable parameters such as nutrition and drug intake. The standard product dose for SPF testing is 2 mg of finalized sunscreen per cm² of skin. SPF is a ratio calculated from the following formula:

$$SPF = \frac{MED \text{ with the tested sunscreen}}{MED \text{ without sunscreen}}$$

This MED-related procedure has the advantage compared to in vitro spectrophotometry to be directly related to the biologic consequences of UV exposure in a given individual. It is based on the individual sensitivity to UVR at a given moment. However, DNA damage and immunosuppression occur even below the erythema threshold dose. These harmful effects are not considered by SPF calculation.[24] At least theoretically, SPF permits to estimate the factor by which sun exposure can be extended in daily practice until erythema threshold: If the recommended dose of 2 mg/cm² is applied (which is in general not the case!) and no external elimination occurs, a SPF10 suncare product permits to stay ten times longer in the sunlight without erythematous reaction than without this protection.

The relation between the percentage of filtered UVB/UVA2 radiation and SPF is a logarithmic and not a linear one (Fig. 4). In recent years cosmetic industry gave a race to higher and higher SPFs and great SPF numbers have become for the consumer the first criterion of choice between different sunscreen products. Indeed UV absorption increases from 0% to 90% between a moisturizer without SPF and a SPF10 sunscreen, but only from 97% to 99% between a SPF30 and a SPF100 product. It has never been demonstrated that SPFs of more than 30 have any clinically relevant impact on the deleterious action of UV exposure in the skin compared to SPF30 sunscreens (which yet absorb almost 97% of erythemogenic UVR). To limit the implicit deception of the consumer by high SPF numbers which can lead to a false hope of "complete" protection and subsequent overexposure to harmful photodamage, several countries have regulated sunscreen labeling: In the European Union sunscreens with SPF of more than 50 have to be labeled "SPF50+". In Australia the SPF scale is limited to 30.

Table 1. Organic and inorganic UV filters marketed in the European Union (positive list of UV filters according to the European Cosmetics Directive, Annex VII)

INCI Name	Abbreviation	IUPAC Name	Max. Auth. Conc.	Trade Name(s)	Abs. Max.	Comments
Pure UVB filters						
PABA	PABA	4-Aminobenzoic acid	5%	PABA®	283 nm	Binding to proteins of the stratum
Octyl Dimethyl PABA = Padimate O	OD-PABA	2-Ethylhexyl p-dimethylamino-benzoate	8%	Eusolex 6007® Escalol 507®	311 nm	corneum ensures good substantivity and good remanence. Photoallergic potential
PEG-25-PABA	PEG-25-PABA	Polyethylene glycol 25 aminobenzoate	10%	Uvinul P25® Unipabol U17®	310 nm	
Octyl Methoxycinnamate = Octinoxate	OMC	2-Ethylhexyl-3-(4-methoxyphenyl) prop-2-enoate	10%	Escalol 557® Eusolex 2292® Neo Heliopan AV® Parsol MCX®	311 nm	Used in combination with other filters as not photostable in pure preparations
Isoamyl p-methoxycinnamate = Cinoxate	IMC	3-Methylbutyl 3-(4-methoxyphenyl) prop-2-enoate	10%	Neo Heliopan E1000® Uvinul N-539®	289 nm	
Camphor Benzalkonium Methosulfate	---		6%	Mexoryl SK®	295 nm	
3-Benzylidene Camphor	BC		2%	Mexoryl SD-20® Unisol-S-22®	295 nm	Good photostability, also permit to stabilize
4-Methylbenzylidene Camphor = (USAN) Enzacamene	MBC	3-(4'-Sulfo)-benzylidene-bornan-2-on	4%	Eusolex 6300® Neo Heliopan MBC® Parsol 500®	305 nm	other UV filters such as cinnamates
Polyacryl-Amidomethyl Benzylidene Camphor	---	N-[2(and 4)-(2-oxoborn-	6%	Mexoryl SW®	295 nm	

continued on next page

Table 1. *Continued*

INCI Name	Abbreviation	IUPAC Name	Max. Auth. Conc.	Trade Name(s)	Abs. Max.	Comments
Homosalate	HMS	3, 3, 5-Trimethyl-cyclohexyl-salicylate	10%	Eusolex HMS® Neo Heliopan®	306 nm	Can reduce photodegradation of oxybenzone and avobenzone
Octylsalicylate	OS	2-Ethylhexylsalicylate	5%	Escalol 587® Neo Heliopan OS®	307 nm	
Phenylbenzimidazole Sulfonic Acid	PBSA	2-Phenylbenzimidazol-5-sulfonic acid	8%	Eusolex 232® Neo Heliopan Hydro® Parsol HS®	308 nm	Hydrophilic filter, can improve photostability of other filters
Dimethicodiethylbenzalmalonate = Polysilicone-15	---	Benzylidene malonate polysiloxane	10%	Parsol SLX®	311 nm	Photostable, used to stabilize BMDBM
Octyl Triazone	OT	2,4,6-tris[p-(ethylhexyl-oxycarbonyl)anilino]-1,3,5-triazine	5%	Uvinul T15®	314 nm	
Octocrylene	OC	2-Ethylhexyl-2-cyano-3, 3-diphenylacrylate	10%	Eusolex OCR® Neo Heliopan 303® Uvinul N-539®	303 nm	Photostable filter, used to stabilize cinnamates
Benzophenone UVB-UVA2 broad spectrum filters						
Benzophenone-3 = Oxybenzone	BENZ-3	2-Hydroxy-4-methoxy-benzophenone	10%	Escalol 567® Eusolex 4360® Neo Heliopan BB® UVAsorb MET/C® Uvinul M40®	288 and 325 nm	Photolabile, important photoallergic potential; warning "contains oxybenzone" to be printed
Benzophenone-4 = Sulisobenzone	BENZ-4	2-Hydroxy-4-methoxy-benzophenone-5-sulfonic acid	5%	Escalol 577® UVAsorb S5® Uvinul MS40®	288 and 366 nm	Good photostability, photoallergic cross-reaction with oxybenzone

continued on next page

Table 1. *Continued*

INCI Name	Abbreviation	IUPAC Name	Max. Auth. Conc.	Trade Name(s)	Abs. Max.	Comments
Pure UVA filters						
Butyl Methoxy-Dibenzoylmethane = Avobenzone	BMDBM	1-(4-tert.	5%	Eusolex 9020® Parsol 1789®	356 nm	Poor photostability in its pure form, needs to be stabilized by association with other filters such as BC, OC or Polysilicone-15
Dioctyl Butamido Triazone	DBT	4,4'-[(6-[4-((1,1-Dimethylethyl)-amino-carbonyl)-phenyl-amino]-1, 3, 5-tri-azine-2, 4-yl)-diimino]-bis-(benzoic acid-2-ethylhexylester)	10%	UVAsorb HEB®	345 nm	
Disodium Phenyl Dibenzimidazole Tetrasulfonate	DPDT	2,2'-(1,	10%	Neo Heliopan AP®	345 nm	hydrosoluble
Diethylamino Hydroxy-benzoyl Hexyl Benzoate	DHHB		10%	Uvinul A Plus®	330 and 370 nm	photostable
Last generation UVB-UVA2-UVA1 broad spectrum filters						
Terephthalidene Dicamphor Sulfonic acid = (USAN) Ecamsule	MSX	3,3'-(1,4-Phenylene-di-methylidene)bis-(7,7-dimethyl-2-oxobicyclo-(2.- 2.1)hep-tane-1-methanesulfonic acid	10%	Mexoryl SX®	345 nm	Hydrosoluble, photostable

continued on next page

Table 1. Continued

INCI Name	Abbreviation	IUPAC Name	Max. Auth. Conc.	Trade Name(s)	Abs. Max.	Comments
Drometrizole Trisiloxane = Silatrizol	MXL	2-(2H-benzotri-azol-2-yl)-4-meth-yl-6-(2-methyl3-(1,-,3,3-tetramethy-l-1-(trimethyl-	10%	Mexoryl XL®	303 and 344 nm	Liposoluble, photostable
Methylene bis-Benzotriazolyl Tetramethyl-butylphenol = (USAN) Bisoctrizole	MBBT	2,2'-Methy-lene-bis-6-(2H-benzo-triazol-2-yl)-4-(1,1,3,3-tetramethylbutyl)-phe-nol	10%	Tinosorb M®	306 and 360 nm	Very photostable, UV absorption and reflection, hydrosoluble
Bis-Ethylhexyloxyphenol Methoxyphenyltriazine = Anisotriazine = (USAN) Bemotrizinol	BEMT		10%	Tinosorb S®	305 and 345 nm	Excellent photostability, oil soluble, water resistant
Inorganic filters						
Titanium Dioxide (micronized)	TiO₂		25%		Depending on particle size:	Excellent UVB and UVA2 coverage, less in UVA1
Zinc Oxide (micronized)	ZnO		25%		UVB-UVA-visible light	Good UVA1 coverage, less effective in UVB

Abbreviations: INCI = International Nomenclature of Cosmetic Ingredients; IUPAC = International Union of Pure and Applied Chemistry; Max. auth. conc. = Maximum filter concentration authorized by the European Cosmetics Directive for finalized sunscreen products; Abs. Max. = Wavelength at which maximum absorption occurs with the filter; USAN = United States adopted name.

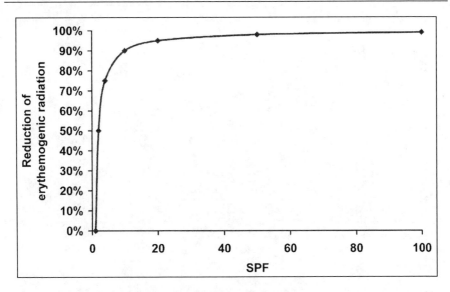

Figure 4. Reduction of erythemogenic UVR by sunscreens.

UVA protection is more difficult to quantify than UVB-SPF, because UVA is few erythemogenic. Currently there is no uniformly accepted standard method for measuring UVA protection by sunscreens. The most commonly used methods are in vivo PPD and critical wavelength assessed in vitro by spectrophotometry. Critical wavelength is defined as the wavelength below which 90% of the sunscreen's UV absorbency occurs as measured in the band region from 290 to 400 nm.[25]

Organic UV Filters

Organic UV filter substances mainly act by absorption of photons in the UV wavelength band. They are aromatic molecules conjugated with carbonyl groups. These chromophores absorb UV photons through electron resonance delocalization in the aromatic compounds that raise the molecule from the electronic ground singlet state S_0 into an excited electronic state S_1 or higher. In most classic UVB absorbers such as PABA this leads to a transitory polarization of the organic molecule (Fig. 5). Organic UV filter molecules capture photons of a more or less specific wavelength λ around their absorption maximum. No organic UV filter, especially not the "classic molecules", cover the entire UV spectrum. For this reason, finalized sunscreen products are in general an association of several filter substances. The absorbed energy is dissipated by vibronic relaxation that delivers heat via collisions with the surrounding medium.[26] A minor part of energy may also be emitted in form of fluorescent radiation ($\lambda = 400\text{-}700$ nm), i.e., visible light, with wavelengths that are longer than those of the initial photon. Although this kind of radiation is harmless, it has to be limited for the cosmetic acceptance of the UV filter. Energy release permits the excited filter molecule to return to its ground state where it is again available to absorb additional photons. Filters that perfectly repeat this cyclical process without undergoing significant chemical change are classified as photostable. Photostable filters can retain their UV-absorbing potency during long exposures.

The excited form of filter molecules after UV absorption has to be very short-lived in order to prevent chemical reactions between the filter and tissular proteins or oxygen which could lead to photoallergic or phototoxic reaction. Unfortunately such reactions, mainly photoallergy, have been described repeatedly with PABA derivatives, cinnamates and benzophenones.[27,28] Several molecules have been withdrawn. The photosensitization to benzophenone-3 (oxybenzone) is particularly severe, because photoallergic cross-reactions are known with benzophenone-4 (another broad

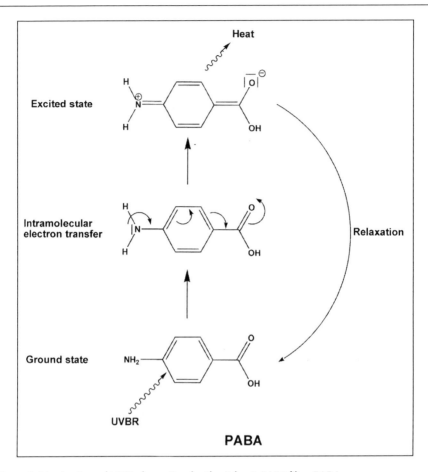

Figure 5. Mechanism of UVB absorption by the "classic" UV filter PABA.

spectrum filter), topically applied ketoprofen and even with systemically administered fenofibrate.[27] Considering the large use of sunscreens, however, these photocontact allergies to UV filters remain relatively rare events. In the case of eczema in sun-exposed skin areas that have been treated with sunscreens, not UV-related contact sensitization to UV filters as well as contact and photocontact allergy to other components of sunscreens besides the filters have to be eliminated.

Some UVB filters such as cinnamates undergo after UV absorption an intramolecular trans to cis isomerization. Others experience definitive structural transformation which alters their protective capacity. This is a major problem with the currently used UVA filter avobenzone which looses considerably of its photoprotective potential after irradiation in its pure form.[29] As photoprotection by sunscreens is tested by single irradiation, the photounstable character of the concerned molecules is not assessed by standard test protocols. Photounstable filters can be stabilized by association with other organic UV filters (see Table 1) or with inorganic filters. In the US an association of avobenzone and oxybenzone with 2-6-diethylhexyl naphtalate, a photostabilizing solvent, has recently been marketed in order to overcome the avobenzone photodegradation problem and to comply with FDA regulations (Helioplex®, Neutrogena). But this combination still suffers from the presence of oxybenzone as a photoallergenic filter with significant systemic absorption.

Indeed classic organic UV filters are little-sized more or less lipophilic molecules. These chemical properties allow easy penetration at least into the deeper layers of the epidermis where the filters encounter living cells (Fig. 6) which explains the incidence of photoallergy as a clinical manifestation of immunologic reaction to filter molecules having formed haptens after photoactivation. Percutaneous systemic absorption of organic UV filters has been reported for several filter molecules: Sarveiya et al found 1% of topically applied oxybenzone in the urine of 48 hours after sunscreen use.[30] Janjua et al detected oxybenzone, octyl-methoxycinnamate (OMC) and 4-methylbenzylidene camphor (MBC), i.e., representative molecules of 3 different families of organic UVB filters, in plasma and urine of healthy volunteers.[31] The penetration of systemically absorbed sunscreens into the organs and their clearance have never been assessed. One study reported an estrogen-like activity of octyl dimethyl PABA (OD-PABA), OMC, homosalate, 4-methylbenzylidene camphor, oxybenzone and avobenzone in vitro in MCF-7 breast cancer cells and in vivo in the immature rat uterotrophic assay.[32] These results were not confirmed in human adults.[31] Sunscreen absorption and endocrine activity have never been examined in prepubertal children who are not only more prone to systemic absorption than adults but are also more sensitive to low levels of hormone action due to their low levels of endogenous reproductive hormones.

For these penetration problems, the use of organic UV filters is not recommended for young children who have an immature stratum corneum and for patients with pre-existing skin lesions that may go along with an impairment of the epidermal barrier function. In these two groups of users, penetration of organic filters is probably yet more important than for the general skin-healthy adult population. They may be exposed to a higher risk of photocontact sensitization to organic filter molecules and to systemic absorption of larger amounts of these substances.

Besides their proper dermal penetration, organic UV filters have been shown to enhance topical penetration of herbicides and insecticides. This has been demonstrated for the herbicides 2,4-dichlorophenoxyacetic acid and paraquat and for the insecticides parathion and malathion.[33] The filters OD-PABA, OMC, homosalate, octyl salicylate, octocrylene, oxybenzone and benzophenone-4 (molecules from 5 different chemical subgroups of organic UVB filters) were tested in a mouse model and in human split skin in vitro:[34] All but octocylene were found to increase cutaneous

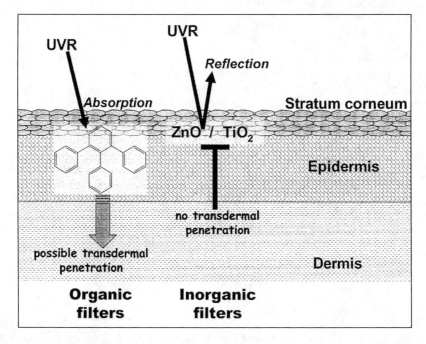

Figure 6. Organic and inorganic UV filters on the skin: mechanism of UV protection and penetration of the filters into the skin.

penetration of the applied herbicides and insecticides. This finding is particularly alarming for agricultural workers using pesticides who are encouraged to wear sunscreens for their outdoor work and for fair-skinned individuals from the temperate zone who seek to protect themselves during a stay in tropical countries from both intense sunlight and insect attack.

By reaction with tissular proteins, DNA or oxygen, photounstable UV filters may cause harmful or even procarcinogenic effects in the skin: In vitro studies found DNA nucleotide dimer formation to be enhanced under PABA treatment,[35] UVR-induced mutagenity to be increased by isoamyl p-methoxycinnamate and tissular radicals to be formed by photo-degraded avobenzone. However, the in vivo significance of these findings is doubtful and a review of available clinical data concluded that UV filters, at least when used occasionally, do not pose a human health concern.[36]

The first sunscreen in the world appeared in 1928 in the United States with the commercial introduction of an emulsion that contained the two organic UVB filters benzyl salicylate and benzyl cinnamate.[1] PABA was patented in 1943. The main concern when the first topical sunscreens were developed was to provide protection from UVB-induced sunburn. During the following decades new chemical filter families with more and more derivatives were developed and optimization of their concentration and combination of several filters with complementary absorption peaks allowed higher SPFs. Up to the 1980s, high SPFs in a cosmetically pleasant galenic presentation were sufficient to satisfy sunscreen users worldwide. Absence of UVA protection was tolerated as it provided desirable tan without risk of sunburn. With increasing evidence about the role of UVAR in the long-term deleterious effects of sun exposure, organic filters with absorption maximum in the UVA band range and benzophenones being the first UVB/UVA2 broad spectrum filters were marketed. But benzophenones provide only insufficient protection in the long-wave UVA1 band region. Because of photolability and dermal penetration of classic organic filters, the above described adverse events—mostly photoallergy and contact dermatitis—were successively reported. Research therefore focused on the development of filter substances providing both a maximum of product safety and an absorbing coverage of the entire UV spectrum, but permitting on the other hand an association with classic UV filters in finalized products.

In 1993 L'Oréal (Clichy, France) introduced the first representative of a new generation of organic broad spectrum UV filters: terephthalidene dicamphor sulfonic acid (Mexoryl® SX, MSX). MSX is a water-soluble filter that is suitable for day wear sunscreen formulations including sunscreen-containing moisturizers and facial formulations. In 1998 the same manufacturer completed its range of products by an oil-soluble substance: drometrizole trisiloxane (Mexoryl® XL, MXL), a hydroxybenzotriazole derivative. This molecule is composed of two different chemical subunits: The 2-hydroxyphenyl benzotriazole subunit contains the UV-absorbing potential over the whole UVB, UVA2 and UVA1 wavelength spectrum with two different absorption peaks, one in the UVB band ($\lambda = 303$ nm) and another one at the limit between UVA2 and UVA1 ($\lambda = 344$ nm). The siloxane subunit of MXL confers to the molecule a lipophilic character that renders it suitable for water-resistant sunscreen formulations, including those worn on the beach and during vigorous physical exercise.[1] Another hydroxybenzotriazole derivative was commercialized in 1999 by Ciba Specialty Chemicals (Basel, Switzerland): The hydrosoluble methylene bis-benzotriazolyl tetramethylbutylphenol (MBBT, Tinosorb® M) covers, with two absorption peaks, the entire UVB and UVA spectrum. This organic filter has the particularity to associate for its UV-protective action both absorbing and reflecting properties. UV reflection is normally only seen with inorganic UV filters. MBBT consists of microfine organic particles that are dispersed in the aqueous phase of sunscreen emulsions.

The latest oil-soluble UV filter is bis-ethylhexyloxyphenol methoxyphenyltriazine (BEMT, Tinosorb® S). It was introduced in 2002. The mechanism of action of BEMT is illustrated in Figure 7: BEMT is a large polyaromatic molecule. Its size impedes dermal penetration in spite of its lipophilic property. The asymmetric structure of the molecule harbors separate absorption sites for UVBR and UVAR. After absorption of UV photons the molecule is promoted into an excited state that undergoes photo-tautomerism with intramolecular proton transfer. The duration of this isomerization is in the order of 10^{-12} second. This extremely short time

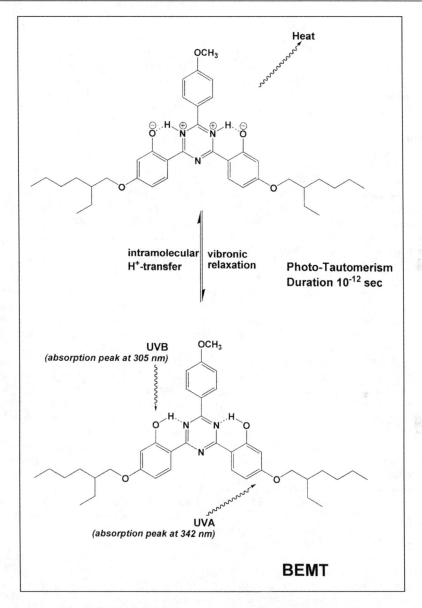

Figure 7. Mechanism of UVA and UVB absorption by bis-ethylhexyloxyphenol methoxy-phenyltriazine (BEMT, Tinosorb® S)[26].

span does not permit any external chemical reaction to be triggered. This prevents the formation of radicals or haptens from the photoexcited BEMT molecule. BEMT returns by vibronic relaxation with heat release into its energetic ground state in chemically unchanged form and is again ready to absorb UVR.[26]

Mexoryls and tinosorbs provide strong absorbency up to the UVA1 range and excellent photostability. Their use in commercial sunscreen preparations permits to achieve significantly better UVA protection as measured by the PPD protocol. In order to obtain high UVB-SPF and

UVA-PF which cannot be achieved with one filter alone, they are nevertheless associated with classic organic filters and inorganic pigments in commercialized sunscreens. They can stabilize photolabile filters such as cinnamates or avobenzone.[37] Percutaneous absorption, photoallergic and phototoxic reactions have not been reported so far with these last generation organic filters. Both MBBT and BEMT do not have estrogenic or androgenic activity in vitro.[38]

Thirteen years after its marketing in most parts of the world, MSX finally obtained FDA approval in July 2006. Tinosorbs are still not available in the United States.

Inorganic UV Filters

Inorganic UV filter substances are chemically inert pigments that stay in the upper layers of the epidermis and stratum corneum. They reflect or scatter radiation (Fig. 6). The degree of reflection and scattering by these pigments is strongly dependent on their particle size and shape. Two inorganic oxides are used for UV protection in humans: zinc oxide (ZnO) and titanium dioxide (TiO_2). In their nonmicronized form, with a particle size of 200 to 500 nm, inorganic filters act as opaque radiation blockers that reflect not only UVR in both the UVB and the UVA spectrum, but also visible light and infrared radiation. In this form they are particularly suitable for protection in visible light-induced photosensitivity diseases such as porphyrias.[39] However, the reflection of visible light makes inorganic sunscreens visible to the eyes and thus cosmetically less acceptable. Iron oxide, a reddish pigment with absorbing capacity in the UVA range, is sometimes added to large sized particle inorganic filter preparations to correct their "white" look. Cosmetic acceptability of inorganic UV filters is improved by micronization of the particle size to 10-50 nm. Decreasing the particle size reduces reflection, mainly of longer wavelengths and shifts protection towards shorter wavelengths by increasing absorbency by micronized filter particles.[1] Microfine ZnO protects over a wide range of UVA, including UVA1, but is less effective against UVBR. It is very photostable and does not react with organic UV filters.[40] Micronized TiO_2 provides good protection in the UVB and UVA2 range, but is insufficient for UVA1. ZnO and TiO_2 are therefore perfectly complementary in one sunscreen preparation. They are frequently associated to organic UV filters for their photostabilizing properties. Although the particle size of micronized TiO_2 is smaller than the one of ZnO, it has a higher reflective index and appears therefore whiter than ZnO.[1,40] Micronized TiO_2 is also more photoreactive than ZnO by UV absorption: The crystalline forms of TiO_2 are semiconductors. UVB or UVA2 photons can promote electrons from the valence band to the conduction band, generating simple electrons and positively charged spaces called holes. After formation, electrons and holes either recombine or migrate rapidly in about 10^{-11} second to the particle surface where they react with the surrounding medium. In aqueous environment, this can lead to formation of ROS and in vitro cellular DNA damage has been reported in one study.[41] As inorganic filters do not penetrate into layers of epidermis containing living cells, this phenomenon does not seem to play a significant role in clinical use of sunscreens. Nevertheless, the photoreactivity of inorganic UV filters reduce their protective efficacy.

For this reason, TiO_2 and ZnO particles are often coated with dimethicone or silica which stabilizes the filter substances.[1] Another possibility is to integrate micronized inorganic UV filters together with organic filters into solid lipid nanoparticles (SLN). In SLN, the inorganic filter pigment is embedded in association with lipophilic organic UV filters such as cinnamates into a drug-carrying solid lipid phase at nanoscale that is coated with triglycerids (Fig. 8). This triglycerid envelope permits to establish two-phase UV filter delivery systems by dispersion of SLN within an aqueous phase by high-pressure homogenization.[42,43] In SLN, organic UV filters and TiO_2 stabilize each other and their association yields higher SPF than the two filters separately. The embedding into a solid lipid matrix inhibits the direct contact between TiO_2 crystals and water and thereby prevents the formation of ROS by TiO_2 photoreactions. It furthermore reduces the intrinsic irritation provoked by TiO_2 and the photoallergenic potential of cinnamate filter molecules.[43]

Inorganic UV filters are characterized by good substantivity by fixation to stratum corneum proteins and little or no penetration into the skin. ZnO in a phenyl trimethicone solution was even shown to inhibit transdermal pesticide penetration, whereas TiO_2 alone had no effect.[33]

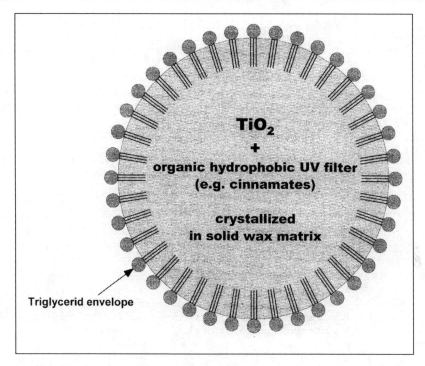

Figure 8. Solid lipid nanoparticles (SLN) for coating of inorganic UV filters.

Immunologic sensitization to inorganic filter pigments has not been reported so far.[1] They are therefore ideal sunscreen agents for young children and patients with pre-existing skin lesions.

Efficacy of Sunscreens

Sunscreen SPF is defined by the product's capacity of protecting from UV-induced erythema. If applied correctly, sunscreens are therefore by definition effective against sunburn.

But today, consumers expect sunscreen use to also protect them from the other harmful effects of UVR that have been developed above. It is difficult to comment on the "real" efficacy of sunscreens for other indications, especially for tumor prevention, for two major reasons:

- Studies on the protective efficacy of sunscreens against skin aging and cutaneous carcinogenesis often use animal models in which these changes are induced within weeks after UV irradiation. However, in human beings, cutaneous carcinogenesis is a multi-step process developing over several decades. As skin tumor formation in humans seems to be a much more complex scenario than in mouse models, the observations obtained in these models can be transferred to the situation in humans only with great caution. In the same way, murine skin aging models do not necessarily reflect the conditions in human skin.
- Skin tumors arising a very long time after irradiation, up to 40 years, the entire epidemiologic data available today was obtained with sunscreen agents commercialized before the introduction of UVA1/UVA2 filters and last generation broad band filters. Although sunscreen use was already wide-spread in the 1980s, the advances in sunscreen development achieved since that time concerning the coverage of the entire UVA spectrum and filter photostability do without any doubt contribute to the long-term efficacy of sunscreens.

Factors affecting the efficacy of sunscreens are essentially inadequate application and external elimination.

Whereas SPF testing protocol is based on an application of 2 mg/cm^2 of sunscreen, under real life conditions users were found to apply rather amounts about 0.5 mg/cm^2. Under these application conditions, a SPF50 sunscreen indeed provides a SPF of only 5.[44] Indeed protection increases exponentially with increasing sunscreen concentration.[45] Some sites such as back, lateral sides of the neck and ears are regularly missed during sunscreen application. Because of their white appearance, inorganic sunscreens are often applied in lesser amounts than organic filters which obviously even more decreases their efficacy compared to the one that could be expected from their UVB-SPF/UVA-PF.[46]

Most people apply sunscreens only occasionally for important and planned sun exposure, mostly during leisure time and holidays. However, as the greatest part of cumulative lifetime UV exposure occurs outside these periods, i.e., through short-time but repeated daily outdoor stays and by UVAR indoor, it is not surprising that daily use of a sunscreen is more protective against UV-induced skin changes than intermittent use of the same product.[47]

When correctly used, sunscreens provide a satisfactory but not complete protection against photodermatoses: Light forms of polymorphous light eruption, actinic herpes labialis, solar urticaria and actinic reticuloid can be prevented by broad spectrum sunscreens.[1,48] Broad-spectrum sunscreens with high UVB-SPF also protect lupus erythematodes patients from flares.[49]

UVAR is the principal responsible for UV-induced skin aging.[50] For this reason, only studies that assess dermal changes after solar simulating irradiation, i.e., containing UVA, are representative of the skin aging process in humans. In reconstructed epidermis,[51] mouse models,[52,53] and humans in vivo,[54] only sunscreens with high protection factors in both the UVB and the UVA spectrum were found to diminish skin aging effects. But even with MXS the protection remained incomplete although the test was performed with little UVA doses and after repeated long-term exposure, elastotic changes appeared even in sunscreen-protected skin areas. Phillips et al emphasized the importance of consequent daily application in prevention of skin aging: They showed that forgetting sunscreen application only every fourth day significantly impairs treatment benefits in long-term use.[47] But the efficacy and safety of sunscreens in skin aging prevention has not been established for long-term use over several years.

To prevent cutaneous photo-immunosuppression, sunscreens must provide protection against both UVBR and UVAR. But even broad spectrum sunscreens can only partially restore Langerhans cell numbers, delayed-type hypersensitivity to recall antigens and contact hypersensitivity (CHS) response to chemical allergens.[24,51,55] A nearly complete conservation of CHS is only obtained with sunscreens offering high UVA-PPD protection with a superiority of mexoryls compared to avobenzone.[51] In humans, sunscreen protection against photoinduced immunosuppression is not correlated to SPF and it is inferior to protection from erythema.[24]

The protective value of sunscreens against photocarcinogenesis is difficult to access because of the long time span between the beginning of UV exposure and the appearance of a clinically perceptible skin tumor in humans. Although sunscreens are widely used since the 1960s, the incidence of melanoma and nonmelanoma skin cancer is steadily increasing. This raises some doubt about the capacity of sunscreens to prevent cutaneous photocarcinogenesis. Two randomized case-control studies, one conducted over only six months[56] and another one conducted over 4.5 years,[57] found a reduced number of new actinic keratoses (AK) and a higher number of remission of pre-existing AK in the group treated with daily sunscreen compared to the placebo group. The benefit of daily sunscreen application was in the order of an average of one AK avoided per person over the 4.5-year study period.[57] Concerning squamous cell carcinoma (SCC), Wulf et al found a delay in the incidence of UV-provoked tumors in a mouse model with sunscreen protection compared to an unprotected control group. But finally, earlier or later even in the sunscreen-protected group nearly all mice developed skin cancer.[58] Although sunscreens seem to have some delaying effect on AK and SCC, a complete protection cannot be achieved even by daily application. But none of these studies examined last generation broad spectrum filters. For the evaluation of this new substance group, only preclinical assays are available to date:

Several studies in mice[59] and in humans[51,60,61] have shown an inhibition by sunscreens of p53 expression increase after UV irradiation, considered as a marker of DNA damage, but no impact on the appearance of p53 mutations. In these studies, TiO_2 was superior to OMC. A product containing MSX, MXL, avobenzone and TiO_2 with an UVA-PF (PPD) of 14 completely suppressed p53 expression in humans whereas another sunscreen having a UVA-PF of 7 and containing only avobenzone and TiO_2 as UVA filters did not.[51] The use of reduced p53 expression as efficacy marker of sunscreens is subject of controversy: Indeed p53 is a pro-apoptotic protein that intervenes in the organism's natural anti-tumor defense. Its suppression is therefore not an ideal criterion for the evaluation of anti-photocarcinogenic activity.

MSX and OMC were found to provide equal protection against pyrimidine dimer formation in mice that were irradiated with a solar simulator. But when polychromatic light was used that contained only UVA and visible light, MSX protected better than OMC.[62] The same workgroup reported that MSX completely abrogated UV-induced DNA fragmentation in a comet assay.[51] In vivo they described a superiority of MSX compared to OMC in preventing tumor formation in mice after UV irradiation.[63] One should notice, however, that all cited studies on MSX activity[51,54,62,63] have been done at the research center of L'Oréal (Clichy, France) who is the manufacturer of mexoryls.

A randomized controlled trial over a 4.5-year period on 1383 adult patients in Australia found a reduced incidence of SCC in the patient group that applied daily a SPF15+ sunscreen compared to the group without photoprotection, but no difference between these two groups in incidence of basal cell carcinomas (BCC).[64] This lack to protect from BCC incidence in adults may be explained by the fact that BCC is probably induced by sun exposure during childhood and adolescence[65] whereas SCC incidence is related to cumulative UV dose including chronic exposure during later phases of life.

The positive or negative role of sunscreens in the development of melanoma has produced major controversy: Some retrospective studies published in the late 1990s concluded that melanoma incidence was higher among sunscreen users and that, paradoxically, sunscreens may induce melanoma.[66-69] These studies were criticized for confounding, e.g., people who are at most risk of burning and most likely to develop melanoma are also most likely to use sunscreens.[70] Two meta-analyses on all data published between 1966 and 2003 did not confirm any relation between sunscreen use and melanoma incidence, neither in positive nor in negative sense.[71,72]

How to explain this confusion? Wavelengths that induce melanoma are not known. The literature emphasizes the role of acute-intermittent sun exposure with sunburn, especially during childhood and adolescence,[73,74] which suggests a role of UVBR in melanoma induction. On the other hand, the augmented melanoma incidence among former PUVA patients[75] demonstrates that UVAR probably also contributes to melanoma initiation. Finally, genetic susceptibility that is not controlled by sun protection habits may play a more important role in melanoma tumorigenesis than previously suspected.

In summary, the to date available epidemiologic data do not prove a protective role of sunscreens against melanoma and BCC, although both tumors are at least partially UV-induced and they show only an incomplete effect against AK, SCC and skin aging. This may have several reasons that are linked under each other:

- The use of sunscreens with insufficient UVB-SPF and lack of coverage in the UVA spectrum: Most data were collected before last generation broad spectrum filters were available. Based on the results of preclinical studies with the new filters, we can expect better protection performance with these sunscreens. But as the time span between UV exposure and skin cancer manifestation in humans is extremely long, incidence numbers will not decrease before several decades.
- The inadequate choice of study population for prospective epidemiologic studies: For both BCC and melanoma, the role of UV exposure especially during the early years of life has been emphasized.[65,74] Studies should therefore focus on protective intervention during this period which makes them yet more difficult to realize as the corresponding tumors arise

about 40 years after critical sun exposure. Gallagher et al reported a randomized controlled intervention trail on white children in which the treatment group that applied a broad spectrum SPF30 sunscreen before each sun exposure over three years developed fewer nevi than the unprotected group. The difference was particularly significant in freckled white children who developed 30% to 40% fewer nevi in the sunscreen-protected group than freckled children assigned to the control group.[76] As high nevus density is recognized as a risk factor of melanoma, this study may indicate a protective potential of broad spectrum sunscreens if they are used regularly during childhood.

- The induction of overexposure behavior by sunscreens protecting effectively against erythema: Autier et al confirmed that sunscreen users usually stay longer in the sunlight than unprotected people.[77] High SPFs suppress the alarm signal of UVB-induced sunburn and induce a false hope of "complete" protection in its users. But DNA damage and photo-immunosuppression are induced already by suberythemal UV doses. Especially if UVA protection of the employed sunscreen is not perfect, overexposure can induce severe photodamage that is not immediately obvious to the sunscreen user.

- The suppression of natural photoprotection mechanisms by the currently marketed sunscreens: Melanine synthesis, release of melanosomes and thickening of stratum corneum are mainly triggered by UVBR that is effectively blocked by modern sunscreens. In the case of repeated sun exposure with a topical photoprotectant having an elevated SPF/PPD (UVB/UVA protection) ratio, the sunscreen user is thus more submitted to the harmful epidermal and dermal effects of UVAR than an unprotected individual who will undergo natural adaptation that protects against both UVBR and UVAR. This is consistent with the observation that people with important chronic UV exposure by occupational outdoor activity, e.g., agricultural workers, who typically have tan and skin thickening in sun-exposed sites, are at a significantly reduced risk of melanoma compared to indoor workers with intermittent UV exposure.[73,74]

Sunscreens and Vitamin D3 Synthesis

Besides its well-known key role in skeletal homeostasis, vitamin D has been reported to have anti-carcinogenic properties. Some studies found an inverse correlation between solar UVB exposure and mortality from cancers, including colon, breast and prostate cancer and between sun exposure and incidence of colon cancer. But these reports failed to eliminate confounding by geographic variations in population genetics or lifestyle behaviors, diet and socioeconomic status of the examined population. Moreover, several other studies did not confirm a role of vitamin D in preventing these cancers (reviewed in ref. 6). An antiproliferative effect for vitamin D is also supported by cell culture and animal model experiments, but the vitamin D concentrations needed to produce these data were generally in the toxic range for humans.

As the cutaneous synthesis of cholecalciferol (vitamin D3) from 7-DHC in cell membranes is exclusively triggered by UVR in the UVB-spectrum (Fig. 1), an interference of high SPF sunscreens with vitamin D3 synthesis seems, at least theoretically, possible. Reduced serum concentration of 25-hydroxyvitamin D has been reported in some persons after regular sunscreen use.[78]

Cutaneous cholecalciferol production is saturated at 10% to 20% of the original epidermal 7-DHC concentration.[79] This threshold amount is achieved by far suberythemal UVB doses in the order of 0.25% DEM to the face and backs of hands 3 times weekly.[6] Additional UVBR transforms previtamin D3 into the biologically inactive metabolites tachysterol and lumisterol.[79] Two prospective controlled studies, one conducted in Australia at a latitude of 37°S with a SPF17 sunscreen and another one done in Spain at a latitude of 41°N with a SPF15 sunscreen, did not find decrease of 25-hydroxyvitamin D serum levels in the protected group compared to the control group, even not in elder individuals of 70 years and older. Secondary hyperparathyroidism and change in markers of bone remodeling were not more frequent in the sunscreen users.[80,81] Another workgroup followed the 25-hydroxyvitamin D serum levels of eight xeroderma pigmentosum (XP) patients who practiced for their severe DNA repair enzyme defect rigorous photoprotection by avoidance, clothing and sunscreens. Over a 6-year study period, the 25-hydroxyvitamin D serum levels remained in the low normal range with normal levels of PTH and calcitriol.[82] Of course, cutaneous vitamin D3 synthesis may be more difficult in countries at higher latitude than those where the cited studies were conducted, especially in the elder population. On the other hand, housebound elderly are certainly not the principal consumers of sunscreens. For the active population who is continuously or intermittently exposed to sunlight, the given data on the impact of UVB filters on photo-induced vitamin D production does not permit to change recommendation for regular sunscreen use. The actual sunscreen use habits providing only an incomplete protection from UVBR, the remaining UVB exposure seems to be widely sufficient to guarantee cutaneous vitamin D3 synthesis. Moreover, alimentary intake of vitamin D3, e.g., in form of fortified milk or orange juice, can help to maintain sufficient plasma levels.[6] For patients at real risk for vitamin D deficiency, dietary supplementation is efficacious and safe.

Alternative Photoprotective Agents

A great number of substances for topical application have been proposed for photoprotective purpose, e.g., antioxidants acting as radical scavengers, DNA repair enzymes, oligonucleotides stimulating natural melanogenesis, vitamin A derivatives and active botanic components. They have anti-erythemogenic effect and they provided DNA and connective tissue protection in mouse models or in vitro assays after UV irradiation.[7] An anticarcinogenic effect in healthy humans has been described with none of these alternative photoprotectants. Some of them, especially α-tocopherol (vitamin E), L-ascorbic acid (vitamin C) and ferulic acid, are sometimes added to sunscreen preparations. Others are still at an experimental state. In a group of XP patients, topical application of phage T_4 endonuclease V (dimericine) during one year resulted in a 30% decrease of BCC incidence and a 70% decrease of AK incidence.[83] Such significant efficacy of dimericine has not been demonstrated so far in individuals without XP.

Antioxidants have also been tested for photoprotection in oral form. The most currently employed substance is β-carotene with a recommended dose of 120 to 180 mg daily. It diminishes photosensitivity in mild forms of photodermatoses and can moderately increase MED in the healthy caucasian population.[84] This systemic antioxidant may cause cosmetical problems in some individuals by induction of brown-reddish skin color. However, oral β-carotene failed to prevent AK, SCC and BCC in a randomized controlled trial over 4.5 years.[57,64]

Although the photoprotective effects of these alternative agents are promising, their anti-erythemogenic and anti-elastotic action is by far inferior to the one of sunscreens and their efficacy in skin tumor prevention is not established. They may complement the photoprotective activity of sunscreens, but they will probably not replace them as first line photoprotective means.

Discussion and Conclusion

80 years after their commercial introduction, sunscreens remain still most effective for what they have originally been made for, i.e., protection against sunburn and other short-term UV effects such as photodermatoses. They have limited effect in preventing skin aging, AK and SCC. Also in some particular conditions such as genetic disorders or post-transplant iatrogenic immunosuppression that expose to important risk of intermediate-term development of multiple skin cancers, benefit from regular sunscreen use has been clinically established. However, based on this review of clinical and epidemiological data, today's sunscreen formulations cannot pretend to provide protection from nonsquamous cell skin cancer for the general adult population. The genetic part in the etiology of these tumors is not sufficient to explain their still rising incidence worldwide despite wide-spread sunscreen use.

This disappointing lack of efficacy may partially be due to inadequate use of suncare products: Users do generally not apply them for daily short-term outdoor stays and indoor exposure to UVAR traversing window glass, although these conditions are responsible of the major part of cumulative life-time UV dose in the general population having rather indoor occupation. However, non-observance of daily application has been shown to cancel the benefit of sunscreens in long-term use. Even for planned UV exposure, sunscreens are usually applied in insufficient quantity compared to the protection factor testing conditions which considerably reduces the effective SPF.[44,45] Moreover, users often omit re-application every two hours that is recommended to compensate external product elimination. On the other hand, a consequent and lifelong use of sunscreens in the recommended amounts is not practicable for time and financial expense and safety raisons: In summer 2007, the price of a good quality broad spectrum sunscreen with SPF50+ and an SPF/PPD <2.5 ratio is about 300 €/kg in France. Before sun exposure on the beach, a man with a body surface area of 1.8 m^2 who respects the recommended sunscreen amounts has to apply 36 g for total body protection which causes costs of 10.80 € for only one application. On the other hand, the innocuousness of sunscreen long-term use in the recommended amounts has never been examined with regard to their irritation potential, interaction with toxic substances in the environment, systemic absorption, endocrine activity and clearance.[31] Another reason for sunscreen inefficacy my be the actual use of inadequate efficacy markers for measuring sunscreen protection potency: Both SPF and currently employed UVA-PF markers such as PPD or critical wavelength are not related to photostability, remanence, genome protection and immunoprotection which are however critical parameters for cancer prevention.[85] For the consumer, sunscreen choice is no easy deal: For lack of standardization in UVA protection testing, UVA-PF is often not indicated even for sunscreens with protective activity in this band region. The efficacy of sunscreens is most of all determined by their UV filter composition. But for ingredient lists, the manufacturer can use INCI, IUPAC and trade names of filters which makes it difficult to the user to identify the respective substances. In Europe the consumer is furthermore confronted to confusing multi-language labeling and ingredient lists containing abbreviations in foreign language.

With regard to this review, physicians should omit messages to their patients suggesting that sunscreens can protect from BCC and melanoma. Dermatologists should be concerned to preserve our discipline's credibility in a context where public information is too much dominated by commercial interest of cosmetic and pharmaceutical industry. Sunscreens in their current form are probably not the key to skin cancer prevention in the general population. More basic, but highly effective measures should still be encouraged. This includes sun avoidance especially during peak UVR between 10:00 A.M. and 4:00 P.M., UV-absorbing window filters, photoprotective clothing and wearing broad-brimmed hats. Sunscreens can perfectly complete these recommendations, but they should never cancel them. Much educational work is yet to be done to overcome the popularity of sunbathing and the tanning ideal that are still wide-spread in our society especially in adolescents and young adults. After 30 years, primary and secondary prevention programs now begin to show positive outcomes in Australia, especially in melanoma incidence and survival.[86]

Nevertheless, the benefit of sunscreens against short-term harmful effects of UVR, in cancer prevention in patients with genetic or pharmacological risk of skin tumors and—to a minor degree—even in prevention of skin aging and SCC in the general population is undeniable. Good sunscreen products afford both high SPF and a well balanced SPF/PPD ratio. At the moment, a SPF/PPD ratio of less than 2.5 should be recommended, but in the future even lower SPF/PPD ratios may become possible. Their regular use at least for unavoidable intermittent UV exposure seems to be safe and efficacious. Alternative topical and systemic photoprotectants such as antioxidants and DNA repair enzymes are still at an experimental state in skin cancer prevention.

Major progress has been made during the past 20 years in the sunscreen domain with the development of potent UVA filters, micronization of inorganic sunscreens and synthesis of new photostable and well-tolerated organic filter molecules. These recent sunprotective products will improve the acceptance of sunscreens and thereby the observation of recommendations. They protect us from sunlight probably better than former UV filters that were used in most epidemiologic studies available today on sunscreen efficacy. Considering the slow development of skin cancer in humans, the benefit of our actual sunscreen market will take years to become clinically and epidemiologically obvious. This review will probably have to be revised when the outcome of long-term studies with recent sunscreens will be available.

References

1. Kullavanijaya P, Lim HW. Photoprotection. J Am Acad Dermatol 2005; 52:937-58.
2. Schaefer H, Moyal D, Fourtanier A. Recent advances in sun protection. Semin Cut Med Surg 1998; 17:266-75.
3. Jeanmougin M. Photodermatoses et photoprotection. Paris: Deltacom, 1983.
4. Young AR. Chromophores in human skin. Phys Med Biol 1997; 42:789-802.
5. Goukassian DA, Eller MS, Yaar M et al. Thymidine dinucleotide mimics the effect of solar-simulated irradiation on p53 and p53-regulated proteins. J Invest Dermatol 1999; 112:25-31.
6. Wolpowitz D, Gilchrest BA. The vitamin D questions: How much do you need and how should you get it? J Am Acad Dermatol 2006; 54:301-17.
7. Pinnell SR. Cutaneous photodamage, oxidative stress and topical antioxidant protection. J Am Acad Dermatol 2003; 48:1-19.
8. Wenczl E, Pool S, Timmerman AJ et al. Physiological doses of ultraviolet irradiation induce DNA strand breaks in cultured human melanocytes, as detected by means of an immunochemical assay. Photochem Photobiol 1997; 66:826-30.
9. Parsons PG, Hayward IP. Inhibition of DNA repair synthesis by sunlight. Photochem Photobiol 1985; 42:287-93.
10. Marrot L, Belaidi JP, Meunier JR et al. The human melanocyte as a particular target for UVA radiation and an endpoint for photoprotection assessment. Photochem Photobiol 1999; 69:686-93.
11. Mouret S, Baudouin C, Charveron M et al. Cyclobutane pyrimidine dimers are predominant DNA lesions in whole skin exposed to UVA radiation. Proc Natl Acad Sci USA 2006; 103:13765-70.
12. Hönigsmann H. Erythema and pigmentation. Photodermatol Photoimmunol Photomed 2002; 18:75-81.
13. Eller MS, Yaar M, Gilchrest BA. DNA damage and melanogenesis. Nature 1994; 372:413-4.
14. Gilchrest BA, Park HY, Eller MS et al. Mechanisms of ultraviolet-induced pigmentation. Photochem Photobiol 1996; 63:1-10.
15. Gange RW, Blackett AD, Matzinger EA et al. Comparative protection efficiency of UVA and UVB-induced tans against erythema and formation of endonuclease-sensitive sites in DNA by UVB in human skin. J Invest Dermatol 1985; 85:362-4.
16. Varani J, Spearman D, Perone P et al. Inhibition of type I procollagen synthesis by damaged collagen in photoaged skin and by collagenase-degraded collagen in vitro. Am J Pathol 2001; 158:931-42.
17. Kawaguchi Y, Tanaka H, Okada T et al. Effect of reactive oxygen species on the elastin mRNA expression in cultured human dermal fibroblasts. Free Radic Biol Med 1997; 23:192-5.
18. Kelly DA, Young AR, McGregor JM et al. Sensitivity to sunburn is associated with susceptibility to UVR-induced suppression of cutaneous cell-mediated immunity. J Exp Med 2000; 191:561-6.
19. Bestak R, Halliday GM. Chronic low-dose UVA irradiation induces local suppression of contact hypersensitivity, Langerhans cell depletion and suppressor cell avtivation in C3H/HeJ mice. Photochem Photobiol 1996; 64:969-74.
20. Nghiem DX, Kazimi N, Clydesdale G et al. Ultraviolet A radiation suppresses an established immune response: implications for sunscreen design. J Invest Dermatol 2001; 117:1193-9.
21. DeBuys HV, Levy SB, Murray JC et al. Modern approaches to photoprotection. Dermatol Clin 2000; 18:577-90.
22. Lacour JP. Carcinogenesis of basal cell carcinomas: genetics and molecular mechanisms. Br J Dermatol 2002; 146 Suppl 61:17-9.
23. Ting WW, Vest CD, Sontheimer R. Practical and experimental consideration of sun protection in dermatology. Int J Dermatol 2003; 42:505-13.
24. Kelly DA, Seed PT, Young AR et al. A commercial sunscreen's protection against ultraviolet radiation-induced immunosuppression is more than 50% lower than protection against sunburn in humans. J Invest Dermatol 2003; 120:65-71.
25. Diffey BL, Tanner PR, Matts PJ et al. In vitro assessment of the broad-spectrum ultraviolet protection of sunscreen products. J Am Acad Dermatol 2000; 43:1024-35.
26. Ciba Specialty Chemicals. Ciba Tinosorb® product brochure. Basel, 2002.
27. Szczurko C, Dompmartin A, Michel M et al. Photocontact allergy to oxybenzone: ten years of experience. Photodermatol Photoimmunol Photomed 1994; 10:144-7.
28. Journé F, Marguery MC, Rakotondrazafy J et al. Sunscreen sensitization: a 5-year-study. Acta Derm Venereol 1999; 79:211-3.
29. Bouillon C. Recent advances in sun protection. J Dermatol Sci 2000; 23 Suppl 1:S57-61.
30. Sarveiya V, Risk S, Benson HAE. Liquid chromatographic assay for common sunscreen agents: application to in vivo assessment of skin penetration and systemic absorption in human volunteers. J Chromatogr B 2004; 803:225-31.

31. Janjua NR, Mogensen B, Andersson AM et al. Systemic absorption of the sunscreens benzophenone-3, octyl-methoxycinnamate and 3-(4-methyl-benzylidene) camphor after whole-body topical application and reproductive hormone levels in humans. J Invest Dermatol 2004; 123:57-61.

32. Schlumpf M, Cotton B, Conscience M et al. In vitro and in vivo estrogenicity of UV screens. Environ Health Perspect 2001; 109:239-44.

33. Brand RM, Pike J, Wilson RM et al. Sunscreens containing physical UV blockers can increase transdermal absorption of pesticides. Toxicol Ind Health 2003; 19:9-16.

34. Pont AR, Charron AR, Brand RM. Active ingredients in sunscreens act as topical penetration enhancers for the herbicide 2,4-dichlorophenoxyacetic acid. Toxicol Appl Pharmacol 2004; 195:348-54.

35. Sutherland JC, Griffin KP. P-aminobenzoic acid can sensitize the formation of pyrimidine dimers in DNA: direct chemical evidence. Photochem Photobiol 1984; 40:391-4.

36. Gasparro FP, Mitchnick M, Nash JF. A review of sunscreen safety and efficacy. Photochem Photobiol 1998; 68:243-56.

37. Chatelain E, Gabard B. Photostabilization of butyl methoxydibenzoylmethane (avobenzone) and ethyl-hexyl methoxycinnamate by bis-ethylhexyloxyphenol methoxyphenyl triazine (Tinosorb S), a new UV broadband filter. Photochem Photobiol 2001; 74:401-6.

38. Ashby J, Tinwell H, Plautz J et al. Lack of binding to isolated estrogen or androgen receptors and inactivity in the immature rat uterotrophic assay, of the ultraviolet sunscreen filters Tinosorb M-active and Tinosorb S. Regul Toxicol Pharmacol 2001; 34:287-91.

39. Moseley H, Cameron H, MacLeod T et al. New sunscreens confer improved protection for photosensitive patients in the blue light region. Br J Dermatol 2001; 145:789-94.

40. Mitchnick MA, Fairhurst D, Pinnell SR. Microfine zinc oxide (Z-cote) as a photostable UVA/UVB sunblock agent. J Am Acad Dermatol 1999; 40:85-90.

41. Nakagawa Y, Wakuri S, Sakamoto K et al. The photogenotoxicity of titanium dioxide particles. Mutat Res 1997; 394:125-32.

42. Müller RH, Mäder K, Gohla S. Solid lipid nanoparticles (SLN) for controlled drug delivery—a review of the state of the art. Eur J Pharm Biopharm 2000; 50:161-71.

43. Villalobos-Hernández JR, Müller-Goymann CC. Sun protection enhancement of titanium dioxide crystals by the use of carnauba wax nanoparticles: The synergistic interaction between organic and inorganic sunscreens at nanoscale. Int J Pharm 2006; 322:161-70.

44. Wulf HC, Stender IM, Lock-Andersen J. Sunscreens used at the beach do not protect against erythema: A new definition of SPF is proposed. Photodermatol Photoimmunol Photomed 1997; 13:129-32.

45. Faurschou A, Wulf HC. The relation between sun protection factor and amount of sunscreen applied in vivo. Br J Dermatol 2007; 156:716-9.

46. Diffey BL, Grice J. The influence of sunscreen type on photoprotection. Br J Dermatol 1997; 137:103-5.

47. Phillips TJ, Bhawan J, Yaar M et al. Effect of daily versus intermittent sunscreen application on solar simulated UV-radiation-induced skin response in humans. J Am Acad Dermatol 2000; 43:618-8.

48. Béani JC. Photoprotection externe. In: Société Française de Photodermatologie, ed. Photodermatologie. Rueil-Malmaison: Arnette, 2003: 131-46.

49. Stege H, Budde MA, Grether-Beck S et al. Evaluation of the capacity of sunscreens to photoprotect lupus erythematosus patients by employing the photoprovocation test. Photodermatol Photoimmunol Photomed 2000; 16:256-9.

50. Kligman LH, Sayre RM. An action spectrum for ultraviolet induced elastosis in hairless mice: quantification of elastosis by image analysis. Photochem Photobiol 1991; 53:237-42.

51. Fourtanier A, Bernerd F, Bouillon C et al. Protection of skin biological targets by different types of sunscreens. Photodermatol Photoimmunol Photomed 2006; 22:22-32.

52. Kligman LH, Agin PP, Sayre RM. Broad-spectrum sunscreens with UVA I and UVA II absorbers provide increased protection against solar simulation radiation-induced damage in hairless mice. J Soc Cosmet Chem 1996; 47:129-55.

53. Tsukahara K, Moriwaki S, Hotta M et al. The effect of sunscreen on skin elastase activity induced by ultraviolet-A irradiation. Biol Pharm Bull 2005; 28:2302-7.

54. Seité S, Moyal D, Richard S et al. Mexoryl SX: a broad absorption UVA filter protects human skin from the effects of repeated suberythemal doses of UVA. J Photochem Photobiol B 1998; 44:69-76.

55. Serre I, Cano JP, Picot MC et al. Immunosuppression induced by acute solar-simulated ultraviolet exposure in humans: prevention by a sunscreen with a sun protection factor of 15 and high UVA protection. J Am Acad Dermatol 1997; 37:187-94.

56. Thompson SC, Jolley D, Marks R. Reduction of solar keratoses by regular sunscreen use. N Engl J Med 1993; 329:1147-51.

57. Darlington S, Williams G, Neale R et al. A randomized controlled trial to assess sunscreen application and beta carotene supplementation in the prevention of solar keratoses. Arch Dermatol 2003; 139:451-5.

58. Wulf HC, Poulsen T, Brodthagen H et al. Sunscreens for delay of ultraviolet induction of skin tumors. J Am Acad Dematol 1982; 7:194-202.
59. Ananthaswamy HN, Loughlin SM, Cox P et al. Sunlight and skin cancer: inhibition of p53 mutations in UV-irradiated mouse skin by sunscreens. Nat Med 1997; 3:510-4.
60. Krekels G, Voorter C, Kuik F et al. DNA-protection by sunscreens: p53-immunostaining. Eur J Dermatol 1997; 7:259-62.
61. Berne B, Ponten J, Ponten F. Decreased p53 expression in chronically sun-exposed human skin after topical photoprotection. Photodermatol Photoimmunol Photomed 1998; 14:148-53.
62. Ley RD, Fourtanier A. Sunscreen protection against ultraviolet radiation-induced pyrimidine dimers in mouse epidermal DNA. Photochem Photobiol 1997; 65:1007-11.
63. Fourtanier A. Mexoryl SX protects against solar-simulated UVR-induced photocarcinogenesis in mice. Photochem Photobiol 1996; 64:688-93.
64. Green A, Williams G, Neale R et al. Daily sunscreen application and betacarotene supplementation in prevention of basal-cell and squamous-cell carcinomas of the skin: a randomized controlled trial. Lancet 1999; 354:723-9.
65. Gallagher RP, Hill GB, Bajdik CD et al. Sunlight exposure, pigmentary factors and risk of nonmelanocytic skin cancer. I. Basal cell carcinoma. Arch Dermatol 1995; 131:157-63.
66. Westerdahl J, Olsson H, Masback A et al. Is the use of sunscreens a risk factor for malignant melanoma? Melanoma Res 1995; 5:59-65.
67. Whiteman DC, Valery P, McWhirter W et al. Risk factors for childhood melanoma in Queensland, Australia. Int J Cancer 1997; 70:26-31.
68. Wolf P, Quehenberger F, Mulegger R et al. Phenotypic markers, sunlight-related factors and sunscreen use in patients with cutaneous melanoma: an Austrian cas-control study. Melanoma Res 1998; 8:370-8.
69. Westerdahl J, Ingvar C, Masback A et al. Sunscreen use and malignant melanoma. Int J Cancer 2000; 87:145-50.
70. Diffey BL. Sunscreens and melanoma: The future looks bright. Br J Dermatol 2005; 153:378-81.
71. Huncharek M, Kupelnick B. Use of topical sunscreens and the risk of malignant melanoma: a meta-analysis of 9067 patients from 11 case-control studies. Am J Public Health 2002; 92:1173-7.
72. Dennis LK, Beane Freeman LE, Van Beek MJ. Sunscreen use and the risk of melanoma: a quantitative review. Ann Intern Med 2003; 139:966-78.
73. Elwood JM, Jopson J. Melanoma and sun exposure: an overview of published studies. Int J Cancer 1997; 73:198-203.
74. Walter SD, King WD, Marrett LD. Association of cutaneous malignant melanoma with intermittent exposure to ultraviolet radiation: results of a case-control study in Ontario, Canada. Int J Epidemiol 1999; 28:418-27.
75. Stern RS; PUVA Follow up study. The risk of melanoma in association with long-term exposure to PUVA. J Am Acad Dermatol 2001; 44:755-61.
76. Gallagher RP, Rivers JK, Lee TK et al. Broad-spectrum sunscreen use and the development of new nevi in white children: A randomized controlled trial. JAMA 2000; 283:2955-60.
77. Autier P, Dore JF, Negrier S et al. Sunscreen use and duration of sun exposure: a double-blind, randomized trial. J Natl Cancer Inst 1999; 91:1304-9.
78. Matsuoka LY, Wortman J, Hanifan N et al. Chronic sunscreen use decreases circulating concentrations of 25-hydroxyvitamin D: a preliminary study. Arch Dermatol 1988; 124:1802-4.
79. MacLaughlin JA, Anderson RR, Holick MF. Spectral character of sunlight modulates photosynthesis of previtamin D3 and its photoisomers in human skin. Science 1982; 216:1001-3.
80. Marks R, Foley PA, Jolley D et al. The effects of regular sunscreen use on vitamin D levels in an Australian population: results of a randomized controlled trial. Arch Dermatol 1995; 131:415-21.
81. Farrerons J, Barnadas M, Rodriguez J et al. Clinically prescribed sunscreen (sun protection factor 15) does not decrease serum vitamin D concentration sufficiently either to induce changes in parathyroid function or in metabolic markers. Br J Dermatol 1998; 139:422-7.
82. Sollitto RB, Kraemer KH, DiGiovanna JJ. Normal vitamin D levels can be maintained despite rigorous photoprotection: six years' experience with xeroderma pigmentosum. J Am Acad Dermatol 1997; 37:942-7.
83. Yarosh D, Klein J, O'Connor A et al. Effect of topically applied T_4 endonuclease V in liposomes on skin cancer in xeroderma pigmentosum: a randomized study. Xeroderma Pigmentosum Study Group. Lancet 2001; 357:926-9.
84. Stahl W, Krutmann J. Systemische Photoprotektion durch Karotinoide. Hautarzt 2006; 57:281-5.
85. Leroy D. Les crèmes solaires. Ann Dermatol Venereol 1999; 126:357-63.
86. McCarthy WH. The Australian experience in sun protection and screening for melanoma. J Surg Oncol 2004; 86:236-45.

CHAPTER 13

UV Damage and DNA Repair in Malignant Melanoma and Nonmelanoma Skin Cancer

Knuth Rass* and Jörg Reichrath

Abstract

Exposition of the skin with solar ultraviolet radiation (UV) is the main cause of skin cancer development. The consistently increasing incidences of melanocytic and nonmelanocytic skin tumors are believed to be at least in part associated with recreational sun exposure. Epidemiological data indicate that excessive or cumulative sunlight exposition takes place years and decades before the resulting malignancies arise. The most important defense mechanisms that protect human skin against UV radiation involve melanin synthesis and active repair mechanisms. DNA is the major target of direct or indirect UV-induced cellular damage. Low pigmentation capacity in white Caucasians and rare congenital defects in DNA repair are mainly responsible for protection failures. The important function of nucleotide excision DNA repair (NER) to protect against skin cancer becomes obvious by the rare genetic disease xeroderma pigmentosum, in which diverse NER genes are mutated.

In animal models, it has been demonstrated that UVB is more effective to induce skin cancer than UVA. UV-induced DNA photoproducts are able to cause specific mutations (UV-signature) in susceptible genes for squamous cell carcinoma (SCC) and basal cell carcinoma (BCC). In SCC development, UV-signature mutations in the p53 tumor suppressor gene are the most common event, as precancerous lesions reveal ~80% and SCCs >90% UV-specific p53 mutations. Mutations in Hedgehog pathway related genes, especially PTCH1, are well known to represent the most significant pathogenic event in BCC. However, specific UV-induced mutations can be found only in ~50% of sporadic BCCs. Thus, cumulative UVB radiation can not be considered to be the single etiologic risk factor for BCC development.

During the last decades, experimental animal models, including genetically engineered mice, the Xiphophorus hybrid fish, the south american oppossum and human skin xenografts, have further elucidated the important role of the DNA repair system in the multi-step process of UV-induced melanomagenesis. An increasing body of evidence now indicates that nucleotide excision repair is not the only DNA repair pathway that is involved in UV-induced tumorigenesis of melanoma and nonmelanoma skin cancer. An interesting new perspective in DNA damage and repair research lies in the participation of mammalian mismatch repair (MMR) in UV damage correction. As MMR enzyme hMSH2 displays a p53 target gene, is induced by UVB radiation and is involved in NER pathways, studies have now been initiated to elucidate the physiological and pathophysiological role of MMR in malignant melanoma and nonmelanoma skin cancer development.

*Corresponding Author: Knuth Rass—Clinic for Dermatology, Venerology and Allergology, The Saarland University Hospital, 66421 Homburg/Saar, Germany. Email: knuth.rass@uks.eu

Sunlight, Vitamin D and Skin Cancer, edited by Jörg Reichrath. ©2008 Landes Bioscience and Springer Science+Business Media.

Introduction

Sunlight is an indispensable requirement for life on earth by spending the essential thermal energy and facilitating photosynthesis in plants, which in turn supplies our atmosphere with oxygen. On the other hand, ultraviolet radiation of sunlight (UV) can be assumed to be the most important and ubiquitously occurring physical carcinogen inducing melanocytic and nonmelanocytic skin cancer with increasing incidences. The solar UV spectrum consists of UVC (wavelengths below 280 nm), UVB (280-315 nm) and UVA bands (315-400 nm). The predominant part of the short-wave, high-energy and destructive UV spectrum cannot reach the earth's surface: the ozone layer of the outer earth atmosphere absorbs the shorter wavelengths up to ~310 nm (UVC and main part of UVB radiation). The remaining transmitted UV spectrum, i.e., a small UVB and the complete UVA band, is responsible for biological effects in human skin.

UV light does not penetrate the body any deeper than the skin and is absorbed by the different skin layers in a wavelength-dependent manner: UVB is almost completely absorbed by the epidermis; only 10-20% of UVB energy reaches the epidermal stratum basale and the dermal stratum papillare. In contrast, UVA penetrates deeper into the dermis and deposits 30-50% of its energy in the dermal stratum papillare. These absorption characteristics in human skin explain why UVB effects have to be expected predominantly in the epidermis (skin cancer development) and UVA effects in the dermis (solar elastosis, skin ageing). As human skin is continuously exposed to solar UV light, protection strategies that include melanin synthesis and active repair mechanisms were developed to avoid structural damage of the most important UV target molecule, the DNA. DNA is a major epidermal chromophore with an absorption maximum of 260 nm and a continuous absorption-decrease over the UVB and UVA spectra. Excessive or continuing chronic sun exposure, low pigmentation capacity in white Caucasians and rare congenital defects are important factors that may be responsible for failures of these adaptive defense mechanisms.

UVB-and far less UVA-are able to cause molecular DNA rearrangements with formation of specific photoproducts, which are known to be mutagenic. The genotoxic potential of UVA is predominantly due to oxidative DNA damage. If UV-induced mutations concern particular genes involved in signaling pathways of cell cycle control, proliferation, apoptosis or DNA repair, a malignant tumour can emerge. The fact that skin cancer does not occur immediately after sun exposure but with a latency period of years and decades underlines the theory that multiple genomic hits are necessary to establish a malignant phenotype (multistep carcinogenesis). Extending mutations in affected skin cells make it subsequently more probable that these cells gain abilities to progress (activating oncogene mutations) or loose cell growth inhibitory or anti-apoptotic functions (inactivating tumor suppressor gene mutations).

Furthermore, UV radiation displays immunosuppressive effects and is able to generate tolerance against immunogenetic skin tumors. Thus, UV is considered to be a "double-edged sword" causing skin cancer by DNA damage on the one hand and enabling tumor escape from immune surveillance on the other.

In the following essay, the pathogenic role of UV radiation for tumourigenesis of malignant melanoma and nonmelanocytic skin cancer (squamous and basal cell carcinoma) is elucidated, focussing on genotoxic effects of UV radiation and important repair mechanisms to avoid resulting structural DNA damage.

UV Damage and DNA Repair

In 1928 Gates described for the first time that the bactericidal effect of UV radiation is connected with its absorption by prokaryotic DNA.[1] Thirteen years later Hollaender and Emmons observed that the occurrence of mutations in eukaryotic (Fungi) DNA due to UV radiation is wavelength dependent.[2] Thus, the indispensable importance of DNA concerning cell survival and cell transformation on the one hand and the relevance of UV light to induce potentially lethal genomic disruptions on the other was already known in the first half of the last century (for review see refs. 3-5). In the 1960's the essential molecular characteristics of DNA alterations caused directly by UVC and UVB radiation were uncovered:

Beukers and Berends,[6] as well as Setlow and Carrier[7] found covalent interactions between two adjacent pyrimidine bases forming cyclobutane pyrimidine dimers (CPD: thymine dimers, cytosine dimers); later on Varghese und Patrick[8] described another typical dimer formation at di-pyrimidine sites, the 6-4 photoproducts (6-4 PP: thymine-cytosine dimers).

UVC is completely absorbed by the atmospheric ozone layer. Nevertheless, if UVC would reach the earth surface-in consideration of an increasing ozone dismantling-its short wavelength spectrum would hardly allow to penetrate into the human epidermal stratum basale with an effective dose. On the other hand, it has been shown that squamous cell carcinomas (SCC) and fibrosarcomas could be generated by 254 nm UVC irradiation in mice.[9] Thus, it is not clear at present, to what extent UVC would be relevant for the induction of skin cancer in humans if ozone dismantling would continue.

The biological effects of UVA on DNA are different from UVB/UVC and are predominantly indirect: UVA energy is mainly absorbed by chromophores other than DNA. The energetic activation of those chromophores-endogenous or exogenous "photosensitizers" like NADH or different drugs (psoralen, tetracyclines)-causes reactive oxygen species (ROS) by photochemical interactions in vitro. The energy-enhanced photosensitizers themselves (type I) or the aggressive oxygen molecules (type II) in turn react with the DNA molecule leading to DNA single strand breaks and DNA-to-protein crosslinks.[10] The relevance of these findings for carcinogenesis were confirmed by different animal experiments, which demonstrate the induction of SCC's, melanomas and other tumors by UVA alone and an enhancement of the carcinogenic UVB effect by UVA.[11-13] Beside the indirect effects of UVA on DNA, a small part of the UVA spectrum (315-327 nm) is considered to be able to generate CPD's and 6-4 PP directly. Between 328 and 347 nm UVA irradiation can induce both, direct and indirect reaction types of DNA damage (Fig. 1).[14]

UV-induced DNA lesions influence cellular death, aging, mutagenesis and carcinogenesis, if they are not completely rejected by the nuclear DNA repair machinery. The ability to erase DNA photoproducts from bacterial DNA, a process nowadays known as nucleotide excision repair (NER), was discovered in 1964.[15] NER is the main repair system responsible for correcting directly UV-induced DNA damage. Oxidized (indirect) DNA base lesions are removed by essentially two types of activity: base excision repair (BER), involving removal of single lesions by a glycosylase action and NER. In contrast to NER, disruptions in BER as a principle for cancer development are not known so far.

NER failure or exceeding of its repair capacity is one important pathogenic step in UV associated skin cancer development as suggested by the rare autosomal recessive disease xeroderma pigmentosum (XP, Fig. 2): Patients suffering from XP are extremely sun-sensitive with severe sunburns in childhood, are characterized by photo-aged freckled skin and are very prone to sunlight-induced skin tumors (keratoacanthoma, SCC, basal cell carcinoma, melanoma) occurring early in life (childhood-adolescence). As compared to unaffected individuals, skin cancer incidence in XP patients is appr. 2000-fold elevated.[16,17] In 1968 Cleaver[18] initially uncovered the etiology of XP as caused by deficient NER. As a consequence of deficient NER, UV-induced photoproducts accumulate in XP and subsequent mutations can result in malignant phenotypes. Seven different types (complementation groups A-G) and a variant form of XP have been revealed so far. Besides skin cancer development, XP is associated with internal malignancies, neurological and ocular abnormalities. Each complementation group is defined by underlying mutations in genes encoding different NER proteins (XPA-XPG, XPV; Table 1). In short, NER functions as follows: DNA photoproducts were recognized by different protein complexes, CSA/CSB in transcription-coupled repair (TCR) and XPC/hHR23B in global genome repair (GGR), whereas XPA, replication protein A (RPA) and damaged DNA binding protein (DDB)/XPE/p48 join the recognition complex both in TCR and GGR. The complexes combine with TFIIH, a transcription factor containing XPB and XPD, which reveal helicase activity in both DNA directions (3'→5' and 5'→3') and are important for unwinding the double strand DNA. After recognition of CPD or 6-4 PP and unwinding the DNA, two endonucleases (XPF-ERCC1 and XPG) incise 5' and 3' from the lesion releasing a 25-27 nucleotide fragment containing the photoproduct. The following

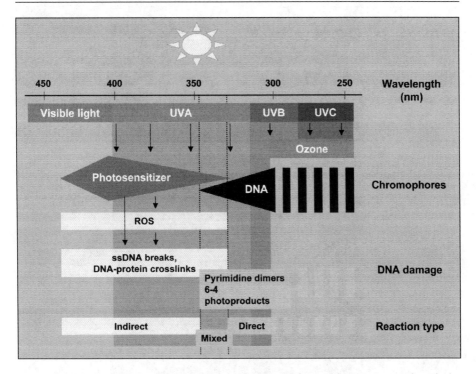

Figure 1. UV-induced DNA damage. The reaction type of DNA damage is wavelength-dependent: direct induction of DNA photoproducts (CPD, 6-4 PP) by UVB/UVC and shortwave UVA spectrum (315-327 nm); indirect induction of oxidative DNA disruptions (ssDNA breaks, DNA-protein crosslinks) by longwave UVA spectrum (347-400 nm); mixed reaction type with direct and indirect effects by UVA wavelength 327-347 nm. Oxidative DNA damage is mediated by photosensitizers (Type I reaction) or by photosensitizer-induced reactive oxygen species (ROS, Type II reaction).

so-called "unscheduled" DNA synthesis fills the resulting gaps involving DNA polymerases ε/δ, proliferating cell nuclear antigen (PCNA), replication factor C (RFC) and DNA ligase I. Lesions in actively transcribed DNA are repaired faster and more accurately by TCR compared to those in the global genome or in the nontranscribed strand of active genes; 6-4 PP are removed faster than CPD (for review, see ref. 19).

Apart from XP, most DNA photoproducts are eliminated in NER competent cells following UV-exposure. However, mutations may occur when the repair capacity is exceeded (for instance by repetitive UV expositions without adequate repair intervals). They can be identified as UV specific C→T transitions at dipyrimidine sites or CC→TT base changes (UV-signature, -fingerprint, Fig. 3).[17,20] Interestingly, neighboring thymines do not appear to yield a mutation, because non-informative bases on the template DNA strand were substituted by an adenine on the opposite DNA strand, the so called A-rule.[21] Thymine dimers will therefore be regularly substituted by two thymines corresponding to the opposite DNA strand by NER. When UV-induced mutations affect critical genes encoding proteins or enzymes contributing to DNA repair, cell cycle control or apoptosis, it is likely that cumulative or subsequent DNA alterations are not sufficiently eradicated. Disrupted functions of such regulative proteins are strongly connected with early stages of skin carcinogenesis.[22] Thus, UV-fingerprint mutations can be abundantly detected in the well characterized and pathogenically important tumor suppressor gene p53 from squamous[17] and basal cell carcinoma[23] of human skin.

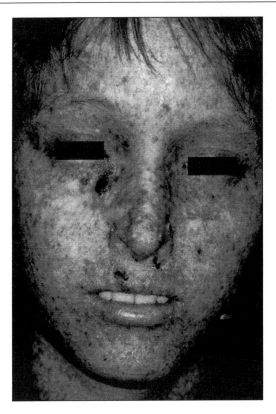

Figure 2. 9-year-old boy with xeroderma pigmentosum presenting with typical poikilodermia in the light-exposed skin, multiple actinic keratoses, actinic cheilitis, squamous cell carcinoma (bridge of nose) and basal cell carcinomas (right nose-canthus region, upper lip).

More recent observations suggest that another DNA repair system-the methyl-derived mammalian mismatch repair (MMR)-may also be attributable to the multistep tumorigenesis of UV-associated skin cancer. Microsatellite instability (MSI), caused by replication errors of small repetitive DNA sequences can be detected in epithelial and melanocytic skin tumours[24] and is characterized by length changes at those repetitive loci scattered throughout the genome.[25,26] Tumor cells that display MSI are typically defective in posttranscriptional MMR providing a direct link between insufficient mispairing DNA repair and genetic instability.[27,28] Concomitant replication errors in different tumor suppressor and growth regulatory genes are supposed to be the genetic mechanism of tumorigenesis in those cells.

Mutations in MMR genes are etiologically responsible for hereditary nonpolyposis colon cancer (for review, see ref. 29). Functional MMR alterations are furthermore associated with visceral malignancies and the occurrence of sebaceous skin tumors, keratoacanthomas and less frequently squamous cell carcinomas in the rare autosomal dominant Muir-Torre syndrome. Underlying mutations were found in the hMSH2 and hMLH1 gene.[30-32]

MMR and NER seem to be functionally connected: Mellon and Champe[33] demonstrated, that disruptions of the bacterial DNA mismatch repair genes mutS and mutL reduces NER of the lactose operon in E. coli. Human cells with mutations in particular MMR genes were likewise found to have a deficiency in the repair of UV-induced pyrimidine dimers.[34] Furthermore specific binding of MSH2/MSH6 (human homologs of mutS) heterodimers to DNA incorporating thymine- or uracil-containing UV light photoproducts[35] and UV-induced activation of transcription

Table 1. Xeroderma pigmentosum: complementation groups, genetics, clinical features and distribution

Complementation Group	Unscheduled DNA Synthesis (% of Normal)	Skin Cancer	Neurological Abnormalities	Number of Reported Cases[16,19]	Gene
A	<10%	+	+	377 (48,7%)	XPA
B	3-7%	+	+	3 (0,4%)	XPB/ERCC3
C	10-20%	+	–	71 (9,2%)	XPC
D	25-50%	+	+	60 (7,8%)	XPD/ERCC2
E	40-50%	+	–	22 (2,8%)	DDB2/XPE/p48
F	10-20%	+	–	44 (5,7%)	XPF/ERCC4
G	<5-25%	+	+	8 (1,0%)	XPG/ERCC5
Variant	75-100%	+	–	189 (24,4%)	XPV/hRAD30
Total				774 (100%)	

of hMSH2 via p53 and c-Jun[36] seem to confirm a significance of MMR pathways for the repair of UV-induced DNA damage. On the other hand Rochette et al[37] previously reported that human cells with homozygous mutations in the DNA mismatch repair genes hMLH1 (homologs of mutL) or hMSH2 were proficient in NER. Thus the relevance of MMR concerning UV-induced DNA disruptions remains controversial.

UV-Induced Carcinogenesis in Squamous Cell Carcinoma (SCC)

The interfollicular epidermal basal keratinocyte is assumed to represent the precursor cell of SCC and its precancerous progenitor, the actinic keratosis (AK). AK and SCC are strongly related to solar UV exposure, because predilection sites were the regularly sun exposed skin areas (head, forehead, back of nose, ears, back of hands) in about 90% and the lifetime risk to develop a SCC correlates very closely with the individual cumulative UV dose.[38]

Historically, the connection between sunlight and epithelial skin cancer was initially described by Unna[39] and Dubreuilh[40] in the last decade of the 19th century. They observed AK and SCC in chronically sun-exposed skin from sailors and vineyard workers. The carcinogenic potential of solar UV radiation, substantiating the clinical observations by Unna and Dubreuilh, has been proved by animal experiments in the 1920's.[41] 40 years later hairless mice became available and thus an excellent animal model to investigate skin cancer induction by UV with similarity to human skin has been established. By means of hairless mice SCC with AK as precancerous lesion could be generated by UV and later on de Grujil demonstrated a wavelength dependency due to SCC induction effecivity: the murine UV action spectrum peaks at ~300 nm in the UVB band and continuously decreases among the UVA band with a smaller peak at ~380 nm.[42] Thereupon these findings were applied to human skin estimating the differences in UV transmission characteristics between murine and human skin and it was demonstrated that the relative efficacy to induce SCC by 300 nm UVB irradiaton is appr. 1000-fold higher as compared to UVA at 380 nm.[43] The estimated human UV action spectrum correlates very closely with the measured concentration of CPD's in human skin in situ following UV radiation with a single peak at ~315 nm.[5,44] In contrast to UVC and UVB, the amount of inducible CPD by UVA irradiation is rather low.[44] On the other hand it is meanwhile well established that UVA is also able, but less effective than UVB, to induce SCC, at least in mice.[45] The small ~380 nm peak in de Grujil's action spectrum can be explained by the above mentioned UVA mediated indirect DNA damage: UVA predominantly causes photosensitizer-mediated oxidative DNA damage. In a teratocarcinoma cell line it has been demonstrated that the greatest amount of DNA-protein crosslinks and single strand breaks are generated by wavelengths between 334 and 405 nm with a peak at 365 nm.[10] As in this part

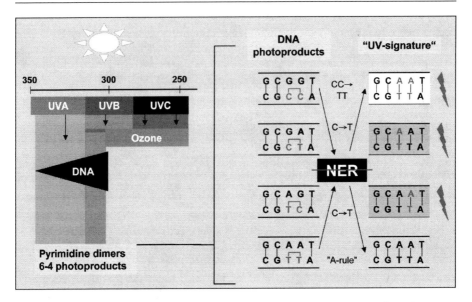

Figure 3. UV-induced specific mutations: UV-signature mutations (#) resulting from 6-4 photoproducts can be identified as C→T transitions at dipyrimidine sites (cytosine-thymine, thymine-cytosine); cytosine cyclobutane dimers result in CC→TT tandem transitions. Thymine cyclobutane dimers do not yield a mutation, because non-informative bases on the template DNA strand were substituted by an adenine on the opposite DNA strand ("A-rule").

of the UVA spectrum (347-400 nm) direct DNA damage is not observed, it can be assumed that the indirect oxidative UVA effects contribute to the mutagenic potential of UVA in the above mentioned wavelength range.[46]

Finally, all these findings convincingly demonstrate that UVB is more powerful than UVA to induce AK and SCC and has to be considered as the predominant carcinogen of solar UV exposure. This is furthermore confirmed by the mutation characteristics in AK and SCC as described below.

Numerous studies have verified the multistep carcinogenesis model of SCC, as precancerous AK can be found in up to 97% adjacent to SCC's.[47] The necessity of further mutational events establishing an invasive SCC from an AK is reflected by the fact that not all AK, which are reversible, result in invasive SCC: the 10-year risk for the development of AK into SCC is not more than 16%.[48]

The most important protein involved in early UV-induced carcinogenesis of SCC appears to be the tumor suppressor p53. p53 is an essential and well defined transcription factor regulating cell cycle control and apotosis.[49] The most well known function is activation of the G1 checkpoint which is believed to provide time for DNA repair prior to entry into S-phase.[50] If the extent of DNA damage exceeds repair capacity and therefore is irreversible, p53 activates pro-apoptotic factors inducing programmed cell death independent from cell cycle control.[51] UV-radiation is known to strongly induce p53 posttranslational stabilization and transcriptional activity by protection of protein degradation via MDM2 oncoprotein inhibition.[52,53] Mutations of the p53 gene were found in various tumors and play a general role for carcinogenesis.[54] Thus, UV specific p53 mutations can be found in 75-80% of AK[22] and in more than 90% of cutaneous squamous cell carcinoma.[17,55] These UV-fingerprint mutations of p53 mutations appear to correspond predominantly to UVB radiation, as UVA-induced carcinomas in hairless mice reveal p53 mutations only in 15%.[45]

The important role of p53 for the protection against UV-induced cancer is furthermore demonstrated by p53-deficient mice: these knockout animals lacking a functional p53 reveal an enormously increased sensitivity to skin cancer by UVB radiation.[56]

The p53 gene is located on chromosome 17 (17p13.1).[57] Dysfunction of the p53 protein, similar to other tumor suppressor proteins, depends on truncating mutations in both alleles. As only few dipyrimidine hot spot areas in the p53 gene are susceptible for UV mutations (codons 177, 196, 278, 294 and 342), the probability for corresponding mutations on both alleles is appropriate.[55] Moreover, loss of heterozygosity (LOH) in several chromosomes, including 17p, have been commonly found in AK.[58] In vitro abrogation of both p53 alleles causes aneuploidy and uncontrolled gene amplification.[55] Such additional events and further unknown UV accumulative mutations in susceptible genes encoding for example other growth control factors or DNA repair enzymes may be responsible for the multistep carcinogenesis from sunburn cells to AK and ultimately to SCC.

Recent data suggest that the MMR protein hMSH2 is a novel p53 regulated target gene indicating a direct involvement of p53 in DNA repair mechanisms. Scherer et al cloned the promoter region of hMSH2 and could detect a site with homology to the p53 consensus binding sequence.[59] Furthermore, they demonstrated that purified p53 binds specifically to this hMSH2 motif.[60] As our group and others were previously able to demonstrate that functionally active MMR protein hMSH2 is detectable in normal human skin, melanocytic and nonmelanocytic tumors, a link between UV radiation, DNA repair and carcinogenesis of skin cancer was supposed.[61-63] Recently, Liang et al reported that hMSH2 expression is elevated in precancerous skin lesions (AK, Bowen's disease), but not in SCC compared to adjacent normal skin.[62] These observations have been confirmed by our group (Fig. 4a-b)[64] and underline the above mentioned physiological importance of MMR due to UV-induced DNA damage in precancerous skin lesions; diminished hMSH2 expression in SCC could reflect the malignant transformation associated with DNA repair deficiencies following p53 dysfunction (second allelic hit, see above). The question whether down-regulation of hMSH2 is just a side effect or essential for the carcinogenesis of SCC is yet unsolved.

UV-Induced Carcinogenesis in Basal Cell Carcinoma (BCC)

BCC is the most common malignancy in white people with a worldwide increasing incidence. Exposure to UV radiation is assumed to be the main causative pathogenic factor for BCCs as well, but the precise relation between amount, timing and pattern of UV exposure and BCC risk is still discussed. Compared to SCC, the correlation of UV with basal cell carcinogenesis is far less obvious and epidemiological data are not completely in line with an impact of cumulative UV dose. Some studies revealed a link between cumulative UV dose and BCC risk, although the relative risks were small with odds ratios of 1.0 to 1.5.[65,66] Other investigations failed to demonstrate such an association.[67] Thereupon the predilection sites of BCC do not exactly correspond with the "sun terraces" as it has been shown for SCC; BCC predominantly affect the seborrhoical central parts of the face (root of nose-canthus region, nasal flaring, nasolabial fold), the head, the trunk and lower limbs; BCCs on the backs of the hands are absolutely rare. Thus, the anatomic distribution is not exclusively explainable with cumulative solar UV exposition. Parallel to melanoma, sunburns in childhood and adolescence may contribute more to BCC and recreational sun exposure in childhood seems to be an important risk factor.[67,68] In this context, it has been recently demonstrated, that in adulthood sunscreens protect against new formation of SCCs but not against formation of BCCs.[69] Another facet underlines, that cumulative UV cannot be the decisive causative agent in BCC: Patients with BCC have a three year risk to develop a subsequent BCC between 33% and 77%, but only a 6% risk to develop a SCC.[70]

The BCC precursor cell is less well defined than in SCC and is supposed to stem from interfollicular epidermal basal keratinocytes with retained basal morphology, from follicular outer root sheath or sebaceous gland derived keratinocytes.[71] The deeper anatomic localization of the BCC originating cells in hair follicles and sebaceous glands may be one explanation for differences in the carcinogenesis of BCC and SCC.

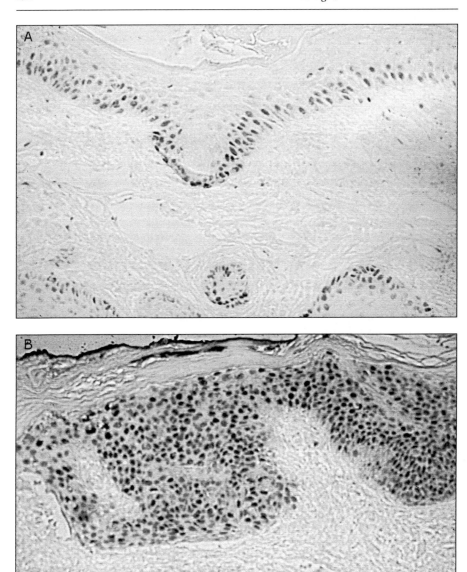

Figure 4. Immunohistochemical detection of hMSH2 protein in initial actinic keratosis (A) and Bowen's disease (B). Notice moderate staining for hMSH2 in basal cell layers of an initial actinic keratosis compared to strong and homogenous staining for hMSH2 in Bowen's disease. HMSH2 expression in SCC in turn is diminished and might reflect the malignant transformation associated with DNA repair deficiencies following complete p53 dysfunction (not shown).

BCC's are predominantly sporadic, or appear in persons suffering from rare hereditary disorders like nevoid basal cell carcinoma syndrome (NBCCS; Gorlin's syndrome) or XP (see above). NBCCS is an autosomal dominant neurocutaneous disorder characterized by multiple BCCs occurring early in life, development of other tumors (medulloblastoma, ovarian fibroma), jaw cysts, calcification of falx cerebri, skeletal defects, pitting of the palms and the soles of the feet and other abnormalities.[72] Mutations in the human homologue of Drosophila segment polarity gene *patched* (PTCH1) are responsible for Gorlin's syndrome[73,74] and UV exposition does not play a main role for BCC development in this complex disease. Physiologically, PTCH1 plays a crucial role in embryonic patterning and is a member of the so-called Hedgehog (Hh) signaling pathway.[75]

In sporadic BCC, genetic mapping reveals only few chromosomal regions with LOH apart from chromosome 9q22. This region harbors the PTCH1 tumor suppressor gene and inactivating mutations of PTCH1 in the second allele are described in BCC.[76] Thereupon significant mutations concern the p53 gene on the one hand and PTCH1 related genes involved in the Hh pathway (mutations of Sonic Hedgehog, Smoothened gene (SMO), PTCH2; up-regulation of Gli 1 zinc finger protein) on the other. The common effect of the latter genes consists in a constitutive Hh pathway target gene induction. Target genes are, among others, again PTCH, which was found overexpessed in all BCCs (familial and sporadic) investigated in one study.[77] So, it has to be assumed, that the Hh pathway is the common key to BCC establishment. Finally, Hh pathway activation results in a positive effect of cell cycle progression and hence it stimulates cell growth.[78] UV fingerprint mutations occur rarely in sporadic BCC compared to SCC: p53 mutations can be observed in appr. 56% of all BCCs and specific C→T transitions and/or CC→TT tandem mutations are present in appr. 65% of them.[79] PTCH1 mutations are less frequent with 30-40% and a UV signature rate of 41%.[80] The frequency of UV specific mutations in other Hedgehog related genes in sporadic BCC is still unknown. Thus, overall UVB associated mutations can be detected only in appr. 50%.

In XP the NER dysfunction contributes to a predominant UV dependency of carcinogenesis in those patients, as described in detail above. XP related BCCs are even stronger UVB associated compared to sporadic and familial BCCs: PTCH gene mutations were detected in 73% of BCCs from XP patients and 50% reveal both p53 and PTCH gene mutations with a high amount of UV-specific alterations (appr. 80%).[81-83] Furthermore activating UV-specific mutations in the SMO gene have been found in 30% of XP BCCs.[81] As mutations in genes participating in the Hh pathway are frequently found in BCC, but not in SCC, it can be speculated, that those are specific for BCC (amongst UV-induced skin cancer) and probably not directly involved in SCC formation.[83-85] Interestingly, recent findings indicate that other factors that influence the risk to develop BCC or SCC include distinct variants of the melanocortin 1 receptor.[86]

Role of DNA Repair for UV-Induced Carcinogenesis in Malignant Melanoma (MM)

Epidemiologic and in vitro studies have shown that solar UV-exposure is not exclusively an etiologic agent for the development of SCC and BCC, but also for the development of malignant melanoma.[87,88] Although great efforts are being made in understanding the underlying genetic basis of melanoma, fundamental questions concerning UV radiation and the mechanisms by which it induces DNA damage and interacts with the DNA repair machinery remain unresolved, compromising efforts to develop effective sun protection strategies and antimelanoma therapy. Recently developed experimental animal models, including genetically engineered mice, the Xiphophorus hybrid fish, the south american opposum and human skin xenografts, constitute novel platforms upon which to build strategies designed to further elucidate the pathogenesis of UV-induced melanomagenesis.[88] Important new informations were obtained analyzing UV-inducible melanogenesis in the HGF/SF transgenic mouse.[89,90] Using this model, it was demonstrated that dermal melanomas arise in untreated mice with a mean onset age of approximately 21 months, a latency that was not overtly altered in response to chronic suberythemal, or skin nonreddening UV irradiation.[89,90] In contrast, a single erythemal dose to 3.5-day-old-neonatal HGF/SF mice induced cutaneous melanoma with significantly reduced latency.[89,90] (Fig. 5) Moreover, the UV-induced murine melanomas frequently resembled their human counterparts with respect to histopathological appearance and graded progression. Exposure of HGF/SF transgenic neonates to a second erythemal dose of UV-irradiation did not accelerate melanomagenesis, however, the dual exposure did significantly increase the number of melanocytic lesions arising per mouse.[89,90] (Fig. 5) The important role of the DNA repair system in the multi-step process of melanoma tumourigenesis is suggested by the autosomal recessive disease xeroderma pigmentosum, in which the development of multiple skin malignancies including malignant melanomas early in life is associated with deficient nucleotide excision repair of pyrimidine dimers induced by UV irradiation.[16,18,91] DNA repair plays a fundamental role in the maintenance of genomic integrity and decreased DNA repair has been associated with increased risk of several human cancers, including melanoma.[92] A variety of somatic genetic alterations occur in malignant melanoma, including mutations that are associated with exposure to UV radiation.[93] Various epidemiological studies have previously examined a putative association between individual DNA repair capacity (DRC) and melanoma risk [for review,[92,94]]. Hsu et al[95] reported a higher level of bleomycin-induced DNA breaks in melanoma patients compared with controls. Roth et al[96] observed increased loss of thymine dimer antigenicity in melanoma patients compared with controls. Wei et al[97] and Landi et al[98] used the host cell reactivation assay to evaluate repair of UV-induced DNA damage using lymphocytes from melanoma patients and cancer-free controls. Wei et al[97] found that patients with melanoma had significantly reduced mean DRC as compared to controls. Landi et al[98] did not find an overall case–control difference in DRC, but DRC was reduced among melanoma patients with low tanning ability and dysplastic nevi as compared to the corresponding controls. Recently, an

HGF/SF Transgenic Mice	UV-Treatment	Melanoma Outcome
Neonate	Single erythemal exposure	Melanomas with junctional activity arise with significant reduction in latency
Juvenile	Dual erythemal exposure	No change from single exposure exept for increased multiplicity
Adult	Chronic sub-erythemal exposure	No change from untreated mice
Adult	None	Dermal melanomas arise in aged mice

Figure 5. UV-induced melanomagenesis in the HGF/SF transgenic mouse.[89,90] Dermal melanomas arise in untreated mice with a mean onset age of approximately 21 months, a latency that is not overtly altered in response to chronic suberythemal, or skin nonreddening UV irradiation.[89,90] In contrast, a single erythemal dose to 3.5-day-old-neonatal HGF/SF mice induces cutaneous melanoma with significantly reduced latency.[89,90] Note that the UV-induced murine melanomas frequently resemble their human counterparts with respect to histopathological appearance and graded progression. Exposure of HGF/SF transgenic neonates to a second erythemal dose of UV-irradiation does not accelerate melanomagenesis, however, the dual exposure significantly increases the number of melanocytic lesions arising per mouse.[89,90]

association of a polymorphism in the melanocortin receptor 1 gene, that is associated with a distinct skin type, with reduced DRC and an increased risk for the development of malignant melanoma has been reported.[99-102] There are only a few studies that analyze a putative assoziation of NER genotypes and melanoma risk and these studies do not provide consistent results. Winsey et al[103] demonstrated an increased frequency of the *XPF* nt 2063 T/T genotype in melanoma patients compared with controls. These authors also reported a slightly increased frequency of the *XPD* codon 312 Asn/Asn and codon 751 Gln/Gln genotypes in melanoma patients compared with controls. Tomescu et al[104] found an increased frequency of the *XPD* codon 751 Lys/Lys genotype in melanoma patients as compared to controls. These authors also reported positive associations for *XPD* markers in exon 6 and exon 22. Baccarelli et al[105] reported no overall association between *XPD* codon 312 and 751 genotypes and melanoma, but noted stronger associations for both variant *XPD* genotypes and melanoma at older ages. The authors also reported that DRC, as measured by the host cell reactivation assay, was lower in participants carrying the *XPD* codon 751 Gln allele. Blankenburg et al[106] reported no association for *XPG* codon 1104 genotype and malignant melanoma and no association for three markers in *XPC*: T1601C, G2166A and C3507G. In the same study population, these authors found positive associations for three other *XPC* markers: intron 9 PAT, intron 11 C-6A and codon 939 Lys/Gln.[108] In the Nurses' Health Study Cohort, Han et al[107] reported modest inverse associations between *XPD* codon 312 Asn/Asn and codon 751 Gln/Gln genotypes and risk of malignant melanoma, but the results were not statistically significant. Interactions were observed between *XPD* genotypes and solar UV-exposure.[107] Taken together, the results of these studies suggested that *XPD* genotypes may play a role in the etiology of melanoma, but further studies are needed to determine which alleles are associated with increased risk. In a well-done recent analysis, it was found that when genotypes across six NER genes (*XPD, HR23B, XPG, XPC, XPF* and *ERCC6*) were combined, malignant melanoma cases showed a statistically significant trend toward more variant alleles compared with controls, although the magnitude of the trend was very small.[101] These data provide preliminary evidence in support of a multigenic model for melanoma that includes NER genes. However, additional studies that incorporate a large number of NER genes are urgently needed to clarify the role of NER genes for pathogenesis of malignant melanoma.

However, as pointed out above, an increasing body of evidence now indicates that nucleotide excision repair represents not the only DNA repair pathway that is involved in UV-induced melanomagenesis. Human cells with mutations in particular mismatch repair genes were found to have a deficiency in transcription-coupled repair of UV-induced pyrimidine dimers[33,34] as well. The significance of mismatch repair pathways for the repair of UV light-induced DNA damage was confirmed by demonstrating specific binding of human MSH-2/MSH-6 heterodimers to DNA incorporating thymine- or uracil-containing UV light photoproducts[35] and by UV-induced activation of transcription of *h*MSH-2 via p53 and c-Jun.[36] These observations lead to the hypothesis, that defective mismatch repair may be a risk factor for the multistep tumourigenesis of skin cancer, including malignant melanoma. However, the mechanism how hMSH2 is involved in the complex response mechanisms to DNA damage induced by UV or other agents are not completely clear. It was suggested that the mismatch repair system is an initial step of the damage signaling and repair cascade.[109] Additionally, increasing evidence indicate an important function of MSH2 for other pathways that are of importance for UV-induced melanomagenesis, including cell cycle regulation and modulating the apoptotic response of cells following UV-exposure.[109] As outlined above, the mechanisms by which MSH2 contributes to repair of UV-B-induced DNA damage are not completely understood. It has been hypothesized that MMR may indirectly facilitate removal of UV-induced adducts through cell cycle arrest,[109-112] thus suppressing mutagenesis. It has been demonstrated that MSH2 modulates UV-B-induced cell cycle progression in melanoma cells. Additionally, it has been reported that in melanoma cells, MSH2 modulates the post-UV protective cellular response of UV-B-induced apoptosis. These results were in contrast to findings in MSH2-null primary mouse embryonic fibroblasts where deletion of MSH2 resulted in significantly reduced sensitivity to UV-B-induced apoptosis as compared to wild-type control cells and it has been concluded that the apoptosis-inducing effect of MSH2 is uncoupled in melanoma cells and that this mechanism may be of importance for the UV-induced melanomagenesis.

MMR has been shown to facilitate cell cycle arrest in the G_2—M transition in response to DNA damage.[109-112] Therefore, depending on the type of DNA damage, loss of MMR may result in loss of cell cycle control and/or resistance to apoptosis, both of which promote neoplastic transformation. The ability of MMR to contribute to the postreplicative repair of single base mismatches and loops, to contribute to the removal of some endogenous and exogenous DNA lesions, as well as to influence cell cycle arrest and apoptosis in response to some exogenous DNA damage illustrates the versatility of MMR for the maintenance of genomic integrity.

We have analyzed previously the immunohistochemical staining pattern of hMSH2 in malignant melanoma, demonstrating increased immunoreactivity for MSH2 in primary cutaneous malignant melanomas and metastases as compared to acquired melanocytic nevi.[113] Additionally, it has been reported that MSH2 RNA levels are increased in primary cutaneous malignant melanomas and metastases as compared to acquired melanocytic nevi. Consistent with these findings, increased MSH2 RNA levels were found in melanoma cell lines as compared to cultured normal melanocytes. Additionally, it has been demonstrated that MSH2 RNA levels in melanoma cell lines are modulated following UV-B-treatment.[113] The complex mechanisms that are involved in the regulation of MSH2 gene expression in mammalian cells are only beginning to be elucidated. Recently, the hMSH2 gene has been identified as a possible novel p53 regulated target gene, indicating a direct involvement of p53 in repair mechanisms via DNA-binding of a mismatch repair gene.

Conclusions

Sunlight-induced DNA damage and its repair are of high importance for skin cancer development and its defense. UVB is significantly more powerful to induce non melanoma skin cancer than UVA. The unique role of NER to avoid melanocytic and nonmelanocytic tumors is graphically illustrated by the rare genetic disorder XP. An interesting new perspective in DNA damage and repair research, as recent publications suggest, lies in the participation of MMR in DNA photodamage correction; however, its clear function in DNA repair pathways and in skin carcinogenesis has to be elucidated in further investigations.

UVB radiation is the predominant carcinogen responsible for the induction of SCC, xeroderma pigmentosum related BCC and to a lower degree of sporadic BCC. Epidemiological and experimental data obviously demonstrate that cumulative UVB radiation is the main carcinogenic factor in AK and SCC. In BCC, the pathogenic role of UV is not that transparent and it seems that intensive sun expositions in childhood contribute to an elevated BCC risk. UV-specific mutations in the p53 tumor suppressor gene are the common and pathogenically important event in AK and SCC. Mutations in Hedgehog related genes, especially PTCH1, which are only partially UV-specific, represent the most significant pathogenic event in BCC.

Solar UV-exposure is widely regarded as the critical environmental risk factor for cutaneous malignant melanoma. Although great efforts are being made in understanding the underlying genetic basis of melanoma, fundamental questions concerning UV radiation and the mechanisms by which it induces DNA damage and interacts with the DNA repair machinery remain unresolved, compromising efforts to develop effective sun protection strategies and antimelanoma therapy. These circumstances have been fueled, at least in part, by the lack of a suitable genetically tractable, UV-dependent animal model for human melanoma. During the last decades, a number of animal melanoma models have been described, however, the histopathological appearance and graded progression of the arising melanocytic malignancies are, for most animal models, distinct from human melanoma.

Recently, in vitro and in vivo laboratory investigations have shown that the DNA repair machinery modulates in melanoma cells UV-B-induced DNA repair, cell cycle progression and apoptosis. These findings point at an important role of the DNA repair machinery for pathogenesis, progression and therapy of malignant melanoma.

References

1. Gates FL. On nuclear derivatives and lethal action of ultraviolet light. Science 1928; 68:479-480.
2. Hollaender A, Emmons CW. Wavelength dependence of mutation production in the ultraviolet with special emphasis on fungi. Cold Spring Harbor Symp Quand Biol 1941; 9:179-186.
3. Setlow RB. DNA damage and repair: a photobiological odyssey. Photochem Photobiol 1997; 65S:119S-122S.
4. Coohill TP. Historical aspects of ultraviolet action spectroscopy. Photochem Photobiol 1997; 65S:123S-128S.
5. De Grujil FR. Skin cancer and solar uv radiation. Eur J Cancer 1999; 35:2003-2009.
6. Beukers R, Berends W. Isolation and identification of the irradiation product of thymine. Biochim Biophys Acta 1960; 41:550-551.
7. Setlow RB, Carrier WL. Pyrimidine dimers in ultraviolet-irradiated DNA's. J Mol Biol 1966; 17:237-254.
8. Varghese AJ, Patrick MH. Cytosine derived heteroadduct formation in ultraviolet-irradiated DNA. Nature 1969; 223:299-300.
9. Lill PH. Latent period and antigenicity of murine tumors induced in C3H mice by short-wavelength ultraviolet radiation. J Invest Dermatol 1983; 81:342-6.
10. Peak JG, Peak MJ. Comparison of initial yields of DNA-to-protein crosslinks and single-strand breaks induced in cultured human cells by far- and near-ultraviolet light, blue light and X-rays. Mutation Res 1991; 246:187-191.
11. Van Weelden H, Van der Putte SCJ, Toonstra J et al. UVA-induced tumours in pigmented hairless mice and the carcinogenic risks of tanning with UVA. Arch Dermatol 1990; 282:289-294.
12. Staberg B, Wulf HC, Klemp P et al. The carcinogenic effect of UV-A irradiation. J Invest Dermatol 1983; 81:517-519.
13. Talve L, Stenbaeck TL, Jansen CT. UVA irradiation increases the incidence of epithelial tumors in UVB-irradiated hairless mice. Photodermatol Photoimmunol Photomed 1990; 7:109-115.
14. Peak MJ, Peak JG. Molecular photobiology of UVA. In: Urbach F, Gange RW, eds. The biological effects of UVA irradiation. New York: Praeger, 1986; 42-52.
15. Setlow RB, Carrier WL. The disappearance of thymine dimers from DNA: an error-correcting mechanism. Proc Natl Acad Sci USA 1964; 51:226-231.
16. Kraemer KH, Lee MM, Scotto J. Xeroderma pigmentosum. Cutaneous, ocular and neurologic abnormalities in 830 published cases (review article). Arch Dermatol 1987; 123:241-250.
17. Brash ED, Rudolph JA, Simon JA et al. A role for sunlight in skin cancer: UV-induced p53 mutations in squamous cell carcinoma. Proc Natl Acad Sci USA 1991; 88:10124-10128.
18. Cleaver JE. Defective repair replication of DNA in xeroderma pigmentosum. Nature 1968; 218:652-656.
19. Moriwaki SI, Kraemer KH. Xeroderma pigmentosum-bridging a gap between clinic and laboratory. Photodermatol Photoimmunol Photomed 2001; 17:47-54.
20. Sarasin A. The molecular pathways of ultraviolet-induced carcinogenesis. Mutat Res 1999; 428:5-10.
21. Strauss B, Rabkin S, Sagher D et al. The role of DNA polymerase in base substitution mutagenesis on non-instructional templates. Biochimie 1982; 64:829-838.
22. Ortonne JP. From actinic keratosis to squamous cell carcinoma. Br J Dermatol 2002; 146(Suppl. 61):20-23.
23. Ziegler AD, Leffel DJ, Kunala S et al. Mutation hotspots due to sunlight in the p53 gene of nonmelanoma skin cancers. Proc Natl Acad Sci USA 1993; 90:4216-4220.
24. Quinn AG, Healy E, Rehman I et al. Microsatellite instability in human nonmelanoma and melanoma skin cancer. J Invest Dermatol 1995; 104:309-312.
25. Fishel R, Lescoe MK, Rao MR et al. The human mutator gene homolog MSH2 and its association with hereditary nonpolyposis colon cancer. Cell 1993; 75:1027-1038.
26. Loeb LA. Microsatellite instability: marker of a mutator phenotype in cancer. Cancer Res 1994; 54:5059-5063.
27. Peltomäki P, Aaltonen LA, Sistonen P et al. Genetic mapping of a locus predisposing to human colorectal cancer. Science 1993; 260:810-812.
28. Palombo F, Hughes M, Jiricny J et al. Mismatch repair and cancer. Nature 1994; 367:417.
29. Peltomäki P. Deficient DNA mismatch repair: a common etiologic factor for colon cancer. Hum Mol Genet 2001; 10:735-740.
30. Kruse R, Rutten A, Lamberti C et al. Muir-Torre phenotype has a frequency of DNA mismatch-repair-gene mutations similar to that in hereditary nonpolyposis colorectal cancer families defined by the Amsterdam criteria. Am J Hum Genet 1998; 63:63-70.
31. Suspiro A, Fidalgo P, Cravo M et al. The Muir-Torre syndrome: a rare variant of hereditary nonpolyposis colorectal cancer associated with hMSH2 mutation. Am J Gastroenterol 1998; 93:1572-4.

32. Mathiak M, Rutten A, Mangold E et al. Loss of DNA mismatch repair proteins in skin tumors from patients with Muir-Torre syndrome and MSH2 or MLH1 germline mutations: establishment of immunohistochemical analysis as a screening test. Am J Surg Pathol 2002; 26:338-43.

33. Mellon I, Champe GN. Products of DNA mismatch repair genes mutS and mutL are required for transcription-coupled nucleotide-excision repair of the lactose operon in Escherichia coli. Proc Natl Acad Sci USA 1996; 93:1292-1297.

34. Mellon I, Rajpal DK, Koi M et al. Transcription-coupled repair deficiency and mutations in human mismatch repair genes. Science 1996; 272:557-560.

35. Wang H, Lawrence CW, Li GM et al. Specific binding of human MSH2/MSH6 mismatch-repair protein heterodimers to DNA incorporating thymine- or uracil-containing UV light photoproducts opposite mismatched bases. J Biol Chem 1999; 274:16894-16900.

36. Scherer SJ, Maier SM, Seifert M et al. P53 and c-Jun functionally synergize in the regulation of the DNA repair gene hMSH2 in response to UV. J Biol Chem 2000; 275:37469-73.

37. Rochette PJ, Bastien N, McKay BC et al. Human cells bearing homozygous mutations in the DNA mismatch repair genes hMLH1 or hMSH2 are fully proficient in transcription-coupled nucleotide excision repair. Oncogene 2002; 21:5743-52.

38. Vitasa BC, Taylor HR, Strickland PJ et al. Association of nonmelanoma skin cancer and actinic keratosis with cumulative solar ultraviolet exposure in Maryland Watermen. Cancer 1990; 65:2811-2817.

39. Unna PG. Histopathologie der Hautkrankheiten. Berlin, August Hirschwald, 1894.

40. Dubreuilh W. Des hyperkeratoses circonscriptes. Ann Derm et Syph 1896; 7:1158-1204.

41. Findlay GM. Ultraviolet light and skin cancer. Lancet 1928; 2:1070-1073.

42. De Grujil FR, Sterenborg HJCM, Forbes PD et al. Wavelength dependence of skin cancer induction by ultraviolet irradiation of albino hairless mice. Cancer Res 1993; 53:53-60.

43. De Grujil FR, Van der Leun JC. Estimate of the wavelength dependency of ultraviolet carcinogenesis in humans and its relevance to risk assessments of a stratopheric ozone depletion. Health Phys 1994; 67:319-325.

44. Freeman SE, Hacham H, Gange RW et al. Wavelength dependence of pyrimidine dimer formation in DNA of human skin irradiated in situ with ultraviolight light. Proc Natl Acad Sci USA 1989; 86:5605-5609.

45. Van Kranen HJ, De Laat A, Van de Ven J et al. Low incidence of p53 mutations in UVA (365-nm)-induced skin tumours in hairless mice. Cancer Res 1997; 57:1238-1240.

46. Rünger TM. Role of UVA in the pathogenesis of melanoma and nonmelanoma skin cancer. A short review. Photodermatol Photoimmunol Photomed 1999; 15:212-6.

47. Hurwitz RM, Monger LE. Solar keratosis: an evolving squamous cell carcinoma. Benign or malignant? Dermatol Surg 1995; 21:184.

48. Babilas P, Landthaler M, Szeimies RM. Actinic keratoses. Hautarzt 2003; 54:551-562.

49. Vogelstein B, Kinzler KW. P53 function and dysfunction. Cell 1992; 70:523-526.

50. Kuerbitz SJ, Plunkett BS, Walsh WV et al. Wild-type p53 is a cell cycle checkpoint determinant following irradiation. Proc Natl Acad Sci USA 1992; 89:7491-7495.

51. Donehower LA, Bradley A. The tumor suppressor p53. Biochim Biophys Acta 1993; 1155:181-205.

52. Shieh SY, Ikeda M, Taya Y et al. DNA damage-induced phosphorylation of p53 alleviates inhibition by MDM2. Cell 1997; 91:325-334.

53. Freedman DA, Wu L, Levine AJ. Functions of the MDM2 oncoprotein. Cell Mol Life Sci 1999; 55:96-107.

54. Greenblatt MS, Bennett WP, Hollstein M et al. Mutations in the p53 tumor suppressor gene: clues to cancer etiology and molecular pathogenesis. Cancer Res 1994; 54:4855-4878.

55. Brash DE, Ziegler A, Jonason AS et al. Sunlight and sunburn in human skin cancer: p53, apoptosis and tumor promotion. J Invest Dermatol Symp Proc 1996; 1:136-142.

56. Li G, Tron VA, Ho V. Induction of squamous cell carcinoma in p53-deficient mice after ultraviolet irradiation. J Invest Dermatol 1998; 110:72-75.

57. Nigro JM, Baker SJ, Preisinger AC et al. Mutations in the p53 gene occur in diverse human tumour types. Nature 1989; 342:705-708.

58. Rehman I, Quinn AG, Healy E et al. High frequncy of loss of heterozygosity in actinic keratoses, a usually benign disease. Lancet 1994; 344:788-789.

59. Scherer SJ, Welter C, Zang KD et al. Specific in vitro binding of p53 to the promoter region of the human mismatch repair gene hMSH2. Biochem Biophys Res Commun 1996; 221:722-8.

60. Scherer SJ, Seib T, Seitz G et al. Isolation and characterization of the human mismatch repair gene hMSH2 promoter region. Hum Genet 1996; 97:114-116.

61. Rass K, Gutwein P, Müller SM et al. Immunohistochemical analysis of DNA mismatch repair enzyme hMSH2 in normal human skin and basal cell carcinomas. Histochem J 2000; 32:93-97.

62. Liang SB, Furihata M, Takeuchi T et al. Reduced human mismatch repair protein expression in the development of precancerous skin lesions to squamous cell carcinoma. Virchows Arch 2001; 439:622-627.
63. Lage H, Christmann M, Kern MA et al. Expression of DNA repair proteins hMSH2, hMSH6, hMLH1, O6-methylguanine-DNA methyltransferase and N-methylpurine-DNA glycosylase in melanoma cells with acquired drug resistance. Int J Cancer 1999; 80:744-750.
64. Rass K, Gutwein P, Welter C et al. Expression of DNA mismatch repair enzyme hMSH2 in epithelial skin tumours and its induction by ultraviolet B radiation in vitro. Submitted for publication.
65. Zanetti R, Rosso S, Martinez C et al. The multicentre south European study "helios" I: skin characteristics and sunburns in basal cell and squamous cell carcinomas of the skin. Br J Cancer 1996; 73:1440-1446.
66. Rosso S, Zanetti T, Martinez C et al. The multicentre south European study "helios" II: different sun exposure patterns in the etiology of basal and squamous cell carcinomas of the skin. Br J Cancer 1996; 73:1447-1454.
67. Corona R, Dogliotti E, D'Ericco M et al. Risk factors for basal cell carcinoma in a Mediterranean population. Arch Dermatol 2002; 137:1162-1168.
68. Gallagher RP, Hill GB, Bajdik CD et al. Sunlight exposure, pigmentary factors and risk of nonmelanocytic skin cancer. Arch Dermatol 1995; 131:157-163.
69. Green A, Wiliams G, Neale R et al. Daily sunscreen application and betacarotene supplementation in prevention of basal-cell and squamous-cell carcinomas of the skin: a randomised controlled trial. Lancet 1999; 354:723-729.
70. Marcil I, Stern RS. Risk of developing a subsequent nonmelanoma skin cancer in patients with a history of nonmelanoma skin cancer. Arch Dermatol 2000; 136:1524-1530.
71. Kruger K, Blume-Peytavi U, Orfanos CE. Basal cell carcinoma possibly originate from the outer root sheath and/or the bulge region of the vellus hair follicle. Arch Dermatol Res 1999; 291:253-259.
72. Gorlin RJ. Nevoid basal-cell carcinoma syndrome. Medicine 1987; 66:98-113.
73. Hahn H, Wicking C, Zaphiropoulous PG et al. Mutations of the human homolog of Drosophila patched in the nevoid basal cell carcinoma syndrome. Cell 1996; 85:841-851.
74. Johnson RL, Rothman AL, Xie J et al. Human homolog of patched, a candidate gene for the basal cell nevus syndrome. Science 1996; 272:1668-1671.
75. Bale AE, YU KP. The hedgehog pathway and basal cell carcinomas. Hum Mol Genet 2001; 10:757-762.
76. Gailani MR, Stahle-Backdahl M, Leffell DJ et al. The role of the human homologue of Drosophila patched in sporadic cell carcinomas. Nat Genet 1996; 14:79-81.
77. Unden AB, Zaphiropoulos PG, Bruce K et al. Human patched (PTCH) mRNA is overexpressed consistently in tumor cells of both familial and sporadic basal cell carcinoma. J Natl Cancer Inst 1996; 88:349-354.
78. Barnes EA, Kong M, Ollendorff V et al. Patched 1 interacts with cyclin B1 to regulate cell cycle progression. EMBO J 2001; 20:2214-2223.
79. Soehnge H, Ouhtit A, Ananthaswamy HN. Mechanisms of induction of skin cancer by UV radiation. Frontiers Bioscience 1997; 2:538-551.
80. Lacour JP. Carcinogenesis of basal cell carcinomas: genetics and molecular mechanisms. Br J Dermatol 2002; 146(S61):17-19.
81. Couvé-Privat S, Bouadjar B, Avril MF et al. Significantly high levels of ultraviolet-specific mutations in the Smoothened gene in basal cell carcinomas from DNA repair-deficient xeroderma pigmentosum patients. Cancer Res 2002; 62:7186-7189.
82. Bodak N, Queille S, Avril MF et al. High levels of patched gene mutations in basal-cell carcinomas from patients with xeroderma pigmentosum. Proc Natl Acad Sci USA 1999; 96:5117-5222.
83. Eklund LK, Lindström E, Undén AB et al. Mutation analysis of the human homologue of Drosophila patched and the xeroderma pigmentosum complementation group A genes in squamous cell carcinomas of the skin. Mol Carcinog 1998; 21:87-92.
84. Kang SY, Lee KG, Lee W et al. Polymorphisms in the DNA repair gene XRCC1 associated with basal cell carcinoma and squamous cell carcinoma of the skin in a Korean population. Cancer Sci 2007; [Epub ahead of print].
85. Leibeling D, Laspe P, Emmert S. Nucleotide excision repair and cancer. J Mol Histol 2006; 37(5-7):225-38.
86. Han J, Kraft P, Colditz GA et al. Melanocortin 1 receptor variants and skin cancer risk. Int J Cancer 2006; 119(8):1976-84.
87. Markovic SN, Erickson LA, Rao RD et al. Melanoma Study Group of the Mayo Clinic Cancer Center. Malignant melanoma in the 21st century, part 1: epidemiology, risk factors, screening, prevention and diagnosis. Mayo Clin Proc 2007; 82(3):364-80.

88. Jhappan C, Noonan FP, Merlino G. Ultraviolet radiation and cutaneous malignant melanoma. Oncogene 2003; 22(20):3099-112.
89. Noonan FP, Recio JA, Takayama H et al. Neonatal sunburn and melanoma in mice. Nature 2001; 413(6853):271-2.
90. Noonan FP, Otsuka T, Bang S et al. Accelerated ultraviolet radiation-induced carcinogenesis in hepatocyte growth factor/scatter factor transgenic mice. Cancer Res 2000; 60(14):3738-43.
91. Kraemer KH, Lee MM, Andrews AD et al. The role of sunlight and DNA repair in melanoma and nonmelanoma skin cancer. The xeroderma pigmentosum paradigm. Arch Dermatol 1994; 130(8):1018-21.
92. Berwick M, Vineis P. Markers of DNA repair and susceptibility to cancer in humans: an epidemiologic review. J Natl Cancer Inst 2000; 92:874-897.
93. Chin L. The genetics of malignant melanoma: lessons from mouse and man. Nat Rev Cancer 2003; 3:559-570.
94. Neumann A, Sturgis E, Wei Q. Nucleotide excision repair as a marker for susceptibility to tobaccorelated cancers: A review of molecular epidemiological studies. Mol Carcinog 2005; 42:65-92.
95. Hsu TC, Fuen L, Trizna Z et al. Differential sensitivity among three human subpopulations in response to 4-nitroquinoline-1-oxide and to bleomycin. Int J Oncol 1993; 3:827-830.
96. Roth M, Muller H, Boyle JM. Immunochemical determination of an initial step in thymine dimer excision repair in xeroderma pigmentosum variant fibroblasts and biopsy material from the normal population and patients with basal cell carcinoma and melanoma. Carcinogenesis 1987; 8:1301-1307.
97. Wei Q, Lee JE, Gershenwald JE et al. Repair of UV light-induced DNA damage and risk of cutaneous malignant melanoma. J Natl Cancer Inst 2003; 95:308-315.
98. Landi MT, Baccarelli A, Tarone RE et al. DNA repair, dysplastic nevi and sunlight sensitivity in the development of cutaneous malignant melanoma. J Natl Cancer Inst 2002; 94:94-101.
99. Hauser JE, Kadekaro AL, Kavanagh RJ et al. Melanin content and MC1R function independently affect UVR-induced DNA damage in cultured human melanocytes. Pigment Cell Res 2006; 19(4):303-14.
100. Millikan RC, Hummer A, Begg C et al; for the GEM Study Group. Polymorphisms in nucleotide excision repair genes and risk of multiple primary melanoma: the Genes Environment and Melanoma Study. Carcinogenesis 2006; 27(3):610-618.
101. Li C, Hu Z, Liu Z et al. Polymorphisms in the DNA Repair Genes XPC, XPD and XPG and Risk of Cutaneous Melanoma: a Case-Control Analysis. Cancer Epidemiol Biomarkers Prev 2006; 15(12):2526-2532.
102. Debniak T, Scott R, Masojc B et al. MC1R common variants, CDKN2A and their association with melanoma and breast cancer risk. Int J Cancer 2006; 119(11):2597-602.
103. Winsey SL, Haldar NA, Marchs HP et al. A variant within the DNA repair gene XRCC3 is associated with the development of melanoma skin cancer. Cancer Res 2000; 60:5612-5616.
104. Tomescu D, Kavanagh G, Ha T et al. Nucleotide excision repair gene XPD polymorphisms and genetic predisposition to melanoma. Carcinogenesis 2001; 22:403-408.
105. Baccarelli A, Calista D, Minghetti P et al. XPD gene polymorphism and host characteristics in the assocation with cutaneous malignant melanoma risk. Br J Cancer 2004; 90:497-502.
106. Blankenburg S, Konig I, Moessner R et al. No association between three xeroderma pigmentosum group C and one group G gene polymorphisms and risk of cutaneous melanoma. Eur J Hum Genet 2005; 13:253-255.
107. Han J, Colditz GA, Liu JS et al. Genetic variation in XPD, sun exposure and risk of skin cancer. Cancer Epidemiol Biomarkers Prev 2005; 14:1539-1544.
108. Blankenburg S, Konig IR, Moessner R et al. Assessment of 3 xeroderma pigmentosum group C gene polymorphisms and risk of cutaneous melanoma: a case-control study. Carcinogenesis 2005; 26:1085-1090.
109. Seifert M, Böhm M, Löbrich M et al. The DNA-mismatch repair enzyme hMSH2 modulates UV-B-induced cell cycle arrest and apoptosis in melanoma cells. J Invest Dermatol, in press.
110. Hawn MT, Umar A, Carethers JM et al. Evidence for a connection between the mismatch repair system and the G2 cell cycle checkpoint. Cancer Res 1995; 55(17):3721-5.
111. Davis TW, Wilson-van Patten C, Meyers M et al. Defective expression of the DNA mismatch repair protein, MLH1, alters G2-M cell cycle checkpoint arrest following ionizing radiation. Cancer Res 1998; 58(4):767-78.
112. Lan Z, Sever-Chroneos Z, Strobeck MW et al. DNA damage invokes mismatch repair-dependent cyclin D1 attenuation and retinoblastoma signaling pathways to inhibit CDK2. J Biol Chem 2002; 277(10):8372-81.
113. Rass K, Gutwein P, Welter C et al. DNA-mismatch-repair enzyme hMSH-2 in malignant melanoma: increased immunoreactivity as compared to acquired melanocytic nevi and strong mRNA expression in melanoma cell lines. Histochem J 2001; 33:459-467.

CHAPTER 14

Role of Viruses in the Development of Squamous Cell Cancer and Melanoma

Ulrich R. Hengge*

Abstract

In this chapter, the evidence for the role of human papilloma virus (HPV) in the pathogenesis of squamous cell cancer of the skin will be reviewed. Considerable dispute exists questioning the etiological role of HPV. This is due to the low copy number of HPV DNA in skin cancers and additional cofactors such as UV exposure, immunosuppression, light skin color and hyperproliferative skin disease as well as the genetic background of the host. These additional cofactors are probably required because of the weak transforming activity of cutaneous HPV types in contrast to high-risk genital HPV strains.

On a different note, the involvement of viruses in the etiology of melanoma has only recently been suggested. Melanoma-associated retrovirus (MelARV) has been detected in mice and men and was shown to subvert immunosurveillance besides insertional mutagenesis. The state of the art of viral participation in melanomagenesis will be discussed.

Nonmelanoma Skin Cancer

Nonmelanoma skin cancer (NMSC) is the most common cancer of men. Of all NMSC, basal cell carcinoma (BCC) and squamous cell carcinoma (SCC) represent the two most common histological types. Large population-based epidemiologic studies have identified several risk factors such as exposure to UV radiation, skin color and host immune status for the occurrence of skin cancer. The involvement of HPV in human SCC has been first recognized in patients with a rare hereditary disease, called epidermodysplasia verruciformis (EV). This disease is characterized by disseminated, persistent, flat warts and reddish-brown macules or plaques. Individuals affected by EV have a selective immune deficiency in recognizing HPV epitopes of HPV-4 and -7 that cause skin lesions in EV.[1] In addition, HPV types 5 and 8 are also involved. In EV skin lesions, high HPV copy numbers have been demonstrated within a few carcinoma cells by in situ hybridization. When these findings were applied to NMSC in immunocompetent patients, sensitive techniques such as nested polymerase chain reaction have identified HPV DNA in many NMSC lesions.

Role of the Immune System in HPV Carriers

Collectively, in immunosuppressed patients, up to 90% of SCC lesions contain viral DNA. In these individuals, multiple different HPV types, mostly belonging to the EV-associated genus, have been detected; several HPV types may also exist within the same lesion. In general, the HPV load in lesions from immunosuppressed patients generally tends to be higher than in lesions from the general population. Moreover, the lag period from infection through latency to the development of cancer is considerably shorter (2-5 years instead of 15-20 years).

*Ulrich R. Hengge—Department of Dermatology, Heinrich-Heine-University, Moorenstr. 5, D-40225 Düsseldorf, Germany. Email: ulrich.hengge@uni-duesseldorf.de

Sunlight, Vitamin D and Skin Cancer, edited by Jörg Reichrath. ©2008 Landes Bioscience and Springer Science+Business Media.

In contrast, in immunocompetent individuals no single HPV type has been found to predominate in skin cancers and there has also been no evidence for high-risk types in contrast to the occurrence of high-risk type analogues in EV or cervical cancer.[2-4]

Problems in Detection of HPV in Lesional and Normal Skin

Part of the divergent results reported in the literature are attributable to differences in the sensitivity of the detection techniques used.[5,6] In these experiments using various PCR protocols, many new HPV DNA sequences have been identified. Collectively, these novel sequences belong to the supergroup B (cutaneous EV/HPV) of the phylogenetic tree of HPV. Another complicating fact is the finding that HPV DNA is frequently detected in healthy skin specimens or in plucked hairs from healthy individuals in up to 80% of analyzed samples.[7,8] In addition, HPV was detected more frequently in specimens from the forehead than from the arms or thighs, probably being the result of local photoimmunosuppression due to sunlight exposure, resulting in higher production of HPV. However, the detection of viral DNA in skin swabs or skin biopsies may also reflect surface contamination rather than established infection, unless detection is supported by the demonstration of viral gene expression within the epithelium or by seroconversion.

Detection of HPV in SCC and Its Precursor Lesions

Different cutaneous HPV types have been found using hybridization and PCR-based techniques.[9,10] Carcinogenesis of NMSC is thought to occur from individual lesions e.g., actinic keratosis (AK) or in situ carcinoma (M. Bowen), that ultimately may progress to SCC. For comparison, for the development of BCC no such precursor lesions have been described. Several studies have analyzed HPV DNA in AK and NMSC. In one of the first studies by de Villier et al, HPV DNA was found in 65% of AKs, 91% of in situ SCC and 91% of invasive SCC, respectively.[9]

In another trial, HPV detection was associated with the presence of AK (odds ratio: 24.8; 95% CI = 2.3-262.6).[11] A study from Australia reported that HPV-38 was found significantly more often in AKs than in SCC.[12] In this study, a variety of 45 different HPV types was detected in a total of 59 Australian patients with BCC, SCC and AKs. Various HPV types of the B1 group (EV HPV types) were found in 26 of 64 (40%) of the lesions (BCC, SCC and AKs), 44 of 64 (69%) of perilesional swabs and 35 of 59 (59%) buttock swabs, respectively.[12] Similar studies detected HPV DNA in 80% of AK, 46% of SCC and 54% of BCC, respectively.[13] Perilesional skin was positive in 68%.[13] Viral load in SCC, BCC and perilesional tissue was similar. Interestingly, viral loads found in AK were significantly higher than in SCC.[13] The authors concluded that the persistence of HPV is not necessary for the maintenance of the malignant phenotype of individual NMSC cells, suggesting a carcinogenic role of HPV in the early steps of tumor development.[13]

Another recent study determined HPV DNA positivity (analyzed in plucked eyebrow hairs) in 67 of 126 (53%) of AK and 28 of 64 SCC (44%) as well as from 23 of 57 (40%) of tumor-free controls.[14] Interestingly, significant positive associations were observed for overall HPV L1 seropositivity with increasing severity of the lesions accounting for 13, 26 and 37% in controls, AK and SCC patients, respectively.[14] In contrast, antibodies to E6 tended to decline with AK and SCC, especially for HPV-8 (21%, 11% and 2%, respectively). Generally, there was a positive trend between overall HPV DNA positivity and L1 seropositivity, but not E6 seropositivity.

As a major criticism of these studies, HPV DNA was found to be widespread in normal adult skin in 20 of 57 (35%).[15] Another study by the same authors reported that 58 of 67 (87%) renal transplant recipients harbored HPV DNA in normal skin from sun-exposed and non-exposed sites.[15] The authors found a significant association between NMSC and the presence of EV HPV DNA (odds ratio: 6.41 (95% CI: 1.79-22.9). There was no association of HPV DNA from cutaneous or mucosal types and NMSC.[15] In general, there was no difference between the HPV detection in normal appearing skin as compared with NMSC in transplant patients. Only in immunocompetent patients, there was an increased HPV detection in NMSC as compared with normal skin of the same individual.[15]

In addition, the correlation of p16 and pRb expression with HPV detection was described in Bowen's disease in 28 of 32 (88%) of cases.[16] Fifteen percent of analyzed cases contained HPV DNA. Most cases of Bowen's disease were found to express p16, but not pRb. It has been hypothesized that p16 overexpression in Bowen's disease may reflect destruction of the G1/S checkpoint, resulting in unregulated cell cycle progression.[16] In contrast to these findings, an earlier study has failed to demonstrate HPV involvement in Bowen's disease.[17]

NMSC in Organ Transplant Recipients

The incidence of NMSCs is increased in organ transplant patients as has been demonstrated in several reports. One larger recent single-center study reported that transplant patients were about 15 years younger at time of NMSC diagnosis compared to immunocompetent individuals.[18] In addition, tumors in transplant patients often occurred as multiple lesions and in localizations aside from the head. The outcome of transplant SCCs, but not transplant BCCs was worse than in the normal immunocompetent control population.[18] Unfortunately, HPV genotyping was not performed in this study.

Another study from the United Kingdom by Harwood et al reported detectable HPV DNA in 37 of 44 (84.1%) SCC, 18 of 24 (75%) BCC and 15 of 17 (88.2%) AKs from immunosuppressed patients with 27% being detectable in SCC, 36% in BCC and 54% in AKs in the immunocompetent group, respectively.[3] EV HPV types prevailed in all types of lesions from both groups of patients. Moreover, in immunosuppressed individuals cutaneous HPV types could also be identified at high frequency as well as codetection of multiple HPV types within single lesions. This rate of HPV DNA detection is in agreement with earlier findings, where HPV DNA was found in 65% of AKs, 91% of in situ SCC and 91% of invasive SCC.[9] Furthermore, the same set of EV HPV types was detected in malignant lesions.

Detection of HPV-Specific Antibodies

As antibodies to HPV may be detected in more than 50% of serum from children up to 6 years of age, acquisition of HPV may occur very early in life.[19,20] The evidence from seroepidemiologic studies that try to link HPV infections with the occurrence of cutaneous tumors is rather weak.[21] In one of the most convincing studies, the presence of antibodies against HPV-8 viral-like particles (VLP) was associated with large numbers of actinic keratoses after adjusting for gender, age, hair color and sun exposure, showing an odds ratio of 2.3 (95% CI = 1.0-5.3) and with the development of SCC (odds ratio of 3.1 (95% CI = 0.74-13.3).[21]

In a case control study from Italia including 46 patients with cutaneous SCC and 84 matched control subjects, infection with EV HPV types was assessed by serology.[22] Positive serologic findings for HPV type 8 were associated with SCC in immunocompetent individuals (odds ratio: 3.2; 95% CI: 1.3-7.9), independent of other risk factors, whereas positive serology for HPV type-15 was negatively associated with SCC.[22]

Potential Mechanisms of HPV in Skin Carcinogenesis

In vitro studies have shown a rather weak transforming potential of cutaneous HPV.[23,24] The E6 gene of EV-HPV seems to be the most powerful oncogene in rodent cells, leading to altered morphology and anchorage-independent growth; however, tumorigenicity has not been observed in nude mice. The E6 proteins of high-risk HPV-16 and -18 are known to bind cellular p53 and to promote its proteolytic degradation.[25] In addition, E6 proteins of cutaneous HPV types have been demonstrated to reduce the level of the proapoptotic cellular Bak protein independent of p53 function, thereby inhibiting UVB-induced apoptosis.[23]

The E7 gene of HPV type-5/-8 was also able to transform rodent cells in collaboration with an activated H-Ras gene.[25] In addition, the E7 proteins of high-risk HPV types interact with the retinoblastoma protein (pRb).[26] With regard to activation of the transcription of HPV genes upon exposure to UV irradiation, an UV-inducible p53-responsive element has been found in HPV-77 that was isolated from a SCC of a transplant patient.[27]

It should also be noted that potential immunomodulatory functions of E6 and E7 proteins may impair the immunologic elimination of cancer cells.[28] In particular, the secretion of anti-inflammatory cytokines from HPV-positive cells could protect the tumor from the action of the host immune system.

However, a set of experimental data argues against a general role of HPV in skin carcinogenesis (Table 1). First, there were no high-risk HPV types within supergroup B in malignant tumors and second, the low copy number of HPV DNA in skin cancers with only a minority of the tumor cells containing HPV DNA. In addition, there is no experimental proof that HPV DNA and HPV viral activities are acquired for maintaining the malignant phenotype. Therefore, the implication of cutaneous HPV may possibly be important for tumor initiation and progression ("hit-and-run" mechanism of carcinogenesis).

Future Studies

In order to gain more insight into the pathogenetic role of HPV in cutaneous tumors, longitudinal studies of the natural course of cutaneous HPV infections are urgently needed. These studies would have to determine the persistence and the activity of individual HPV types during the year-long process of skin carcinogenesis. Towards this goal, carefully designed case-control studies assessing type-specific humoral immune responses should be assessed over time making use of recombinant viral particles against HPV early antigens. These physiologic responses of the human body bear a higher potential to give the necessary information than the mere detection of HPV DNA with increasingly sensitive techniques. In addition, careful attention should be placed on additional activators and risk factors of HPV transcription and replication.

In addition, exact molecular tools to quantify HPV load and replication are required. HPV viral load quantification is particularly important as most individuals have been infected with various HPV types in childhood and early adulthood.

Role of Retroviruses in Melanomagenesis

In the 1980ies, it has been observed that p16 melanomas derived from C57BL/6 mice express a melanoma-associated antigen (MAA) that is recognized by a particular monoclonal antibody (MM2-9B6).[29] Interestingly, this antibody was highly efficient in eradicating lung and livermetastases of C57BL/6 melanomas.[30] Further immunoelectron microscopy studies have revealed that MMA is closely associated with the surface coat of C-type retroviral particles.[29] More specifically,

---

Table 1. Role of HPV in squamous cell carcinoma of the skin

Pros

- Clinical studies have detected HPV in a substantial fraction of actinic keratoses and SCC in individuals who were also at risk for UV exposure, light skin color and immunosuppression
- Transforming potential of cutaneous HPV has been demonstrated in vitro
- Immunomodulatory functions of E6 and E7 proteins may impair the immunologic elimination of cancer cells

Cons

- No single HPV type has been found to predominate in skin cancers
- No evidence of high-risk HPV in immunocompetent patients with SCC
- Low copy number of HPV DNA
- Highly sensitive techniques detect HPV in lesional and nonlesional skin at similar frequency (contamination vs. infection)
- No experimental proof that HPV DNA and HPV viral activities are acquired for maintaining the malignant phenotype

the MMA is encoded by the *env* gene of this ecotropic retrovirus.[31] Southern blot analysis has suggested that C57BL/6 melanoma cells contain at least four copies of ecotropic retroviruses inserted into different sites of the melanoma genome.[31] One of these proviruses encoded the endogenous N-tropic/ecotropic retrovirus Emv-2 that is replication defective.[32] The other ecotropic retroviruses are novel species that have emerged in melanoma cells during malignant transformation or tumor progression.

In addition, C-type retroviruses have also been found in Cloudman S91 melanoma, which originated in DBA/2 mice and in K1735 melanoma of C3H mice.[29] Consequently, the gene products of these recombinant retroviruses that have emerged in melanomas from DBA/2 and C3H mice are not recognized by the MM2-9B6 monoclonal antibody.

Random Insertion of Retroviruses

C-type retroviruses do not contain oncogenes and may therefore induce malignant transformation only due to insertion into the genome such as has been observed in clinical trials of severe combined immune deficiency syndrome.[33] The insertion site affects the function of various oncogenes or genes involved in the regulation of the cell cycle and ultimately leads to proliferation.

The presence of C-type retroviruses that were initially discovered in murine leukemias raises the question of whether this melanoma-associated retrovirus (MelARV) was activated as a by-product of malignant transformation or whether it played an active role in melanoma formation. Towards this end, the B16 melanoma-derived ecotropic retrovirus MelARV was shown to infect and induce malignant transformation of cultured normal melanocytes.[34] Interestingly, the retroviral insertion sites observed in the immortalized cells was found to occur on chromosome 8 within the *c-maf* proto-oncogene, which encodes a leucine zipper transcription factor related to the AP-1 family that is able to interact with Fos and Jun.[34,35]

Characterization of Melanoma-Associated Retrovirus (MelARV)

Cloning and sequencing of the full-length MelARV genome and its insertion sites has revealed a typical full-length retroviral genome with a high degree of homology (98.5%) to Emv-2.[35] It is probable that MelARV has emerged as a result of recombination within Emv-2 and an endogenous non-ecotropic provirus. The observed differences in the gag and pol regions of MelARV may account for the restoration of productivity and infectivity of a novel retrovirus that has somatically emerged during melanoma formation. MelARV by itself does not contain any oncogenes.

Human Melanoma also Contains Retroviral DNA Sequences

Endogenous retroviral sequences occur in up to 1-2% of the human genome. In human melanoma, the production of retrovirus-like particles that exhibit reverse transcriptase activity has been detected.[36] In addition, these melanoma cells were shown to package sequences homologous to human endogenous retrovirus K (HERV-K) and contain mature forms of the gag and env proteins.[36]

HERV-K is the only known human endogenous retrovirus with open reading frames for the structural enzymes gag, pol and env.[37,38] In addition, HERV-K also encodes a nuclear RNA export factor called rec, a functional homologue of the HIV-1 Rev protein.[39] While the expression of HERVs is usually repressed, exogenous factors such as UV radiation, chemicals, related exogenous retroviruses as well as hormones and cytokines may activate repressed HERVs. Although full-length mRNA expression is detectable in many tissues, protein expression as well as particle production has been demonstrated only in cell lines established from human teratocarcinoma.[37,40] In a recent trial, HERV-K protein expression was detected in 9 of 9 primary melanomas, in 9 of 9 lymph node metastases and in 3 of 3 cutaneous metastases, while it was only detected in 1 of 25 nevi.[36] From these data, it was concluded that expression of retroviral genes and production of retroviral particles were activated during development of melanoma. While these data of detectable retroviral sequences and particles in melanoma cells do not prove their pathogenic role, the question needs to be answered, whether the retroviruses are activated as a by-product of malignant transformation or whether they play an active role in melanoma formation or progression. So far, the detected HERV-K-like viruses were not able to infect normal cultured melanocytes, even under additional UV exposure. Even if melanocytes are nonpermissive for the melanoma-associated viruses, they may have retained important features of replicating retroviruses. Along these lines, de novo insertion by retrotransposition has the same pathogenic impact as insertion by infection, either by loss of function (tumor suppressor genes) or by gain of function (activating oncogenes) mutations.

So far, no infectious HERV-K has been detected, probably due to the lack of env processing, a prerequisite for viral entry into host cells.[41] A recent study suggested that retroviruses associated with melanoma express HERV-K antigens that are targets for cytolytic T-lymphocytes in melanoma patients.[42]

Another study assessed the expression of HERV-K using sets of primers that were able to discriminate between full-length and spliced mRNA and mRNA from deleted and undeleted proviruses.[43] Expression of full-length mRNA from deleted and undeleted proviruses was detected in all human cells investigated. Expression of spliced env and rec was detected in 45% of the metastatic melanoma biopsies and in 44% of the melanoma cell lines.[43] In addition, viral proteins were expressed in primary melanomas, metastases and melanoma cell lines by immunohistochemistry and Western blot analysis.[43] Moreover, 22% (13 of 60) of melanoma patients' sera contained antibodies against the recombinant HERV-K transmembrane envelope protein.

This rather low detection rate is in contrast to the report by Muster et al[36] Along the same lines, HERV-K-specific antibodies against rec and Mp9 were detected in sera of melanoma patients in 14% for rec, but in 0% against Mp9.[44,45] Of note, the generation of HERV-K-specific antibodies indicates the lack of tolerance to this retrovirus and also suggests that expression during oncogenesis does not occur.

As an alternative scenario, the transmembrane envelope protein contains an immunosuppressive domain that inhibits lymphocyte proliferation and modulates cytokine production.[46] Thus, transcription from this endogenous retrovirus during melanoma development/progression will impair the host immune response. However, there are no data that describe an obvious difference in the course of the disease between patients with melanomas that express HERV-K with those that do not. Also, there was no correlation with age, gender, tumor thickness or tumor stage with the expression of spliced HERV-K mRNA.[43] The role of endogenous retroviruses suppressing the host immune response was further supported by a recent report describing that inactivation of endogenous MelARV by RNA interference led to rejection of B16 melanoma cells in immunocompetent mice that usually grow to lethal tumors.[47] In this model, the transformed phenotype of tumor cells was not altered by RNA-mediated knockdown as shown by in vivo studies using immunocompromised mice.[47] The authors described that tumor rejection could be reverted upon adoptive transfer of regulatory T-cells from control melanoma-engrafted mice, as well as from reexpression of the unique transmembrane envelope gene of MelARV.[47] Therefore, it is tempting to speculate that MelARV is directly responsible for the induction of regulatory T-cells that will permit tumor progression.[47,48] The immunodominant epitope was recently identified within the N-protein of MelARV.[49] Such an epitope may in the future be useful for diagnosis and in particular immunotherapy of melanoma.

References

1. Orth G. Genetics of epidermodysplasia verruciformis: Insights into host defense against papillomaviruses. Semin Immunol 2006; 18:362-374.
2. Berkhout RJ, Bouwes Bavinck JN, ter Schegget J. Persistence of human papillomavirus DNA in benign and (pre)malignant skin lesions from renal transplant recipients. J Clin Microbiol 2000; 38:2087-2096.
3. Harwood CA, Surentheran T, McGregor JM et al. Human papillomavirus infection and nonmelanoma skin cancer in immunosuppressed and immunocompetent individuals. J Med Virol 2000; 61:289-297.
4. Wieland U, Ritzkowsky A, Stoltidis M et al. Communication: papillomavirus DNA in basal cell carcinomas of immunocompetent patients: an accidental association? J Invest Dermatol 2000; 115:124-128.
5. Meyer T, Arndt R, Christophers E et al. Frequency and spectrum of HPV types detected in cutaneous squamous-cell carcinomas depend on the HPV detection system: a comparison of four PCR assays. Dermatology 2000; 201:204-211.

6. Strauss S, Desselberger U, Gray JJ. Detection of genital and cutaneous human papillomavirus types: differences in the sensitivity of generic PCRs and consequences for clinical virological diagnosis. Br J Biomed Sci 2000; 57:221-225.
7. Boxman IL, Berkhout RJ, Mulder LH et al. Detection of human papillomavirus DNA in plucked hairs from renal transplant recipients and healthy volunteers. J Invest Dermatol 1997; 108:712-715.
8. Antonsson A, Forslund O, Ekberg H et al. The ubiquity and impressive genomic diversity of human skin papillomaviruses suggest a commensalic nature of these viruses. J Virol 2000; 74:11636-11641.
9. de Villiers EM, Lavergne D, McLaren K et al. Prevailing papillomavirus types in nonmelanoma carcinomas of the skin in renal allograft recipients. Int J Cancer 1997; 73:356-361.
10. de Villiers EM, Fauquet C, Broker TR et al. Classification of papillomaviruses. Virology 2004; 324:17-27.
11. Alotaibi L, Provost N, Gagnon S et al. Diversity of cutaneous human papillomavirus types in individuals with and without skin lesion. J Clin Virol 2006; 36:133-140.
12. Forslund O, Ly H, Reid C et al. A broad spectrum of human papillomavirus types is present in the skin of Australian patients with nonmelanoma skin cancers and solar keratosis. Br J Dermatol 2003; 149:64-73.
13. Weissenborn SJ, Nindl I, Purdie K et al. Human papillomavirus-DNA loads in actinic keratoses exceed those in nonmelanoma skin cancers. J Invest Dermatol 2005; 125:93-97.
14. Struijk L, Hall L, van der Meijden E et al. Markers of cutaneous human papillomavirus infection in individuals with tumor-free skin, actinic keratoses and squamous cell carcinoma. Cancer Epidemiol Biomarkers Prev 2006; 15:529-535.
15. Harwood CA, Surentheran T, Sasieni P et al. Increased risk of skin cancer associated with the presence of epidermodysplasia verruciformis human papillomavirus types in normal skin. Br J Dermatol 2004; 150:949-957.
16. Willman JH, Heinz D, Golitz LE et al. Correlation of p16 and pRb expression with HPV detection in Bowen's disease. J Cutan Pathol 2006; 33:629-633.
17. Lu S, Syrjanen K, Havu VK et al. Failure to demonstrate human papillomavirus (HPV) involvement in Bowen's disease of the skin. Arch Dermatol Res 1996; 289:40-45.
18. Harwood CA, Proby CM, McGregor JM et al. Clinicopathologic features of skin cancer in organ transplant recipients: a retrospective case-control series. J Am Acad Dermatol 2006; 54:290-300.
19. Steger G, Olszewsky M, Stockfleth E et al. Prevalence of antibodies to human papillomavirus type 8 in human sera. J Virol 1990; 64:4399-4406.
20. Stark S, Petridis AK, Ghim SJ et al. Prevalence of antibodies against virus-like particles of Epidermodysplasia verruciformis-associated HPV8 in patients at risk of skin cancer. J Invest Dermatol 1998; 111:696-701.
21. Bouwes Bavinck JN, Stark S, Petridis AK et al. The presence of antibodies against virus-like particles of epidermodysplasia verruciformis-associated humanpapillomavirus type 8 in patients with actinic keratoses. Br J Dermatol 2000; 142:103-109.
22. Masini C, Fuchs PG, Gabrielli F et al. Evidence for the association of human papillomavirus infection and cutaneous squamous cell carcinoma in immunocompetent individuals. Arch Dermatol 2003; 139:890-894.
23. Jackson S, Storey A. E6 proteins from diverse cutaneous HPV types inhibit apoptosis in response to UV damage. Oncogene 2000; 19:592-598.
24. Caldeira S, Zehbe I, Accardi R et al. The E6 and E7 proteins of the cutaneous human papillomavirus type 38 display transforming properties. J Virol 2003; 77:2195-2206.
25. Smola-Hess S, Pfister H. Interaction of papillomaviral oncoproteins with cellular factors. In: Holzenburg A, Bogner E, eds. Structure-Function Relationships of Human Pathogenic Viruses. New York: Kluver Academic/Plenum Publishers, 2002; 431-461.
26. Pfister H, Ter Schegget J. Role of HPV in cutaneous premalignant and malignant tumors. Clin Dermatol 1997; 15:335-347.
27. Purdie KJ, Pennington J, Proby CM et al. The promoter of a novel human papillomavirus (HPV77) associated with skin cancer displays UV responsiveness, which is mediated through a consensus p53 binding sequence. EMBO J 1999; 18:5359-5369.
28. Frazer IH, Thomas R, Zhou J et al. Potential strategies utilised by papillomavirus to evade host immunity. Immunol Rev 1999; 168:131-142.
29. Leong SP, Muller J, Yetter RA et al. Expression and modulation of a retrovirus- associated antigen by murine melanoma cells. Cancer Res 1988; 48:4954-4958.
30. Eisenthal A, Lafreniere R, Lefor AT et al. Effect of anti-B16 melanoma monoclonal antibody on established murine B16 melanoma liver metastases. Cancer Res 1987; 47:2771-2776.

31. Li M, Muller J, Xu F et al. Inhibition of melanoma-associated antigen expression and ecotropic retrovirus production in B16BL/6 melanoma cells transfected with major histocompatibility complex class I genes. Cancer Res 1996; 56:4464-4474.

32. King SR, Berson BJ, Risser R. Mechanism of interaction between endogenous ecotropic murine leukemia viruses in (BALB/c X C57BL/6) hybrid cells. Virology 1988; 162:1-11.

33. Hacein-Bey-Abina S, Von Kalle C, Schmidt M et al. LMO2-associated clonal T-cell proliferation in two patients after gene therapy for SCID-X1. Science 2003; 302:415-419.

34. Li M, Xu F, Muller J et al. Ecotropic C-type retrovirus of B16 melanoma and malignant transformation of normal melanocytes. Int J Cancer 1998; 76:430-436.

35. Li M, Huang X, Zhu Z et al. Sequence and insertion sites of murine melanoma- associated retrovirus. J Virol 1999; 73:9178-9186.

36. Muster T, Waltenberger A, Grassauer A et al. An endogenous retrovirus derived from human melanoma cells. Cancer Res 2003; 63:8735-8741.

37. Lower R, Lower J, Kurth R. The viruses in all of us: characteristics and biological significance of human endogenous retrovirus sequences. Proc Natl Acad Sci USA 1996; 93:5177-5184.

38. Mayer J, Sauter M, Racz A et al. An almost-intact human endogenous retrovirus K on human chromosome 7. Nat Genet 1999; 21:257-258.

39. Yang J, Bogerd HP, Peng S et al. An ancient family of human endogenous retroviruses encodes a functional homolog of the HIV-1 Rev protein. Proc Natl Acad Sci USA 1999; 96:13404-13408.

40. Lower R, Boller K, Hasenmaier B et al. Identification of human endogenous retroviruses with complex mRNA expression and particle formation. Proc Natl Acad Sci USA 1993; 90:4480-4484.

41. Tonjes RR, Czauderna F, Kurth R. Genome-wide screening, cloning, chromosomal assignment and expression of full-length human endogenous retrovirus type K. J Virol 1999; 73:9187-9195.

42. Schiavetti F, Thonnard J, Colau D et al. A human endogenous retroviral sequence encoding an antigen recognized on melanoma by cytolytic T-lymphocytes. Cancer Res 2002; 62:5510-5516.

43. Buscher K, Trefzer U, Hofmann M et al. Expression of human endogenous retrovirus K in melanomas and melanoma cell lines. Cancer Res 2005; 65:4172-4180.

44. Harwood CA, Proby CM. Human papillomaviruses and nonmelanoma skin cancer. Curr Opin Infect Dis 2002; 15:101-114.

45. Buscher K, Hahn S, Hofmann M et al. Expression of the human endogenous retrovirus-K transmembrane envelope, Rec and Np9 proteins in melanomas and melanoma cell lines. Melanoma Res 2006; 16:223-234.

46. Denner J, Norley S, Kurth R. The immunosuppressive peptide of HIV-1: functional domains and immune response in AIDS patients. AIDS 1994; 8:1063-1072.

47. Mangeney M, Pothlichet J, Renard M et al. Endogenous retrovirus expression is required for murine melanoma tumor growth in vivo. Cancer Res 2005; 65:2588-2591.

48. Mangeney M, de Parseval N, Thomas G et al. The full-length envelope of an HERV-H human endogenous retrovirus has immunosuppressive properties. J Gen Virol 2001; 82:2515-2518.

49. Humer J, Waltenberger A, Grassauer A et al. Identification of a melanoma marker derived from melanoma-associated endogenous retroviruses. Cancer Res 2006; 66:1658-1663.

CHAPTER 15

Melanoma and Nonmelanoma Skin Cancers and the Immune System

Diana Santo Domingo and Elma D. Baron*

Introduction

A connection between tumorigenesis and the immune system has been known to exist since the late 1960s. Two pioneers in this concept were Lewis Thomas and F. Macfarlane Burnett. In 1967 Burnett introduced the concept of immunosurveillance.[1] This idea is based on the concept that an intact immune system actively recognizes and rids the body of tumor cells.[2,3] This concept raises several questions. If the body is indeed able to eliminate transformed cells, why do some survive, proliferate and even metastisize? Does neoplastic growth result from a breakdown on the part of the immune system or a coup on the part of the tumor cells? What circumstances lead to spontaneous regression vs. metastatic malignancy? Furthermore, if tumor cells originate from cells that were previously seen as "self" what is the significance of autoimmunity and regulation of these "surveillance" mechanisms?

Knowledge of the relationship between immunology and cancer has evolved and developed through several stages continually increasingly in complexity. Current thinking favors tumor survival when tumor cells are able to shift the chemical signaling milieu towards an environment supporting immunologic tolerance.[4]

Compelling evidence for the overlap of immunology and oncology has been supported by the fact that transplant recipients are known to have an increased risk for developing cancers, especially squamous cell and basal cell carcinomas of the skin. In immune competent individuals, it has been more difficult to demonstrate mechanisms of immune surveillance.[3] In addition, the fact that tumor cells can originate from self makes tolerance to self antigens an obstacle to complete antitumor activity.[5] Over the last two decades advances in methods of experimentation and the rapid surge in developing therapies have revealed the complex and dynamic role played by the immune system in tumorigenesis, tumor survival and tumor proliferation. This chapter will review what is currently known about the immune system and melanoma and nonmelanoma skin cancers.

Epidemiology

Skin Cancer in the General Population

Skin cancer is the most common cancer in the United States effecting approximately one million Americans a year.[6] It is estimated that almost fifty thousand melanoma in situ will be diagnosed in 2006.[7] In immune competent individuals basal cell carcinoma is the most common non melanoma skin cancer with a ratio of BCC to SCC of approximately 4-5:1.[7]

*Corresponding Author: Elma D. Baron—Department of Dermatology, Case Western Reserve University, University Hospitals of Cleveland, 11100 Euclid Ave., Lakeside 3500, and Dermatology Department, Cleveland Veterans Affairs Medical Center, Cleveland, OH, U.S.A. Email: elma.baron@case.edu

Sunlight, Vitamin D and Skin Cancer, edited by Jörg Reichrath. ©2008 Landes Bioscience and Springer Science+Business Media.

Skin Cancer in Organ Transplant Recipients

Skin cancer is the most common cancer to develop in organ transplant patients who are on immune suppressive therapy.[8] Interestingly, organ transplant recipients have an inverse ratio of BCC to SCC (1.2-1.5:1).[9] Melanomas in renal transplant recipients have been reported to occur approximately eight times the rate of the general population.[10] Additionally, the skin cancers seen in organ transplant recipients are more aggressive and more rapidly metastasize than those found in the non-immune suppressed population.[8,11] The risk of developing skin cancer correlates with the degree of immune suppression. For example, cardiac transplant recipients who are on higher levels of immunosuppressive drugs to prevent rejection are most susceptible to developing skin cancer, relative to other organ transplant recipients who receive lower doses of immunosuppressives.[11] Similarly, rates of skin cancer in transplant patients decrease when the immunosuppressive regimen is concurrently decreased.[8] Increased UV exposure remains a contributing factor in this population.[12] The relationship between immune suppression and UV radiation will be discussed in more detail later in the chapter.

It is believed by some that the high incidence of SCC in transplant patients cannot be adequately explained by immune suppression alone or by secondary oncogenic infections. The idea has been raised that indiscriminant immune suppression alone may not be responsible for transplant patients' susceptibility for skin cancers, but in fact, the immunosuppressive agent itself may have direct causative effects. Cyclosporin and tacrolimus in particular have been implicated in this increased cancer risk.[13] Systemic administration of calcineurin inhibitors has been implicated in skin cancer susceptibility by preventing the dephosphorylation of NFAT, a transcription factor necessary for DNA repair and Bcl2a agonist of cell death (BAD). Calcineurin inhibtors also suppress cytochrome C release and therefore prevent apoptosis.[14] Azathioprine and the thiopurines have also been named as contributors to skin carcinogenesis. When exposed to UVA, azathioprine generates reactive oxygen species which cause oxidative stress and DNA damage events known to be a leading cause of carcinogenesis.[15] These insights point to a mechanism of immune-manipulation rather than just suppression occurring to off set the delicate homeostasis of healthy skin and favor development of skin neoplasms.

Skin Cancer in Other Immune Suppressed Individuals

Patients infected with human immunodeficiency virus (HIV) do not show the same predilection for squamous and basal cell carcinomas seen in solid organ transplant patients. However these patients are susceptible to other pathogens such as human herpesvirus 8 and human papilloma virus. These patients frequently develop common warts and Kaposi's sarcoma. Interestingly, viral warts have been implicated as a risk factor for NMSC in transplant recipients.[16] While it is unclear as to what extent these HPV infections in HIV patients do translate into frank NMSCs, an association is not unreasonable. HIV infected individuals do have a higher incidence of BCC than the immune competent population.[17] Furthermore, it is known that when these patients develop SCC and melanoma, the course of their disease is more aggressive than that of an immune competent individual.[18]

UV Light and Immune Suppression

UV from solar radiation is the major environmental influence in the pathogenesis of both melanoma and non melanoma skin cancer. Chronic UV exposure is the main risk factor for development of squamous cell and basal cell carcinoma.[19,20] Although melanoma pathogenesis is less understood, it has been postulated that intermittent intense UV exposure is a risk factor for its development. One way UV light directly promotes tumorigenesis is through DNA damage.[21] DNA absorbs UVB which causes formation of cyclopyrimidine dimers and other photoproducts, which if left unrepaired can result in mutagenesis.[21] UVA may also have consequences on DNA via oxidative pathways resulting in the production of modified bases such as 8-hydroxy-2'deoxyguanosine or OHdG.[22,23] Interestingly, UV-induced DNA damage has been shown to result in upregulation of cytokines with immunosuppressive function.[24-25]

It has been found that over 90% of patients with nonmelanoma skin cancer exhibited depressed immune response or required increased hapten to initiate an immune response in the form of decreased contact hypersensitivity response to cutaneous antigens.[26,27] These results indicate that maintenance of immune responses is essential in preventing tumor growth. There are several mechanisms by which UV radiation induces immunosuppressive effects on the skin. One is through release of immunosuppressive cytokines.[28,29] When stimulated by UV radiation, dermal neutrophils secrete Il-4 and IL-10.[30] These cytokines induce tumor associated macrophages (TAMS) to an M2 tumor favorable state.[31] These M2 TAMS promote tumor progression which will be discussed later. Keratinocytes receive a significant portion of UV radiation. In response to this direct stimulation they release IL-1 and TNF alpha.[32] Another mode of immune suppression is achieved by induction of T-lymphocytes into apoptosis.[33,34] Still another mechanism involves Langerhans cells' presentation of antigens upon UV exposure, which can activate suppressor T-cells.[34,29]

UV radiation suppresses Langerhans cell function and numbers. It does so by affecting their morphology and ATP-ase activity.[35,34] In vitro studies show that low doses of UVB inhibit the capacity of Langerhans cells to produce Th1 but not Th2 type cytokines and in this way UVB disrupts the cytokine milieu towards a Th2 response.[36] In vitro UV exposed CD4+ T-cells produce decreased amounts of IFN gamma and IL2, as well as increased amounts of IL-4 and 5.[37] A link between UV mediated DNA damage and Fas/fasL has been described, indicating that when DNA damaged cyclobutane pyrimidine dimers are presented to CD4+ T-cells, there is down regulation of responding Fas+ T-cells and up regulation of FasL leading to T-cell apoptosis.[34]

In the stratum corneum, urocanic acid (UCA) absorbs UV light and undergoes isomerization from trans to cis forms. The cis but not trans form has been shown in vitro and in vivo to be one factor responsible for UV induced immune suppression through impairment of the antigen presenting ability of dendritic cells.[38] Murine studies have shown a relationship between dermal mast cells and more specifically mast cell derived histamine and the extent of immune suppression induced by UV light.[39,40] M cell degranulation is a response to the isomerization of trans UCA to cis UCA.[41] The same link between mast cells, histamine and decreased immune response is hypothesized to exist in human skin.[42] Keratinocytes perpetuate increased dermal mast cells when activated by UV radiation. They do this through the release of IL-1 and IL-10, which are chemotactic for mast cell migration.[43,44] This relationship between immune suppression and mast cell degranulation provides some explanation for the correlation between a high concentration of dermal mast cells and risk for basal cell carcinoma.[45]

UV radiation is particularly dangerous because it acts as both a tumor initiator and promoter.[46] Overall, UV radiation suppresses both the initiation of immunity (Langerhans cells) as well as long term immunological memory (T-cells). T-cell damage produces what is known as tolerance induction.[47] It unclear whether primary or secondary immune responses are more vital to a tumor cell's escape from the body's surveillance mechanism.[48] What is known, is that UV light is an immune suppressor with a significant and multi-faceted role in carcinogenesis.

Role of the Immune System

The ability of tumor cells to escape detection from the immune system is known as "tumor immune escape".[4] The immune system is traditionally divided into two parts—innate and adaptive. Each part has a distinct function. Innate immunity is mainly responsible for responses that are considered non specific and immediate, such as fighting bacterial and viral pathogens.[49] Alternatively, adaptive immunity is more specific, involving B and T-cells that become activated after contact with unique antigens.[50] The role of B-cells in tumor immunity is still unclear. Recent evidence supports that they may have a role in recruiting mast cells to tumor stroma, but the implications are still unclear. It has been proposed that B-cells play a role in lymphogenesis and metastasis of melanoma cells.[51]

Adaptive immunity was previously thought to be the major contributor to tumor surveillance via T-cells and their receptors. The role of antigen presenting cells and innate immunity was considered minor. It is now believed that both components may be equally vital. Other key factors include a complex play of costimulatory molecules, ligands and cytokines that bring together innate and adaptive elements. This section outlines some of the key elements of both adaptive and innate immunity and ways in which skin tumor cells manipulate protective functions to circumvent elimination and survive.

Inflammation

Acute inflammation causes a cascade of linked events including cytokine proliferation and cell migration. Similarities between wound repair and tumor development are evident. Both are strongly governed by inflammatory cells. During an inflammatory response in wound repair, platelets, neutrophils and mast cells participate by releasing many of the same growth factors and protineases released by tumor cells to initiate angiogenesis and re-epithelialization. However, these signals usually resolve upon re-epitelialization. On the other hand, in tumor tissue the response is chronic and persistent thereby promoting undesirable effects of growth and invasion.[31]

Areas of chronic inflammation have been known since the mid nineteenth century to be common sites for many epithelial cancers.[31] It is now known that inflammation could be serve as a tumor promoting microenvironment..

In the lab several inflammatory chemicals such as 12-O-tetra-decanoylphrobol 13 acetate (TPA) and 7,12-dimethylbenzanthracene (DMBA) are applied to the skin of mice to produce epithelial tumors. In fact, most experimentally used tumor promoters also initiate some inflammatory response.[52] Clinical evidence linking chronic inflammation to skin cancer is evidenced by Marjolin's ulcer[31] and an association with SCC development in non healing wounds and inflammatory disorders such as discoid lupus, osteomyelitis, perineal inflammatory disease and epidermolysis bullosa.[31] Moreover healed wounds with scar tissue are more susceptible to development of SCC and BCC. Interestingly, a transient inflammatory stage was observed during the transformation of actinic keratoses to SCC.[31]

Cells of Innate Immunity

Macrophages

Inflammatory chemokines act on undifferentiated monocytes to generate tumor infiltrating macrophages and dendritic cells.[53] Activated macrophages are subdivided into two main groups. M1 macrophages are capable of inducing nitric oxide synthase, interleukin-12 and tumor necrosis factor (TNF). M2 macrophages produce arginase, IL-10, transforming growth factor beta (TGF beta) and prostaglandin E2 (PGE2). With their respective cytokine repertoire, M1 macrophages promote tumor elimination while M2 macrophages promote angiogenesis and tissue remodeling. M2 macrophages contribute to a tumor permissive environment by restricting the Type 1 response and secreting IL-10. This action perpetuates an M2 state.[54] Their secretion of pro-inflammatory cytokines also perpetuates an inflammatory state.[55] Type I macrophages and antibodies to IL-10 were shown to produce a rapid regression of tumors through IL-12 and TNF as well as release of nitric oxide.[53]

Stat-3 is an oncogenic pathway commonly and constitutively activated in several cancers including those of epithelial origin.[56] Stat 3 macrophages have been shown to have an anti tumor effect by producing IL-12. Enigmatically, Stat 3 was demonstrated to be responsible for incomplete maturation of dendritic cells. Some studies showed that termination of the Stat 3 pathway resulted in an increased immune response which was not seen in Stat-3 positive mice.[56]

Mast Cells

Enhanced recruitment of mast cells has been observed during chemically induced skin carcinomas.[57] In another study using the k14-HPV16 mouse model spontaneous epithelial hyperplasias progressed to SCC in 20% of subjects. Mast cells were seen infiltrating all neoplasms and were found to contribute to activation of a tumor promoting environment, via release of chymase, tryptase and proMMP activators.[58] Mouse models deficient in either mast cells or MMP 9 had decreased incidence of skin tumors. Hence a link was established between mast cells and initial development of SCCs.[59]

NK-Cells

NK-cells are a part of innate immunity's arsenal used against tumor cells.[60,61] NK-cells use direct (perforin) and indirect (production of IFN gamma) methods to achieve their antitumor effect.[62] The function of these cytotoxic cells depends on the balance between activating and suppressive signals within the surrounding environment.[62] Melanoma cells can down regulate MHC class I on T-cells. Under such circumstances NK activity is upregulated.[2,60] Such increased NK-cell activity alone is not sufficient in eradicating tumor cells.

NK-cells participate in tumor surveillance through a variety of receptors and mechanisms.[2,63] A receptor known as the NKG2d appears on both NK-cells and a subset of T-cells (gamma delta and alpha beta T-cells) and therefore links innate and adaptive immunity together in immune surveillance.[2] NKG2D is a primary recognition receptor on suspect cells, such as transformed tumor cells.[62] However tumor cells that express NKG2D escape tumor surveillance, perhaps through suppression of perforin synthesizing signals or resistance to perforin itself.[62] In vitro HLA-G has been shown to inhibit NK activity.[64] Melanoma cells inhibit NK activity by interacting with a specific HLA-G class I molecules and interacting with KIRs.[64]

Dendritic Cells

Initiation of an immune response begins with a signal. In the case of tumor surveillance this signal comes from a transformed cell.[63] One way tumor cells evade the immune system is by failing to initiate an adequate warning signal.[63] This "danger" signal will activate antigen presenting cells (APC).[63] such as Langerhans cells, which are the dendritic cells of the epidermis.[65] Langerhans cells originate in the bone marrow from progenitor cells.[66] They mature and differentiate under the influence of growth and differentiation factors such as granulocyte macrophage colony stimulating factor (G-MCSF) and fms-like tyrosine kinase 3 ligand.[67] They are related to macrophages and monocytes through surface cell markers.[68] They are distinguished by expression of CD1a, E-cadherin and Birbeck granules.[69]

As Langerhans cells mature in skin they migrate to draining lymph nodes.[65] Here they interact with naïve lymphoid T-cells via a CD40-CD40 ligand. This ligand is responsible for the regulation of dendritic cell migration and therefore indirectly affects T-cell activation. CD40 expression on keratinocytes is important in the costimulation of T-cell proliferation. Increased expression of CD40 has been observed in the epidermis associated with BCC. Another important role of dendritic cells is expression of costimulatory molecules and production of cytokines during the differentiation of Th cells after antigen presentation.[63] These events are characterized by the costimulatory molecules CD40, CD80 and CD86 and T-cell priming.[63]

Immature DCs have the ability to dampen the immune response. They can do this two ways, either by decreasing amounts of T-cells or increasing amounts of regulatory T-cells,[70] It has been shown that melanoma cells although unable to effect maturation of differentiated Langerhans cells, were able to inhibit differentiation of early Langerhans cell precursors in vitro. The degree of inhibition was directly related to the aggressiveness of the melanoma line.[71] In fact, some deeply invasive melanomas have found dermal LC to be completely absent.[71] The presence of CD1a+ DCs was not found to be a prognostic indicator for melanoma disease, however the density of mature DCs especially when in the presence of activated T-cells, was found to be a predictor of survival and parameter of functional immune response in melanoma patients.[72]

Indoleamine 2,3-dioxygenase or IDO is an enzyme responsible for the catabolism of tryptophan.[73] This enzyme is known in mice to play a role in the immunogenic tolerance of allogenic fetuses.[74] This molecule is also an inhibitor of T-cell proliferation in vitro[75] and in addition down regulates T-cell responses in vivo.[74] A subset of human monocyte-derived dendritic cells express IDO.[76] It has been speculated that IDO+ APCs may participate in the state of apparent immune responsiveness displayed by many cancer patients toward tumor-associated antigens.[76] Their direct mechanism of action on the immune system is however still undetermined.

Tumor Antigens

Tumor associated antigens or TAAs are present on several tumor types including melanomas.[77] Melanoma cells can express several tumor associated antigens.[77] Antigens such as gp100, tyrosinase related protein (TRP1),[78] TRP2, tyrosinase melanoma antigen recognized by T-cells (MART-1) are melanocyte lineage specific antigens.[79] Other tumor specific T-cell targets are preferentially expressed antigen on melanomas (PRAME),[80] and melanoma antigen 1 (MAGE1). These are antigens derived from genes expressed in other cancers.[79,77] Intuitively, the immune system should be able to eradicate these antigenic tumor cells from the body. Both antigen types have been used as tumor rejection antigens against melanoma with disappointing results. These results may be partially explained by the fact that these tumor antigens behave more like self antigens,[81,4] in which case T-cells respond with lower affinity relative to T-cell response against foreign Ags.[81] Immunogenicity of tumor antigens can be diminished when tumor cells create dysfunctions in processing and presenting or deficiencies in quantity.[82] Additionally, failure of costimulatory molecules on tumor cells to express themselves promotes a tumor tolerant environment.

Cytokines

Cytokines and growth factors control the balance between immune responsiveness and tolerance they play a role in the immunoregulatory function in both melanoma[83,84] and non melanoma skin cancers.[55]

IL-12

IL-12 promotes a Th1 response.[5] IL-12 was originally known as NK stimulatory factor and as cytotoxic lymphocyte maturation factor.[85] IL-12 up regulates proliferation and maturation of T-cells, inhibits angiogenesis and induces the production of IFN gamma.[85] Il-12 is thought of as a bridging cytokine between the adaptive and innate immune response because activation of CD40 ligand on dendritic cells induces Il-12 which goes on to effect $CD8^+$ cells.[85] There is also evidence that IL-12 can stimulate macrophages[85] IL-12 can be produced by a variety of immune cells including dendritic cells, macrophages, B-cells and keratinocytes.[38] IL-12 may interfere with the production of IL-10 in vivo.[86] It can also act synergistically with IL-2 to upregulate Th1 cytokine production. Studies by Brunda et al[87] have shown that transplantable tumors have a significant decrease in size and formation of metastasis when exposed to IL-12.[88] IL-12 also counteracts the immune suppression induced by UV light.[88,29] and was shown in vivo to counteract the suppressive effects of cis-urocanic acid on Langerhans cells[38] IL-12 is also associated with DNA repair that takes place after UV exposure.[89]

IFN Gamma

Interferon gamma (IFN gamma) is produced by CD8, CD4, T-gamma delta cells and NK-cells.[53] This cytokine mediates multiple antitumor effects. It plays a role in melanoma control[90] and is known to inhibit cell proliferation.[91]

TNF Alpha

TNF alpha plays a role in UV induced immune suppression and is also a well studied pro-inflammatory cytokine in skin carcinogeneis and in wound healing. TNF alpha knock-out mice were found to be resistant to the usual carcinogenic effects of DMBA or TPA.[55] Further studies using antibodies to block TNF alpha demonstrate that induction of TNF alpha secretion by skin keratinocytes during the first 0-6 weeks is crucial to skin tumor promotion.[92] Later stages of carcinogenesis are not effected by the absence of TNF alpha.[92]

Interestingly, TNF alpha and IFN gamma are produced by T-cells to increase target cell toxicity.[93] Both have the ability to upregulate intercellular adhesion molecule1 (ICAM 1) which is costimulatory molecule on the surface of APC.[94] Studies looking at BCC tumor cells' response to ICAM-1 in vitro have speculated that a decreased number of IFN gamma receptors on tumor cells and shedding of ICAM-1 is one way that BCC tumor cells survive and evade the antitumor immune responses.[95,94]

Il-6

IL-6 dampens the Th1 response and is a poor prognostic indicator in melanoma.[96] IL-6 has a key role in immune regulation and because of its potency, its production is under strict regulation. IL 6 enhances tumor growth when transfected into human BCCs.[97] Studies done in vitro and in vivo using BCC showed that IL-6 plays a role in the aggressiveness of BCC by decreasing apoptosis via Bcl expression. IL-6 also increases angiogenesis through VEGF and Cox-2.[97] IL-6, along with IL-8 prostaglandin E2, TGF B are melanoma-derived cytokines with direct effects on the body's immune response[98-101]

IL-10

IL-10 is produced by T-lymphocytes, B-lymphocytes and monocytes. It was shown, in vitro, to inhibit antigen specific activation. However, Shin-ichiro et al showed in vivo that high doses of IL-10 in mice activated production of anti tumor mediators IL-2 and IL-4 and activated and protected CD8+ T-cells.[102] IL-10 and IL-4 both considered type 2 or Th2 cytokines are predominant in cutaneous carcinomas.[102] These were shown to be secreted by BCC and SCC tumor cells themselves.[95] In BCC, IL-10 secretion accounts for many of this neoplasm's mechanisms of immune evasion. It is believed to be responsible either directly or indirectly for the absence of HLA, ICAM-1 CD40 and CD80 on BCC in situ.[95]

Cytokines IL-10, TGF-beta and PGE2 and VEGF are all known to suppress the immune response. This occurs via a number of ways, one being their effect on dendritic cells.[103] However IL-6 along with TNF alpha, IL 1 beta and prostaglandin E2 can be used in culture to induce dendritic cell maturation. At the same time PGE2 has been known to impair the production of IL-12 from dendritic cells and polarize naïve CD4 T-cells towards Th1 activity.[104]

TGF Beta

It is difficult to classify TGF beta as tumor promoting or tumor suppressive because it appears to have a role in both. TGF acts on stroma, endothelial cells and immune cells to promote tumor growth. It appears to have a prohibitive effect in the early stage but a tumor supportive effect in the later stage.[105]

TGF beta has been thought to antagonize many of the antitumor effects of IL-12[88] TGF betas form a group of ligands responsible for upregulating and downregulating various multicellular functions. These include apoptosis, decreased cell proliferation, migration, differentiation, induction of MMP production, increased angiogenesis and decreased immune surveillance.[106] In mammals, TGF betas exist as several different isoforms which function through the same receptor signaling systems, although they appear to have distinct modes of action in vivo.[107]

Interestingly, mouse models have shown some cancers (breast) to become hypoplastic in the presence of active TGF beta,[108] while others (lung and skin) have shown enhancement in the presence of this polypeptide ligand.[109] Cui et al demonstrated that abundant expression of TGFB in keratinocytes prevented the development of benign papillomas, whereas the same overexpression of TGF beta in mice with transgenic tumors caused more aggressive tumors and increased metastasis.[110] Mice who are resistant to TGF beta have been shown to mount effective immune responses against tumors.[111] In addition, mice in which the TGF beta pathway has been inhibited have shown effective tumor clearance.[93] Malfunctioning of this cytokine contributes to several aspects of tumor progression including loss of inhibitory control, increased metastasis and evasion of immune surveillance.[112] This evasion of immune surveillance is directly caused by the cytokine's interaction with cytotoxic lymphocytes (CTL). TGFB signals through Smad dependent and independent pathways[113] to inhibit T-cell proliferation. Smad is critical for inhibition of anti CD3 and anti CD28 but not necessary for TGF production of IL-2 nor it's effects on T-cell regulation.[113] TGF betas also effect the perforin and granzyme producing genes of CTL.[93]

Adaptive Immunity

T-Cells

T-cells are a key component of the immune system's ability to reject cancer.[81] They interact with antigen presenting cells through a T-cell receptor (TCR). There are numerous subsets of T-cell populations, including cytotoxic T-cells (CTL), helper T-cells (Th), regulatory T-cells (Treg) which were previously known as T-suppressor cells,[114] and natural killer T-cells which share a common receptor type (α β) with other types of T-cells, but are associated with NK-cells by common molecular markers. NKT-cells have an invariant T-cell receptor (TCR) which are known as iNKT. This receptor works through nonclassical MHC and is important in signaling and maturing DC.[115] Activation of T-cells requires additional costimulation with molecules and ligands. T-cells can also be labeled by their receptor types and costimulatory markers: CD8[+] (cytotoxic), CD4[+] (helper) and CD4[+] CD25[+] (regulatory), CD4[+] CD28[+] (helper with CD28 costimulatory molecule), alpha beta (common T-cells), gamma delta (intraepithelial T-cells) etc.

The development of naïve T-cells into their distinct subgroups is dictated by the predominance of cytokines expressed in their particular environment. Traditionally, these environments are dichotomized into stimulatory (Th1 or Type 1) or regulatory (Th2 or Type 2). Cytokines such a interferon gamma and Interleukin-2 are associated with a Th1 response, whereas Interleukin 4, 5, 6 and 10 are associated with a Th2 response.[116,28] An effective antitumor response requires antigen processing by DC along with specific signaling pathways to initiate a Th1 response.[69] Melanoma cells have been shown to influence PBMCs towards a Th2 profile. Moreover, patients with advanced or progressing melanoma frequently have circulating cytokines reflective of a Th2 environment[117] A sustained Th2 profile allows for immune tolerance of melanoma cells allowing them to proliferate.[114] Interestingly, CD4[+] T-cells can express both Th1 and Th2 cytokines as well as attract and activate other antitumor cells.[50] Furthermore Th1 and Th2 mechanisms are not necessarily always anatagonistic but can work together to produce an effective antitumor effect.[50]

The skin contains a population of T-cells specialized by function and location. These are known as intraepithelial lymphocytes (IELs).[118] In mice the majority of skin IELs are gamma delta T-cells. These cells are extremely specific with regard to antigen interaction in their V region similar to NK-cells of innate immunity, IELs become activated through NKG2d ligand. When skin is exposed to carcinogens, the induction of NKG2d ligands (Rae-1 and H60 in mice and MICA/MICB in humans) is triggered, resulting in eradication of stressed and transformed cells before they can multiply and become tumors.[2]

T-cells along with NK-cells are frequently seen infiltrating skin tumors.[119] Yet surprisingly, T-cell density within BCC SCC or melanoma is no indication for a favorable prognosis. Tumor cells have several ways to manipulate T-cell mediated immunity in order to evade the immune response. Mouse studies have shown that melanoma could encourage the development of hypo responsive T-cells.[81] One mechanism for immune evasion occurs through T-cell receptor manipulation. Tumor cells can evade T-cell detection by causing down regulation of MCH class I molecules, which is a key component needed for antigen recognition and therefore tumor surveillance.[64,120,121,77] This interferes with critical events that generate an optimal interaction between dendritic cell and T-cell.

Additionally, melanoma cells can interact with killing inhibiting receptors (KIR) on TCR signaling. When CD8[+] and CD4[+] cells become activated they express CD28. CD28 is a costimulatory signal needed for proper CD8[+] and CD4[+] functioning. Failure of costimulatory molecules on tumor cells to express themselves has been shown to promote a tumor tolerant environment.[122] The tumor itself can also promote a favorable environment for survival. In patients with certain cancers, including melanoma, tumor cells release endosome derived microvesicles. These microvesicles are armed with various molecules including immunoregulators such as TGF-Beta which has been shown to suppress effective T-cell function against the tumor and generate myeloid suppressor cells (MSCs) thereby inhibiting the host immune response. Unlike interaction with receptor signaling these microvesicles function without cell to cell contact.[123] Additionally, these (MSCs) are found in higher numbers in melanoma patients when compared to normal controls.[124]

CD8 Cells

Cytotoxic T-cells are killer cells that attack viruses and tumors. They are known to play a protective role against melanoma. For this reason they have been used experimentally to treat the cancers. In human studies, CD8[+] cells were induced by self/tumor antigens in significant quantities thought to be sufficient to produce tumor regression. However, despite the generation of these protective cells, tumor regression was not observed.[125] Another suspected way that melanoma tumors evade immune attack is by effecting the maturation of CD8[+] T-cells.[124] This theory is supported by the finding that T-cells from PBMCs of melanoma patients are unable to release perforin and other lytic enzymes necessary for cytotoxic activity.[126]

Human studies looking at melanoma specific T-cells showed that proliferation and induction of antigen specific CD8[+] T-cells takes place later during the advanced stage of the disease and may be due to tumor growth and spread rather than an attempt at rejection. This suggests that T-cells generated during antitumor response may be distinct from those melanoma specific CD8[+] T-cells found in late stage melanomas.[77]

In several murine studies, vitiligo corresponded with melanoma regression.[127] Yet some patients whose tumors exhibit large amounts of tumor antigen positive T-cells fail to demonstrate either vitiligo or regression. Other studies in mice have shown that CD8[+] T-cells were necessary for the vitiligo response and concurrent tumor rejection.[127] This is evidence for either a different type of T-cell or a different mechanism. While mice models have been vital to unraveling the complexities of immune surveillance, it is more important to keep in mind that a difference exists between the immunogenicity of the cancer cells seen in mice vs. humans.[5]

CD4 Cells

For effective and long term tumor eradication, the action of both CD8[+] and CD4[+] T-cells is required. This has been demonstrated using T-cell subset depletion studies, in which antibodies to CD4[+] T-cells given to mice prior to tumor challenge showed that they were unable to mount an adequate anti tumor response.[50] Although the role of CD4[+] T-cells takes place during the priming phase,[53] CD4[+] T helper cells are needed for both the induction and maintenance of antitumor immunity.[128] Additionally cytokines released by these helper T-cells promote migration and activation of macrophages and eosinophils,[50] priming them to produce the nitric oxide and superoxides needed as part of the immunologic attack.[128] Cancer patients with progressive disease in general have decreased CD4[+] counts. Interestingly, decreased CD4[+] cells are found in tumor deposits of patients who failed therapy.[114]

Murine studies by Willimsky et al[129] raise the possibility that tumor cells do not just evade detection but actually induce T-cell tolerance, by decreasing IFN gamma and increasing TGF beta.

T-Reg Cells

CD4[+] 25[+] suppressor cells known as regulatory T-cells play a role in regulating immunity and maintaining peripheral self-tolerance.[130,5] Murine studies demonstrated that removal of these cells using antibodies along with addition of IL-12 had a potent antimelanoma effect.[5] Conversely when CD8[+] cells or NK-cells were blocked, tumor regression did not occur. In another study using melanoma B16, Turk et al found that this tumor was significantly more immunogenic in mice lacking T-reg cells than in mice with an intact T-reg population, indicating their importance in dampening the immune response to tumor antigens.[130]

Other Factors that Interact with the Immune Mechanisms in Tumorigenesis and Tumor Invasion

Apoptosis

Apoptosis, or programmed cell death is important for maintaining homeostasis. Cancer cells survive because of resistance to apoptosis. T-cells mediate cell death in two ways: (1) secretion of granzymes and perforin, (2)via interaction of Fas and fas ligand. Fas-fasL plays an immunogenic role. It is responsible for discontinuing the T-cell response when no longer needed, decreasing clonal

T-cell population and promoting periphral tolerance to self Ags.[131] Tumor cells can manipulate this pathway by becoming resistant to both the fas/fasl killing and the ERK1/2 mitogen activated kinase pathway.[132] Ironically, the Fas- ligand (FasL) is also expressed by tumor cells and can be used by them to kill T-cells.[133] Therefore through this mechanism of acquired immortality and T-cell attack, tumor cells are able not only to evade the immune response but manipulate it to their advantage.[132] This attack by tumor cells does not eliminate all T-cells. It has been shown[134] that an unquantified subset of CD4+ and CD+ T-cells exisits that is not sensitive to Fas-fasL apoptosis. These T-cells kill tumor cells through a fas independent mechanism.[134]

Ligands

CD80 which is found on T-and other cells is also known as B7-1. The B7H ligands are a family of tumor associated molecules found on stimulated macrophages, DCs and T-cells as well as some epithelial and endothelial cells. Depending on receptor interaction they can have CD-28, ICOS (stimulating) or PD-L1 (supressive) effects. When interaction with PD-L1 takes place these ligands induce apoptosis of activated tumor reactive T-cells.[135,136] PD-L1 expression by tumor cells is one way for them to develop T-cell immunity.[137] Antibodies used to block B7-H1 were shown to have therapeutic antitumor effects and increase the efficacy of adoptive T-cell therapy of squamous cell carcinoma of the head and neck in vivo.[138] This study also demonstrated that B7-H1 can be upregulated by IFN gamma. This is significant because it suggests induction of B7-H1 may be used by tumor cells to decrease T-cell population and avoid elimination.[138] BH-71 also selectively costimulates the production of IL-10 and IFN gamma.[139]

Tumor necrosis factor related apoptosis inducing ligand (TRAIL) is a member of the tumor necrosis factor family that preferentially induces apoptosis in transformed but not normal cells.[140] TRAIL is expressed in the skin.[140] It is known to bind to two receptors TRAIL-R1 and TRAIL-R2. It is speculated that the high expression of TRAIL within the epidermis is protective against the development of skin cancer. TRAIL expression is decreased in elderly or chronically UV exposed skin as well as actinic keratoses and absent in squamous and basal cell carcinoma.[140]

MMP

Immune suppression can be associated with increased matrix metalloproteinase (MMP) expression. The MMP family of proteinases are able to break down components of the extracellular matrix (ECM) and basement membrane (BM) and therefore promote tumor invasion.[32] A study found that MMP expression from SCC in immune compromised patients was greater compared to that of SCC in immune competent individuals. MMPs can activate regulatory molecules including growth factors and cytokines, such as TGF beta.[141,32]

Therapies and Future Work

As mechanisms of tumor surveillance and survival become better understood, novel therapies attempting to manipulate these mechanisms to the host's favor are developed. Melanoma vaccines using tumor antigens have been tested with limited clinical outcome. Adoptive immunotherapy has also been attempted with mixed results.[124] Despite the various melanoma antigens only a small fraction (10-15) have been used in either type of therapy,[124] and methods to increase their immunogenicity are continually being examined.[142]

Other potential immunotherapies take advantage of stimulating cytokines.[143] For example, interferon gamma and IL-2 have been shown to produce remissions and eradication of melanomas.[144] IL-12 IL-2 pulse was also shown to enhance both Fas-fasL gene expression within the local tumor cite through an IFN gamma dependant mechanism.[144] IL 12 has cytotoxic effects which occur in a dose dependant relationship.[5] Administering a plasmid encoding IL-12 with electro-corporation has been shown to be therapeutic on both primary and metastatic tumors.[145] Current studies are looking into the effects of various cytokines including IFN [90,146] and Il-2.[143]

Other strategies include attempts to block signaling pathways that lead to decreased melanoma expression and loss of antigenecity.[147] Use of recombinant viruses and proteins encoding cancer Ags, immunization with whole tumor cells and Ag-loaded dendritic cells have also been studied.[67]

These therapies initially showed promising results during phase I and II trials but were not able to replicate their success in phase III randomized trials.[124] However, dendritic cells continue to be studied as an important entity in melanoma therapy.[84,148]

Other research has attempted to manipulate T-cell functions. In one study specific toll like receptors on CD8[+] T-lymphocytes were utilized for their secretion of tumoricidal cytokines to cause rejection of melanoma in mice.[149] Monoclonal antibodies against T-cell regulators as well a manipulation of tumor genes that effect T-cells are also being investigated with some success.[124]

While no therapy has provided a complete success these trials provide insight and inspire novel strategies to counteract the intricate immunological pathways responsible for tumor surveillance escape mechanisms.[124]

Conclusion

The immune system actively attempts to eradicate transformed cells from the body. During this response a complex interplay between tumor cells, stimulatory molecules, ligands and immune cells takes place in an attempt to tip the balance of the surrounding cytokines and stroma between tumor eradication or immune escape. As the intricacies of these interactions are uncovered conventional models are replaced with a more fluid model of the immune system where cellular and molecular roles are not firmly defined and instead adjust according to the specific surroundings. As novel therapies are developed the dynamic nature of this relationship becomes increasingly apparent.

References

1. Burnet M. Concepts of autoimmune disease and their implications for therapy. Perspect Biol Med 1967 Winter; 10(2):141-151.
2. Pardoll DM. Immunology. Stress, NK receptors and immune surveillance. Science 2001; 294(5542):534-536.
3. Dunn GP, Old LJ, Schreiber RD. The immunobiology of cancer immunosurveillance and immunoediting. Immunity 2004; 21(2):137-148.
4. Pardoll D. Does the immune system see tumors as foreign or self? Annu Rev Immunol 2003; 21:807-839.
5. Nagai H, Horikawa T, Hara I et al. In vivo elimination of CD25[+] regulatory T-cells leads to tumor rejection of B16F10 melanoma, when combined with interleukin-12 gene transfer. Exp Dermatol 2004; 13(10):613-620.
6. Han J, Colditz GA, Hunter DJ. Risk factors for skin cancers: a nested case-control study within the Nurses' Health Study. Int J Epidemiol 2006.
7. Veness MJ. Defining patients with high-risk cutaneous squamous cell carcinoma. Australas J Dermatol 2006; 47(1):28-33.
8. Jemec GB, Holm EA. Nonmelanoma skin cancer in organ transplant patients. Transplantation 2003; 75(3):253-257.
9. Nguyen TH, Ho DQ. Nonmelanoma skin cancer. Curr Treat Options Oncol 2002; 3(3):193-203.
10. Le Mire L, Hollowood K, Gray D et al. Melanomas in renal transplant recipients. Br J Dermatol 2006; 154(3):472-477.
11. Euvrard S, Kanitakis J, Decullier E et al. Subsequent skin cancers in kidney and heart transplant recipients after the first squamous cell carcinoma. Transplantation 2006; 81(8):1093-1100.
12. Boyle J, MacKie RM, Briggs JD et al. Cancer, warts and sunshine in renal transplant patients. A case-control study. Lancet 1984; 1(8379):702-705.
13. Tiu J, Li H, Rassekh C et al. Molecular basis of posttransplant squamous cell carcinoma: the potential role of cyclosporine a in carcinogenesis. Laryngoscope 2006; 116(5):762-769.
14. Yarosh DB, Pena AV, Nay SLV et al. Calcineurin inhibitors decrease DNA repair and apoptosis in human keratinocytes following ultraviolet B irradiation. J Invest Dermatol 2005; 125(5):1020-1025.
15. O'Donovan P, Perrett CM, Zhang X et al. Azathioprine and UVA light generate mutagenic oxidative DNA damage. Science 2005; 309(5742):1871-1874.
16. Ramsay HM, Fryer AA, Reece S et al. Clinical risk factors associated with nonmelanoma skin cancer in renal transplant recipients. Am J Kidney Dis 2000; 36(1):167-176.
17. Wilkins K, Turner R, Dolev JC et al. Cutaneous malignancy and human immunodeficiency virus disease. J Am Acad Dermatol 2006; 54(2):189-206, quiz 207-10.
18. Nguyen P, Vin-Christian K, Ming ME et al. Aggressive squamous cell carcinomas in persons infected with the human immunodeficiency virus. Arch Dermatol 2002; 138(6):758-763.
19. Armstrong BK, Kricker A. The epidemiology of UV induced skin cancer. J Photochem Photobiol B 2001; 63(1-3):8-18.

20. Melnikova VO, Ananthaswamy HN. Cellular and molecular events leading to the development of skin cancer. Mutat Res 2005; 571(1-2):91-106.
21. Yarosh DB. DNA repair, immunosuppression and skin cancer. Cutis 2004; 74(5 Suppl):10-13.
22. Hattori Y, Nishigori C, Tanaka T et al. 8-hydroxy-2'-deoxyguanosine is increased in epidermal cells of hairless mice after chronic ultraviolet B exposure. J Invest Dermatol 1996; 107(5):733-737.
23. Zhang X, Wu RS, Fu W et al. Production of reactive oxygen species and 8-hydroxy-2'deoxyguanosine in KB cells co-exposed to benzo[a]pyrene and UV-A radiation. Chemosphere 2004; 55(10):1303-1308.
24. Schwarz T. Mechanisms of UV-induced immunosuppression. Keio J Med 2005; 54(4):165-171.
25. Cooper KD. Cell-mediated immunosuppressive mechanisms induced by UV radiation. Photochem Photobiol 1996; 63(4):400-406.
26. Yoshikawa T, Rae V, Bruins-Slot W et al. Susceptibility to effects of UVB radiation on induction of contact hypersensitivity as a risk factor for skin cancer in humans. J Invest Dermatol 1990; 95(5):530-536.
27. Streilein JW, Taylor JR, Vincek V et al. Relationship between ultraviolet radiation-induced immunosuppression and carcinogenesis. J Invest Dermatol 1994; 103(5 Suppl):107S-111S.
28. Rivas JM, Ullrich SE. Systemic suppression of delayed-type hypersensitivity by supernatants from UV-irradiated keratinocytes. An essential role for keratinocyte-derived IL-10. J Immunol 1992; 149(12):3865-3871.
29. Nghiem DX, Kazimi N, Mitchell DL et al. Mechanisms underlying the suppression of established immune responses by ultraviolet radiation. J Invest Dermatol 2002; 119(3):600-608.
30. Noonan FP, De Fabo EC, Kripke ML. Suppression of contact hypersensitivity by UV radiation and its relationship to UV-induced suppression of tumor immunity. Photochem Photobiol 1981; 34(6):683-689.
31. Mueller MM. Inflammation in epithelial skin tumours: old stories and new ideas. Eur J Cancer 2006; 42(6):735-744.
32. Shellman YG, Makela M, Norris DA. Induction of secreted matrix metalloproteinase-9 activity in human melanoma cells by extracellular matrix proteins and cytokines. Melanoma Res 2006; 16(3):207-211.
33. Ozawa H, Aiba S, Nakagawa et al. Interferon-gamma and interleukin-10 inhibit antigen presentation by Langerhans cells for T helper type 1 cells by suppressing their CD80 (B7-1) expression. Eur J Immunol 1996; 26(3):648-652.
34. Hill LL, Shreedhar VK, Kripke ML et al. A critical role for Fas ligand in the active suppression of systemic immune responses by ultraviolet radiation. J Exp Med 1999; 189(8):1285-1294.
35. Toews GB, Bergstresser PR, Streilein JW. Langerhans cells: sentinels of skin associated lymphoid tissue. J Invest Dermatol 1980; 75(1):78-82.
36. Simon JC, Cruz PD, Jr, Bergstresser PR et al. Low dose ultraviolet B-irradiated Langerhans cells preferentially activate CD4+ cells of the T helper 2 subset. J Immunol 1990; 145(7):2087-2091.
37. Araneo BA, Dowell T, Moon HB et al. Regulation of murine lymphokine production in vivo. Ultraviolet radiation exposure depresses IL-2 and enhances IL-4 production by T-cells through an IL-1-dependent mechanism. J Immunol 1989; 143(6):1737-1744.
38. Beissert S, Ruhlemann D, Mohammad T et al. IL-12 prevents the inhibitory effects of cis-urocanic acid on tumor antigen presentation by Langerhans cells: implications for photocarcinogenesis. J Immunol 2001; 167(11):6232-6238.
39. Hart PH, Jaksic A, Swift G et al. Histamine involvement in UVB- and cis-urocanic acid-induced systemic suppression of contact hypersensitivity responses. Immunology 1997; 91(4):601-608.
40. Hart PH, Grimbaldeston MA, Swift GJ et al. Dermal mast cells determine susceptibility to ultraviolet B-induced systemic suppression of contact hypersensitivity responses in mice. J Exp Med 1998; 187(12):2045-2053.
41. Khalil Z, Townley SL, Grimbaldeston MA et al. cis-Urocanic acid stimulates neuropeptide release from peripheral sensory nerves. J Invest Dermatol 2001; 117(4):886-891.
42. Grimbaldeston MA, Skov L, Finlay-Jones JJ et al. Increased dermal mast cell prevalence and susceptibility to development of basal cell carcinoma in humans. Methods 2002; 28(1):90-96.
43. Piccinni MP, Maggi E, Romagnani S. Environmental factors favoring the allergen-specific Th2 response in allergic subjects. Ann NY Acad Sci 2000; 917:844-852.
44. Kameyoshi Y, Morita E, Tanaka T et al. Interleukin-1 alpha enhances mast cell growth by a fibroblast-dependent mechanism. Arch Dermatol Res 2000; 292(5):240-247.
45. Grimbaldeston MA, Skov L, Baadsgaard O et al. Communications: high dermal mast cell prevalence is a predisposing factor for basal cell carcinoma in humans. J Invest Dermatol 2000; 115(2):317-320.
46. Ziegler A, Leffell DJ, Kunala S et al. Mutation hotspots due to sunlight in the p53 gene of nonmelanoma skin cancers. Proc Natl Acad Sci USA 1993; 90(9):4216-4220.
47. Schwarz T. Mechanisms of UV-induced immunosuppression. Link between UV-induced tolerance and apoptosis. Eur J Dermatol 1998; 8(3):196-197.

48. Byrne SN, Spinks N, Halliday GM. The induction of immunity to a protein antigen using an adjuvant is significantly compromised by ultraviolet A radiation. J Photochem Photobiol B 2006; 84(2):128-134.
49. Schiller M, Metze D, Luger TA et al. Immune response modifiers—mode of action. Exp Dermatol 2006; 15(5):331-341.
50. Hung K, Hayashi R, Lafond-Walker A et al. The central role of CD4($^+$) T-cells in the antitumor immune response. J Exp Med 1998; 188(12):2357-2368.
51. Harrell MI, Iritani BM, Ruddell A. Tumor-induced sentinel lymph node lymphangiogenesis and increased lymph flow precede melanoma metastasis. Am J Pathol 2007; 170(2):774-786.
52. Poland A, Palen D, Glover E. Tumour promotion by TCDD in skin of HRS/J hairless mice. Nature 1982; 300(5889):271-273.
53. Guiducci C, Valzasina B, Dislich H et al. CD40/CD40L interaction regulates CD4$^+$ CD25$^+$ T-reg homeostasis through dendritic cell-produced IL-2. Eur J Immunol 2005; 35(2):557-567.
54. Moore KW, de Waal Malefyt R, Coffman RL et al. Interleukin-10 and the interleukin-10 receptor. Annu Rev Immunol 2001; 19:683-765.
55. Mueller MM. Inflammation in epithelial skin tumours: old stories and new ideas. Eur J Cancer 2006; 42(6):735-744.
56. Wang T, Niu G, Kortylewski M et al. Regulation of the innate and adaptive immune responses by Stat-3 signaling in tumor cells. Nat Med 2004; 10(1):48-54.
57. Farnoush A, Mackenzie IC. Sequential histological changes and mast cell response in skin during chemically-induced carcinogenesis. J Oral Pathol 1983; 12(4):300-306.
58. Coussens LM, Werb Z. Matrix metalloproteinases and the development of cancer. Chem Biol 1996; 3(11):895-904.
59. Coussens LM, Tinkle CL, Hanahan D et al. MMP-9 supplied by bone marrow-derived cells contributes to skin carcinogenesis. Cell 2000; 103(3):481-490.
60. Trinchieri G. Biology of natural killer cells. Adv Immunol 1989; 47:187-376.
61. Smyth MJ, Thia KY, Cretney E et al. Perforin is a major contributor to NK-cell control of tumor metastasis. J Immunol 1999; 162(11):6658-6662.
62. Hayakawa Y, Kelly JM, Westwood JA et al. Cutting edge: tumor rejection mediated by NKG2D receptor-ligand interaction is dependent upon perforin. J Immunol 2002; 169(10):5377-5381.
63. Smyth MJ, Godfrey DI, Trapani JA. A fresh look at tumor immunosurveillance and immunotherapy. Nat Immunol 2001; 2(4):293-299.
64. Paul P, Rouas-Freiss N, Khalil-Daher I et al. HLA-G expression in melanoma: a way for tumor cells to escape from immunosurveillance. Proc Natl Acad Sci USA 1998; 95(8):4510-4515.
65. Caux C, Massacrier C, Dezutter-Dambuyant C et al. Human dendritic Langerhans cells generated in vitro from CD34$^+$ progenitors can prime naive CD4$^+$ T-cells and process soluble antigen. J Immunol 1995; 155(11):5427-5435.
66. Katz SI, Tamaki K, Sachs DH. Epidermal Langerhans cells are derived from cells originating in bone marrow. Nature 1979; 282(5736):324-326.
67. O'Neill DW, Adams S, Bhardwaj N. Manipulating dendritic cell biology for the active immunotherapy of cancer. Blood 2004; 104(8):2235-2246.
68. Kripke ML. Effects of UV radiation on tumor immunity. J Natl Cancer Inst 1990; 82(17):1392-1396.
69. Banchereau J, Steinman RM. Dendritic cells and the control of immunity. Nature 1998; 392(6673):245-252.
70. Figdor CG, de Vries IJ, Lesterhuis WJ et al. Dendritic cell immunotherapy: mapping the way. Nat Med 2004; 10(5):475-480.
71. Stene MA, Babajanians M, Bhuta S et al. Quantitative alterations in cutaneous Langerhans cells during the evolution of malignant melanoma of the skin. J Invest Dermatol 1988; 91(2):125-128.
72. Ladanyi A, Kiss J, Somlai B et al. Density of DC-LAMP(+) mature dendritic cells in combination with activated T-lymphocytes infiltrating primary cutaneous melanoma is a strong independent prognostic factor. Cancer Immunol Immunother 2007.
73. Mellor AL, Keskin DB, Johnson T et al. Cells expressing indoleamine 2,3-dioxygenase inhibit T-cell responses. J Immunol 2002; 168(8):3771-3776.
74. Munn DH, Zhou M, Attwood JT et al. Prevention of allogeneic fetal rejection by tryptophan catabolism. Science 1998; 281(5380):1191-1193.
75. Munn DH, Shafizadeh E, Attwood JT et al. Inhibition of T-cell proliferation by macrophage tryptophan catabolism. J Exp Med 1999; 189(9):1363-1372.
76. Munn DH, Sharma MD, Lee JR et al. Potential regulatory function of human dendritic cells expressing indoleamine 2,3-dioxygenase. Science 2002; 297(5588):1867-1870.
77. van Oijen M, Bins A, Elias S et al. On the role of melanoma-specific CD8$^+$ T-cell immunity in disease progression of advanced-stage melanoma patients. Clin Cancer Res 2004; 10(14):4754-4760.

78. Boczkowski D, Nair SK, Nam JH et al. Induction of tumor immunity and cytotoxic T-lymphocyte responses using dendritic cells transfected with messenger RNA amplified from tumor cells. Cancer Res 2000; 60(4):1028-1034.

79. Anichini A, Mortarini R, Maccalli C et al. Cytotoxic T-cells directed to tumor antigens not expressed on normal melanocytes dominate HLA-A2.1-restricted immune repertoire to melanoma. J Immunol 1996; 156(1):208-217.

80. Griffioen M, Kessler JH, Borghi M et al. Detection and functional analysis of CD8⁺ T-cells specific for PRAME: a target for T-cell therapy. Clin Cancer Res 2006; 12(10):3130-3136.

81. McWilliams JA, McGurran SM, Dow SW et al. A modified tyrosinase-related protein 2 epitope generates high-affinity tumor-specific T-cells but does not mediate therapeutic efficacy in an intradermal tumor model. J Immunol 2006; 177(1):155-161.

82. Bennink JR anderson R, Bacik I et al. Antigen processing: where tumor-specific T-cell responses begin. J Immunother 1993; 14(3):202-208.

83. Konjevic G, Mirjacic Martinovic K, Vuletic A et al. Low expression of CD161 and NKG2D activating NK receptor is associated with impaired NK-cell cytotoxicity in metastatic melanoma patients. Clin Exp Metastasis 2007.

84. Lee TH, Cho YH, Lee MG. Larger numbers of immature dendritic cells augment an antitumor effect against established murine melanoma cells. Biotechnol Lett 2007; 29(3):351-357.

85. Brunda MJ, Gately MK. Antitumor activity of interleukin-12. Clin Immunol Immunopathol 1994; 71(3):253-255.

86. Nghiem DX, Kazimi N, Mitchell DL et al. Mechanisms underlying the suppression of established immune responses by ultraviolet radiation. J Invest Dermatol 2002; 119(3):600-608.

87. Brunda MJ, Luistro L, Warrier RR et al. Antitumor and antimetastatic activity of interleukin 12 against murine tumors. J Exp Med 1993; 178(4):1223-1230.

88. Germann T, Rude E, Schmitt E. The influence of IL12 on the development of Th1 and Th2 cells and its adjuvant effect for humoral immune responses. Res Immunol 1995; 146(7-8):481-486.

89. Maeda A, Schneider SW, Kojima M et al. Enhanced photocarcinogenesis in interleukin-12-deficient mice. Cancer Res 2006; 66(6):2962-2969.

90. Baron S, Hernandez J, Bekisz J et al. Clinical model: interferons activate human monocytes to an eradicative tumor cell level in vitro. J Interferon Cytokine Res 2007; 27(2):157-164.

91. Billiau A. Interferon-gamma: biology and role in pathogenesis. Adv Immunol 1996; 62:61-130.

92. Moore RJ, Owens DM, Stamp G et al. Mice deficient in tumor necrosis factor-alpha are resistant to skin carcinogenesis. Nat Med 1999; 5(7):828-831.

93. Thomas DA, Massague J. TGF-beta directly targets cytotoxic T-cell functions during tumor evasion of immune surveillance. Cancer Cell 2005; 8(5):369-380.

94. Kooy AJ, Prens EP, Van Heukelum A et al. Interferon-gamma-induced ICAM-1 and CD40 expression, complete lack of HLA-DR and CD80 (B7.1) and inconsistent HLA-ABC expression in basal cell carcinoma: a possible role for interleukin-10? J Pathol 1999; 187(3):351-357.

95. Kooy AJ, Tank B, Vuzevski VD et al. Expression of interferon-gamma receptors and interferon-gamma-induced up-regulation of intercellular adhesion molecule-1 in basal cell carcinoma; decreased expression of IFN-gamma R and shedding of ICAM-1 as a means to escape immune surveillance. J Pathol 1998; 184(2):169-176.

96. Mouawad R, Rixe O, Meric JB et al. Serum interleukin-6 concentrations as predictive factor of time to progression in metastatic malignant melanoma patients treated by biochemotherapy: a retrospective study. Cytokines Cell Mol Ther 2002; 7(4):151-156.

97. Jee SH, Shen SC, Chiu HC et al. Overexpression of interleukin-6 in human basal cell carcinoma cell lines increases anti-apoptotic activity and tumorigenic potency. Oncogene 2001; 20(2):198-208.

98. Biggs MW, Eiselein JE. Suppression of immune surveillance in melanoma. Med Hypotheses 2001; 56(6):648-652.

99. Ijland SA, Jager MJ, Heijdra BM et al. Expression of angiogenic and immunosuppressive factors by uveal melanoma cell lines. Melanoma Res 1999; 9(5):445-450.

100. Redondo P, Sanchez-Carpintero I, Bauza A et al. Immunologic escape and angiogenesis in human malignant melanoma. J Am Acad Dermatol 2003; 49(2):255-263.

101. Ugurel S, Rappl G, Tilgen W et al. Increased serum concentration of angiogenic factors in malignant melanoma patients correlates with tumor progression and survival. J Clin Oncol 2001; 19(2):577-583.

102. Kim J, Modlin RL, Moy RL et al. IL-10 production in cutaneous basal and squamous cell carcinomas. A mechanism for evading the local T-cell immune response. J Immunol 1995; 155(4):2240-2247.

103. Guiducci C, Vicari AP, Sangaletti S et al. Redirecting in vivo elicited tumor infiltrating macrophages and dendritic cells towards tumor rejection. Cancer Res 2005; 65(8):3437-3446.

104. Luft T, Jefford M, Luetjens P et al. Functionally distinct dendritic cell (DC) populations induced by physiologic stimuli: prostaglandin E(2) regulates the migratory capacity of specific DC subsets. Blood 2002; 100(4):1362-1372.
105. Derynck R, Akhurst RJ, Balmain A. TGF-beta signaling in tumor suppression and cancer progression. Nat Genet 2001; 29(2):117-129.
106. Dumont N, Arteaga CL. Targeting the TGF beta signaling network in human neoplasia. Cancer Cell 2003; 3(6):531-536.
107. Massague J. TGF-beta signal transduction. Annu Rev Biochem 1998; 67:753-791.
108. Pierce DF Jr, Johnson MD, Matsui Y et al. Inhibition of mammary duct development but not alveolar outgrowth during pregnancy in transgenic mice expressing active TGF-beta 1. Genes Dev 1993; 7(12A):2308-2317.
109. Bottinger EP, Jakubczak JL, Haines DC et al. Transgenic mice overexpressing a dominant-negative mutant type II transforming growth factor beta receptor show enhanced tumorigenesis in the mammary gland and lung in response to the carcinogen 7, 12-dimethylbenz-[a]-anthracene. Cancer Res 1997; 57(24):5564-5570.
110. Cui W, Fowlis DJ, Bryson S et al. TGFbeta1 inhibits the formation of benign skin tumors, but enhances progression to invasive spindle carcinomas in transgenic mice. Cell 1996; 86(4):531-542.
111. Gorelik L, Flavell RA. Transforming growth factor-beta in T-cell biology. Nat Rev Immunol 2002; 2(1):46-53.
112. Derynck R, Akhurst RJ, Balmain A. TGF-beta signaling in tumor suppression and cancer progression. Nat Genet 2001; 29(2):117-129.
113. McKarns SC, Schwartz RH, Kaminski NE. Smad3 is essential for TGF-beta 1 to suppress IL-2 production and TCR-induced proliferation, but not IL-2-induced proliferation. J Immunol 2004; 172(7):4275-4284.
114. McCarter M, Clarke J, Richter D et al. Melanoma skews dendritic cells to facilitate a T helper 2 profile. Surgery 2005; 138(2):321-328.
115. Hermans IF, Silk JD, Gileadi U et al. NKT cells enhance CD4+ and CD8+ T-cell responses to soluble antigen in vivo through direct interaction with dendritic cells. J Immunol 2003; 171(10):5140-5147.
116. Pulendran B. Modulating TH1/TH2 responses with microbes, dendritic cells and pathogen recognition receptors. Immunol Res 2004; 29(1-3):187-196.
117. Lauerova L, Dusek L, Simickova M et al. Malignant melanoma associates with Th1/Th2 imbalance that coincides with disease progression and immunotherapy response. Neoplasma 2002; 49(3):159-166.
118. Girardi M, Oppenheim DE, Steele CR et al. Regulation of cutaneous malignancy by gammadelta T-cells. Science 2001; 294(5542):605-609.
119. Tefany FJ, Barnetson RS, Halliday GM et al. Immunocytochemical analysis of the cellular infiltrate in primary regressing and nonregressing malignant melanoma. J Invest Dermatol 1991; 97(2):197-202.
120. Ferrone S, Marincola FM. Loss of HLA class I antigens by melanoma cells: molecular mechanisms, functional significance and clinical relevance. Immunol Today 1995; 16(10):487-494.
121. Garrido F, Ruiz-Cabello F, Cabrera T et al. Implications for immunosurveillance of altered HLA class I phenotypes in human tumours. Immunol Today 1997; 18(2):89-95.
122. Chen C, Nabavi N. In vitro induction of T-cell anergy by blocking B7 and early T-cell costimulatory molecule ETC-1/B7-2. Immunity 1994; 1(2):147-154.
123. Valenti R, Huber V, Filipazzi P et al. Human tumor-released microvesicles promote the differentiation of myeloid cells with transforming growth factor-beta-mediated suppressive activity on T-lymphocytes. Cancer Res 2006; 66(18):9290-9298.
124. Parmiani G, Castelli C, Santinami M et al. Melanoma immunology: past, present and future. Curr Opin Oncol 2007; 19(2):121-127.
125. Rosenberg SA, Sherry RM, Morton KE et al. Tumor progression can occur despite the induction of very high levels of self/tumor antigen-specific CD8+ T-cells in patients with melanoma. J Immunol 2005; 175(9):6169-6176.
126. Mortarini R, Piris A, Maurichi A et al. Lack of terminally differentiated tumor-specific CD8+ T-cells at tumor site in spite of antitumor immunity to self-antigens in human metastatic melanoma. Cancer Res 2003; 63(10):2535-2545.
127. Lengagne R, Le Gal FA, Garcette M et al. Spontaneous vitiligo in an animal model for human melanoma: role of tumor-specific CD8+ T-cells. Cancer Res 2004; 64(4):1496-1501.
128. Pardoll DM, Topalian SL. The role of CD4+ T-cell responses in antitumor immunity. Curr Opin Immunol 1998; 10(5):588-594.
129. Willimsky G, Blankenstein T. Sporadic immunogenic tumours avoid destruction by inducing T-cell tolerance. Nature 2005; 437(7055):141-146.
130. Turk MJ, Guevara-Patino JA, Rizzuto GA et al. Concomitant tumor immunity to a poorly immunogenic melanoma is prevented by regulatory T-cells. J Exp Med 2004; 200(6):771-782.

131. Abbas AK. Die and let live: eliminating dangerous lymphocytes. Cell 1996; 84(5):655-657.
132. Walker PR, Saas P, Dietrich PY. Role of Fas ligand (CD95L) in immune escape: the tumor cell strikes back. J Immunol 1997; 158(10):4521-4524.
133. Hahne M, Rimoldi D, Schroter M et al. Melanoma cell expression of Fas(Apo-1/CD95) ligand: implications for tumor immune escape. Science 1996; 274(5291):1363-1366.
134. Rivoltini L, Radrizzani M, Accornero P et al. Human melanoma-reactive CD4+ and CD8+ CTL clones resist Fas ligand-induced apoptosis and use Fas/Fas ligand-independent mechanisms for tumor killing. J Immunol 1998; 161(3):1220-1230.
135. Dong H, Zhu G, Tamada K et al. B7-H1, a third member of the B7 family, costimulates T-cell proliferation and interleukin-10 secretion. Nat Med 1999; 5(12):1365-1369.
136. Dong H, Strome SE, Salomao DR et al. Tumor-associated B7-H1 promotes T-cell apoptosis: a potential mechanism of immune evasion. Nat Med 2002; 8(8):793-800.
137. Iwai Y, Ishida M, Tanaka Y et al. Involvement of PD-L1 on tumor cells in the escape from host immune system and tumor immunotherapy by PD-L1 blockade. Proc Natl Acad Sci USA 2002; 99(19):12293-12297.
138. Strome SE, Dong H, Tamura H et al. B7-H1 blockade augments adoptive T-cell immunotherapy for squamous cell carcinoma. Cancer Res 2003; 63(19):6501-6505.
139. Tamura H, Dong H, Zhu G et al. B7-H1 costimulation preferentially enhances CD28-independent T-helper cell function. Blood 2001; 97(6):1809-1816.
140. Stander S, Schwarz T. Tumor necrosis factor-related apoptosis-inducing ligand (TRAIL) is expressed in normal skin and cutaneous inflammatory diseases, but not in chronically UV-exposed skin and nonmelanoma skin cancer. Am J Dermatopathol 2005; 27(2):116-121.
141. Chebassier N, Leroy S, Tenaud I et al. Overexpression of MMP-2 and MMP-9 in squamous cell carcinomas of immunosuppressed patients. Arch Dermatol Res 2002; 294(3):124-126.
142. Guo J, Zhu J, Sheng X et al. Intratumoral injection of dendritic cells in combination with local hyperthermia induces systemic antitumor effect in patients with advanced melanoma. Int J Cancer 2007.
143. Ribas A. Update on immunotherapy for melanoma. J Natl Compr Canc Netw 2006; 4(7):687-694.
144. Wigginton JM, Gruys E, Geiselhart L et al. IFN-gamma and Fas/FasL are required for the antitumor and antiangiogenic effects of IL-12/pulse IL-2 therapy. J Clin Invest 2001; 108(1):51-62.
145. Lucas ML, Heller R. IL-12 gene therapy using an electrically mediated nonviral approach reduces metastatic growth of melanoma. DNA Cell Biol 2003; 22(12):755-763.
146. Marshall JA, Forster TH, Purdie DM et al. Immunological characteristics correlating with clinical response to immunotherapy in patients with advanced metastatic melanoma. Immunol Cell Biol 2006; 84(3):295-302.
147. Kono M, Dunn IS, Durda PJ et al. Role of the mitogen-activated protein kinase signaling pathway in the regulation of human melanocytic antigen expression. Mol Cancer Res 2006; 4(10):779-792.
148. Schuler G, Schuler-Thurner B, Steinman RM. The use of dendritic cells in cancer immunotherapy. Curr Opin Immunol 2003; 15(2):138-147.
149. Tormo D, Ferrer A, Bosch P et al. Therapeutic efficacy of antigen-specific vaccination and toll-like receptor stimulation against established transplanted and autochthonous melanoma in mice. Cancer Res 2006; 66(10):5427-5435.

CHAPTER 16

Solar UV-Radiation, Vitamin D and Skin Cancer Surveillance in Organ Transplant Recipients (OTRs)

Jörg Reichrath* and Bernd Nürnberg

Introduction

During the last decades, the annual numbers of performed solid organ transplants continuously increase world-wide. For example in the United States of America (US) alone, it has been reported by the United Network for Organ Sharing, that over 25,000 solid organ transplantations were performed in 2003 (based on OPTN data as of January 1, 2004).[1] It is now well recognized, that solid organ transplant recipients (OTR) have an increased risk to develop malignancies, with skin cancer representing the most common malignancy.[2] Additionally, OTR in general develop a more aggressive form of these malignancies. Therefore, dermatologic surveillance is of high importance for OTR and these patients represent an increasing and significant challenge to clinicians including dermatologists. In OTRs, patient and organ survival have increased considerably and continuously over the past two decades as a result of better immunosuppressive regimens and better posttransplant care. However, it now has become evident that the more effective immunosuppression regimens have as an unintended consequence resulted in more frequent and aggressive skin cancers.[3-6] It has been convincingly demonstrated that the incidence of skin cancer increases with survival time after transplantation.[3] The biological behavior of these malignant skin tumors demonstrates a much more aggressive profile when compared to the non-immunosuppressed population, leading to considerable cutaneous morbidity, mortality and decrease in quality of life.

The First Challenge: Increased Incidence and Prevalence of Nonmelanoma Skin Cancer (NMSC) in Solid Organ Transplant Recipients

Nonmelanoma skin cancer (NMSC), most importantly basal cell carcinomas (BCC) and cutaneous squamous cell carcinomas (SCC) represent the single most commonly diagnosed malignancy in the Caucasian population. In the US alone, an estimated 1 million new cases are reported each year.[7] Cutaneous SCCs are in general easily managed in immunocompetent individuals where they rarely grow aggressively or metastasize. However, when SCCs develop in patients who have been immunosuppressed over long time periods (e.g., in solid OTRs), they grow aggressively and are a difficult management problem with substantial morbidity and mortality. It has now been convincingly demonstrated that NMSC accounts for appr. 90% of all skin cancers in

*Corresponding Author: Jörg Reichrath—Clinic for Dermatology, Venerology and Allergology, The Saarland University Hospital, 66421 Homburg/Saar, Germany.
Email: hajrei@uniklinik-saarland.de

Sunlight, Vitamin D and Skin Cancer, edited by Jörg Reichrath. ©2008 Landes Bioscience and Springer Science+Business Media.

transplant recipients.[8-10] While SCC has been reported to represent the most common skin cancer in transplant recipients occurring up to 250 times as frequently as in the general population, the incidence of BCC is increased by a factor of appr. 10 in solid OTRs.[10] Following transplantation, the usual BCC/SCC ratio in the general population (4:1 in higher latitude, respectively 2,5:1 in lower latitude)[11] reverses in favor of SCC up to rates > 3:1.[12] These differences are most likely markedly caused by differences in genetic backgrounds, skin types and sun exposure habits at different latitudes.[13]

In recent yeas, it has been convincingly shown that the incidence of NMSC increases continuously with the duration of the time period after transplantation and with the level of immunosuppression. Additionally, recent data indicate that solar and artificial UV-exposure both before and after organ transplantation increase the risk to develop skin cancer and that the incidence of NMSC varies with the type and dose of immunosuppressive medication used. As an example, it has been reported that in Australia, NMSCs occur in appr. 3% of renal transplant recipients by 1 year after transplantation, approximately 25% by 5 years and appr. 44% by 9 years posttransplantation.[14] Patients from the Netherlands, United Kingdom and Italy were demonstrated to have a 10-15% incidence of skin cancer 10 years after solid organ transplantation. In the United States, a study from Oregon reported a 35% incidence of skin cancer 10 years after transplantation.[15]

Several independent pathogenetic mechanisms that mostly involve the cutaneous immune system were discussed to cause these clinical findings, including dysfunction of antigen presentation, induction of immunosuppressive cytokines (e.g., IL-10, TNF-α), isomerization of trans-urocanic acid to cis-urocanic acid and formation of reactive oxygen species.[16]

The Second Challenge: The Aggressive Behavior of Nonmelanoma Skin Cancer in Transplant Recipients

The biologic behavior of cutaneous SCC, including local growth and metastasizing behaviour, is more aggressive in solid OTRs as compared to the general population. In OTRs, SCCs develop at younger ages, starting 3-5 years after transplantation. In OTRs, SCCs are also characterized by a more aggressive behaviour, with a high frequency of local recurrence (13.4%) during the first 6 months after excision and with a high frequency of lymph node metastasis (7%) during the second year after excision.[17] In OTRs, these tumors in general grow rapidly to a large size (>2 cm diameter) and have an aggressive histological growth pattern (Broders grade 3 or 4), that is often associated with perineural invasion or invasion of cartilage, fat, or bone.[17] Metastatic SCCs have a poor prognosis with a 3-year disease specific survival of 56%.[17] Patients with a history of NMSC prior to transplant are at an increased risk of metastatic NMSC, most likely because of genetic factors. As long-term survival after organ transplantation is increasing, partly because of better immunosuppressive regimens and posttransplant care, dermatologists including dermatologic oncologists will continue to be challenged in the optimal care of potentially life threatening NMSC in the posttransplant period.[18]

Risk Factors Associated with the Development of Nonmelanoma Skin Cancer in Transplant Recipients

Several risk factors have been identified that lead to an increased risk of skin cancer in transplant patients. Some factors, such as Fitzpatrick skin types I or II, significant exposure to ultraviolet (UV) radiation and age lead to an increased risk of NMSC in the general population, as well as in transplant recipients.[19,20] Other risk factors, including type, dosage and duration of immunosuppressive medication, are more specifically associated with the transplant recipient population. Patients with a history of melanoma or NMSC are at higher risk to develop aggressive and potentially life-threatening skin cancer posttransplantation. Penn et al found that 62% of patients who had a history of NMSC developed additional NMSC after transplantation. They also noted that 30% of the patients who had malignant melanoma developed melanoma metastases and subsequently died from metastatic melanoma.[21] Increased number of actinic keratoses (AK) also leads to a higher risk of developing NMSC.[22] It has to be emphasized that the management and treatment of AKs is of high importance in OTRs. Other major risk factors for the development of skin cancer after transplantation are the level and the duration of immunosuppression. More intensive and longer regimens lead to an increased risk for the development of AKs and skin cancer.[8,23-25] Infection with human papillomavirus (HPV) may be another risk factor for the development of NMSC, especially in immunosuppressed patients including OTRs. It has been speculated that cutaneous infections with HPV types 5 and 8 (HPV5, HPV8) may cause an increased risk for SCC development in transplant recipients.[26] Local and systemic immunodeficiencies in general promote the proliferation and activity of HPV, which acts as a cocarcinogen. Therefore, the presence of HPV-induced verrucous lesions in OTRs is associated with an increased risk of NMSC. Recent studies have shown the presence of HPV DNA in up to 70-90% of cutaneous SCCs.[23,24,27,28] The incidence of HPV in AKs and NMSC has also been shown to be higher in OTRs as compared to non-immunosuppressed patients.[29,30] It is well known that heart transplant recipients have the greatest risk to develop skin cancer posttransplantation, followed by kidney and liver transplant recipients. It has now been shown that recipients of cardiac transplantation have a threefold higher increase in the incidence of NMSC that occurs earlier after transplantation (mean: 2 years) as compared to recipients of renal transplants, most likely because of a more profound immunosuppression.[26,31]

In contrast, gender of the recipient, type of donor (cadaveric or live) and duration of dialysis do not appear to affect the incidence of posttransplantation skin cancer.[12,32,33]

Organ Allograft Recipients Are at Increased Risk for Malignant Melanoma

Interestingly, epidemiologic studies indicate that organ allograft recipients are at a 2- to 8-fold increased incidence of de novo melanoma after transplantation.[34] It has to be noted that a surprisingly high proportion of posttransplant melanomas arise in dysplastic nevi. This observation suggests that immunosuppression in a host with a melanoma precursor confers a particular susceptibility to neoplastic transformation. Interestingly, the sudden appearance of both benign and neoplastic nevi in transplant recipients has been reported.[21] Obviously, OTRs with de novo primary cutaneous malignant melanomas are unable to react with an appropriate cellular immune response to these neoplastic cells, permitting rapid evolution of the malignant tumor. In addition to the de novo development of melanoma post-transplant, one has to be aware of the concern of donor-derived melanoma, which frequently has been shown to affect the allograft, metastasizes rapidly in OTRs and in many cases results in the death of the recipient within months.[21]

Increased Incidence and Prevalence of Other Types of Skin Cancer in Solid Organ Transplant Recipients

The immunosuppressed state and other factors lead in solid OTRs to an increased incidence of other types of cutaneous malignancies besides SCC, BCC and malignant melanoma. In agree with this observation, Kaposi's sarcoma (KS) has been reported to have an appr. 84-fold increased incidence in solid OTRs as compared to the general population[9] and Merkel cell carcinoma also appears to be more common in OTRs.[35,36] Other tumors, such as atypical fibroxanthoma, dermatofibrosarcoma protuberans, angiosarcoma, verrucous carcinoma, leiomyosarcoma and cutaneous T-cell lymphoma, are suspected to also have an increased incidence and more aggressive growth behaviour in OTRs. However, it has to be noted that this opinion has to be confirmed. For no large-scale studies have been performed the actual incidence of these rare malignancies in OTRs is unknown and available data are based solely on case reports.[37-38]

Immunosuppressive Treatment: A Double-Edged Sword

After solid organ transplantation, patients usually have to take a lifelong immunosuppressive medication which is accused to play an important role in the cancerogenesis of NMSC and various other malignancies. It is well documented by the literature that the intensity and duration of immunosuppression is positively correlated with the development of cancer.[8,25] However, it has to be noted that the relative risk of individual immunosuppressive therapy modalities for cancerogenesis of NMSC is still unclear.

Actually, four different classes of immunosuppressive medications can be distinguished according to their different sites of cellular and molecular action: inhibitors of cell proliferation, amplification signals, STATs (Signal transducers and activators of transcription) or DNA synthesis.[39] As a result of their relatively early introduction into clinical medicine, most retrospective data exist for azathioprine and ciclosporine. Azathioprine is an antimetabolite that acts via inhibition of the de-novo synthesis of purins. Cyclosporine belongs to the group of calcineurin inhibitors that were shown to modulate the amplification of intracellular signals. More recently, biologics and other very effective immunosuppressive drugs were introduced into clinical practice such as muromonab-CD$_3$ (orthoclonal OKT$_3$), basiliximab, daclizumab, mycophenolate mofetil (MMF), tacrolimus, everolimus and sirolimus.[40,41] However, it has to be noted that in general, the causality between a single immunosuppressive medication and the development of cancer is difficult to analyze because usually a combination of different immunosuppressive drugs is used and changes in individual immunosuppressive therapy modalities including changes in dose rates are common practice in transplantation medicine.

Consequently, the association of individual immunosuppressive therapy modalities and cancer incidence has been analyzed. Jensen et al demonstrated in 1999 that kidney transplant recipients receiving cyclosporine, azathioprine and prednisolone had a 2.8 times increased risk of developing cutaneous SCC as compared to to kidney transplant recipients that received only azathioprine and prednisolone.[9] Dantal et al showed in a randomized comparison of two cyclosporine regiments in kidney graft recipients that the dosis of cyclosporine significantly modulates the risk for the development of cancer. In this study, the low dose regiment was associated with a reduced incidence of malignancies as compared to the high dose regiment.[42]

Results of the studies analyzing the association of cancer risk with immunosuppressive therapies are still a matter of dicussion. Penn et al concluded 1999 that skin cancers occurred more frequently in recipients receiving azathioprine (40,6%) and azathioprine combined with cyclosporine (34,2%) compared with those treated with a monotherapy of cyclosporine (25,1%),[43] although he depicted that cyclosporin A accelerates the development of de novo malignancies (after 26 month) in comparision to azathioprine and prednisolone (after 64 months).[43] Similar results were presented by Thiel et al in a comparision of kidney transplant recipients receiving cyclosporine versus a treatment with azathioprine and prednisolone.[44]

Immunosuppressive agents are also accused to influence the growth behaviour, including the agility and invasiveness of tumor cells in a direct cellular way. In agreement with this, Hojo et al demonstrated in 1999 a direct cyclosporine A-induced TGF-beta dependent tumor progression in SCID mice.[45] Stallone showed in 2005 that sirolimus blocks the progression of dermal Kaposi's sarcoma in kidney-transplant recipients resulting in a complete tumor regression within 3 month.[46]

Only a few studies analysed the potentially carcinogenic side-effects of immunosuppressive therapy modalities. Krupp et al investigated the side-effect profile of cyclosporin A in patients with severe psoriasis: skin cancer occurred in 0,7% and the SCC/BCC ratio was 6:1 which was suggested to be at least in part be caused by previous treatment with PUVA and/or methotrexate.[47]

Vitamin D Deficiency in Solid Organ Transplant Recipients: An Underrecognized Risk Factor for a Broad Variety of Severe Diseases

It is well known that, due to immunosuppression, OTRs are at increased risk for UV-induced NMSC. As a result, OTRs are advised to protect themselves from exposure to solar UV radiation. Since sunlight is the major source of vitamin D for most humans, OTRs, who avoid the sun or wear sun protection, therefore are at risk of developing vitamin D deficiency. Vitamin D deficiency is not only associated with increased risk for metabolic bone disease, but is associated with other severe health problems including various types of internal malignancies (e.g., colon, prostate- and breast cancer).[48-50] In consideration of these negative effects screening for vitamin D deficiency in OTRs is warranted. Serum levels of 1,25-dihydroxyvitamin D$_3$ [1,25(OH)$_2$D, calcitriol] have been monitored in renal transplant patients since it was realized that the kidneys were responsible for the conversion of 25-hydroxyvitamin D_3 [25(OH)D] to 1,25(OH)$_2$D. Patients with bone disease after kidney transplantation are often monitored for their serum 1,25(OH)$_2$D levels. 1,25(OH)$_2$D and its active analogs such as alfacalcidiol and paracalcitol have been shown to be effective in prevention of post transplantation bone loss.[51-53] However, serum levels of 1,25-dihydroxyvitamin D_3 in the normal range do not protect against the broad variety of independent diseases that are associated with deficient or insufficient 25(OH)D serum levels. We have recently analyzed the serum levels of 25(OH)D, which is the major circulating form of vitamin D and is used to determine the vitamin D status of patients in OTRs.[54,55] These patients need to protect themselves for medical reasons from sun exposure and therefore are at risk to develop vitamin D deficiency. Serum 25(OH)D levels were analyzed in renal transplant patients with adequate renal function and in an age- and gender-matched control group at the end of winter.[55] All renal transplant patients had practised solar UV protection after transplantation. Serum 25(OH)D levels were significantly lower in renal transplant patients as compared to controls (p = 0.007).[55] Geometric mean (with 95% confidence interval) in renal transplant patients was 10.9 ng/ml (8.2-14.3) compared to 20.0 ng/ml (15.7-25.5) in the control group.[55] In 10 of the 31 renal transplant patients serum 25(OH)D levels were undetectable (<4 ng/ml). Five additional patients had 25(OH)D levels <15 ng/ml. In renal transplant recipients, serum creatinine levels were ≤4 mg/dl post transplantation [mean: 1.7 mg/dl, normal range: 0.7-1.2 mg/dl (male), 0.5-0.9 mg/dl (female)]; parathyroid hormone ranging from 37 to 1058 pg/ml [mean: 198.7 pg/ml, normal range: 15-55 pg/ml].[55] To investigate whether vitamin D deficiency is characteristic for OTRs or can be found in other sunlight-deprived risk groups as well, we have analysed basal 25(OH)D_3 serum levels in a small group of patients with Xeroderma Pigmentosum (XP, n = 3) and basal cell nevus syndrome (BCNS, n = 1) at the end of wintertime (February/March).[56] 25(OH)D_3 levels in all four patients were markedly decreased with a mean value of 9.5 ng/ml (normal range: 15.0-90.0 ng/ml).[56] In conclusion, we demonstrated reduced serum 25(OH)D_3 levels in OTRs and other sunlight-deprived risk groups.[54,56]

A Paradigm Shift in the Diagnosis and Management of Skin Malignancies in Solid Organ Transplant Recipients

General Principles

It has now become evident that the most important element of preventive management of skin cancer in transplant recipients is patient education and rigorous sun protection.[57] Historically, patients were referred to dermatology or to dermatologic surgery only after having developed significant skin neoplasms. However, in recent years, a paradigm shift occurred and multidisciplinary approaches to patient care have been increasingly implemented with the integration of multiple services, including dermatology, dermatologic surgery and Mohs' micrographic surgery, transplant surgery, nephrology, cardiology and hepatology. The clinical paradigm is now one of preventive education, early intervention and administration of prophylactic regimens against cutaneous malignancies.

To realize this paradigm shift and to implement such an intervention, dermatology clinics are established onsite in some academic centers, within the transplant unit. The existence of a dermatology clinic within the transplant center greatly facilitates patient education regarding protection against artificial and solar UV-radiation, prevention of skin cancer in general and surveillance in the time period after transplantation. Guidelines of care for OTRs include education in sun protection and self-examination; risk assessment based on skin type, history of skin cancer, standard follow-up intervals and prophylaxis for high-risk groups. Additionally, patients are evaluated and assessed on risk of skin cancer development after receiving an organ transplant. Skin cancers have to be treated consequently according to their aggressive growth behaviour, emphasizing rapid and direct access to dermatology.

The implementation of a specialty dermatology clinic within the transplant center also allows the appropriate supervision of aggressively growing SCC and enable the evaluation of the role of sentinel lymph node biopsies and new immunosuppressive therapies in the management of NMSC. Additionally, the implementation of a specialty dermatology clinic within the transplant center also strengthens communication with transplant surgery on the development of a strategic approach toward reduction of immunosuppression in high-risk patients.

All OTRs should be evaluated for skin cancer and educated on prevention as soon as possible after transplant. Very low-risk patients can be followed by their transplant physician on a regular basis and referred to the dermatology clinic in longer time intervals or if concern over any skin lesions arises. Any OTR who has multiple risk factors for the development of skin cancer after transplantation should be seen by a dermatologist either before transplantation or as soon as possible after receiving a transplant. In addition, they should be followed regularly by the dermatologist for a full-body skin examination. On the first visit with the dermatologist, OTRs should be educated on recognizing premalignant and cancerous skin lesions and encouraged to seek medical attention early if suspicious skin lesions develop. Patients should also be advised to perform skin self-examination on a regular (monthly) basis.

Sun Protection

All OTRs should be continually advised to use appropriate sun protection because of their increased risk of developing skin cancer. Patients should be counseled to avoid solar and artificial UV-exposure whenever possible. Use of sunscreens containing titanium dioxide should be advised to provide a physical block from solar UV-radiation. The sunscreen should be rated with a sun protection factor (SPF) of 30 or greater. Sunscreen should be applied every day to all solar UV-radiation-exposed skin and it is helpful to encourage OTRs to keep multiple bottles of sunscreen in the car or elsewhere to guarantee continuous protection. It should be recommended that sunscreen should be applied every day, not just when solar UV-radiation exposure is expected. Protective clothing is also an important means of skin cancer prevention. OTRs should be advised to wear a wide-brimmed hat with a four-inch brim on all sides when they are out in the sun. Wearing tightly woven long-sleeve shirts and long pants of darker color is also protective and should be recommended. Use of appropriate solar UV-radiation protection should be recommended at every follow-up visit with the dermatologist.

Types of Skin Lesions

Actinic Keratosis

Actinic keratoses (AK) have the same clinical appearance in OTRs as in the general population; however, they may be more numerous in the former. They appear on chronically solar UV-radiation exposed sites such at the face, scalp, extensor forearms and dorsum of the hands. The lesions may appear as single or multiple discrete dry, rough, scaly plaques. Palpation may be helpful in the diagnosis of this type of lesion. Aks may progress to hypertrophic AKs or cutaneous horns characterized by a macular or papular base with a white, black, or yellowish keratotic cap. AKs are considered precancerous lesions that may progress to SCC if left untreated. Histologically, AKs in OTRs have been found statistically more likely to demonstrate bacterial colonization, confluent parakeratosis, hyperkeratosis, increased mitotic activity and verrucous changes.[58] Because of the increased risk of developing SCC in OTRs, AKs should be managed consequently and treated aggressively. Follow-up visits for OTRs with AKs should be scheduled at least every 6 months.[18] Treatment regiments include cryotherapy, topical 5-fluorouracil (5-FU), electrodessication with curettage, topical treatment with imiquimod or photodynamic therapy (PDT). Any lesion that persists after appropriate therapy should be biopsied or excised to rule out progression to SCC. Patients with multiple AKs may also be treated with topical medication, e.g., imiquimod, which has been approved for the treatment of AKs. It has to be noted that to date, there is no evidence that topical treatment with imiquimod confers risk to the transplanted organ.

Recently, the efficacy of topical PDT with 5-FU in clearing epidermal dysplasia in organ transplant recipients was compared, showing a greater efficacy of PDT in achieving complete resolution of lesions, its superior cosmetic outcome and patient preference over 5-FU, despite the initially higher levels of pain associated with PDT treatment.[59]

While a number of studies demonstrated successful treatment of epidermal dysplasia in immunocompetent patients using topical PDT (with clearance rates ranging from 69-100%),[60-68] previous studies had clearly indicated reduced clearance rates in OTRs. Dragieva et al[69] treated epidermal dysplasia (AK, CIS) in 20 OTRs and 20 controls with topical PDT using 5-ALA and in a second study compared MAL PDT with placebo in the treatment of 129 AKs in 17 OTRs.[70] In the first study, the overall CRR in OTRs at 4, 12 and 48 weeks was 86%, 68% and 48% respectively, whilst in the second study, the overall CRR at 4 months was 90% (56 of 62) for PDT and 0 (0 of 67) for placebo. Schleier et al[71] treated a total of 32 cutaneous lesions, comprising AKs, BCCs, keratoacanthomas and SCCs, in five OTRs and reported a CRR of 75% at 3 months. It has been speculated that the apparent decline in efficacy with time following PDT[69] may be due to either recurrence of inadequately treated lesions, or the appearance of new lesions at the treated site. Interestingly, de Graaf et al[72] reported a randomized controlled trial in 40 OTRs where PDT showed no statistically significant effect on reduction of keratotic skin lesions on the arm treated with either one or two cycles of PDT. More recently however, Perrett et al reported that topical MAL PDT was more effective than topical 5-FU in the treatment of epidermal dysplasia in OTRs.[59] The clearance rate of 89% at 6 months for topical PDT in that study was comparable to that reported in most existing open studies in both immunocompetent[60-68] and OTRs.[69-71] A number of possible explanations may account for why the efficacy of PDT was lower in the study of de Graaf et al in OTRs.[72] as compared to the study of Perrett et al,[59] including: (i) the treated keratotic lesions in the study by de Graaf and colleagues were not histologically confirmed and were not all necessarily areas of epidermal dysplasia; (ii) violet light (400-450 nm) was used in the study of de Graaf et al,[72] which has reduced penetration compared with the red light (600-700 nm) used by Perrett et al;[59] (iii) failure to remove lesional hyperkeratotic scale and crust before treatment may have prevented adequate penetration of photosensitizer in the study of de Graaf et al;[72] (iv) 5-ALA was used by de Graaf et al which penetrates less deeply than MAL that was used by Perrett et al;[59] (v) the treatment protocol of the study of de Graaf et al[72] may not have been optimal with only half of the lesions treated twice but with a 6-month gap in between rather than 1 week; and (vi) the study sample of Perrett et al,[59] was small. Interestingly, Perrett et al[59] did not experience a decline in CRR with time for PDT-treated lesions as reported by Dragieva et al[69] and, once again, different methods may have partly accounted for this. It has been emphasized that such practical considerations may be of particular relevance in optimizing PDT for immunosuppressed individuals.[73] In the study of Perrett et al[59] the improved outcome for PDT vs. 5-FU appears, at least in part, to reflect a poorer than expected clearance of epidermal dysplasia with 5-FU in the patient group. From data in immunocompetent patients, a 90% clearance rate should have been expected, as compared with the 11% CRR that we observed at 6 months. It was concluded that 5-FU regimens recommended for treatment of immunocompetent patients may not be appropriate for OTRs.[59]

SCC

An important step for the management of SCC in OTRs was the publication of guidelines by the International Transplant-Skin Cancer Collaborative (ITSCC). Based on this report, patients should be divided into low-risk and high-risk categories based on aggressive growth characteristics of the SCC.

Low-Risk SCC

First, any lesion suspicious for SCC should be biopsied or excised. Electrodessication and curettage (ED&C) may be performed at the time of biopsy for those lesions that are clinically determined to be less aggressive.[59] For lesions judged to be low risk based on histology as well, treatment options include: cryosurgery with curettage, ED&C, surgical excision, or Mohs' micrographic surgery.[59] For those areas where conservation of tissue is a priority or for sites that are in anatomic areas of moderate risk, Mohs' micrographic surgery is the best option.[59]

Aggressive SCC

For skin lesions that are determined to be aggressively growing based on clinical characteristics or histologic features, destructive techniques are not recommended. Aggressively growing SCC should be treated with excisional techniques, particularly Mohs' micrographic surgery. Other recommended options for complete excision include surgery with intraoperative frozen section evaluation, or excision with postoperative margin assessment. Margins should include the subcutaneous fat and 6-10 mm beyond any surrounding erythema.[74] If there is evidence of perineural involvement, invasion of surrounding bones or glands, unclear margins, or if the lesion persists after excision, then further evaluation is necessary. Radiation therapy should be considered in cases where there is perineural involvement or where there is inability to achieve clear margins.[59] Sentinel lymph node biopsy (SLNB) has been shown in small studies to be effective in identifying nodal disease in patients with SCC of the lip.[59,75] This option should be considered for patients with high risk SCC. The decision to decrease immunosuppressive therapy should be discussed with the patient's transplant team.

Metastatic SCC

Any patient with metastatic nodal spread should be evaluated for excision with therapeutic lymphadenectomy or primary radiation therapy (XRT). Patients with in-transit cutaneous metastasis who do not have lymph nodes that are positive for metastatic spread should have excision of the primary and satellite lesions. In these patients, Mohs' surgery is recommended. Chemotherapy, the use of systemic retinoids and the reduction of immunosuppressive medication are other additional options that should be considered in patients with nodal spread or satellite lesions.[59]

Multiple NMSC

Application of prophylactic topical retinoids or episodic 5-FU may be used in patients who develop multiple AKs or NMSC. In OTRs who develop more than five NMSCs in 1 year, prophylactic administration of systemic retinoids should be considered. It has been reported that the administration of systemic acitretin (30 mg/day) leads to a reduction in the incidence of SCC.[76] However, chemoprophylaxis with retinoids is problematic in OTRs because of the need for long-term therapy. Well known side effects include hyperlipidemia, which should be treated consequently in OTRs. Any patient receiving systemic retinoids should have liver function tests and lipids checked on a regular basis. A rebound effect after discontinuation of retinoids, resulting in an increase in the number of skin cancers, has been observed.[18,59] Dermatologists should discuss the possibility of a reduction of the immunosuppressive medication with the transplant team for patients with more than 5-10 NMSC per year.[77] Recently, it has been analyzed whether common known polymorphisms in the regulatory region of the cyclooxygenase-2 (COX-2) gene (PTGS2) can be associated with NMSC predisposition after organ transplantation and whether cancer risks are associated with specific COX-2 gene haplotypes containing these polymorphisms.[78] In that study, it was demonstrated that COX-2 common variants -765G—>C and -1195A—>G appear to be associated with risk of NMSC, although in different ways in the SCC and BCC subgroups, indicating that environmental and genetic risk factors may play different roles in the outcome leading to these two phenotypes.[78] Recently, a comprehensive literature review was carried out to discuss relevant genetic polymorphism for the development of NMSC in organ transplant recipients.[79] These include genetic polymorphisms in glutathione S-transferase, interleukin-10, retinoblastoma and p53 genes. Additionally, genetic polymorphisms in the folate pathway, melanocortin 1 receptor and vitamin D receptor were discussed. The authors concluded that no single factor is causative in cutaneous carcinogenesis in transplant recipients and that most likely interactions of some of the above mechanisms with known environmental factors lead to increased risk.[79]

Keratoacanthoma

Keratoacanthomas (KA) also have a similar clinical appearance in solid organ transplant recipients as in the general population. Clinically, they appear as dome-shaped nodules or papules with a central keratotic plug. They occur on solar UV-radiation exposed areas and can grow very rapidly. OTRs may have multiple KAs on solar UV-radiation exposed areas. KAs may not always be clinically distinguished from SCC and therefore should be treated with surgical excision. For OTRs with multiple KAs, systemic retinoids may be used.

BCC

BCC has the same clinical appearance in OTRs as in normal hosts. It presents as a pearly telean-giectatic papule or as a crusted, atrophic or ulcerated lesion. In contrast to the general population, OTRs have much higher incidence rates of SCC compared to BCC. BCC can be treated with various therapeutic modalities, including ED&C, surgical excision, or Mohs' surgery depending on the size of the lesion, its location and whether it is recurrent. Topical imiquimod has also been approved for the treatment of superficial BCC in non-immunocompromised patients. Use of topical imiquimod in OTRs for superficial BCC has only been reported in a limited number of cases, but preliminary results are encouraging.

Malignant Melanoma

Malignant melanoma (MM) has the same clinical appearance in transplant recipients as in normal hosts, but has a slightly higher incidence in transplant recipients. It has been recommended that surveillance for MM should be more aggressive in OTRs. Many centers have utilized full-body photography and dermatoscopy to follow patients with multiple pigmented nevi. Any lesion that is suspicious for MM should be biopsied or excised. Localized lesions should be treated with wide local surgical excision. In OTRs with MM that are more than 1 mm thick or that are ulcerated, sentinel lymph node biopsy may be useful. For kidney or pancreas allograft patients with metastatic MM, discontinuation of immunosuppressive medication should be considered.[77]

Follow-up

OTRs with a history of one NMSC should be seen every 6 months by a dermatologist. OTRs with a history of multiple NMSC, high risk NMSC or MM, should be seen at least every 3 months. Sites of any previous cutaneous malignancy should be reevaluated at every examination. Regional lymph node exam should also be performed. If there is any suspicion of metastatic disease, further evaluation that may include laboratory or radiologic studies has to be performed.[59]

Summary

The introduction of organ transplantation in clinical medicine has resulted in a constantly increasing, large population of patients that are chronically on immunosuppressive medication. It is well known that skin cancer, especially SCC, in this population has higher incidence rates, behaves more aggressively and has higher rates of metastasis. OTRs who have been treated for many years with immunosuppressive medication are at the highest risk for developing malignant skin tumors. Therefore, the intensity of surveillance for cutaneous lesions is of high importance in OTRs. A full-body skin exam at least once a year and more frequently if skin cancer or precancerous cutaneous lesions develop is recommended. Clinicians should not hesitate to biopsy or to surgically excise any suspicious skin lesion. Of high importance is also the education of OTRs about their increased risk. Protection against solar and artificial UV-radiation and monthly self-examinations are good ways to prevent and to recognize any new suspicious skin lesions. Patients are advised to always wear solar UV-radiation protection (e.g., clothing, sunscreen) before going outdoors. However, investigations have revealed that solar UV-B-exposure and serum 25(OH)D levels positively correlate with decreased risk for various internal malignancies (e.g., breast, colon, prostate and ovarian cancer) and other severe diseases. As we have shown previously, renal transplant recipients are at high risk of vitamin D deficiency. A sunscreen with a sun protection factor (SPF)-8 reduces the skin's production of vitamin D by 95%. Clothing completely blocks all solar UVB-radiation and this prevents any vitamin D production. Therefore, it is important to detect and treat vitamin D deficiency in solid organ transplant recipients. Optimal manage-ment of these patients requires communication between the transplant teams and the treating dermatologist and other clinicians. For advanced or metastatic disease, collaboration between clinicians of different disciplines, including the transplant team, dermatologists and radiation oncologists is also essential. In the future, dermatology clinics that are integrated into transplant centers may make it easier to manage and to treat OTRs, may make an interdisciplinary approach more effective and may thereby improve the clinical outcome in OTRs.

References

1. Traywick C, O'Reilly FM. Management of skin cancer in solid organ transplant recipients. Dermatol Ther 2005; 18(1):12-8.
2. Greenlee RT, Murray T, Bolden S et al. Cancer statistics. CA Cancer J Clin 2000; 50:7-33.
3. Sheil AG. Development of malignancy following renal transplantation in Australia and New Zealand. Transplant Proc 1992; 24:1275-1279.
4. Edwards NM, Rajasinghe HA, John R et al. Cardiac transplantation in over 1000 patients: a single institution experience from Columbia University. Clin Transplan 1999; 249-261.
5. Penn I. Posttransplant malignancy: the role of immunosuppression. Drug Saf 2000; 23:101-113.
6. Moloney FJ et al. Maintenance versus reduction of immunosuppression in renal transplant recipients with aggressive squamous cell carcinomas. Derm Surg 2004; 30(4):674-678.
7. Penn I. Incidence and treatment of neoplasia after transplantation. J Heart Lung Transplant 1993; 12: S328-36.
8. Euvrard S, Kanitakis J, Claudy A. Skin cancers after organ transplantation. N Engl J Med 2003; 348:1681-91.
9. Jensen P, Hansen S, Moller B et al. Skin cancer in kidney and heart transplant recipients and different long-term immunosuppressive therapy regimens. J Am Acad Dermatol 1999; 40:177-86.
10. Hartevelt MM, Bavinck JN, Koote AM et al. Incidence of skin cancer after renal transplantation in the Netherlands. Transplantation 1990; 49:506-9.
11. Giles GG, Marks R, Foley P. Incidence of nonmelanocytic skin cancer treated in Australia. Br Med J (Clin Res Ed) 1988; 296(6614):13-7.
12. Ramsay HM, Fryer AA, Reece S et al. Clinical risk factors associated with nonmelanoma skin cancer in renal transplant recipients. Am J Kidney Dis 2000; 36(1):167-76.
13. Molony FJ, Comber H, O'Lorcain P et al. A population-based study of skin cancer incidence and prevalence in renal transplant recipients. Br J Dermatol 2006; 154(3):498-504.
14. Bouwes-Bavinck JN, Hardie DR, Green A. The risk of skin cancer in renal transplant recipients in Queensland, Australia. A follow-up study. Transplantation 1996; 61:715-21.
15. Lampros TD, Cobanoglu A, Parker P et al. Squamous and basal cell carcinomas in heart transplant recipients. J Heart Lung Transplant 1998; 17:586-591.
16. Granstein RD, Matsui MS. UV-radiation-induced immunosuppression and skin cancer. Cutis 2004; 74(5 Suppl):4-9.
17. Carucci JA, Martinez JC, Zeitouni N et al. In-transit metastasis from primary cutaneous squamous cell carcinoma in organ transplant recipients and nonimmunosuppressed patients: clinical characteristics, management and outcome in a series of 21 patients. Derm Surg 2004; 30(4):651-655.
18. Stasko T, Brown MD, Carucci J et al. Guidelines for the management of squamous cell carcinoma in organ transplant recipients. Derm Surg 2004; 30(4):642-650.
19. Ferrandiz C, Fuente MJ, Ribera M et al. Epidermal dysplasia and neoplasia in kidney transplant recipients. J Am Acad Dermatol 1995; 33:590-596.
20. Ramsay HM, Fryer AA, Reece S et al. Clinical risk factors associated with nonmelanoma skin cancer in renal transplant recipients. Am J Kidney Dis 2000; 36:167-176.
21. Penn I. Malignant melanoma in organ allograft recipients. Transplantation 1996; 61:274-278.
22. Bavnick JN, DeBoer A, Vermeer BJ et al. Sunlight, keratotic lesions and skin cancer in renal transplant recipients. Br J Dermatol 1993; 129:242-249.
23. Harwood CA, Surentheran T, McGregor JM et al. Human papillomavirus infection and nonmelanoma skin cancer in immunosuppressed and immunocompetent individuals. J Med Virol 2000; 61:289-297.
24. Berkhout RJM, Bouwes-Bavinck JN, ter Schegget J. Persistence of human papillomavirus DNA in benign and (pre) malignant skin lesions from renal transplant recipients. J Clin Microbiol 2000; 38:2087-2096.
25. Hampton T. Skin cancer's ranks rise: immunosuppression to blame. JAMA. 2005. 28; 294(12):1476-80.
26. Gjersvik P, Hansen S, Moller B et al. Are heart transplant recipients more likely to develop skin cancer than kidney transplant recipients? Transpl Int 2003; 13 Suppl 1:S. 380-1.
27. De Villiers EM, Lavergne D, McLaren KM et al. Prevailing papillomavirus types in nonmelanoma carcinomas of the skin in renal allograft recipients. Int J Cancer 1997; 73:356-361.

28. Meyer T, Arndt R, Christophers E et al. Importance of human papillomaviruses for the development of skin cancer. Cancer Detect Prev 2001; 25:533-547.
29. Shamanin V, zur Hausen H, Lavergne D et al. Human papillomavirus infections in nonmelanoma skin cancers from renal transplant recipients and nonimmunosuppressed patients. J Natl Cancer Inst 1996; 88:802-811.
30. Stockfleth E, Nindl I. Wolfram et al. Human papillomaviruses in transplant associated skin cancers. Dermatologic Surg 2004; 30:604-609.
31. Adamson R, Obispo E, Dychter S et al. High incidence and clinical course of aggressive skin cancer in heart transplant recipients: a single-center study. Transplant Proc 1996; 1124-1126.
32. London NJ, Farmery SM, Will EJ et al. Risk of neoplasia in renal transplant patients. Lancet 1995; 346:403-406.
33. Roeger LS, Sheil AGR, Disney APS et al. Risk factors associatedwith the development of squamous cell carcinomas in immunosuppressed renal transplant recipients. Clin Transplant 1992; 6:202-211.
34. Le Mire L, Hollowood K, Gray D et al. Melanomas in renal transplant recipients. Br J Dermatol 2006; 154(3):472-7.
35. Douds AC, Mellotte GJ, Morgan SH. Fatal Merkel-cell tumour (cutaneous neuroendocrine carcinoma) complicating renal transplantation. Nephrol Dial Transplant 1995; 10:2436-2438.
36. Penn I, First MR. Merkel's cell carcinoma in organ recipients: report of 41 cases. Transplantation 1999; 58(11):1717-21.
37. Hafner J, Kunzi W, Weinreich T. Malignant fibrous histiocytoma and atypical fibroxanthoma in renal transplant recipients. Dermatology 1999; 198:29-32.
38. Wehril BM, Janzen DL, Shokeir O et al. Epitheliod angiosarcoma arising in surgically constructed arteriovenous fistula: a rare complication of chronic immunosuppression in the setting of renal transplantation. Am J Surg Pathol 1998; 22:1154-1159.
39. Stallone G, Infante B, Gesualdo L. Immunosuppressive drugs and renal transplantation. G Ital Nefrol 2005; 22 Suppl 33:S.76-9.
40. Nashan B, Moore R, Amlot P et al. Randomised trial of basiliximab versus placebo for control of acute cellular rejection in renal allograft recipients. Lancet 1997; 350:1193-1198.
41. Nashan B. Maximizing clinical outcomes with mTOR inhibitors in the renal transplant recipients: what role for calcineurin inhibitors? Transpl Int 2004; 17:279-285.
42. Dantal J, Hourmant M, Cantarovich D et al. Effect of long-term immunosuppression in kidney-graft recipients on cancer incidence: randomised comparison of two cyclosporin regimens. Lancet 1998; 351(9103):623-8.
43. Penn I. Cancers in cyclosporin treated vs azathioprin-treated patients. Transplant Proc 1996; 28:876-878.
44. Thiel G, Bock A, Spöndlin M et al. Long-term benefits and risks of cyclosporin A (sandimmun)—an analysis at 10 years. Transplant Proc 1994; 26(5):2493-8.
45. Hojo M, Morimoto T, Maluccio M et al. Cyclosporine induces cancer progression by a cell-autonomous mechanism. Nature 1999; 397(6719):530-4.
46. Stallone G, Shena A, Infante B et al. Sirolimus for Kaposi's sarcoma in renal-transplant recipients. N Engl J Med 2005; 352:1317-1323.
47. Krupp P, Monka C. Side-effect profile of cyclosporin A in patients treated for psoriasis. Br J Dermatol 1990; 122 Suppl; 36:47-56.
48. Garland CF, Comstock GW, Garland FC et al. Serum 25-hydroxyvitamin D and colon cancer: eight year prospective study. Lancet 1989; 1176-8.
49. Grant WB. An ecologic study of dietary and solar ultraviolet-B links to breast carcinoma mortality rates. Cancer 2002; 94:272-81.
50. Grant WB. An estimate of premature cancer mortality in the US due to inadequate doses of solar ultraviolet-B radiation. Cancer 2002; 94:1867-75.
51. Massenkeil G, Fiene C, Rosen O et al. Loss of bone mass and vitamin D deficiency after hematopoietic stem cell transplantation: standard prophylactic measures fail to prevent osteoporosis. Leukemia 2001; 15(11):1701-5.
52. Jeffery JR, Leslie WD, Karpinski ME et al. Prevalence and treatment of decreased bone density in renal transplant recipients : a randomized prospective trial of calcitriol versus alendronate. Transplantation 2003; 76(10):1498-502.
53. El-Agroudy AE, El-Husseini AA, El-Sayed M et al. Preventing bone loss in renal transplant recipients with vitamin D. J Am Soc Nephrol 2003; 14(11):2975-9.
54. Segal E, Baruch Y, Kramsky R et al. Vitamin D deficiency in liver transplant patients in Israel. Transplantation Proceedings 2001; 33(6):2955-56.
55. Querings K, Girndt M, Geisel J et al. 25-Hydroxyvitamin D-deficiency in renal transplant recipients: an underrecognized health problem. J Clin Endocrinol Metab 2006; 91(2):526-9.

56. Querings K, Reichrath J. A plea for the analysis of Vitamin-D levels in patients under photoprotection, including patients with xeroderma pigmentosum (XP) and basal cell nevus syndrome (BCNS). Cancer Causes Control 2004; 15(2):219.

57. Robinson JR, Rigel DS. Sun protection attitudes and behaviors of solid-organ transplant recipients. Derm Surg 2004; 30(4):610-615.

58. Boyd AS. Histologic features of actinic keratoses in solid organ transplant recipients and healthy controls. J Am Acad Dermatol 2001; 45:217-221.

59. Perrett CM, McGregor JM, Warwick J et al. Treatment of posttransplant premalignant skin disease: a randomized intrapatient comparative study of 5-fluorouracil cream and topical photodynamic therapy British Journal of Dermatology 2007; 156(2):320-328.

60. Szeimies RM, Karrer S, Sauerwald A et al. Photodynamic therapy with topical application of 5-aminolevulinic acid in the treatment of actinic keratoses: an initial clinical study. Dermatology 1996; 192:246-51.

61. Szeimies RM, Karrer S, Radakovic-Fijan A et al. Photodynamic therapy using topical methyl 5-aminolevulinate compared with cryotherapy for actinic keratosis: a prospective, randomized study. J Am Acad Dermatol 2002; 47:258-62.

62. Pariser DM, Lowe NJ, Stewart DM et al. Photodynamic therapy with topical methyl aminolevulinate for actinic keratosis: results of a prospective randomized multicenter trial. J Am Acad Dermatol 2003; 48:227-32.

63. Freeman M, Vinciullo C, Francis D et al. A comparison of photodynamic therapy using topical methyl aminolevulinate (Metvix) with single cycle cryotherapy in patients with actinic keratosis: a prospective, randomized study. J Dermatol Treat 2003; 14:99-106.

64. Varma S, Wilson H, Kurwa HA et al. Bowen's disease, solar keratoses and superficial basal cell carcinomas treated by photodynamic therapy using a large-field incoherent light source. Br J Dermatol 2001; 144:567-74.

65. Salim A, Leman JA, McColl JH et al. Randomized comparison of photodynamic therapy with topical 5-fluorouracil in Bowen's disease. Br J Dermatol 2003; 148:539-43.

66. Cairnduff F, Stringer MR, Hudson EJ et al. Superficial photodynamic therapy with topical 5-aminolaevulinic acid for superficial primary and secondary skin cancer. Br J Cancer 1994; 69:605-8.

67. Morton CA, Whitehurst C, Moore JV et al. Comparison of red and green light in the treatment of Bowen's disease by photodynamic therapy. Br J Dermatol 2000; 143:767-72.

68. Morton CA, Whitehurst C, Moseley H et al. Comparison of photodynamic therapy with cryotherapy in the treatment of Bowen's disease. Br J Dermatol 1996; 135:766-71.

69. Dragieva G, Hafner J, Reinhard D et al. Topical photodynamic therapy in the treatment of actinic keratoses and Bowen's disease in transplant recipients. Transplantation 2004; 77:115-21.

70. Dragieva G, Prinz BM, Hafner J et al. A randomized controlled clinical trial of topical photodynamic therapy with methyl aminolaevulinate in the treatment of actinic keratoses in transplant recipients. Br J Dermatol 2004; 151:196-200.

71. Schleier P, Hyckel P, Berndt A et al. Photodynamic therapy of virus-associated epithelial tumours of the face in organ transplant recipients. J Cancer Res Clin Oncol 2004; 130:279-84.

72. de Graaf YG, Kennedy C, Wolterbeek R et al. Photodynamic therapy does not prevent cutaneous squamous cell carcinoma in organ-transplant recipients: results of a randomised-controlled trial. J Invest Dermatol 2006; 126:569-74.

73. Oseroff A. PDT as a cytotoxic agent and biological response modifier: implications for cancer prevention and treatment in immunocompromised and immunocompetent patients. J Invest Dermatol 2006; 126:542-4.

74. Rowe DE, Carroll RJ, Day CL Jr. Prognostic factors for local recurrence, metastasis and survival rates in squamous cell carcinoma of the skin, ear and lip. Implications for treatment modality selection. J Am Acad Dermatol 1992; 26:976-990.

75. Altinyollar H, Berberoglu U, Celen O. Lymphatic mapping and sentinel node biopsy in squamous cell carcinoma of the lower lip. Eur J Surg Oncol 2002 ; 28:72-74.

76. Bavinck JN, Tieben LM, Van der Woude FJ et al. Prevention of skin cancer and reduction of keratotic skin lesions during acitretin therapy in renal transplant recipients: a double-blind, placebo-controlled study. J Clin Oncol 1995; 13:1933-1938.

77. Berg D, Otley C. Skin cancer in organ transplant recipients: epidemiology, pathogenesis and management. J Am Acad Dermatol 2002; 47:1-17.

78. Lira MG, Mazzola S, Tessari G et al. Association of functional gene variants in the regulatory regions of COX-2 gene (PTGS2) with nonmelanoma skin cancer after organ transplantation. Br J Dermatol 2007; 157(1):49-57.

79. Laing ME, Kay E, Conlon P et al. Genetic factors associated with skin cancer in renal transplant patients. Photodermatol Photoimmunol Photomed 2007; 23(2-3):62-7.

CHAPTER 17

Histology of Melanoma and Nonmelanoma Skin Cancer

Cornelia S.L. Mueller* and Jörg Reichrath

Squamous Cell Cancer, In Situ Carcinomas, Actinic Keratosis (AK)

According to the WHO classification of skin tumours from 2006 actinic keratoses are very common intraepidermal neoplasm of sun-damaged skin with variable atypia of the epidermal keratinocytes. Main cause of these changes is chronical exposition to UVB light, but Aks are also observed following long term PUVA-treatments as well as exposure to arsenic.[1] The actinic keratoses can be considered to represent early squamous cell carcinomas in situ,[2,3] respectively possess a striking potential to progress to fully developed neoplasms.[4] But only small portions of actinic keratoses will develop into an invasive squamous cell carcinoma. Regression of some cases of actinic keratoses have been reported, most likely as a result of immune mechanisms.[5] Metastases after transformation of actinic keratoses into invasive squamous cell carcinomas are very rare except for those tumours that arise on the ear, lip, anus and vulva, which have been reported to be often associated with a more aggressive behaviour.[6] It has been widely accepted, that actinic keratoses are a clinical manifestation of UV-induced neoplastic transformation of keratinocytes representing a continuum with progress to a fully developed squamous cell carcinomas.[7] Cockerell observed the same cytological features of keratinocytic atypia in actinic keratoses than in epidermal or metastatic SCCs.[8] Like current nomenclature of cervical intraepidermal neoplasia (CIN) Cockerell therefore recommends the use of the term "keratinocytic intraepidermal neoplasia" to illustrate the biological nature of these lesions.[7]

Histopathologically, the actinic keratoses are classified into six groups: hypertrophic, atrophic, bowenoid, acantholytic, pigmented and lichenoid. All of these subtypes collective is a partial thickness atypia of crowded keratinocytes with overlying parakeratosis and sparing of acrotrichia and acrosyringia extensions with overlying orthokeratosis. This characteristical pattern of alternating ortho- and parakeratosis is often referred to as "flag sign" or "pink and blue pattern".[7] The cytologic atypia include nuclear enlargement and prominence, hyperchromasia, pleomorphism, mitotic activity and dyskeratosis. Constantly associated dermal changes are solar elastosis and a sometimes dense lymphocytic infiltrate and an increased vascularity.

Bowen's Disease

Clinically Bowen's disease represents a slow growing malignancy which most often arises in sun-damaged skin of the elderly.[9,10] In Bowen's disease, the epidermis usually shows localized full thickness atypia resembling carcinoma in situ and it is seen as a distinct clinicopathologic entity of the skin and the mucocutaneous junction. Typically, a completely disordered architechture, abnormal mitosis, dyskeratoses, involvement of the pilosebaceous unit with an intact epidermal junction is seen.[11] Synonyms of the same entity are: squamous carcinoma in situ, intraepidermal

*Corresponding Author: Cornelia S.L. Mueller—The Saarland University Hospital, Dermatology Clinic, Kirrbergerstr., 66421 Homburg/Saar, Germany. Email: hacmue@uniklinikum-saarland.de

Sunlight, Vitamin D and Skin Cancer, edited by Jörg Reichrath. ©2008 Landes Bioscience and Springer Science+Business Media.

carcinoma, bowenoid dysplasia and bowenoid squamous carcinoma in situ. The most common causation of Bowen's disease is, likewise for the actinic keratoses, chronic exposition to UVB-light. Histopathologically characteristical, hyperkeratosis, parakeratosis, hypo- or hypergranulosis and plaque-like acanthosis with an increased cellularity is seen, as well as a complete loss of epidermal polarity and keratinocytic maturation are found (Fig.1). Typically, crowding of atypical kera-tinocytes with pleomorphism, multinucleated or vacuolated cells with hyperchromatism and dyskeratosis appear. In addition, very large atypical cells (Fig.2) and bizzar mitoses are usually found. In Bowen's disease typically the follicular epithelium is involved. Morphological variants have been described, including clear-cell, pagetoid and pigmented forms.[12] As in actinic keratoses dermal changes are composed of solar elastosis, a lymphocytic and plasma cell- rich infiltrate in the papillary dermis and ectatic vessels. Bowen's disease affecting the penis is referred as Erythroplasia Queyrat.[13] The histologically features of lesions on the glans or shaft of the penis are identical to those at other sites of the skin.[11]

Invasive Squamous Cell Carcinoma (SCC)

SCCs are the most frequent form of skin cancer among blacks and the second one in the white population. The average age of patients is about 70 years and males are more frequently affected than females.[14] Even genodermatoses such as Xeroderma pigmentosum, albinism and Epidermodysplasia verruciformis are at increased risk for SCCs.[14] Main factors associated with an increased risk of developing an invasive squamous cell carcinoma are UVB-exposition, viral HPV-infections, therapeutic immunosuppression for allogenic organ transplants, arsenic exposure, ionizing radiation and chronic dermatoses, e.g., lichen sclerosus genitalis.[11]

By definition a SCC is a malignant neoplasia of epidermal (and mucous membrane) kerati-nocytes in which the component cells show variable squamous differentiation[12] and the ability of local infiltration and tissue destruction.[14] Mostly seen in elderly people, they arise on chronically

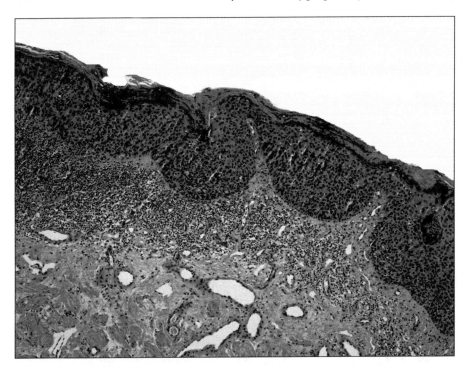

Figure 1. Bowen's disease. All images are available in color online at www.Eurekah.com.

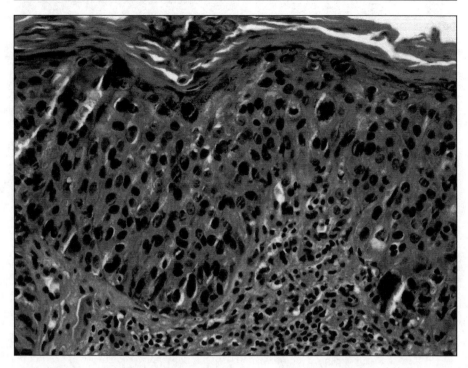

Figure 2. Bowen's disease; "monster cells".

sun-damaged skin sites. Histologically SCCs are composed of nests, sheets or strands of squamous epithelial cells arising from the epidermis and extending into the dermis in a variable degree. Initially developing as carcinoma in situ, they later become invasive, infiltrating dermis, subcutis, musculature, cartilage or bone and may also lead to regional lymph node disease and distant metastatic spread.[14] Typically, horn pearl formation and central keratinization are seen, depending on the degree of differentiation of the tumour. Immunohistochemically these atypical cells are positive for epithelial membrane antigen (EMA) and cytokeratins.

Actually, multiple classification systems exist, mostly historically developed:
- Classification into "well", "moderately" and "poorly" differentiated types.
- Broder's system of classification, based on four grades of differentiation
  grade 1: 75% or more of the lesion is well differentiated
  grade 2: 50%-75% or more well differentiated
  grade 3: 25-50% well differentiated tumour cells
  grade 4: less than 25% well differentiated tumour cells.[15]
- WHO classification system distinction between in situ carcinomas and invasive carcinomas with the following variants: SCCs with horn pearl formation, spindle cell SCCs, lymphoepithelial carcinoma, acantholytic SCCs, SCCs arising from Bowen's disease and the verrucous carcinoma.[14]
- Additionally, there are a lot of rare variants of SCCs known, including clear-cell, signet-ring, pigmented, basaloid, inflammatory, infiltrative, desmoplastic, verrucous and rhabdoid types.[14,16]

Though there are numerous classification systems, only little is known about the behaviour with respect to local recurrence and metastasis. In general, poorly differentiated tumours recur and metastasize more frequently than well differentiated variants.[17] Neurotropism is associated with high recurrence and metastasis rate. Perineural spread is particularly common in tumours arising on head and neck, especially lips and mid-face. The clinical outcome of SCCs of the skin depends on the microscopic parameters of thickness and histologic grade. Additional, attention should be paid to the histologic subtype because the individual SCCs forms vary considerably in prognosis. Based on a proposal of Cassarino et al the above mentioned forms of SCCs should be classified upon their malignancy behaviour and prognostic factors into four groups: low risk (less than 2% metastatic rate), intermediate (3-10%), high (greater than 10%) and the intermediate behaviour.[10]

- Low risk SCCs: actinic keratoses, HPV associated SCCs, tricholemmal carcinomas, spindle cell SCCs not associated with radiation.
- Intermediate risk SCCs: acantholytic SCCs, intraepidermal epithelioma with invasion, lymphoepithelioma-like carcinoma of the skin.
- High risk SCCs: de novo SCCs, SCCs arising in association with radiation, burn scars, immunosuppression, invasive Bowen's disease, adenosquamous carcinoma, malignant proliferating pilar tumours.
- Indeterminate behaviour SCCs: singnet-ring-cell, follicular and papillary SCCs, SCCs arising in adnexal cysts, eccrine ductal carcinomas, clear-cell SCCs.

In addition to the above mentioned classification systems prognostic relevant factors such as tumor size, differentiation, depth of invasion, perineural invasion should be announced when diagnosing a squamous cell carcinoma.[10]

Keratoakanthoma (KA)

Clinically, keratoakanthomas appear as usually solitary dome-shaped nodules with a central keratin plug, fastly growing and often spontaneously regressing. Severel clinical subtypes are known, as the giant KA, keratoakanthoma centrifugum marginatum or subungual types. Even multiple and eruptive cases are described, occuring mostly in immunosuppressed patients and within the Muir-Torre syndrome as well as at posttraumatic sites.[12] Rare cases of perineural invasion[18] and intravascular spread[19] have been reported, often occuring in the facial region. In most cases, these tumours affect sun-exposed hair follicle bearing skin of elderly individuals and they mimic clinically and histopathologically well-differentiated squamous cell carcinomas. Keratoakanthomas can therefore be considered as a histologic variant of squamous cell carcinoma with distinct clinical and pathologic attributes.[20] Histologically, they are exophytic squamoproliferative nodules with central keratin plug. Typically, the lesions appear symmetrical with a mixed inflammatory cell infiltrate, including eosinophils and neutrophils, with exocytosis of inflammatory cells[12] (Fig. 3). The center of the tumour presents as a crater filled with eosinophilic laminated orthokeratotic scales. This central crater most often is partially encoled by a well defined lip that forms the superficial border of the neoplasm (Fig. 3). The epithelium of this lip may be hyperplastic, but there is usually no evidence of dysplasia or actinic keratosis in the epithelium adjacent to th tumour.[20-22] Nearly impossible is the differential diagnosis of squamous cell carcinoma in superficial shaves or punch biopsies.[12]

Basal Cell Carcinoma

Basal cell carcinomas are tumours with in general nonmetastasizing behaviour that derive from undifferentiated pluripotent epithelial stem "germinative" cell. They are typically characterized by a fibrous stroma surrounding islands of dependent tumour cells that resembles keratinocytes of the basal layer of the epidermis or hair follicle. Usually, these tumour cells are fairly regular with rounded haematoxiphilic nuclei and little cytoplasm. Typically, the proliferating cell component of the tumour is found predominantly in so called peripheral "palisades" of cells around the margin of each tumour nest (Fig. 4). It has been shown that this phenomenon corresponds to the way, in which basal cell carcinomas grow by slow progressive, local invasion.[23] Basal cell carcinomas show a distinct tumour stroma, that is usually loose and mucin-rich (predominantly hyaluronic acid). A very typical sign of basal cell carcinoma is the presence of a constant retraction artefact; the seperation of the tumour cells from the underlying stroma. Five variants of basal cell carcinomas can be

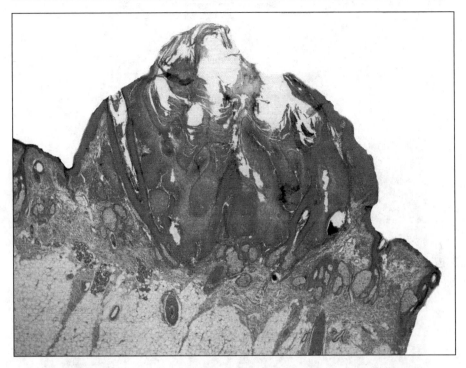

Figure 3. Keratoakanthoma.

distinguished: nodular/ulcerative (solid) with 45-60% (Fig. 4); diffuse (infiltrating, sclerosing) 4-17% (Fig. 5), superficial multicentric 15-35% , pigmented varaients 1-7% and the fibroepithelioma of Pinkus. Rare basal cell carcinomas have been referred to as metatypical carcinomas.[22]

Melanoma Skin Cancer

In this topic a great variety of neoplasms with distinct clinical, morphological and genetic profiles are included. Because of their often fatal biological behaviour they are the most important group of skin cancer. The major environmental risk factor is intermittant high-dose UV radiation, aggravated by the combination with endogenous factors, such as skin types I and II or genetic susceptibility.[12] Most important prognostic factor in malignant melanoma is Breslow's tumour thickness measured from the top of the granular layer of the epidermis to the deepest point of invasion in the dermis. Accordant to the sequence of development of invasive epithelial neoplasias starting with actinic keratoses, Bowen's disease and finally, fully developed invasive carcinoma, the melanoma skin cancer also does show an evolutionary sequence with early lesions, as melanoma in situ or historically named lentigo maligna to fully developed invasive malignant melanomas.

In Situ Melanoma (Syn Lentigo Maligna)

Clinically these early melanomas present as flat, pigmented macules, mostly seen in chronically light-exposed skin sites. The clinical differential diagnoses include lentigo simplex, junctional melanocytic nevus as well as nonmelanocytic lesions, as seborrhoic keratoses and basal cell carcinomas. Changes in preexisting melanocytic lesions or development of a new pigmented lesion later in life should be a striking hint to development of an early melanoma.

Histologically, a melanoma in situ is characterized by linear and nested proliferations of atypical melanocytes predominantly along the dermo-epidermal junction and extending the adnexal epithelium.[12] Later on, single atypical melanocytes can be found in higher layers of the epidermis.[24]

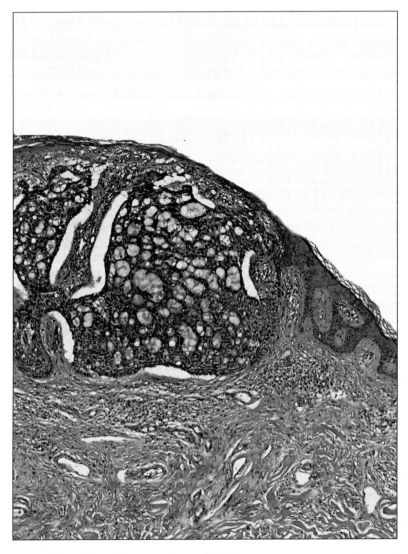

Figure 4. Basal cell carcinoma, solid type.

Characteristically, in early melanomas the neoplastic melanocytes are localized within the epidermis. Dermal changes such as severe solar elastosis, ectatic vessels and a lymphocytic infiltrate but also epidermal atrophy are seen. The lentigo maligna is broadly accepted as in situ variant of the lentigo maligna melanoma, in which the dermis is infiltrated by atypical melanocytes.

Invasive Melanoma

Based on proposals by Clark and Mc Govern[15] the clinicopathological classification of malignant melanoma has evolved into 4 main groups: the lentigo maligna melanoma, the superficial spreading melanoma, the nodular and the acral lentiginous melanoma. The relative incidence of these subtypes vary in different areas of the world. The concept of the radial and vertical growth phase of melanomas is mainly accepted. A progressive centrifugal spread of flat pigmented areas

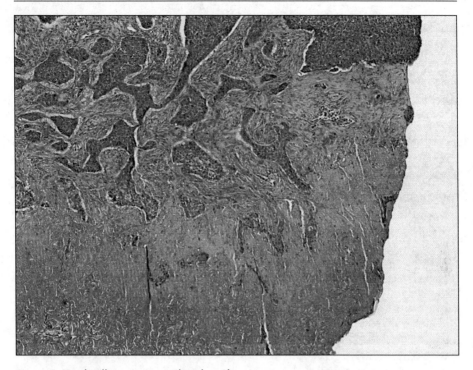

Figure 5. Basal cell carcinoma, sclerodermiformic type.

characterized by intraepidermal proliferating melanocytes labels the radial growth phase. In most cases of lentigo maligna, superficial spreading and nodular melanoma the radial growth phase precedes the vertical growth phase, where the dermis gets infiltrated by melanocytic tumor cells. Associated with the development of the vertical phase is angiogenesis and the expression of vascular endothelial growth factor.[12,25]

Superficial Spreading Melanoma

Proliferating single or nested melanocytic cells with cytological atypias in all levels of the epidermis characterizes this type of melanoma. The superficial adnexial structures usually are involved. Dermal tumour masses contain lymphoid, epithelial, spindle-shaped melanocytic tumours cells with variable degree of pigmentation. Typically, maturation of melanocytic tumour cells in the deeper compartments is missing. Clinically superficial spreading malignant melanomas appear on any part of the body as wells as at any age. Not uncommon are areas of regression mostly caused by immune mechanisms.[25]

Lentigo Maligna Melanoma

Basal proliferations of atypical melanocytes, singly or nested, focally aggregating to crowding conglomerates characterizes this type of melanoma. The deep adnexial epithelium is regularly involved and heavy cellular pleomorphism and cellular atypia are seen. Often there is a moderate to severe solar elastosis of the papillary dermis, but this is not a prerequisit of the lentigo maligna melanoma. Only little pagetoid spreading of atypical cells into higher levels of the epidermis is seen and there are quite often multinucleated tumor cells (Fig. 6). Microinvasive foci are strikingly ignored, in those cases highlightning these areas with S100 and HMB45 is a useful tool. Most of the lentigo maligna melanomas appear in the face and other sun-exposed areas of elderly people.[25]

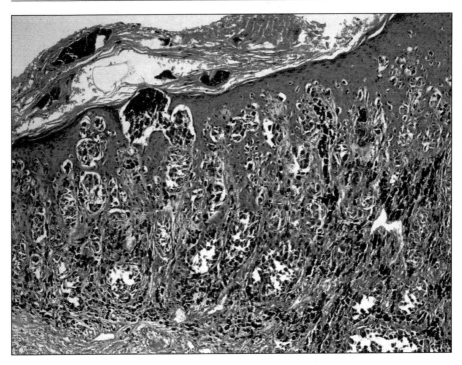

Figure 6. Superficial spreading malignant melanoma; intraepidermal pagetoid spread of atypical melanocytic cells.

Nodular Melanoma

These melanomas do not have any radial growth phase,[25] but show exclusively an vertical proliferation direction. The clinical feature is therefore nodular, polypoid and sometimes pedunculated (Fig. 8). Amelanotic and ulcerated variants do exist. Typically, there is mostly no or little intraepidermal component of atypical melanocytes. Mostly the tumour cells in the dermal part are round to oval with hyperchomatic nuclei[25] and an often epitheloid feature. The cell population mostly appears monomorphous.[12] Failure of deep dermal maturation is a strong hint to the malignant behaviour of this type of melanoma. Characteristically, S100, HMB45 and Melan-A as the typical melanocytic markers are expressed here.

Akral Lentiginous Melanoma

The acral lentiginous melanomas arise on nonhair bearing palmar, plantar and subungual skin sites.[12] It has a characteristical but not distinct histology with marked acanthosis, expanded cornified layer, elongated rete ridges and a lentiginous proliferation of atypical melanocytes in the radial growth phase, with a dominant intraepidermal component (Fig. 7). In the vertical growth phase mostly spindle-shaped tumour cells and a desmoplastic stroma form a nodular tumour.[25]

Variants and Specialities

Malignant melanoma is very well known for the wide range of histological variability and the ability of mimicking a variity of other malignancies. Besides the above mentioned classical forms there are a lot of different variants described, accountable for the often difficult recognition, even by expert dermatopathologists. Smoller and Rongiolette favour a classification of these melanoma variants into four groups corresponding to the architectural patterns, cytologic features, stromal changes and combinations of these three.[26] This description is not only suggestive for pedogogic

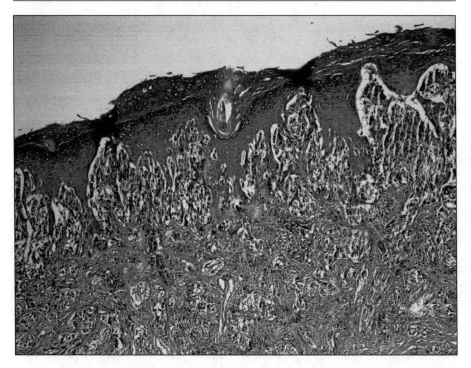

Figure 7. Malignant melanoma, akro-lentiginous type.

and nosologic values, but also important for the possible prognostic correlations. So espeacilly desmoplastic melanomas tend to local recurrence after surgery, angiotropic and ballon cell melanomas tend to skin metastasis whereas signet ring cell melanomas are of poor prognostic sign. In the following the most important variants of malignant melanomas concerning to the above mentioned classification are accounted.

Architectural Patterns

Here polypoid, verrucous, angiomatoid, angiotropic, primary dermal bullous and pseudopapillary/adenoid- cystic melanomas are outlined (Fig. 8). The polypoid malignant melanoma is marked of a distinct exophytic growth pattern with a nodule connecting the underlaying skin by a pedicle. Bulky proliferations of atypical melanocytes fill the nodule. Later on infiltration of these melanoma cells through the pedicle in the underlying skin is seen. The verrucous melanoma is often been misdiagnosed clinically as benign lesions, such as dermal nevus or seborrhoic keratoses. Histologically strikingly at scanning magnification is the prominent papillomatous epidermal component, e.g., hyperkeratosis, parakeratosis and pseudoeptheliomatous pattern. The other mentioned variants of architectural forms of melanomas are extremely rare entities, e.g., only 2 cases of bullous melanomas, with floating melanoma cells in a pigmented epidermal blister are described.[27] In contrast it is not that uncommenly to see subepidermal blistering within classical melanomas.

Stromal Features

In this fraction the desmoplastic or neurotropic melanoma is the most common representative. Among the classical forms desmoplastic melanomas are only seen in 3% of all melanomas.[26] But also the myxoid and ossifying/chondroid melanoma has to be mentioned here. The myxoid pattern is often observed in elderly people and clinically presents as pigmented nodules on the trunk and extremities. Strikingly other mucin-containing neoplasms can be misdiagnosed. A strong positivity

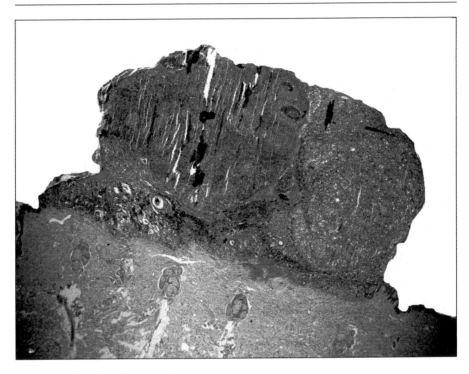

Figure 8. Polypoid malignant melanoma.

for S100 and NSE is observed, whereas Melan A or HMB45 are commonly negative. The osteocartilagineous metaplasia is a very rare histological phenomenon in melanomas.[28] Especially in akral and primary mucosal melanomas this pattern is seen.[29]

Clinically desmoplastic melanomas present as indurated, pigmented or nonpigmented plaques, often associated to lentigo maligna.[30] Histologically, spindle cell proliferations diffusely infiltrating the dermis and/or subcutis associated with a abundent stromal collagen are seen. In the conventional H&E stain these lesions mimick a scar or dermatofibroma. At higher magnification cytologic atypias are observed. The overlaying epidermis often shows lentiginous proliferations of atypical melanocytes. The spindled cells are mostly amelanotic. Concerning to an often strong neurotropism frequently recurrence of demsoplastic melanomas is a common feature after surgery.[31]

Cytological Features

A great variety of melanomas subforms are condensed in this fractions: ballon-cell, spindle-cell, signet-ring-cell, small-cell, animal-type, amelanotic, spitzoid, rhabdoid, schwannoid, ganglioblastic, plasmacytoid, merkel-cell-like and actin-rich melanoma. Mostly they have no distinct clinical features, but are very often difficult not to be misdiagnosed histologically. It shows the capacious spectrum of morphological variants of melanocytes and their atypical forms.

Variants of Combined Patterns

Sometimes the above mentioned architectural and cytological features are associated and form histologically arrestingly melanoma variants. The malignant blue nevus, malignant peripheral nerve sheath tumor like melanoma, clear cell sarcoma (melanoma of the soft parts), the nevoid and minimal deviation melanoma are summarized here. Confusingly is the nomenclature spectrum of the so called nevoid melanomas: Reed 2000 called them minimal deviation melanoma, but also pseudonevoid, small diameter and small cell melanomas often mean the same histological entity.[32] All these forms and terms in commen is the feature that tumor cells mimic nevus cells, with the broad morphological spectrum of nevus cells. Clinically preferential sites are lower extremities and the trunk of middle- aged men and women.[26]

Childhood Melanoma

Childhood melanoma is a very rare and fatal entitiy, with only 1-3% of all childhood malignancies[33] occuring with a slight female predominance. Per definition, these melanomas occur in individuals prior to puberty and can be further subcatagorized as:
- Congenital melanomas (onset in utero to birth)
- Infantile melanomas (birth- to one year of age)
- Childhood melanoma (one year to onset of puberty)

They must be further distinguished from simulants of melanomas, as Spitz naevi and atypical nodular proliferations developing in congenital naevi in infants and young children. Childhood melanomas can be further subcatagorized into three principal groups[12]:

Conventional Melanomas

In about 40 to 50% of childhood melanomas are similar in histology to those in adults. The lentigo maligna melanomas are not seen in this age group, but pagetoid spreading of atypical cells intraepidermal and nested or lentiginous proliferations of melanocytes are seen.[33]

Small Cell Melanomas

They are composed of monomorphous small cells reminiscent such cells as in lymphomas or melanocytic nevi. These cells are arranged in sheets or organoid configurations and they usually appear de novo or develop in congenital naevus. Striking Breslow index and a poor prognosis with a fatal outcome are often seen.

Melanomas Simulating Spitz naevus

These melanomas exhibit features strongly suggesting a Spitz naevus. Characteristically, wedge-shaped configuration, epidermal hyperplasia, epidermal clefting about intraepidermal nests with large epithelioid cells and spindle cells are seen.

Approximately 50% of childhood melanoma arise in association with preexisting lesions (congenital melanocytic nevus but also other aquired melanocytic nevi).[33] Criteria for distinguishing childhood melanomas from nevi or Spitz naevus are: ulceration, high mitotic rate of more than 4 mitosis/ mm^2, large size of mor than 7 milimeters asymmetry, poorly demarked lateral borders, lack of maturation and marked nuclear polymorphism. It is suggested that melanocytic lesions that cannot been classified sufficient as melanomas should be designated as biologically intermediate.

References

1. Brash DE et al. Sunlight and sunburn in human skin cancer: p53 apoptosis and tumor promotion. J Investig Dermatol Symp Proc 1996; 1(2):136-42.
2. Ackerman AB. Solar keratosis is squamous cell carcinoma. Arch Dermatol 2003; 139(9):1216-7.
3. Fu W and CJ. Cockerell. The actinic (solar) keratosis: a 21st-century perspective. Arch Dermatol 2003; 139(1):66-70.
4. Ehrig T et al. Actinic keratoses and the incidence of occult squamous cell carcinoma: a clinical-histopathologic correlation. Dermatol Surg 2006; 32(10):1261-5.
5. Marks R et al. Spontaneous remission of solar keratoses: the case for conservative management. Br J Dermatol 1986; 115(6):649-55.
6. Marks R, G Rennie and TS Selwood. Malignant transformation of solar keratoses to squamous cell carcinoma. Lancet 1988; 1(8589):795-7.
7. Cockerell CJ. Pathology and pathobiology of the actinic (solar) keratosis. Br J Dermatol, 2003; 149 Suppl 66: 34-6.
8. Lebwohl M. Actinic keratosis: epidemiology and progression to squamous cell carcinoma. Br J Dermatol 2003; 149 Suppl 66:31-3.
9. Cassarino DS, DP Derienzo and RJ Barr. Cutaneous squamous cell carcinoma: a comprehensive clinicopathologic classification. Part one. J Cutan Pathol 2006; 33(3):191-206.
10. Cassarino DS, DP Derienzo and RJ Barr. Cutaneous squamous cell carcinoma: a comprehensive clinicopathologic classification—part two. J Cutan Pathol 2006; 33(4):261-79.

11. Arlette JP. Treatment of Bowen's disease and erythroplasia of Queyrat. Br J Dermatol 2003; 149 Suppl 66:43-9.
12. LeBoit P et al. eds. Pathology and Genetics of Skin Tumours. World Health Organization Classification of Tumours. Pathology and Genetics of Skin Tumours 2006, IARC Press: Lyon.
13. Kaye V et al. Carcinoma in situ of penis. Is distinction between erythroplasia of Queyrat and Bowen's disease relevant? Urology 1990; 36(6):479-82.
14. Petter G and UF Haustein. Histologic subtyping and malignancy assessment of cutaneous squamous cell carcinoma. Dermatol Surg 2000; 26(6):521-30.
15. Goyanna R, ET Torres and AC Broders. [Histological grading of malignant tumors; Broder's method.] Hospital (Rio J) 1951; 39(6):791-818.
16. Petter G and UF Haustein. [Rare and newly described histological variants of cutaneous squamous epithelial carcinoma. Classification by histopathology, cytomorphology and malignant potential]. Hautarzt 2001; 52(4):288-97.
17. McKee P, ed. Tumours of the surface epithelium. 2nd ed. Pathology of the skin. 1999, Mosby International London, Philadelphia, St. Louis, Sydney, Tokyo.
18. Godbolt AM, JJ Sullivan and D Weedon. Keratoacanthoma with perineural invasion: a report of 40 cases. Australas J Dermatol 2001; 42(3):168-71.
19. Gottfarstein-Maruani A et al. [Keratoacanthoma: two cases with intravascular spread]. Ann Pathol 2003; 23(5):438-42.
20. Kane CL et al. Histopathology of cutaneous squamous cell carcinoma and its variants. Semin Cutan Med Surg 2004; 23(1):54-61.
21. Stadler R and C Hartig. Epidermale Tumoren. 1st ed. Histopathologie der Haut, ed. G. Kerl, Cerroni, Wolff. 2003, Berlin, Heidelberg, New York: Springer.
22. Murphy G. and D Elder. Nonmelanocytic tumors of the skin. Atlas of tumour pathology, ed. S. Rosai. 1991, Washington, DC: American Registry of Pathology.
23. Grimwood RE et al. Proliferating cells of human basal cell carcinoma are located on the periphery of tumor nodules. J Invest Dermatol 1986; 86(2):191-4.
24. Takata M and T Saida. Early cancers of the skin: clinical, histopathological and molecular characteristics. Int J Clin Oncol 2005; 10(6):391-7.
25. Weedon D. The Skin: The Skin Systemic Pathology Vol. 9. 1993: Churchill Livingstone.
26. Rongioletti F and BR Smoller. Unusual histological variants of cutaneous malignant melanoma with some clinical and possible prognostic correlations. J Cutan Pathol 2005; 32(9):589-603.
27. Vogt T et al. Bullous malignant melanoma: an unusual differential diagnosis of a hemorrhagic friction blister. Dermatol Surg 2003; 29(1):102-4.
28. Banerjee SS et al. Diagnostic lessons of mucosal melanoma with osteocartilaginous differentiation. Histopathology 1998; 33(3):255-60.
29. Moreno A et al. Osteoid and bone formation in desmoplastic malignant melanoma. J Cutan Pathol 1986; 13(2):128-34.
30. Anstey A, P McKee and EW Jones. Desmoplastic malignant melanoma: a clinicopathological study of 25 cases. Br J Dermatol, 1993; 129(4):359-71.
31. Smithers BM, GR McLeod and JH Little. Desmoplastic melanoma: patterns of recurrence. World J Surg 1992; 16(2):186-90.
32. Reed RJ. Minimal deviation melanoma. Borderline and intermediate melanocytic neoplasia. Clin Lab Med 2000; 20(4):745-58.
33. Huynh PM, JM Grant-Kels and CM Grin. Childhood melanoma: update and treatment. Int J Dermatol 2005; 44(9):715-23.

CHAPTER 18

Cytogenetics of Melanoma and Nonmelanoma Skin Cancer

Melanie A. Carless and Lyn R. Griffiths*

Abstract

Cytogenetic analysis of melanoma and nonmelanoma skin cancers has revealed recurrent aberrations, the frequency of which is reflective of malignant potential. Highly aberrant karyotypes are seen in melanoma, squamous cell carcinoma, solar keratosis and Merkel cell carcinoma with more stable karyotypes seen in basal cell carcinoma, keratoacanthoma, Bowen's disease, dermatofibrosarcoma protuberans and cutaneous lymphomas. Some aberrations were common amongst a number of skin cancer types including rearrangements and numerical abnormalities of chromosome 1, −3p, +3q, partial or entire trisomy 6, trisomy 7, +8q, −9p, +9q, partial or entire loss of chromosome 10, −17p, +17q and partial or entire gain of chromosome 20. Combination of cytogenetic analysis with other molecular genetic techniques has enabled the identification of not only aberrant chromosomal regions, but also the genes that contribute to a malignant phenotype. This review provides a comprehensive summary of the pertinent cytogenetic aberrations associated with a variety of melanoma and nonmelanoma skin cancers.

Introduction

Skin cancer represents an accumulation of genetic abnormalities, inherent and/or sporadic, that alter the cells in such a way that normal function is impaired and a tumor arises. Malignant melanoma originates from aberrant melanocytes located in the basal (innermost) layer of the epidermis, whereas nonmelanoma skin cancer (NMSC) is due to abnormalities of other cell types. The two most common forms of NMSC are basal cell carcinoma (BCC) and squamous cell carcinoma (SCC), arising from keratinocytes in the basal and squamous (2nd innermost) layers, respectively.[1] Other NMSCs include those developing from keratinocytes: solar keratosis (SK), SCC in situ (Bowen's disease; BD) and keratoacanthoma (KA)[2]; and those arising from other cells within the skin or associated with the skin, such as: eccrine carcinomas, apocrine and sebaceous gland carcinomas, Kaposi sarcoma, liposarcoma, malignant fibrous histiocytoma, cutaneous lymphoma, Merkel cell carcinoma (MCC), extramammary Paget's disease, leiomyosarcoma, epithelioid sarcoma, malignant schwannoma, malignant granular cell tumor and dermatofibrosarcoma protuberans (DFSP).[2]

Although the development of both melanocytic and nonmelanocytic skin cancers is strongly reliant upon genetic factors, such as skin type, familial incidence (including inherited disorders), race and gender, it is also heavily influenced by environmental factors, most specifically ultraviolet (UV) radiation.[3,4] UV radiation is known to induce DNA point mutations and small deletions.[5,6] Also, Emri and colleagues detected the formation of micronuclei, cytogenetic indicators of chromosomal damage, in melanocytes and fibroblasts exposed to UVB radiation and to a lesser extent

*Corresponding Author: Lyn R. Griffiths—Genomics Research Centre, School of Health Science, Griffith University Gold Coast, PMB 50 Gold Coast Mail Centre, Bundall, QLD, Australia.
Email: l.griffiths@griffith.edu.au

Sunlight, Vitamin D and Skin Cancer, edited by Jörg Reichrath. ©2008 Landes Bioscience and Springer Science+Business Media.

in fibroblasts exposed to UVA radiation.[7] This study indicated that at physiological doses of UV radiation, gross chromosomal aberrations can be induced.[7]

Cytogenetic analysis is a powerful tool used in the identification of chromosomal aberrations with applications ranging from identification of prenatal birth defects to detection and prognostic evaluation of diseases associated with sporadic or inherent karyotypic abnormalities. A wide variety of karyotypic abnormalities are associated with diseases, including changes in karyotypic number, size and structure. In particular, cytogenetic analysis has given invaluable insight into abnormalities associated with hematological malignancies and solid tumors. An important consideration in cytogenetic analysis of solid tumors is clonal derivation as tumors may be of monoclonal (tumors evolve from changes in a single cell) or polyclonal (tumors evolve from multiple cells, each with distinct mutations) origin. Thus, cytogenetic reports often refer to changes associated with different clonal populations and also to random mutations, which are not clonal changes. Particularly relevant to skin cancers is field cancerization, a process where a large epithelial area may have undergone preneoplastic change after prolonged mutagenic exposure resulting in multiple independent tumor foci.[8] As such, there is an increased risk of additional tumor development after the emergence of a tumor and consequently these tumors, although distinct entities, may share similar cytogenetic abnormalities.[8]

Aneuploidy, or abnormal DNA content, is a consequence of defects in the mitotic checkpoint and is the most common characteristic of solid tumors.[9] In fact, the frequency of aneuploidy in tumors suggests that it either contributes to or drives tumorigenesis, as well as indicating malignant potential.[9,10] Aneuploidy is typically detected by flow cytometry or image analysis, with these techniques showing high concordance (>90%) and comparisons with cytogenetic analysis also showing high concordance (>80%).[11,12] DNA aneuploidy and tetraploidy in cancer cells has been associated with poor prognosis, advanced staging and poor histologic differentiation in a variety of solid tumors.[13,14]

Direct analysis of tumor karyotypes allows the detection of various structural and copy number changes that may be a cause or consequence of tumorigenesis. Analyses of hematological malignancies have shown nonrandom, recurrent karyotypic abnormalities that are often highly specific to one or more cancer types.[15] In particular, the Philadelphia chromosome, arising from a reciprocal translocation, t(9; 22)(q34; q11.2), was the first consistent abnormality identified in human cancer and some believe that it should be the defining characteristic of chronic myeloid leukemia.[15] The analysis of solid tumors has been more problematic due to the culture of cells, which may lead to differential cell type selection, subclone selection and cell bias.[16-18] Studies of NMSC cultures have shown fibroblastic rather than the expected epithelial growth pattern, potentially indicating preferential growth of contaminating stromal fibroblasts.[16] Analysis of eight cell lines derived from malignant melanoma demonstrated selection of a subclone and subsequent emergence of its own subclones in each of the lines such that no long-term culture was identical to its line of origin.[17] Additionally, cell culture can be biased toward selection of tumor cells that have a high mitotic index, therefore the culture may not represent the entire tumor specimen.[18] Each of these studies demonstrate inadequacy in some cytogenetic analyses of solid tumors, including skin cancers. As such, caution is warranted in the interpretation of results in studies involving cell culture of skin tumors, particularly long-term culture.

Comparative genomic hybridization (CGH) and fluorescence in situ hybridization (FISH) are fluorescence based molecular tools used for the detection of molecular aberrations. CGH involves hybridization of differentially labeled tumor and reference DNA to normal metaphase spreads to globally screen for gross (>20 mb) copy number aberrations.[19] Imbalances are detected by changes in fluorescence values of the tumor DNA relative to the reference DNA and as such, it does not require the interpretation of complex tumor karyotypes or prior knowledge of aberrations for probe design.[19,20] Although CGH only reveals relatively large numerical or unbalanced aberrations, it identifies previously unknown DNA copy number changes of regions that may harbor tumor suppressor genes or oncogenes associated with cancer development. FISH also allows the identification of copy number changes, both large (up to whole chromosomes) and small (as low as 1-200 kb), as well as detecting translocations and inversions that are difficult to determine using standard karyotyping techniques.[20-22] As probes designed for FISH analysis are of a known, specific sequence, they can be hybridized to cells in interphase, making FISH a useful technique in the identification of aberrations in archival material such as frozen or paraffin embedded samples.[20]

Each technique used for cytogenetic analysis has both advantages and disadvantages, however a combination of these cytogenetic techniques in addition to other molecular genetic techniques can provide a comprehensive overview of abnormalities that drive tumorigenesis and may even predict outcome of the disease. Although not strictly a cytogenetic technique, loss of heterozygosity (LOH) is often used in conjunction with cytogenetic analysis to confirm loss of regions or genes involved in tumorigenesis. Using highly polymorphic markers, or specific genes, a comparison of alleles from normal and tumor DNA of an individual is made; a loss of an allele in the tumor tissue identifies or confirms a deleted chromosomal region.[23] These regions of genetic loss may harbor one or more putative tumor suppressor genes pivotal in cancer development. Also, gene expression analysis can be useful in determining if aberrant regions correlate to transcriptional activity. Using cDNA microarrays, overexpression of several genes has been found to correlate with breakpoint or amplified regions,[24,25] although others suggest this rate of association is quite low (3.8%).[26] The aim of this review is to present a comprehensive summary of cytogenetic and associated abnormalities involved in melanocytic and nonmelanocytic skin cancer development.

Melanocytic Derived Skin Cancers and Their Precursors

Malignant melanoma is the most fatal of the skin cancers, arising from the malignant transformation of cells (melanocytes) found within the basal layer of the epidermis.[27,28] Lifetime risk for melanoma has been estimated at 2.04% for men and 1.45% for women in the US, with rates as high as 8.33% and 5.88% in Queensland, Australia for men and women, respectively.[28,29] Melanoma can be classified into two major groups based on location of the lesion; cutaneous (skin; CMM) and uveal (eye), both of which have numerous chromosomal abnormalities.[4] Melanoma stages I-IV are typically defined by level of invasion (Clark microstaging levels I-V) and tumor thickness (Breslow microstaging).[30-32] Melanoma stages I and II refer to primary lesions yet to metastasize, stage III refers to lesions that have invaded the regional lymph nodes and stage IV refers to lesions that have metastasized to distant sites.[30] Dysplastic nevi are considered a precursor to CMM and although most are biologically stable, their presence has been associated with 100% of familial and 60% of sporadic CMM cases.[33]

In a study of 34 nevi and 53 melanoma, aneuploidy was observed in 2.94% of nevi, 0% of level I-III melanoma, 34.48% of level IV melanoma and 100% of level V melanoma (Clark microstaging) and was associated lesion thickness (0% in lesions <0.76 and 83% in lesions >3.0 mm).[34] Additionally, in a follow-up examination of a sub-group of patients 90% of aneuploid tumors showed recurrence, whereas only 17.39% of diploid tumors recurred; of the 15.09% of tumors that regressed during the study, all were diploid.[34] A study by Kheir and colleagues retrospectively examined 177 stage I cutaneous melanomas, including those in the previously mentioned study and found aneuploidy to be highly predictive of both recurrence and shorter disease-free survival.[35] Aneuploidy (as opposed to diploidy) was associated with increased thickness (8% of tumors <1.5 mm; 39% of tumors ≥3.0 mm), Clark's level (11% of tumors level I, II or III; 31% of tumors level IV or V), ulceration (11% of nonulcerated tumors; 35% of ulcerated tumors), vertical growth (0% of tumors with no growth; 26% of tumors with vertical growth), cell type (17% of epithelioid tumors; 30% of other tumors) and location (12% of tumors of head, neck and trunk; 32% of tumors at extremities).[35]

Many studies have investigated karyotypic abnormalities associated with CMM and a recent comprehensive review of all previously published karyotypes outlined the identified recurrent aberrations.[4] Höglund and colleagues used the Mitelman Database of Chromosome Aberrations in Cancer[36] to identify recurrent imbalances, including deletions, additions, isochrome formation and somy changes associated with 92 cases of cutaneous melanoma.[4] The most common aberrations detected were –10 (59%), –6q10-q27 (42%), –9p10-p24, –21 (37%), +7, –16 (36%), –14, +1q24-q44, –4, –15 (33%), –5 (32%), –1p10-p36, –11q23-q25 (28%), –12q13–q24, +20 (27%),

−17p, +18 (26%), −8p10-p23, +8q10-q24 (25%), −3 (24%), −22, −X (23%), +6p21-p25, −18 (22%), +3 (18%), −19 (17%), +9q22-q34 (15%), +19 (14%), +13, +17q10-q25 (12%), +2, +15, +21 and +22 (11%).[4] Two major karyotypic pathways were detected; the first involved +6p, −6q and possibly −16 as early cytogenetic changes and the second involved −3 and either +8q or −8p as early changes.[4] In addition to these imbalances, balanced translocations involving regions on 1q, 6q, 14q and 19p have been identified in a smaller percentage of cases.[36]

Some studies have investigated cytogenetic changes associated with dysplastic nevi, a precursor lesion to melanoma. One of these studies found loss of chromosome 9 in 2 of 4 dysplastic nevi, suggesting this may be a primary event in the transformation of melanocytes.[37] Another study investigating three nevi from a single patient with a family history of melanoma found simple translocations in each of the nevi, including one with a 6q13 breakpoint (t(6;15)(q13;q21)), a region implicated in CMM.[36,38] An investigation of eight benign nevi also revealed single occurrences of reciprocal translocations involving t(6;15), t(10;15), t(15;20) and t(4;5).[39] This demonstrates that even in benign lesions, chromosomal instability may have already begun and could potentially signify lesions that undergo malignant transformation.

Bastian et al analyzed 132 melanomas and 54 benign nevi by CGH and found that although 96.2% of melanomas exhibited copy number aberrations, only 13% of the nevi displayed aberrations.[40] Specifically, of the seven nevi that exhibited aberration, six of these showed a gain of the entire 11p arm, which was not found in any of the melanomas.[40] In the melanomas studied, regions of recurrent gain included 6p (37%), 1q (33%), 7p, 7q (32%), 8q (25%), 17q (24%) and 20q (22%), with regions of recurrent loss including 9p (64%), 9q, 10q (36%), 10p (30%), 6q (26%) and 11q (21%).[40] An earlier study on a smaller number of melanomas (16) also included analysis of metastatic tumors (12) and found similar aberrations as those listed above for both lesions. Additionally, gains of 5p, 5q21-q23, 10p and 18q and losses of 2p21-pter, 11q13-q23, 12q24. 1-qter, 19q13.1-qter and 22qter were detected in metastatic lesions but not in primary lesions and losses involving 9p and 17 occurred at a higher frequency in metastatic tumors.[41] Specifically, investigation of primary and metastatic lesions excised from the same patient (4 patients) showed additional aberrations associated with metastases, although none were determined to be recurrent.[41]

FISH analysis of melanoma has verified aberrations of: extra copies (89%) and translocations (25%) of chromosome 20 (whole chromosome painting);[42] extra *cyclin D* copies in primary (47%) and metastatic (35%) lesions;[43] higher rates of trisomy seven in metastatic lesions (25%) compared to primary lesions (8%);[44] extra copies of *c-myc* in nodular (61%) and superficial spreading (27%) melanomas;[45] and copy number gains of 7 (40.9%), 6, 17 (27%), 9 and 10 (23%) as well as monosomies of 10 (55%), 9 (37%), 6 (27%), 17 (23%), 1 and 7 (18%) in malignant melanoma (14 primary and 8 metastatic).[46] LOH has been detected for at least one locus at 9p22 (31%), 10q11 (31%) and 1p36 (15%) in early stage CMM (13 cases),[47] and further analysis comparing benign and dysplastic nevi to CMM have shown higher frequency of 1p and 9p LOH in CMM (29% and 50% at most frequently lost loci) compared to dysplastic nevi (12% and 27% at corresponding loci) with complete absence of LOH in benign nevi.[48] Figure 1 summarizes recurrent aberrations (>10%) detected in CMM samples using a combination of karyotypic analysis, CGH and LOH studies.

Keratinocytic Derived Skin Cancers and Their Precursors

Basal cell carcinomas are the most common form of NMSC, with an estimated lifetime risk between 28% and 33%.[49] Although they are locally invasive and highly destructive, BCCs rarely metastasize with an estimated metastatic potential of 0.0028-0.55%.[50] Squamous cell carcinoma is the second most common form of nonmelanoma skin cancer and also the most metastatic, accounting for about 20% of all cutaneous malignancies with a lifetime risk estimated at 7-11%.[51,52] The metastatic potential of SCC is highly variable from as low as 3.6% to 30% depending on the site and etiology of the lesion.[53] Solar keratosis (SK) is a lesion commonly described as a biomarker for both melanoma and nonmelanoma skin cancer, with prevalence ranging from 11% to as high as 80%.[54,55] They are known to undergo progression to SCC (0.1-10%) and it has been proposed

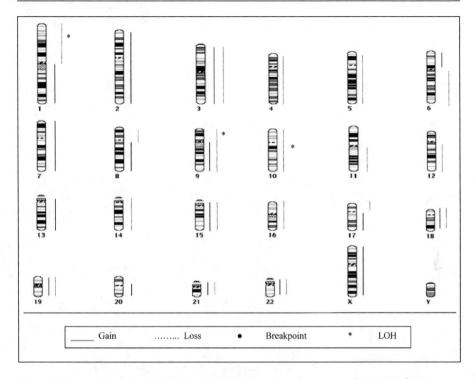

Figure 1. Summary of recurrent genomic aberrations in cutaneous malignant melanoma.

that all SCC are derived from SK, implicating these lesions as the first recognizable stage of NMSC.[54,56,57] Additionally, up to 25% of lesions spontaneously regress.[55] SCC in situ, commonly known as Bowen's disease, is a lesion that infrequently progresses to SCC (about 2-5%) and has limited metastatic ability.[58,59] Keratoacanthoma (KA) is arguably classified as either a distinct lesion or a subtype of SCC, with typical solitary lesions displaying a pattern of growth, maturation and spontaneous regression.[53] As SCC is considered to be the most aggressive form of NMSC, it might be expected that they exhibit a large degree of chromosomal instability. In turn, precursors of SCC or less aggressive forms of skin cancer such as SK, BD and KA and also BCC, would likely show less severe instability.

The incidence of DNA aneuploidy in BCC is fairly low (9-40%), which is indicative of its stability.[13,60,61] However, variability in aneuploidy rates has been seen in specific subgroups with rates of 80% for keratotic, 58% for metatypical, 24% for adenoid and 12% for solid and cystic forms.[62] Aneuploidy rates are estimated to be higher in SCC (25-80%), concurring with the malignant spectrum.[13,61,63] A study by Pilch and colleagues also detected differences between well (46%) and moderately (75%) differentiated SCC.[63] Aneuploidy rates for SK, BD and KA have been estimated at 69%, 89-92% and 4%, respectively.[63-65] Aneuploidy rates for SCC in situ (89-92%) are higher than those reported for both cutaneous SCC and SK and as such Kawara and colleagues have suggested that DNA aneuploidy may not be a good prognostic marker of cutaneous SCC.[64,65] However, aside from these discrepancies in BD data, aneuploidy rates in tumors appears to be indicative of malignant potential with rates for SCC similar to or higher than its precursor lesion, SK, and also higher than rates for most forms of BCC.

A number of recurrent numerical and structural alterations have been detected in BCC, although much of this has been done in short-term cultures, which allows for contamination of other cell types, subclone selection and cell bias. Using a chemically defined media for selection

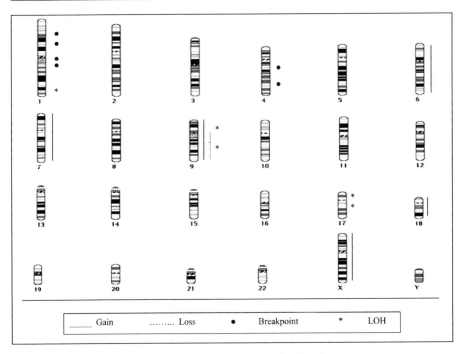

Figure 2. Summary of recurrent genomic aberrations in basal cell carcinoma.

of epithelial cells, Jin and colleagues investigated 69 new and previously published short-term (5-10 days) BCC cultures and identified numerical aberrations of +18 (30%), +7, +X (17%) and +9 (14%) as well as rearrangements of 9q (24%) and breakpoints involving 1p32, 1p22, 1q11, 1q21, 4q21and 4q31 (10%).[66,67] Less frequent breakpoints were also detected. Most of the cultures investigated had simple aberrant karyotypes consisting of only 1 to 3 aberrations, suggesting that these tumors are still relatively genetically stable compared to most other tumor types.[66,67] Casalone and colleagues studied both direct preparations (24 hours; 73 samples) and short-term (10-28 days) cultures and showed inconsistencies in the aberrations detected in each of the techniques.[68] In direct preparations, the most recurrent and nonrandom change observed was +6 (in a small number of cases).[68] Confirmatory FISH analysis detected +6 in a further 8 (of 21) cases where trisomy six was not observed cytogenetically, although this aberration was not detected in any of the short-term cultures.[68] Similar to data found by Jin et al a number of other studies have identified structural abnormalities, such as translocations and inversions involving 9q as a common event in BCCs.[16,69,70]

CGH analysis has also confirmed that there is a reasonable degree of genomic stability associated with BCC, finding that loss of genetic material is generally confined to 9q (33%), a region implicated in karyotypic analysis.[71] This loss was verified by LOH analysis, further defining the region to 9q22.3 in 53% of cases.[71] Regions of recurrent genetic gain were also detected using CGH analysis at 6p (47%), 6q, 9p (20%), 7 and X (13%).[71] The gain of 6p is also consistent with karyotypic and FISH analysis, which have identified trisomy six as a frequent aberration associated with BCC.[68] LOH studies in a Greek population have demonstrated losses of 9p21-p22 (55%), 17q21 (34%) and 17p13 (11%).[72] Quinn et al investigated LOH of BCC using a panel of microsatellite markers, finding loss at 9q (60%) and 1q (14%).[73] Other studies have also verified LOH at 9q22 in 46-60% of cases.[74,75] A summary of recurrent aberrations (>10%) detected in BCC samples by karyotypic analysis, CGH and LOH can be seen in Figure 2.

In a study of short-term cultures of 13 primary cutaneous SCC and review of 10 previously published cases, Jin and colleagues detected recurrent numerical gains of +7p (32%) and +8q (27%) and losses of −21 (41%), −8p (36%), −4p, −11p, −Y (32%), −13, −18q (27%), −10p, −X (23%) and −9p (18%).[8] They also detected various anomalies in the form of isochromes: i(1p10), i(1q10), i(5p10), i(8q10), i(9p10), i(9q10), (all <20%); with i(8q) and i(9q) believed to be early genetic events.[8] Casalone et al examined direct preparations of three primary cutaneous SCC finding aberrations that had not been previously considered recurrent in short-term cultures; these included −1, +6, +8, +9, +11, −14, +16 and +21.[68] However, as only three SCCs were investigated, these regions cannot be classified as recurrent. Most other cytogenetic studies have examined only small numbers of cultured SCCs or examined SCCs from Xeroderma Pigmentosum patients and have not revealed any additional information. Available cytogenetic data on other keratinocytic tumors is somewhat limited. Short-term culture of three SKs and two cases of SK with SCC in situ has identified numerical changes of +7 and +20 (40%) and structural rearrangements involving chromosomes 1 (100%) and 4 (75%), however these numbers are too low to be considered informative.[76] Heim et al investigated short-term cultures from a single SCC in situ and although early passages revealed various aberrant clones, passages 7-11 were dominated by a single clone with a sole anomaly of t(12;17)(p13;q21).[77] Analysis of KA in two studies (1 lesion each) has identified 2p13 alterations in both lesions, although the type of aberration was different in the two lesions; no other anomalies were shared.[78,79]

Early CGH studies have investigated single cases of SCC and their related recurrences and metastases and although they found many copy number aberrations, including anomalies unique to metastatic lesions, recurrent aberrations could not be defined. Our laboratory has investigated SCCs and SKs finding a similar pattern of aberrations in the two lesions, supporting their close relationship. Aberrations in SCC included gains of 3q (47%), 17q (40%), 14q, Xq (33%), 4p, 8q (27%), 1q, 5p, 7q, 9q, 10q and 20q (20%) and losses at 3p (53%), 18q (47%), 17p (33%), 4q (27%), 5q, 8p, 11p, 13q and 18p (20%).[80] For SK, gains were seen at 3q, 4p, 17q (33%), 5p, 9q and 17p (25%) and losses at 9p, 13q (53%), 3p, 4q, 11p and 17p (25%).[80] The loss of 18q in 47% of SCCs was specific to this lesion (P = 0.04) and could likely harbor one or more genes that contribute to malignant progression.[80] Clausen and colleagues performed initial CGH analysis on KA lesions, mostly from immunosuppressed organ transplant recipients and found copy number aberrations in 36% of KAs. Recurrent gains were detected at 8q (20%), 1p and 9q (16%) with losses at 3p, 9p, 19p (20%) and 19q (16%).[81] Their second study examined differences between KA and SCC and found gains of 1p, 14q, 16q, 20q and losses of 4p were significantly more frequent in SCC (P values ≤0.03), whereas a loss of 9p was significantly more frequent in KA (P = 0.04), supporting the theory that SCC and KA are distinct forms of NMSC.[82] CGH studies suggest that both SKs and SCCs are more genetically unstable than BCCs and KAs, showing a significantly higher number of aberrations indicative of a higher malignant potential.

Frequent LOH has been observed in SCC (including BD lesions) at 17q (43%), 13q (38%), 17p (34%), 9p (32%), 3p (26%) and 2q (20%).[73] A higher frequency of LOH has been observed in SK compared to SCC, with losses detected at 17p (64%), 13q (52%), 17q (46%), 9p (39%), 9q (22%) and 3p (31%), a pattern similar to that seen in SCC.[83] Individual analysis of a small number of BD has also revealed recurrent loss of *TP53* in a Korean population (27%).[84] Also, LOH of the region encoding *CDKN2A* occurs in 21% of SK and 46% of SCC, indicating a possible role for *CDKN2A* inactivation in progression towards SCC.[85] LOH is rare in KA, with isolated losses detected at 9p, 9q and 10q.[86] This low frequency of LOH further supports the theory that KA is a distinct lesion rather than a subtype of SCC. Figure 3 presents a summary of recurrent aberrations (>10%) detected in SCC samples by karyotypic analysis, CGH and LOH.

Rare Cancers of the Skin

In addition to the most common forms of skin cancer, a number of rare benign and malignant lesions exist that arise from cells within the skin or are associated with tumor formation in the skin. Merkel cell carcinoma is a rare aggressive skin cancer arising from the neuroendocrine system.[87]

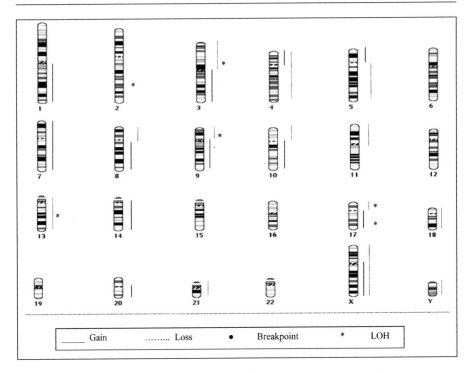

Figure 3. Summary of recurrent genomic aberrations in squamous cell carcinoma.

Dermatofibrosarcoma protuberans is a rare cutaneous disease arising from spindle cells with a histology that may be fibroblastic, histiocytic or neural in origin.[88] Cutaneous T-cell lymphoma (CTCL) and cutaneous B-cell lymphoma (CBCL) arise from the lymphatic system. Subtypes include mycosis fungoides (MF) and Sezary syndrome (SS) for CTCL; and follicular lymphoma (FL), marginal zone B-cell lymphoma and large B-cell lymphoma for CBCL.[89,90]

Even though these tumors are rare, a considerable amount of cytogenetic analysis has been performed on many of them. Table 1 summarizes some of the more pertinent studies that have been performed on these cutaneous lesions. Although other cytogenetic based analyses have been performed on additional rare skin tumors, Table 1 is generally limited to select tumors that have been investigated in multiple studies.

Implications of Cytogenetic Findings

Cytogenetic analysis is an extremely powerful tool to aid in the detection of chromosomal abnormalities involved in neoplastic development and when combined with other molecular techniques, putative genes related to the progression and often outcome of cancer can be identified. Skin cancer results from the accumulation of genetic aberrations that arise within cells of the skin. Malignant melanoma is a particularly aggressive form of skin cancer with high probability of metastasis, whereas nonmelanoma skin cancer is typically less aggressive, although it does show a wide spectrum of clinical outcomes. Additionally, rare skin cancers display a range of clinical behaviors. As genomic instability is a hallmark of cancer aggressiveness, cytogenetic analysis of skin cancer has proven invaluable in detecting changes associated with malignancy and on occasion can be predictive of clinical outcome.

Analysis of aneuploidy in skin cancer is a simple method to detect abnormal chromosomal content. In CMM aneuploidy rates can be up to 100% in advanced disease and associations have been made with various adverse clinical parameters, including advanced disease indicators, disease

Table 1. Common chromosomal aberrations associated with rare tumors of the skin

Tumor	Major Findings	Number of Cases
MCC	Karyotype: rearrangement of 1, −13 (67%), +11, −22 (33%)[91]	6 cases
	CGH: +19q (63%), +19p (50%), +1p (54%), −3p (46%), +1q, +X (42%), +5p, +8q (38%), −10, +3q, −13q (33%), +20p (29%), +7p, −17p, +20q (25%), −5q, +6q, +7q, −8p, +13q, + 18q (21%), −11q, +21 (17%); the average number of imbalances differed in patients surviving >24 months (6.6) and <24 months (11.2)[87]	34 cases (24 patients)
	CGH: +6 (42%), +1q11-q31, +5p (32%), +1q32-qter (26%), +1p33-pter, +12, −13q13-q31 (21%), −4q (16%)[92]	19 cases
	LOH: deletion of 10q23 (43%); unlikely involvement of *PTEN*[93]	18 informative cases
	LOH: deletion of 1p35–36 (70%)[94]	10 cases
DFSP	Karyotype/FISH: t(17;22)(q22;q13), which fuses *COL1A1* and *PDGFB;* often involves formation of ring chromosomes including sequences from these chromosomes (≈70%)[88]	Review of published cases
	CGH: +17q21-qter (100%), +22pter-q13 (82%), +5 (27%)[95] CGH: +17q22-qter (83%), +22q13 (75%), 8q24.1-qter (25%)[96]	11 cases; 12 cases
	CGH: +17q21-qter (100%), +22pter-q13 (70%), +5 (40%), +1 (40%), +12p, +12q23-qter, +21 (30%), +8, +20, −X (20%)[95]	10 cases (fibrosarcomatous transformation)
	Array CGH (pooled analysis): +8q24.3, +17q21.33-qter, +22cen-q13.1 (recurrent)[88]	10 cases
CTCL	Karyotype (SS subtype): structural aberrations affecting 10, 17 (28%), 1p (22%), 6q, 14q (17%) CGH: −1p (38%), −17p (21%), +4/4q (18%), −10q/10, +18, −19 (15%), +17q/17 (12%) FISH (SS subtype): rearrangements of 1p, 17p (33%), 10 (27%)[97]	18 cases (SS subtype); 16 cases (MF subtype)
	LOH (SS subtype): deletion of 9p (46%), 17p (42%), 10q, 2p (14%) LOH (MF subtype): deletion of 9p (16%), 10q (12%), 1p, 17p (10%)[89]	15 cases (SS subtype); 51 cases (MF subtype)
CBCL	FISH: translocations involving *IGH* (52%), *BCL2* (41%) and *BCL6* (7%)[98]	27 cases (FL subtype)
	FISH: translocations involving *IGH* (50%), MYC (43%), BCL6 (36%)[99]	14 cases (large B-cell subtype)
	CGH (secondary large CBCL, 5 cases): −17p (60%) CGH (primary large CBCL, 9 cases): +2q, +7q, +12, +13, −17p, +18, −19 CGH (FL subtype): +3q, +4, +7q[100]	14 cases (large B-cell subtype); 4 cases (FL subtype)

recurrence and shorter disease-free survival. Aneuploidy rates are fairly low in BCC, higher for SK and even higher for SCC, indicating increased rates with malignant potential. Supporting this is an exceptionally low aneuploidy rate for KA, which are well known for their regression. However, aneuploidy rates for BD are typically very high, which is not reflective of their low metastatic potential. Aside from this exception, aneuploidy in skin cancer appears to associate with malignant potential. Additionally, highly aberrant karyotypes were associated with CMM, SCC, SK and MCC, each of these exhibiting more aggressive biologic behaviors.

There were a number of aberrations that were very common amongst the different forms of skin cancer, including: rearrangements and numerical abnormalities of 1 (CMM, BCC, SCC, SK, KA, MCC, DFSP, CTCL); –3p (SCC, SK, KA, MCC); +3q (SCC, SK, MCC, CBCL); trisomy of all or part of 6 (CMM, BCC, SCC, MCC); trisomy 7 (CMM, BCC, SCC, SK, MCC and 7q of CBCL); +8q (CMM, SCC, KA, MCC, DFSP); –9p (dysplastic nevi, CMM, BCC, SCC, SK, KA, CTLC); +9q (CMM, SCC, SK, KA); loss of part or all of 10 (CMM, SCC, MCC, CTCL); –17p (CMM, BCC, SCC, SK, BD, MCC, CTCL, CBCL); +17q (CMM, SCC, SK, DFSP); and gain of all or part of 20 (CMM, SCC, SK, MCC, DFSP). Certain aberrations were contradictory in some cancers, showing amplifications and deletions with similar frequencies in the same region. Such examples include chromosomes 9q, 15, 18, 19, 21 and 22 in melanoma and 4q and 9q in SK. Such regions could be indicative of genomic instability and may not represent aberrations associated with malignancy, or may contain both tumor suppressor genes and oncogenes related to tumor development and progression. Studies have shown that amplified regions contain genes that are both over- and under-expressed, thus gross chromosomal aberrations do not reflect all changes at the gene level.[26]

However, identification of commonly aberrant regions in skin cancer has led to the speculation and even identification of putative tumor suppressor genes and oncogenes involved in malignant progression. Of particular importance is loss of 9p, which occurs in various skin cancers with some studies implicating a higher rate of 9p21-p22 loss in more progressive stages of disease including metastatic melanoma versus CMM versus dysplastic nevi[41,48] and SCC versus SK.[85] This region harbors the *CDKN2A* tumor suppressor gene, a known susceptibility gene for hereditary forms of melanoma and it seems likely that loss of function of this gene is associated with malignant progression.[33,85] However, various studies have been unable to find mutations in *CDKN2A* associated with all cases of loss and some studies have even indicated that there are two additional regions of interest that harbor tumor suppressor genes.[28,72] Other potential tumor suppressor genes and oncogenes include: *FHIT* (3p14.2), loss associated with MCC and lung cancer development;[87] *LAZ3* and *BCL6* (3q26-q27);[87] *E2F3* (6p22.3), over-expressed in retinoblastoma and bladder cancer;[101] *GPNMB* (7p15), over-expressed in melanoma;[25] *CDK6* (7q21) and *NRCAM* (7q31), over-expressed in melanoma;[25] *MYCC* (8q24), amplified in lung cancer and over-expressed in uveal melanoma;[87] *PTEN* (10q23.3), loss of function mutations associated with Cowden disease, an autosomal dominant cancer-predisposition syndrome;[102] *TP53* (17p13), present in about half of all human cancers;[72] *E2F1* (20q11), over-expressed in melanoma.[25] Additionally, many other tumor suppressor genes and oncogenes exist in these regions and novel genes responsible for cancer development may yet to be discovered.

Cytogenetic analysis has also implicated different regions in specific skin cancers, with some of the more pertinent aberrations following. Loss of 18q was found to be significantly higher in SCC compared to SK and may harbor genes responsible for transformation to a more malignant phenotype. 18q21 harbors a number of tumor suppressor genes, with *Smad2* or *Smad4* being likely candidates as they have been implicated in malignant progression in other diseases.[103,104] Analysis has implicated 9q22 in sporadic BCC development, a region which contains the *PTCH* tumor suppressor gene. *PTCH* functions to protect epithelial cells against a variety of genetic hits and had originally been identified in Gorlin's syndrome, an autosomal dominant disorder associated with propensity for BCC development.[23,71] Various cytogenetic techniques have now implicated the same region in sporadic BCC development. Translocation involving 17q22 and 22q13 is a hallmark of DFSP lesions, often involving the formation of supernumerary rings. This translocation creates a characteristic gene fusion between *COL1A1* and *PDGFB*, resulting in aberrant expression of *PDGFB*.[88]

In summary, cytogenetic analysis of melanoma and nonmelanoma skin cancer has revealed a number of recurrent abnormalities. It is interesting to note that a large number of aberrations are common amongst different skin cancers, although whether the genes associated with these abnormalities are common is yet to be determined. Because much of cytogenetic analysis focuses on large aberrations, implicated regions may not always be responsible for malignant progression but may be a result of the genomic instability associated with cancer development. However, it has become clear that a number of regions implicated by cytogenetic analysis harbor tumor suppressor genes and oncogenes involved in tumorigenesis. LOH, mutational and methylation studies may aid in the identification of putative cancer related genes and gene expression analysis can give direct evidence of transcriptional activity associated with implicated genes. A combination of cytogenetic analysis with other molecular techniques has implicated a number of chromosomal regions and associated genes in melanoma and nonmelanoma skin cancer development and will continue to advance our knowledge in this area.

References

1. Albert MR, Weinstock MA. Keratinocyte carcinoma. CA Cancer J Clin 2003; 53(5):292-302.
2. Weinstock MA. Epidemiology of nonmelanoma skin cancer: clinical issues, definitions and classification. J Invest Dermatol 1994; 102(6):4S-5S.
3. Gloster HM, Jr. Brodland DG. The epidemiology of skin cancer. Dermatol Surg 1996; 22(3):217-226.
4. Hoglund M, Gisselsson D, Hansen GB et al. Dissecting karyotypic patterns in malignant melanomas: temporal clustering of losses and gains in melanoma karyotypic evolution. Int J Cancer 2004; 108(1):57-65.
5. Sarasin A. The molecular pathways of ultraviolet-induced carcinogenesis. Mutat Res 1999; 428(1-2):5-10.
6. Matsumura Y, Ananthaswamy HN. Toxic effects of ultraviolet radiation on the skin. Toxicol Appl Pharmacol 2004; 195(3):298-308.
7. Emri G, Wenczl E, Van Erp P et al. Low doses of UVB or UVA induce chromosomal aberrations in cultured human skin cells. J Invest Dermatol 2000; 115(3):435-440.
8. Jin Y, Martins C, Jin C et al. Nonrandom karyotypic features in squamous cell carcinomas of the skin. Genes Chromosomes Cancer 1999; 26(4):295-303.
9. Kops GJ, Weaver BA, Cleveland DW. On the road to cancer: aneuploidy and the mitotic checkpoint. Nat Rev Cancer 2005; 5(10):773-785.
10. Duesberg P, Rasnick D. Aneuploidy, the somatic mutation that makes cancer a species of its own. Cell Motil Cytoskeleton 2000; 47(2):81-107.
11. Klapperstuck T, Wohlrab W. DNA image cytometry on sections as compared with image cytometry on smears and flow cytometry in melanoma. Cytometry 1996; 25(1):82-89.
12. Rapi S, Caldini A, Fanelli A et al. Flow cytometric measurement of DNA content in human solid tumors: a comparison with cytogenetics. Cytometry 1996; 26(3):192-197.
13. Robinson JK, Rademaker AW, Goolsby C et al. DNA ploidy in nonmelanoma skin cancer. Cancer 1996; 77(2):284-291.
14. Williams NN, Daly JM. Flow cytometry and prognostic implications in patients with solid tumors. Surg Gynecol Obstet 1990; 171(3):257-266.
15. Chen Z, Sandberg AA. Molecular cytogenetic aspects of hematological malignancies: clinical implications. Am J Med Genet 2002; 115(3):130-141.
16. Mertens F, Heim S, Mandahl N et al. Cytogenetic analysis of 33 basal cell carcinomas. Cancer Res 1991; 51(3):954-957.
17. Lotem M, Yehuda-Gafni O, Butnaryu E et al. Cytogenetic analysis of melanoma cell lines: subclone selection in long-term melanoma cell cultures. Cancer Genet Cytogenet 2003; 142(2):87-91.
18. James L, Varley J. Advances in cytogenetic analysis of solid tumours. Chromosome Res 1996; 4(7):479-485.
19. Kallioniemi OP, Kallioniemi A, Piper J et al. Optimizing comparative genomic hybridization for analysis of DNA sequence copy number changes in solid tumors. Genes Chromosomes Cancer 1994; 10(4):231-243.
20. Kallioniemi A, Visakorpi T, Karhu R et al. Gene Copy Number Analysis by Fluorescence in Situ Hybridization and Comparative Genomic Hybridization. Methods 1996; 9(1):113-121.
21. Thompson CT, Gray JW. Cytogenetic profiling using fluorescence in situ hybridization (FISH) and comparative genomic hybridization (CGH). J Cell Biochem Suppl 1993; 17G:139-143.

22. Varella-Garcia M. Molecular cytogenetics in solid tumors: laboratorial tool for diagnosis, prognosis and therapy. Oncologist 2003; 8(1):45-58.
23. Happle R. Loss of heterozygosity in human skin. J Am Acad Dermatol 1999; 41(2 Pt 1):143-164.
24. Forozan F, Mahlamaki EH, Monni O et al. Comparative genomic hybridization analysis of 38 breast cancer cell lines: a basis for interpreting complementary DNA microarray data. Cancer Res 2000; 60(16):4519-4525.
25. Okamoto I, Pirker C, Bilban M et al. Seven novel and stable translocations associated with oncogenic gene expression in malignant melanoma. Neoplasia 2005; 7(4):303-311.
26. Platzer P, Upender MB, Wilson K et al. Silence of chromosomal amplifications in colon cancer. Cancer Res 2002; 62(4):1134-1138.
27. Chudnovsky Y, Khavari PA, Adams AE. Melanoma genetics and the development of rational therapeutics. J Clin Invest 2005; 115(4):813-824.
28. Pollock PM, Welch J, Hayward NK. Evidence for three tumor suppressor loci on chromosome 9p involved in melanoma development. Cancer Res 2001; 61(3):1154-1161.
29. Rager EL, Bridgeford EP, Ollila DW. Cutaneous melanoma: update on prevention, screening, diagnosis and treatment. Am Fam Physician 2005; 72(2):269-276.
30. Skin Cancer Foundation. The Stages of Melanoma. http://www.skincancer.org/content/view/17/3/1/3/. Accessed 2/3/2007, 2007.
31. Clark WH, Jr. From L, Bernardino EA et al. The histogenesis and biologic behavior of primary human malignant melanomas of the skin. Cancer Res 1969; 29(3):705-727.
32. Breslow A. Thickness, cross-sectional areas and depth of invasion in the prognosis of cutaneous melanoma. Ann Surg 1970; 172(5):902-908.
33. Hussein MR, Wood GS. Molecular aspects of melanocytic dysplastic nevi. J Mol Diagn 2002; 4(2):71-80.
34. von Roenn JH, Kheir SM, Wolter JM et al. Significance of DNA abnormalities in primary malignant melanoma and nevi, a retrospective flow cytometric study. Cancer Res 1986; 46(6):3192-3195.
35. Kheir SM, Bines SD, Vonroenn JH et al. Prognostic significance of DNA aneuploidy in stage I cutaneous melanoma. Ann Surg 1988; 207(4):455-461.
36. Mitelman Database of Chromosome Aberrations in Cancer. In:Mitelman F, Johansson B, Mertens F. eds. 2006. http://cgap.nci.nih.gov/chromosomes/mitelman.
37. Cowan JM, Francke U. Cytogenetic analysis in melanoma and nevi. Cancer Treat Res 1991;54:3-16.
38. Marras S, Faa G, Dettori T et al. Chromosomal changes in dysplastic nevi. Cancer Genet Cytogenet 1999; 113(2):177-179.
39. Richmond A, Fine R, Murray D et al. Growth factor and cytogenetic abnormalities in cultured nevi and malignant melanomas. J Invest Dermatol 1986; 86(3):295-302.
40. Bastian BC, Olshen AB, LeBoit PE et al. Classifying melanocytic tumors based on DNA copy number changes. Am J Pathol 2003; 163(5):1765-1770.
41. Balazs M, Adam Z, Treszl A et al. Chromosomal imbalances in primary and metastatic melanomas revealed by comparative genomic hybridization. Cytometry 2001; 46(4):222-232.
42. Barks JH, Thompson FH, Taetle R et al. Increased chromosome 20 copy number detected by fluorescence in situ hybridization (FISH) in malignant melanoma. Genes Chromosomes Cancer 1997; 19(4):278-285.
43. Utikal J, Udart M, Leiter U et al. Additional Cyclin D(1) gene copies associated with chromosome 11 aberrations in cutaneous malignant melanoma. Int J Oncol 2005; 26(3):597-605.
44. Udart M, Utikal J, Krahn GM et al. Chromosome 7 aneusomy. A marker for metastatic melanoma? Expression of the epidermal growth factor receptor gene and chromosome 7 aneusomy in nevi, primary malignant melanomas and metastases. Neoplasia 2001; 3(3):245-254.
45. Treszl A, Adany R, Rakosy Z et al. Extra copies of c-myc are more pronounced in nodular melanomas than in superficial spreading melanomas as revealed by fluorescence in situ hybridisation. Cytometry B Clin Cytom 2004; 60(1):37-46.
46. Matsuta M, Imamura Y, Matsuta M et al. Detection of numerical chromosomal aberrations in malignant melanomas using fluorescence in situ hybridization. J Cutan Pathol 1997; 24(4):201-205.
47. Hussein MR, Sun M, Roggero E et al. Loss of heterozygosity, microsatellite instability and mismatch repair protein alterations in the radial growth phase of cutaneous malignant melanomas. Mol Carcinog 2002; 34(1):35-44.
48. Hussein MR, Roggero E, Tuthill RJ et al. Identification of novel deletion Loci at 1p36 and 9p22-21 in melanocytic dysplastic nevi and cutaneous malignant melanomas. Arch Dermatol 2003; 139(6):816-817.
49. Miller DL, Weinstock MA. Nonmelanoma skin cancer in the United States: incidence. J Am Acad Dermatol 1994; 30(5 Pt 1):774-778.
50. Wong CS, Strange RC, Lear JT. Basal cell carcinoma. Bmj 2003; 327(7418):794-798.

51. Bernstein SC, Lim KK, Brodland DG et al. The many faces of squamous cell carcinoma. Dermatol Surg 1996; 22(3):243-254.
52. Diepgen TL, Mahler V. The epidemiology of skin cancer. Br J Dermatol 2002; 146(Suppl 61):1-6.
53. Skidmore RA, Jr. Flowers FP. Nonmelanoma skin cancer. Med Clin North Am 1998; 82(6):1309-1323, vi.
54. Salasche SJ. Epidemiology of actinic keratoses and squamous cell carcinoma. J Am Acad Dermatol 2000; 42(1 Pt 2):4-7.
55. Frost C, Williams G, Green A. High incidence and regression rates of solar keratoses in a queensland community. J Invest Dermatol 2000; 115(2):273-277.
56. Marks R, Rennie G, Selwood TS. Malignant transformation of solar keratoses to squamous cell carcinoma. Lancet 1988; 1(8589):795-797.
57. Evans C, Cockerell CJ. Actinic keratosis: time to call a spade a spade. South Med J 2000; 93(7):734-736.
58. Ramrakha-Jones VS, Herd RM. Treating Bowen's disease: a cost-minimization study. Br J Dermatol 2003; 148(6):1167-1172.
59. Cohen PR. Bowen's disease: squamous cell carcinoma in situ. Am Fam Physician 1991; 44(4):1325-1329.
60. Staibano S, Lo Muzio L, Pannone G et al. DNA ploidy and cyclin D1 expression in basal cell carcinoma of the head and neck. Am J Clin Pathol 2001; 115(6):805-813.
61. Frentz G, Moller U. Clonal heterogeneity in curetted human epidermal cancers and precancers analysed by flow cytometry and compared with histology. Br J Dermatol 1983; 109(2):173-181.
62. Fortier-Beaulieu M, Laquerriere A, Thomine E et al. DNA flow-cytometric analysis of basal cell carcinomas and its relevance to their morphological differentiation: a retrospective study. Dermatology 1994; 188(2):94-99.
63. Pilch H, Weiss J, Heubner C et al. Differential diagnosis of keratoacanthomas and squamous cell carcinomas: diagnostic value of DNA image cytometry and p53 expression. J Cutan Pathol 1994; 21(6):507-513.
64. Biesterfeld S, Pennings K, Grussendorf-Conen EI et al. Aneuploidy in actinic keratosis and Bowen's disease—increased risk for invasive squamous cell carcinoma? Br J Dermatol 1995; 133(4):557-560.
65. Kawara S, Takata M, Takehara K. High frequency of DNA aneuploidy detected by DNA flow cytometry in Bowen's disease. J Dermatol Sci 1999; 21(1):23-26.
66. Jin Y, Mertens F, Persson B et al. Nonrandom numerical chromosome abnormalities in basal cell carcinomas. Cancer Genet Cytogenet 1998; 103(1):35-42.
67. Jin Y, Martins C, Salemark L et al. Nonrandom karyotypic features in basal cell carcinomas of the skin. Cancer Genet Cytogenet 2001; 131(2):109-119.
68. Casalone R, Mazzola D, Righi R et al. Cytogenetic and interphase FISH analyses of 73 basal cell and three squamous cell carcinomas: different findings in direct preparations and short-term cell cultures. Cancer Genet Cytogenet 2000; 118(2):136-143.
69. Jin Y, Merterns F, Persson B et al. The reciprocal translocation t(9;16)(q22;p13) is a primary chromosome abnormality in basal cell carcinomas. Cancer Res 1997; 57(3):404-406.
70. Kawasaki-Oyama RS, Andre FS, Caldeira LF et al. Cytogenetic findings in two basal cell carcinomas. Cancer Genet Cytogenet 1994; 73(2):152-156.
71. Ashton KJ, Weinstein SR, Maguire DJ et al. Molecular cytogenetic analysis of basal cell carcinoma DNA using comparative genomic hybridization. J Invest Dermatol 2001; 117(3):683-686.
72. Saridaki Z, Koumantaki E, Liloglou T et al. High frequency of loss of heterozygosity on chromosome region 9p21-p22 but lack of p16INK4a/p19ARF mutations in greek patients with basal cell carcinoma of the skin. J Invest Dermatol 2000;115(4):719-725.
73. Quinn AG, Sikkink S, Rees JL. Basal cell carcinomas and squamous cell carcinomas of human skin show distinct patterns of chromosome loss. Cancer Res 1994; 54(17):4756-4759.
74. Shen T, Park WS, Boni R et al. Detection of loss of heterozygosity on chromosome 9q22.3 in microdissected sporadic basal cell carcinoma. Hum Pathol 1999; 30(3):284-287.
75. Shanley SM, Dawkins H, Wainwright BJ et al. Fine deletion mapping on the long arm of chromosome 9 in sporadic and familial basal cell carcinomas. Hum Mol Genet 1995; 4(1):129-133.
76. Jin Y, Jin C, Salemark L et al. Clonal chromosome abnormalities in premalignant lesions of the skin. Cancer Genet Cytogenet 2002; 136(1):48-52.
77. Heim S, Caron M, Jin Y et al. Genetic convergence during serial in vitro passage of a polyclonal squamous cell carcinoma. Cytogenet Cell Genet 1989; 52(3-4):133-135.
78. Kim DK, Kim JY, Kim HT et al. A specific chromosome aberration in a keratoacanthoma. Cancer Genet Cytogenet 2003; 142(1):70-72.
79. Mertens F, Heim S, Mandahl N et al. Clonal chromosome aberrations in a keratoacanthoma and a basal cell papilloma. Cancer Genet Cytogenet 1989; 39(2):227-232.
80. Ashton KJ, Weinstein SR, Maguire DJ et al. Chromosomal aberrations in squamous cell carcinoma and solar keratoses revealed by comparative genomic hybridization. Arch Dermatol 2003; 139(7):876-882.

81. Clausen OP, Beigi M, Bolund L et al. Keratoacanthomas frequently show chromosomal aberrations as assessed by comparative genomic hybridization. J Invest Dermatol 2002; 119(6):1367-1372.

82. Clausen OP, Aass HC, Beigi M et al. Are keratoacanthomas variants of squamous cell carcinomas? A comparison of chromosomal aberrations by comparative genomic hybridization. J Invest Dermatol 2006; 126(10):2308-2315.

83. Rehman I, Takata M, Wu YY et al. Genetic change in actinic keratoses. Oncogene 1996; 12(12):2483-2490.

84. Lee HJ, Kim JS, Ha SJ et al. p53 gene mutations in Bowen's disease in Koreans: clustering in exon 5 and multiple mutations. Cancer Lett 2000; 158(1):27-33.

85. Mortier L, Marchetti P, Delaporte E et al. Progression of actinic keratosis to squamous cell carcinoma of the skin correlates with deletion of the 9p21 region encoding the p16(INK4a) tumor suppressor. Cancer Lett 2002;176(2):205-214.

86. Waring AJ, Takata M, Rehman I et al. Loss of heterozygosity analysis of keratoacanthoma reveals multiple differences from cutaneous squamous cell carcinoma. Br J Cancer 1996; 73(5):649-653.

87. Van Gele M, Speleman F, Vandesompele J et al. Characteristic pattern of chromosomal gains and losses in Merkel cell carcinoma detected by comparative genomic hybridization. Cancer Res 1998;58(7):1503-1508.

88. Kaur S, Vauhkonen H, Bohling T et al. Gene copy number changes in dermatofibrosarcoma protuberans-a fine-resolution study using array comparative genomic hybridization. Cytogenet Genome Res 2006; 115(3-4):283-288.

89. Scarisbrick JJ, Woolford AJ, Russell-Jones R et al. Allelotyping in mycosis fungoides and Sezary syndrome: common regions of allelic loss identified on 9p, 10q and 17p. J Invest Dermatol 2001; 117(3):663-670.

90. Hoefnagel JJ, Dijkman R, Basso K et al. Distinct types of primary cutaneous large B-cell lymphoma identified by gene expression profiling. Blood 2005; 105(9):3671-3678.

91. Leonard JH, Leonard P, Kearsley JH. Chromosomes 1, 11 and 13 are frequently involved in karyotypic abnormalities in metastatic Merkel cell carcinoma. Cancer Genet Cytogenet 1993; 67(1):65-70.

92. Larramendy ML, Koljonen V, Bohling T et al. Recurrent DNA copy number changes revealed by comparative genomic hybridization in primary Merkel cell carcinomas. Mod Pathol 2004; 17(5):561-567.

93. Van Gele M, Leonard JH, Van Roy N et al. Frequent allelic loss at 10q23 but low incidence of PTEN mutations in Merkel cell carcinoma. Int J Cancer 2001; 92(3):409-413.

94. Vortmeyer AO, Merino MJ, Boni R et al. Genetic changes associated with primary Merkel cell carcinoma. Am J Clin Pathol 1998; 109(5):565-570.

95. Kiuru-Kuhlefelt S, El-Rifai W, Fanburg-Smith J et al. Concomitant DNA copy number amplification at 17q and 22q in dermatofibrosarcoma protuberans. Cytogenet Cell Genet 2001; 92(3-4):192-195.

96. Nishio J, Iwasaki H, Ohjimi Y et al. Overrepresentation of 17q22-qter and 22q13 in dermatofibrosarcoma protuberans but not in dermatofibroma: a comparative genomic hybridization study. Cancer Genet Cytogenet 2002;132(2):102-108.

97. Mao X, Lillington D, Scarisbrick JJ et al. Molecular cytogenetic analysis of cutaneous T-cell lymphomas: identification of common genetic alterations in Sezary syndrome and mycosis fungoides. Br J Dermatol 2002; 147(3):464-475.

98. Streubel B, Scheucher B, Valencak J et al. Molecular cytogenetic evidence of t(14;18)(IGH;BCL2) in a substantial proportion of primary cutaneous follicle center lymphomas. Am J Surg Pathol 2006; 30(4):529-536.

99. Hallermann C, Kaune KM, Gesk S et al. Molecular cytogenetic analysis of chromosomal breakpoints in the IGH, MYC, BCL6 and MALT1 gene loci in primary cutaneous B-cell lymphomas. J Invest Dermatol 2004; 123(1):213-219.

100. Gimenez S, Costa C, Espinet B et al. Comparative genomic hybridization analysis of cutaneous large B-cell lymphomas. Exp Dermatol 2005; 14(12):883-890.

101. Santos GC, Zielenska M, Prasad M et al. Chromosome 6p amplification and cancer progression. J Clin Pathol 2007; 60(1):1-7.

102. Scarisbrick JJ, Woolford AJ, Russell-Jones R et al. Loss of heterozygosity on 10q and microsatellite instability in advanced stages of primary cutaneous T-cell lymphoma and possible association with homozygous deletion of PTEN. Blood 2000; 95(9):2937-2942.

103. Miyaki M, Kuroki T. Role of Smad4 (DPC4) inactivation in human cancer. Biochem Biophys Res Commun 2003; 306(4):799-804.

104. Tian F, DaCosta Byfield S, Parks WT et al. Reduction in Smad2/3 signaling enhances tumorigenesis but suppresses metastasis of breast cancer cell lines. Cancer Res 2003; 63(23):8284-8292.

CHAPTER 19

Molecular Biology of Basal and Squamous Cell Carcinomas

Jingwu Xie*

Abstract

Basal cell carcinomas and Squamous cell carcinomas are the two most common human cancers. The incidence of these two types of cancer is estimated to double within 20 years. Identification of the key molecular events is critical in helping us design novel strategies to treat and to prevent these cancers. For example, identification of hedgehog signaling activation has opened up many opportunities for targeted therapy and prevention of basal cell carcinomas. Significant progress has also been made in our understanding of squamous cell carcinomas of the skin. In this chapter, we will focus on major recent developments in our understanding of basal cell carcinomas and squamous cell carcinomas at the molecular levels and their clinical implications.

Introduction

The incidence of nonmelanoma skin cancer doubles every 15 to 20 years due to many factors, including an aging population, changes in behavior towards sun exposure and increased UV light fluency at the earth surface with increasing ozone depletion. In particular, the incidence of these cancers in people less than 40 years has significantly increased in the last few decades.[1] In 2007, about 1.2 million Americans are estimated to have nonmelanoma skin cancer, most of which are basal cell carcinomas (BCCs, with estimated incidence about 90,000 in 2007) and squamous cell carcinomas (SCCs, with about 30,000 in 2007) (American Cancer Society Facts and Figures, 2007, http://www.cancer.org), whereas the combined incidence from all other cancer types is around 1.4 millions.[2] Despite the high incidence of nonmelanoma skin cancer, less than 2,000 Americans are estimated to die from them. Consequently, the actual incidence of these cancers is often under-estimated. For the same reason, research of nonmelanoma skin cancers, particularly BCCs, is under-funded. However, growth of these cancers often causes facial destruction and scars following surgery. It is estimated that at least over 2 billion dollars of medical costs are directly associated with BCCs and SCCs in the US alone. In the last few years, significant progress has been made in our understanding of BCCs and SCCs, some of which contributed to cancer syndrome studies.

Activation of the Hedgehog Pathway in BCCs

The major breakthrough in our understanding of Hh signaling in human cancers came from the discovery that mutations of human homologue of the drosophila patched gene (PTCH1) are associated with a rare hereditary form of BCC- Basal Cell Nevus Syndrome (also called Gorlin syndrome).[3-5] PTCH1 is the receptor for hedgehog proteins and previous studies indicated that PTCH1 mainly functions in embryonic development.

*Jingwu Xie—Department of Pharmacology and Toxicology, Sealy Center for Cancer Cell Biology, University of Texas Medical Branch, Galveston, TX 77555-1048, U.S.A. Email: jinxie@utmb.edu

Sunlight, Vitamin D and Skin Cancer, edited by Jörg Reichrath. ©2008 Landes Bioscience and Springer Science+Business Media.

The Hedgehog Pathway

The hedgehog pathway, initially identified in drosophila, is a master regulator of cell proliferation, tissue differentiation and tissue polarity. The current understanding of the hedgehog pathway is as follows (see Fig. 1). Hedgehog proteins are a group of secreted proteins whose active forms are derived from a unique protein cleavage process and following posttranslational modifications.[6] Secreted Hh molecules bind to the receptor PTC, thereby alleviating PTC-mediated suppression of *smoothened* (SMO). Expression of *hedgehogs* (Shh, Ihh and Dhh) is suggested to stabilize SMO protein possibly through posttranslational modification of SMO. This effect of hedgehog molecules can be inhibited by hedgehog-interacting protein (HIP) through competitive association with PTC.[7] In *Drosophila*, SMO stabilization triggers complex formation with Costal-2, Fused and Gli homologue CI, which prevents CI degradation and formation of a transcriptional repressor.[8] However, such a mechanism has not been established in mammalian cells. Recent studies suggest an essential role of cilia components in transmitting SMO signaling[9,10] SMO ultimately activates transcription factors of the Gli family. There is genetic evidence indicating that several proteins link SMO to Gli. These signal transducers include Fu, Su(Fu), Rab23 and protein kinase A (PKA).[11] As transcriptional factors, Gli molecules can regulate target gene expression by direct association with a consensus binding site (5′-tttggttgca-3′) located in the promoter region of target genes.

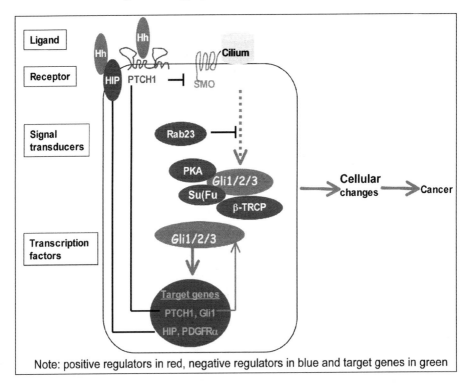

Note: positive regulators in red, negative regulators in blue and target genes in green

Figure 1. A diagram of the vertebrate hedgehog signaling pathway. The hedgehog (Hh) pathway is consisted of ligands (Sonic hedgehog, Indian hedgehog and Desert hedgehog), receptors [Patched-1 (PTCH1) and Patched-2], signaling transducers and signaling intermediates [smoothened (SMO), rab23, protein kinase A (PKA), β-TRCP and Su(Fu)] and transcription factors (Gli1, Gli2 and Gli3). Target genes of this pathway include PTCH1, Gli1 and hedgehog-interacting protein (HIP), which maintain the Hh signaling at an appropriate level in a given cell.

There are several feedback regulatory loops in this pathway (see Fig. 1). PTC, Gli1 and HIP, which are components of this pathway, are also the target genes. PTC and HIP provide negative feedback mechanisms to maintain the pathway activity at an appropriate level in a given cell. In contrast, Gli1 forms a positive regulatory loop. Alteration of these loops will result in abnormal signaling of this pathway.

Mutations of PTCH1 in Basal Cell Nevus Syndrome

Loss-of-function mutations of the *patched* gene (PTCH1) are the cause of basal cell nevus syndrome. This autosomal dominant disorder is characterized by development of benign and malignant tumors (including multiple BCCs, medulloblastomas and ovarian fibromas and less frequently fibrosarcomas, meningiomas, rhabdomyosarcomas and cardiac fibromas) as well as developmental defects (such as pits of the palms and soles, keratocysts of the jaw and other dental malformations, cleft palate, calcification of the falx cerebri, spina bifida occulta and other spine anomalies, bifid ribs and other rib anomalies).[12-14] The clinical feature of this syndrome was carefully characterized by Dr. Robert Gorlin and this syndrome is also called the Gorlin syndrome.

Analysis of the distribution of BCCs in affected individuals in multiple families suggested that the underlying defect might be mutation in a tumor suppressor gene. The gene was later mapped to chromosome 9q22-31, which is also frequently deleted in sporadic BCCs.[15] Positional cloning and candidate gene approaches identified the human homolog of *Drosophila patched* as a candidate gene.[3,4,16] Vertebrate patched was known to function in the development of the organs with abnormalities in Basal Cell Nevus Syndrome, such as neural tube, somites and limb buds,[17] making *PTCH1* a good candidate gene for this syndrome. Screening of the *patched* coding region revealed a wide spectrum of mutations in Gorlin syndrome patients, with the majority predicted to result in premature protein truncation. *PTCH* mutations are mainly clustered into the predicted two large extracellular loops and the large intracellular loop.[18] Different kindreds with identical mutations differ dramatically in the extent of clinical features, suggesting that genetic background or environmental factors may have an important role in modifying the spectrum of both developmental and neoplastic traits.[19]

The tumor suppressor role of PTCH1 has been further demonstrated in mice. Mice heterozygous for a PTCH1 null mutation exhibit the essential features in basal cell nevus syndrome patients, such as tumor development such as (medulloblastomas, rhabdomyosarcomas and BCCs) and developmental defects (such as spina bifida occulta).[20-22] The mouse studies confirm that PTCH1 functions as a tumor suppressor.

Activation of the Hedgehog Pathway in Sporadic BCCs

BCC, the most common human cancer, consistently has abnormalities of the hedgehog pathway and often has lost the function of PTCH1 via point mutations and loss of the remaining allele. Most PTCH1 mutations lead to loss of the protein function. Mice heterozygous for a PTCH1 null mutation develop BCCs following UV irradiation or ion radiation. Currently, Ptch1$^{+/-}$ mice represent the most practical model of UV-mediated BCC formation.[22]

The PTCH1 gene region is lost in more than 50% human sporadic BCCs whereas the hedgehog pathway is activated in almost all BCCs, suggesting alteration of additional genes in the hedgehog pathway in this type of skin cancer. Indeed, mutations of SMO are found in about 10% of sporadic BCCs.[23-27] Unlike wild type SMO, expression of activated SMO molecules in mouse skin results in formation of BCC-like tumors.[23] These findings provide additional insights into the role of the hedgehog pathway in human cancer. It is also reported that Su(Fu) is mutated in some BCCs.[25] Unlike PTCH1, no LOH in the Su(Fu) gene region are detected in sporadic BCCs, suggesting that Su(Fu) loss is not a major somatic change. Taking all the mutation data into account, there are still about 30% of BCCs without the underlying molecular basis for the activated hedgehog signaling. Thus, we predict that mutations of additional genes in the hedgehog pathway are yet to be discovered in sporadic BCCs.

We have shown that activated hedgehog signaling in BCCs, leads to cell proliferation through elevated expression of PDGFRα,[28] whereas targeted inhibition of hedgehog signaling causes apoptosis via Fas induction.[29]

Perspectives of Using Hedgehog Signaling Inhibitors for BCC Treatment

The findings that hyperactivation of the hedgehog pathway is responsible for most sporadic BCCs prompt translational studies using hedgehog signaling inhibitors. Cyclopamine, a plant-derived steroidal alkaloid, binds directly to the transmembrane helices of SMO and inhibits Hh signaling. The discovery of small molecule antagonists of SMO such as cyclopamine has opened up exciting new prospects for molecularly targeted BCC therapy and prevention.

Oral cyclopamine can block the growth of UV-induced BCCs in *Ptch1*[+/−] mice by 50%, perhaps by increasing Fas-induced apoptosis.[29] Furthermore, cyclopamine treatment in this mouse model prevents formation of additional microscopic BCCs, implying a potential use of cyclopamine for BCC prevention. Cyclopamine administration reduced BCCs, but not SCCs or fibrosarcomas in these mice, highlighting the specificity of cyclopamine for the hedgehog pathway.[29] Using murine BCC cell lines derived from this mouse model, cyclopamine is shown to inhibit cell proliferation, possibly through down-regulation of growth factor receptor PDGFRα. Other synthetic SMO antagonists, such as CUR61414 from Curis/Genentech, have also been found to be effective in reducing BCCs from *Ptch1*[+/−] mice. Using an ex vivo model of BCC, CUR61414 causes the regression of UV-induced basaltic lesions in punch biopsies taken from *Ptch1*[+/−] mice.[30] Since then, a topical formulation of this compound was tested against sporadic BCCs in a Phase I clinical trial. However, this clinical trial failed to show effects on Hh target gene expression by the compound and the reason is not clear. In addition, several other synthetic compounds have been identified to bind directly to SMO and with no structural similarity to cyclopamine.

Recent studies indicate that vitamin D3, the secretion of which can be facilitated by PTCH1, can inhibit SMO signaling through direct binding to SMO. This finding raises a possibility to treat BCCs with nutrition supplements.[31]

Crosstalk between the Hedgehog Pathway and Other Pathways

Several signaling pathways have been identified to regulate the hedgehog signaling pathway. The modulation of Hh signaling by other signaling pathways is context dependent, occurring in some tissues or cell lines but not in others. Recent studies indicate that downstream signaling of Ras, PI3K and MEK, enhances Hh signaling.[32-35] We have shown a few years ago that hedgehog signaling activation in BCC cells results in elevated expression and phosphorylation of PDGFRα, which is required for hedgehog-mediated cell proliferation in BCCs.[28] Later, it was shown in HaCaT keratinocytes that Shh induces EGFR signaling, which is required for matrix invasion of HaCaT cells.[36] More extensive studies of the synergetic interactions between hedgehog signaling and EGF have been performed using primary human keratinocytes.[32] It was found that both EGF and sonic hedgehog regulate different sets of target genes when added separately in culture. In the presence of both EGF and sonic hedgehog, another set of genes are induced. In several of these genes, the sites in the promoter have been identified. Similar studies in other cell types also indicate that both AKT and MEK signaling argument Gli1-mediated transcriptional activities.[33,37] The detailed mechanisms of this regulation remain to be identified. Recent studies indicate that Ras can increase the stability of Gli molecules, possibly through regulation of Gli degradation.[38] Since constitutive activation of the hedgehog pathway is the most significant abnormality in BCCs, Ras mutation will not be required to activate hedgehog signaling since most BCCs have gene alterations in the hedgehog pathway. We thus predict that BCCs with Ras mutations are the tumors without mutations in PTCH1, SMO or Su(Fu), which can be tested in a large cohort study.

Protein kinase A (PKA) was first identified as an inhibitory component of the Hh pathway in *Drosophila*. We found in mammalian cells that the cAMP/PKA signaling axis regulates Gli1 protein localization, in part, through regulation phosphorylation of Gli1 at Thr[374], which is near the nuclear localization signal.[39] Other crosstalk includes regulation of sonic hedgehog expression by p63,[40] enhancement of hedgehog-mediated carcinogenesis by p53 loss.[41] Figure 2 summarizes the current understanding of the crosstalk. Recent studies also suggest an interaction between the hedgehog pathway and the Ras pathway in melanomas.

Studies of the crosstalk between hedgehog signaling and other pathways have significant clinical implications. A recent study using hedgehog signaling inhibitor cyclopamine and EGFR inhibitor gefitinib in prostate cancer suggests that a treatment combining the two inhibitors is more effective than single treatment alone.[42] In combination with docetaxel, the synergetic tumor inhibitory effects of cyclopamine and gefitinib are more evident.[42] Thus, combination chemotherapy of cyclopamine with other specific pathway inhibitors in selected tumors has a promising clinical application.

Major Molecular Alterations in SCCs

Major Genetic Alterations in SCC

SCCs are different from SCCs in many aspects (see Table 1). While BCCs develop de novo, formation of skin SCC is a multiple-step process. Actinic keratoses (AK), are precancerous skin

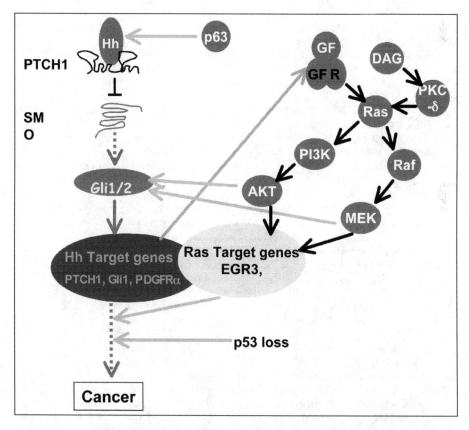

Figure 2. A diagram showing the cross-talks between the hedgehog pathway and other pathways. Bi-directional interactions between hedgehog signaling and the Ras pathway is noticed. On the one hand, hedgehog signaling can activate the Ras pathway through up-regulation of PDGFRα. On the other hand, the growth factor (GF)-growth factor receptor (GFR)-Ras pathway can interact with Gli molecules through PI3K or MEK. Furthermore, p53 family members are known to regulate expression of sonic hedgehog or promote hedgehog-mediated tumorigenesis.

Table 1. Comparison of BCC and SCC

		BCC	SCC
Risk factor	UV irradiation immunosuppression	intermitent 20X	cumulative 200X
Predisposition		PTCH1	Polymorphisms: 53 (Codon 72) or H-ras (Codon 27)
Somatic mutations		Hedgehog pathway [PTCH1, SMO, Su(Fu)] p53	Loss of p53, Loss of p16 or Rb Activation of Ras, C-MYC, STAT
Precancerous stages		no	Actinic keratoses

lesions of SCC.[43] It is estimated that ~1% of these sun-induced lesions will develop into skin SCCs. AK can occur at multiple sites as well as in the vicinity of SCC, supporting the field cancerization hypothesis.[44-47] Infection of human papillomavirus (HPV) is a significant risk factor of SCCs, but not BCCs.[45] The major function of HPV is to immortalize keratinocytes through blocking the functions of p53 (via E6 viral oncogene) and Rb (through E7 viral oncogene). Transgenic mice expressing HPV-16 under the control of keratin 14 promoter is a reproducible mouse model for SCC progression.[48] The biggest genetic change between BCCs and SCCs is loss of chromosome 9p21 (containing the p16/Arf locus) in SCCs.[49-51] The p16/Arf locus contains two genes: p16INK4 as a cyclin kinase inhibitor linked to cell cycle regulation and p14ARF as a negative regulator for p53 (see Fig. 3). Mutations of p16 are more frequently identified in SCCs, suggesting a significant role of p16 in skin SCCs.[52] Loss of p16 or Rb not only allows cells to cycle out of control, but also promotes chromosome aberrations in cancer.[46,53-55]

Despite the differences between SCCs and BCCs, both tumor types harbor mutations in p53 and Ras. UV signature mutation of the p53 gene occurs frequently in both copies of p53 in BCCs and SCCs although specific mutations of p53 are suggested for BCCs (codon 177) and SCCs (codon 278).[56-59] In contrast, cancer of internal organs, such as colorectal cancers, often harbors LOH near the p53 gene region in one copy and p53 mutation in the remaining copy. One major function of p53 is to regulate cell cycle and apoptosis (see Fig. 3). As the guardian of the genome, mutation of p53 is clearly linked to elevated genomic instability.[60-63]

In addition, C-MYC over-expression and activation of STAT signaling occur frequently in skin SCCs although the mechanisms of these changes in SCC progression remain largely unknown.[45,64-66] C-MYC is known to be able to mediate tumor angiogenesis in mouse models through elevating expression of VEGF.[67] In the chemical carcinogenesis model, STAT activation is a major alteration through stimulation of cytokine secretion, resulting in progression of SCCs.

The role of NFkB in SCCs is still controversial.[47,68-70] The NFkB pathway is a highly conserved pathway involved in regulation of inflammation, apoptosis, differentiation and proliferation. The NFkB/Rel transcriptional factors share a large Rel homology domain involving DNA binding and protein-protein interaction. The pathway can be activated by a variety of cytokines through the upstream IKKs and inhibited by IkB proteins, which are designated to protein degradation via proteosome upon phosphorylation of IKKs. Several studies indicate activation of NFkB plays a critical role in human SCCs and in mouse SCCs from the two-stage chemical carcinogenesis protocol whereas suppression of NFkB signaling enhances Ras-mediated SCCs in mice. In head/neck squamous cell carcinoma cells, expression of a dominant negative form of IkB inhibits cell survival, proinflammatory cytokine expression and tumor growth in vivo. In the two stage SCC model, expression of p50/p52 NFkB transcription factors, particularly p52, is induced in papillomas and tumors. In contrast, suppression of the NFkB pathway in mice appears to promote

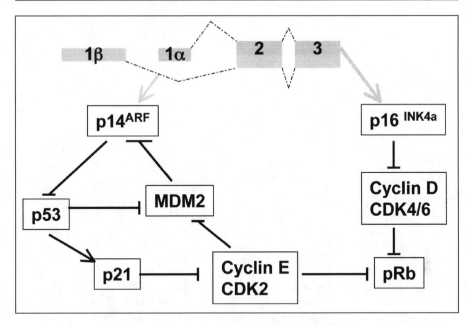

Figure 3. A diagram of the INK4/ARF locus, the gene products and their functions. The p16INK4a and p14ARF proteins are encoded by the INK4/ARF locus on human chromosome 9. As a CDK inhibitor, the p16INK4a protein inhibits the Rb functions via inactivation of the CDK4/6-cyclin D complex. The p14ARF protein, on the other hand, inhibits p53 functions.

Ras-mediated SCC progression, which is in clear contrast with the role of the NFkB pathway in other types of tumors. One explanation of these contradicted results is that maintenance of a certain level of NFkB at a certain stage during carcinogenesis is necessary for normal growth of keratinocytes. Disruption of this fine balance throughout carcinogenesis will result in abnormal cell proliferation.

Sequence of Molecular Events during Development of SCCs

The sequence of these alterations in SCCs has been studied in human specimens. In studies of human specimens, stabilization of p53 is one of the earliest markers of abnormal epidermis, which can be detected even in morphologically normal epidermis.[44] Mutant p53 can be detected by immunohistochemistry with specific monoclonal antibodies (Pab240) recognizing only the mutant form of p53. Some of the p53 positive patches (foci) can develop into AK. UV signature mutations (C to T or CC to TT) are frequently found in p53 in AK as well as in SCCs. About one in 1000 AKs develops into a SCC. AK harbors mostly random p53 mutations whereas SCCs often contain hotspot p53 mutations. In addition, LOH at the p53 locus is frequently found in SCCs, but not in AKs. Progression from AKs to SCCs is accompanied by loss of p16INK4a. Mutation of H-Ras or N-Ras is also observed in SCCs, with a frequency of 30-50%. Invasive SCCs contain multiple changes in different signaling pathways, including angiogenesis factors, cytokines and chemokines, leading to activation of the STAT pathway. However, the exact roles of these molecules in the progression of SCCs are not entirely clear.

Several mouse models have been used to study the molecular events during SCC development and progression. The two-stage skin carcinogenesis using di-methyl-benzanthracene (DMBA) followed by the phorbole ester (TPA) has been on the forefront for providing clues regarding the cellular, biochemical and genetic events linked to the initiation, promotion and progression steps of skin cancer formation.[71-74] In this model, SCCs development requires three steps.[74] In tumor initiation step, Ras activation is the key event. During tumor promotion, loss of p16 (or Rb) and p53 inactivation takes place. For tumor progression and metastasis, loss of TGFβ response is critical. However, the order of genetic events in this model is quite different from those in human SCCs, raising questions about human relevance of this mouse model.

UV irradiation of SKH1 hairless mice represents a closer model for UV-induced SCCs in the humans.[75] In this model, p53 mutations appear before formation of SCCs, just like the human SCCs. The density of p53 positive patches is highly associated with the risk to develop SCCs in this model. Most mutations of p53 are UV related (c to T or CC to TT). Not to our surprise, development of SCCs in this model is dependent on UV irradiation doses.[76] As predicted, deficiency in DNA repair (XPC null mice) accelerates formation of SCCs.[76] Activation of STAT signaling is also observed in this mouse model.[77] However, additional molecular events during SCC development have not been thoroughly studied in this model.

SCC Susceptibility and PTCH1 Polymorphism

It is known that different genetic background determines the susceptibility to cancer, which is best illustrated in cutaneous carcinogenesis studies. For example, C57B/6 mice are more resistant to SCC development either by the two-stage carcinogenesis protocol or following expression of the Ras oncogene, whereas FVB/N mice are more susceptible to SCC formation. It is recently discovered that a Ptch1 polymorphism, which causes N1267T mutation in the c-terminal of Ptch1, is responsible for the resistance of SCC development in C57B/6 mice.[78] Transgenic mice in C57B/6 background expressing the Ptch1 of FVB/N mice under the K14 promoter become susceptible to SCC development. N1267 amino acid is highly conserved residue. From these studies, it is suggested that despite a need of Ptch1 functions during early stages of SCC development, Ptch1 loss is not required for SCC progression. In contrast, a high level of Ptch1 expression may be required for SCC formation.

Therapeutic Implications of Human SCCs

Although significant progress has been made in our understanding of molecular events during SCC development, no clear therapeutic applications have been established. One important reason is that multiple causes for this type of tumor have been identified and their carcinogenesis mechanisms may be different from different risk factors. However, several therapeutic targets may be used in considering SCC therapeutics.

One important target in SCCs is inactivation of the p53 gene.[79-81] Several small molecule compounds have been developed to rescue the effects from inactivation of the p53 gene.[82] Alternatively, expression of wild type p53 can be achieved through adenovirus.[79] Furthermore, adenoviruses have been engineered to selectively kill only cancer cells with p53 mutations.[80] Another therapeutic target is p16 gene.[83,84] The most effective approaches to reduce the medical burden of SCCs are to reduce the risk factors. For example, HPV vaccines have proven to be effective in reducing the incidence of cervical SCCs.[85] While more effective therapies are being developed, effective sun screen, avoidance of extensive sun exposure and other preventive measures are still the best advice to reduce SCCs.

Summary

Major advances have been made in the last few years in our understanding of BCCs and SCCs. Activation of the hedgehog pathway is the most important abnormality in BCCs. Thus, effective inhibition of hedgehog signaling using small molecules should be promising in shrinking BCCs. Development of SCCs is complicated by the existence of many risk factors and multiple genetic alterations. Through further understanding in each genetic change at the molecular levels, it will be possible to design strategies to treat or prevent SCCs. The advantage in skin cancer therapeutics is that topic application of drugs is very effective, which will avoid many unexpected physiological and pathological side effects from systemic drug delivery.

Acknowledgement

This work was supported in part by National Institute of Health (NIH) grant R01- CA94160 and Department of Defense grant PC030429. Due to space limitation, only selected references are listed in this review.

References

1. Christenson LJ, Borrowman TA, Vachon CM et al. Incidence of basal cell and squamous cell carcinomas in a population younger than 40 years. JAMA 2005; 294:681-90.
2. Jemal A, Siegel R, Ward E et al. Cancer statistics, 2007. CA Cancer J Clin 2007; 57:43-66.
3. Hahn H, Wicking C, Zaphiropoulous PG et al. Mutations of the human homolog of Drosophila patched in the nevoid basal cell carcinoma syndrome. Cell 1996; 85:841-51.
4. Johnson RL, Rothman AL, Xie J et al. Human homolog of patched, a candidate gene for the basal cell nevus syndrome. Science 1996; 272:1668-71.
5. Epstein E. Genetic determinants of basal cell carcinoma risk. Med Pediatr Oncol 2001; 36:555-8.
6. Taipale J, Beachy PA. The Hedgehog and Wnt signalling pathways in cancer. Nature 2001; 411:349-54.
7. Chuang PT, McMahon AP. Vertebrate Hedgehog signalling modulated by induction of a Hedgehog-binding protein. Nature 1999; 397:617-21.
8. Jia J, Jiang J. Decoding the Hedgehog signal in animal development. Cell Mol Life Sci 2006; 63:1249-65.
9. Rohatgi R, Milenkovic L, Scott MP. Patched1 regulates hedgehog signaling at the primary cilium. Science 2007; 317:372-6.
10. Corbit KC, Aanstad P, Singla V et al. Vertebrate Smoothened functions at the primary cilium. Nature 2005; 437:1018-21.
11. Pasca di Magliano M, Hebrok M. Hedgehog signalling in cancer formation and maintenance. Nat Rev Cancer 2003; 3:903-11.
12. Gorlin RJ. Nevoid basal-cell carcinoma syndrome. Medicine (Baltimore) 1987; 66:98-113.
13. Gorlin RJ. Living history-biography: from oral pathology to craniofacial genetics. Am J Med Genet 1993; 46:317-34.
14. Gorlin RJ, Goltz RW. Multiple nevoid basal-cell epithelioma, jaw cysts and bifid rib. A syndrome. N Engl J Med 1960; 262:908-12.
15. Gailani MR, Bale SJ, Leffell DJ et al. Developmental defects in Gorlin syndrome related to a putative tumor suppressor gene on chromosome 9. Cell 1992; 69:111-7.
16. Gailani MR, Stahle-Backdahl M, Leffell DJ et al. The role of the human homologue of Drosophila patched in sporadic basal cell carcinomas. Nat Genet 1996; 14:78-81.
17. Goodrich LV, Johnson RL, Milenkovic L et al. Conservation of the hedgehog/patched signaling pathway from flies to mice: induction of a mouse patched gene by Hedgehog. Genes Dev 1996; 10:301-12.
18. Lindstrom E, Shimokawa T, Toftgard R et al. PTCH mutations: distribution and analyses. Hum Mutat 2006; 27:215-9.
19. Bale AE, Yu, KP. The hedgehog pathway and basal cell carcinomas. Hum Mol Genet 2001; 10:757-62.
20. Goodrich LV, Milenkovic L, Higgins KM et al. Altered neural cell fates and medulloblastoma in mouse patched mutants. Science 1997; 277:1109-13.
21. Hahn H, Wojnowski L, Zimmer AM et al. Rhabdomyosarcomas and radiation hypersensitivity in a mouse model of Gorlin syndrome. Nat Med 1998; 4:619-22.
22. Aszterbaum M, Beech J, Epstein EH. Ultraviolet radiation mutagenesis of hedgehog pathway genes in basal cell carcinomas. J Investig Dermatol Symp Proc 1999; 4:41-5.
23. Xie J, Murone M, Luoh SM et al. Activating Smoothened mutations in sporadic basal-cell carcinoma. Nature 1998; 391:90-2.
24. Lam CW, Xie J, To KF et al. A frequent activated smoothened mutation in sporadic basal cell carcinomas. Oncogene 1999; 18:833-6.
25. Reifenberger J, Wolter M, Knobbe CB et al. Somatic mutations in the PTCH, SMOH, SUFUH and TP53 genes in sporadic basal cell carcinomas. Br J Dermatol 2005; 152:43-51.
26. Reifenberger J, Wolter M, Weber RG et al. Missense mutations in SMOH in sporadic basal cell carcinomas of the skin and primitive neuroectodermal tumors of the central nervous system. Cancer Res 1998; 58:1798-803.
27. Couve-Privat S, Bouadjar B, Avril MF et al. Significantly high levels of ultraviolet-specific mutations in the smoothened gene in basal cell carcinomas from DNA repair-deficient xeroderma pigmentosum patients. Cancer Res 2002; 62:7186-9.

28. Xie J, Aszterbaum M, Zhang X et al. A role of PDGFRalpha in basal cell carcinoma proliferation. Proc Natl Acad Sci USA 2001; 98:9255-9.
29. Athar M, Li C, Tang X et al. Inhibition of smoothened signaling prevents ultraviolet B-induced basal cell carcinomas through regulation of Fas expression and apoptosis. Cancer Res 2004; 64:7545-52.
30. Williams JA, Guicherit OM, Zaharian BI et al. Identification of a small molecule inhibitor of the hedgehog signaling pathway: effects on basal cell carcinoma-like lesions. Proc Natl Acad Sci USA 2003; 100:4616-21.
31. Bijlsma MF, Spek CA, Zivkovic D et al. Repression of smoothened by patched-dependent (pro-)vitamin D3 secretion. PLoS Biol 2006; 4:e232.
32. Kasper M, Schnidar H, Neill GW et al. Selective modulation of Hedgehog/GLI target gene expression by epidermal growth factor signaling in human keratinocytes. Mol Cell Biol 2006; 26:6283-98.
33. Riobo NA, Haines GM, Emerson CP. Protein kinase C-delta and mitogen-activated protein/extracellular signal-regulated kinase-1 control GLI activation in hedgehog signaling. Cancer Res 2006; 66:839-45.
34. Riobo NA, Lu K, Ai X et al. Phosphoinositide 3-kinase and Akt are essential for Sonic Hedgehog signaling. Proc Natl Acad Sci USA 2006; 103:4505-10.
35. Kenney AM, Widlund HR, Rowitch DH. Hedgehog and PI-3 kinase signaling converge on Nmyc1 to promote cell cycle progression in cerebellar neuronal precursors. Development 2004; 131:217-28.
36. Bigelow RL, Jen EY, Delehedde M et al. Sonic hedgehog induces epidermal growth factor dependent matrix infiltration in HaCaT keratinocytes. J Invest Dermatol 2005; 124:457-65.
37. Riobo NA, Lu K, Emerson CP. Hedgehog signal transduction: signal integration and cross talk in development and cancer. Cell Cycle 2006; 5:1612-5.
38. Ji Z, Mei FC, Xie J et al. Oncogenic kras supresses GLI1 degradation and activates hedgehog signaling pathway in pancreatic cancer cells. J Biol Chem 2007.
39. Sheng T, Chi S, Zhang X et al. Regulation of Gli1 localization by the cAMP/protein kinase A signaling axis through a site near the nuclear localization signal. J Biol Chem 2006; 281:9-12.
40. Caserta TM, Kommagani R, Yuan Z et al. p63 overexpression induces the expression of Sonic Hedgehog. Mol Cancer Res 2006; 4:759-68.
41. Uziel T, Zindy F, Xie S et al. The tumor suppressors Ink4c and p53 collaborate independently with Patched to suppress medulloblastoma formation. Genes Dev 2005; 19:2656-67.
42. Mimeault M, Johansson SL, Vankatraman G et al. Combined targeting of epidermal growth factor receptor and hedgehog signaling by gefitinib and cyclopamine cooperatively improves the cytotoxic effects of docetaxel on metastatic prostate cancer cells. Mol Cancer Ther 2007; 6:967-78.
43. Quaedvlieg PJ, Tirsi E, Thissen MR et al. Actinic keratosis: how to differentiate the good from the bad ones? Eur J Dermatol 2006; 16:335-9.
44. Takata M, Saida T. Early cancers of the skin: clinical, histopathological and molecular characteristics. Int J Clin Oncol 2005; 10:391-7.
45. Boukamp P. Nonmelanoma skin cancer: what drives tumor development and progression? Carcinogenesis 2005; 26:1657-67.
46. Tsai KY, Tsao H. The genetics of skin cancer. Am J Med Genet C Semin Med Genet 2004; 131C:82-92.
47. Ridky TW, Khavari PA. Pathways sufficient to induce epidermal carcinogenesis. Cell Cycle 2004; 3:621-4.
48. Smith-McCune K, Zhu YH, Hanahan D et al. Cross-species comparison of angiogenesis during the premalignant stages of squamous carcinogenesis in the human cervix and K14-HPV16 transgenic mice. Cancer Res 1997; 57:1294-300.
49. Brown VL, Harwood CA, Crook T et al. p16INK4a and p14ARF tumor suppressor genes are commonly inactivated in cutaneous squamous cell carcinoma. J Invest Dermatol 2004; 122:1284-92.
50. Blokx WA, Ruiter DJ, Verdijk MA et al. INK4-ARF and p53 mutations in metastatic cutaneous squamous cell carcinoma: case report and archival study on the use of Ink4a-ARF and p53 mutation analysis in identification of the corresponding primary tumor. Am J Surg Pathol 2005; 29:125-30.
51. Blokx WA, de Jong EM, de Wilde PC et al. P16 and p53 expression in (pre)malignant epidermal tumors of renal transplant recipients and immunocompetent individuals. Mod Pathol 2003; 16:869-78.
52. Saridaki Z, Liloglou T, Zafiropoulos A et al. Mutational analysis of CDKN2A genes in patients with squamous cell carcinoma of the skin. Br J Dermatol 2003; 148:638-48.
53. Classon M, Harlow E. The retinoblastoma tumour suppressor in development and cancer. Nat Rev Cancer 2002; 2:910-7.
54. Pickering MT, Kowalik TF. Rb inactivation leads to E2F1-mediated DNA double-strand break accumulation. Oncogene 2006; 25:746-55.
55. Soufir N, Moles JP, Vilmer C et al. P16 UV mutations in human skin epithelial tumors. Oncogene 1999; 18:5477-81.
56. Giglia-Mari G, Sarasin A. TP53 mutations in human skin cancers. Hum Mutat 2003; 21:217-28.

57. Bolshakov S, Walker CM, Strom SS et al. p53 mutations in human aggressive and nonaggressive basal and squamous cell carcinomas. Clin Cancer Res 2003; 9:228-34.
58. Kim MY, Park HJ, Baek SC et al. Mutations of the p53 and PTCH gene in basal cell carcinomas: UV mutation signature and strand bias. J Dermatol Sci 2002; 29:1-9.
59. Ansarin H, Daliri M, Soltani-Arabshahi R. Expression of p53 in aggressive and non-aggressive histologic variants of basal cell carcinoma. Eur J Dermatol 2006; 16:543-7.
60. D'Errico M, Calcagnile AS, Corona R et al. p53 mutations and chromosome instability in basal cell carcinomas developed at an early or late age. Cancer Res 1997; 57:747-52.
61. Wiseman SM, Stoler DL, Anderson GR. The role of genomic instability in the pathogenesis of squamous cell carcinoma of the head and neck. Surg Oncol Clin N Am 2004; 13:1-11.
62. Perez-Losada J, Mao JH, Balmain A. Control of genomic instability and epithelial tumor development by the p53-Fbxw7/Cdc4 pathway. Cancer Res 2005; 65:6488-92.
63. Duensing A, Duensing S. Guilt by association? p53 and the development of aneuploidy in cancer. Biochem Biophys Res Commun 2005; 331:694-700.
64. Pelisson I, Soler C, Chardonnet Y et al. A possible role for human papillomaviruses and c-myc, c-Ha-ras and p53 gene alterations in malignant cutaneous lesions from renal transplant recipients. Cancer Detect Prev 1996; 20:20-30.
65. Aziz MH, Manoharan HT, Verma AK. Protein kinase C epsilon, which sensitizes skin to sun's UV radiation-induced cutaneous damage and development of squamous cell carcinomas, associates with Stat3. Cancer Res 2007; 67:1385-94.
66. Quadros MR, Peruzzi F, Kari C et al. Complex regulation of signal transducers and activators of transcription 3 activation in normal and malignant keratinocytes. Cancer Res 2004; 64:3934-9.
67. Dudley AC, Thomas D, Best J et al. A VEGF/JAK2/STAT5 axis may partially mediate endothelial cell tolerance to hypoxia. Biochem J 2005; 390:427-36.
68. Budunova IV, Perez P, Vaden VR et al. Increased expression of p50-NF-kappaB and constitutive activation of NF-kappaB transcription factors during mouse skin carcinogenesis. Oncogene 1999; 18:7423-31.
69. Loercher A, Lee TL, Ricker JL et al. Nuclear factor-kappaB is an important modulator of the altered gene expression profile and malignant phenotype in squamous cell carcinoma. Cancer Res 2004; 64:6511-23.
70. Duffey DC, Chen Z, Dong G et al. Expression of a dominant-negative mutant inhibitor-kappaBalpha of nuclear factor-kappaB in human head and neck squamous cell carcinoma inhibits survival, proinflammatory cytokine expression and tumor growth in vivo. Cancer Res 1999; 59:3468-74.
71. Verma AK, Wheeler DL, Aziz MH et al. Protein kinase Cepsilon and development of squamous cell carcinoma, the nonmelanoma human skin cancer. Mol Carcinog 2006; 45:381-8.
72. Bremner R, Kemp CJ, Balmain A. Induction of different genetic changes by different classes of chemical carcinogens during progression of mouse skin tumors. Mol Carcinog 1994; 11:90-7.
73. DiGiovanni J. Genetic factors controlling responsiveness to skin tumor promotion in mice. Prog Clin Biol Res 1995; 391:195-212.
74. Hirst GL, Balmain A. Forty years of cancer modelling in the mouse. Eur J Cancer 2004; 40:1974-80.
75. Rebel H, Mosnier LO, Berg RJ et al. Early p53-positive foci as indicators of tumor risk in ultraviolet-exposed hairless mice: kinetics of induction, effects of DNA repair deficiency and p53 heterozygosity. Cancer Res 2001; 61:977-83.
76. Rebel H, Kram N, Westerman A et al. Relationship between UV-induced mutant p53 patches and skin tumours, analysed by mutation spectra and by induction kinetics in various DNA-repair-deficient mice. Carcinogenesis 2005; 26:2123-30.
77. Ahsan H, Aziz MH, Ahmad N. Ultraviolet B exposure activates Stat3 signaling via phosphorylation at tyrosine705 in skin of SKH1 hairless mouse: a target for the management of skin cancer? Biochem Biophys Res Commun 2005; 333:241-6.
78. Wakabayashi Y, Mao JH, Brown K et al. Promotion of Hras-induced squamous carcinomas by a polymorphic variant of the Patched gene in FVB mice. Nature 2007; 445:761-5.
79. Roth JA. Adenovirus p53 gene therapy. Expert Opin Biol Ther 2006; 6:55-61.
80. McCormick F. Cancer-specific viruses and the development of ONYX-015. Cancer Biol Ther 2003; 2:S157-60.
81. Lane DP, Lain S. Therapeutic exploitation of the p53 pathway. Trends Mol Med 2002; 8;S38-42.
82. Vassilev LT. p53 Activation by small molecules: application in oncology. J Med Chem 2005; 48:4491-9.
83. Sherr CJ, McCormick F. The RB and p53 pathways in cancer. Cancer Cell 2002; 2:103-12.
84. Green CL, Khavari PA. Targets for molecular therapy of skin cancer. Semin Cancer Biol 2004; 14:63-9.
85. Ozols RF, Herbst RS, Colson YL et al. Clinical cancer advances 2006: major research advances in cancer treatment, prevention and screening—a report from the American Society of Clinical Oncology. J Clin Oncol 2007; 25:146-62.

CHAPTER 20

Molecular Biology of Malignant Melanoma

Mar Pons, Pablo Mancheño-Corvo, Pilar Martín-Duque and Miguel Quintanilla*

Abstract

The incidence of melanoma has increased more rapidly than any other type of cancer. In this review, we summarize the most important genetic alterations that contribute to the development of malignant melanoma. Our knowledge of the genetic and biological events involved in the genesis and progression of this disease has been benefited from the evolvement of a wealth of genetically engineered animal models. Hopefully, the understanding generated by all these studies will contribute to develop new therapeutic strategies to handle this fatal malignancy.

Introduction

Melanoma probably is the most aggressive cancer in humans. When melanoma reaches a critical thickness (of about 4 mm), presents a high risk of metastasis and then treatment options as well as cure and survival rates decrease dramatically. Melanomas derive from melanocytes, the pigment-producing cells that mainly reside in the skin, although they can also arise from melanocytes residing in noncutaneous tissues; i.e., retinal pigmented epithelium. Both genetic predisposition and exposure to environmental agents are risk factors for melanoma development. It is belived that the UV component of sunlight; i.e., UV-A (wavelength 320-400 nm) and UV-B (wavelength 290-320 nm), is the main risk factor for cutaneous melanoma. In contrast to other common skin tumors, such as basal cell carcinoma and squamous cell carcinoma that are derived from epidermal keratinocytes, melanoma results from intense rather than cumulative sun exposure, particularly during childhood.[1,2] Primary cutaneous melanoma have been classified into several histopathological stages:[3] superficial spreading melanoma is the most common form of melanoma in Caucasians, lentigo malignant melanoma typically occurs on chronically exposed skin of the elderly, acral lentiginous melanoma is the predominant form of this disease in individuals with darker skin and nodular melanoma is characterized by vertical growth of transformed melanocytes. However, this classification has been questioned by some authors (see refs. 4 and 5 for reviews). The majority of melanoma subtypes are observed to progress from a radial growth phase (RGP) to a vertical growth phase (VGP). RGP melanoma grows laterally and remains largely confined to the epidermis, while VGP melanoma invades the upper layers of the epidermis and penetrates into the underlying dermis and subcutaneous tissue forming expansile nodules of malignant cells. The crucial step in the evolution to malignant melanoma appears to be the transition from RGP to VGP melanoma.[6,7]

*Corresponding Author: Miguel Quintanilla—Instituto de Investigaciones Biomédicas Alberto Sols, Departamento de Biotecnologia, Universidad Francisco de Vitoria, CSIC-UAM, Arturo Duperier 4, 28029-Madrid, Spain. Email: mquintanilla@iib.uam.es

Sunlight, Vitamin D and Skin Cancer, edited by Jörg Reichrath. ©2008 Landes Bioscience and Springer Science+Business Media.

Genetic Predisposition to Malignant Melanoma

It is well known how physical characteristics, such as fair-skin, red or blond hair, the inability to tan and a freckling phenotype, correlate with increased risk for melanoma development. Since certain melanocortin-1 receptor (MC1R) polymorphic variants are associated with these characteristics and with a diminished ability of the epidermis to respond to UV damage, this pigment regulating gene is seen as a risk modifier of melanoma.[8,9] A predisposition to skin cancer is also associated with the rare hereditary syndrome xeroderma pigmentosum (XP). Individuals with XP carry a nucleotide excision DNA repair defect associated with an acute photosensitivity. The most significant characteristic of XP patients is a predisposition to develop multiple skin cancers, mostly squamous cell carcinomas but also basal cell carcinomas and malignant melanomas.[10] Nonetheless, the most significant risk factor for melanoma occurs in individuals with familial melanoma history.[11]

MSH/MC1R Signalling

When the α-melanocyte-stimulating hormone (αMSH) binds to its seven-transmembrane G-protein-coupled receptor MC1R, which is present on epidermal melanocytes, it triggers an intracellular signalling pathway that is considered the most important regulator of pigmentation.[11] This pathway involves activation of adenylate cyclase and production of cyclic AMP (cAMP). Elevated cAMP levels leads to phosphorylation and activation of the cAMP responsive element binding (CREB) family of transcription factors. A critical CREB target gene is that encoding the microphthalmia associated transcription factor[12,13] (Mitf), a basic helix-loop-helix leucine zipper (b-HLH-Zip) factor that in turn regulates the transcription of genes encoding enzymes that are essential for melanin synthesis, such as tyrosinase, tyrosinase-related protein-1 (TRP-1) and

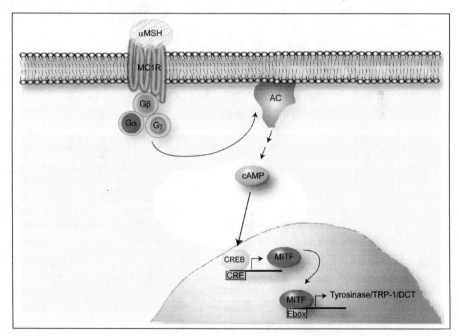

Figure 1. MC1R signalling. Binding of α-MSH to MC1R stimulates adenylate cyclase (AC) through a heterotrimeric G-protein complex. AC catalyzes the production of cAMP that triggers (via several intermediate steps) the phosphorylation of CREB transcription factors family. Activated CREB recruits CBP/p300 coactivators triggering transcriptional activation of multiple genes. *MITF* is a critical CREB target in melanocytes. The *MITF* transcription factor regulates genes involved in pigmentation and differentiation.

dopachrome tautomerase (DCT) (Fig. 1). MC1R is highly polymorphic in the human population. MC1R variants are associated with the Red Hair Color phenotype (RHC), characteristic
of individuals with red hair, fair skin, resistance to tan and freckle tendency, synthesize increased
amounts of the potentially dangerous pheomelanin (reddish-yellow pigment) instead of the
photoreactive black-brown pigment eumelanin. In addition to its diminished UV-light protective
capacity, pheomelanin produce cytotoxic and mutagenic metabolites and presumably contributes
to increase melanoma risk.[8,9,11] In general, those MC1R variants that produce weak or absent cAMP
response to MSH signals are associated with the RHC phenotype.[14]

Familial Melanoma. The CDKN2A Locus

Familial melanomas represent about 8-12% of all melanoma cases. Linkage analysis studies of
families with high melanoma incidence led to the identification of a locus at 9p21 in which the
first melanoma susceptibility gene, *CDKN2A*, was identified.[15,16] *CDKN2A* encodes two unrelated
proteins: p16INK4a and p14ARF (also called p19ARF in mice) via a combination of alternative

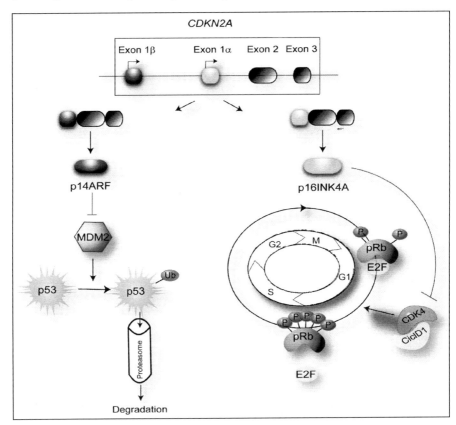

Figure 2. The *CDKN2A* locus. The *CDKN2A* gene encodes two proteins p16INK4a and
p14ARF. Each has a unique first exon (1β or 1α) that then splices to a common second and
third exon, but in alternating reading frames. p16INK4a binds and inhibits the activities of the
cyclin-dependent kinases CDK4 and CDK6, ensuring that pRb remains in a hypophosphorylated state in complex with E2F transcription factor, leading to G1 arrest. p14ARF stabilizes
and enhances p53 levels by inhibiting MDM2-mediated p53 ubiquitylation and degradation
through the proteasome. p53 accumulation leads to either cell cycle arrest or cellular apoptosis.
Adapted from Pons and Quintanilla. Clin. Transl. Oncol. 2006; 8:466-474.

splicing and alternative reading frames (Fig. 2). Both *CDKN2A* products are potent tumor suppressors involved in cell cycle regulation. p16INK4a specifically inhibits G1 cyclin-dependent kinases Cdk4/Cdk6-mediated phosphorylation of the retinoblastoma protein (pRb), arresting cell cycle progression through G1-S.[17] p14ARF, on the other hand, enhances apoptosis and blocks oncogenic transformation by stabilizing p53 levels through inhibition of Mdm2-mediated p53 ubiquitination.[18-21] Therefore, loss of p16INK4a function promotes hyperphosphorylation and inactivation of pRb, leading to unrestricted cell cycle progression, while loss of p14ARF inactivates p53.

Overall, germline *CDKN2A* mutations have been found in 20-40% of familiar melanomas. They comprise missense mutations found in exons 1α and exon 2, as well as in the 5' untranslated region and introns (see ref. 11 for review). As *p16INK4a* shares exon 2 with *p14ARF* (see Fig. 2), many *CDKN2A* mutations affect both proteins confounding the specific role of each gene in the genesis of melanoma. However, mutations affecting only *p14ARF* have been described in some melanoma families,[22-24] thus pointing to *p14ARF* as a melanoma susceptibility gene that is independent of *p16INK4a*. In fact, genetically mouse models have provided convincing evidence that both *p14ARF* and *p16INK4a* are tumor suppressor genes in melanoma development (see below). *MC1R* variants associated with the RHC phenotype increase melanoma penetrance in individuals harbouring *CDKN2A* germline mutations.[25,26]

A second melanoma susceptibility gene, *CDK4*, was found at 12q14.[27-29] Germline and sporadic mutations in *CDK4* abrogating binding of Cdk4 to p16INK4a (see Fig. 2) have been found associated with melanoma pathogenesis. Thus, mutations in this gene have a similar impact to those in *p16INK4a* and the phenotypic characteristics of families carrying *CDK4* germline mutations do not differ from those families affected in the *CDKN2A* locus.[30,31] Consistent with the human data, mice expressing a mutant form of *Cdk4* are predisposed to develop melanoma after carcinogen treatment.[32] An additional evidence that links the entire p16INK4a-Cdk4/6-pRb pathway to melanoma is the observation that hereditary retinoblastoma patients with germline inactivation of the retinoblastoma (*RB1*) gene are predisposed to melanoma.[33,34]

Of note, many reports have described the occurrence of cancers other than melanoma, such as pancreatic cancer, in families carrying *CDKN2A* mutations.[35] However, the precise relationship between pancreatic cancer and the *CDKN2A* locus remains elusive.

Sporadic Melanoma

Despite its important role in melanoma predisposition, mutations in *CDKN2A* are rarely found in sporadic primary melanomas. In contrast, *CDKN2A* mutations are found frequently in melanoma cell lines (reviewed in ref. 31). This discrepancy could reflect a selective event imposed by cell culturing due to the critical role of p16INK4a in senescence, as cells that lose p16INK4a escape senescence and become immortalized. Nevertheless, genetic and molecular studies have identified several important molecules and signalling pathways besides pRb and p53 whose altered regulation appears to be crucial for melanoma development.

RAF, RAS and the Mitogen-Activated Protein Kinase (MAPK) Signalling Pathway

In melanocytic lesions, the most frequent activating mutations found in protooncogenes are those leading to constitutive activation of the mitogen-activated protein kinase (MAPK) signalling cascade. Strikingly, mutations in *BRAF* resulting in constitutive activation of this serine/threonine kinase have been found frequently (27-70%) in melanoma.[36-38] Raf proteins are the primary mediators of Ras signalling, which links extracellular mitogenic stimuli to transcription of genes that regulate cell growth, differentiation, survival, senescence, cell shape and cell migration, via the MAPK pathway[39] (Fig. 3). Most of these *BRAF* mutations occur at a single site (T-A transversion) leading to the substitution of glutamic acid for valine (V600E) at the kinase domain, which confers constitutive activation.[40] This point mutation is not classically associated with UV damage,[10] rising the question of the role of sun exposure on *BRAF* mutations occurring in melanoma.[11] *BRAF* mutations are common in benign and dysplastic nevi,[36,41] pointing to a potential initiating role of

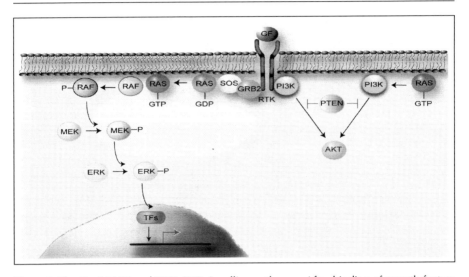

Figure 3. The Ras/MAPK and PI3K-AKT signalling pathways. After binding of growth factors to their respective RTKs, activation of RTKs leads to binding of SOS (a cytosolic protein in close proximity to Ras on the plasma membrane) to the GDP-bound inactive form of Ras. Like other G-proteins, Ras cycles between the GDP-bound inactive form and the GTP-bound active form. The binding of SOS to Ras induces a conformational change that leads to the dissociation of GDP and binding of GTP. The best characterized Ras effector pathway proceeds via a kinase cascade that involves phosphorylation of RAF. RAF in turn phosphorylates MEK which then phosphorylates ERK MAPKs. Activated ERKs translocate into the nucleus where they phosphorylate specific transcription factors that are involved in the regulation of various cellular responses, particularly in promoting cell proliferation. Activated Ras can also bind PI3K, stabilizing its membrane localization and activating its catalytic domain. PI3K catalyse the phosphorylation of phosphatidylinositols (PtdIns) at their 3-position and converts PtdIns(4, 5)P_2 (PIP$_2$) into PtdIns(3, 4, 5)P_3 (PIP$_3$). PIP$_3$ anchors AKT to the membrane allowing to its activation (by phosphorylation with the phosphoinositide-dependent kinases PDK1 and PDK2). Activated AKT mediates the activation and inhibition of several targets, resulting in cell growth, proliferation and inhibition of apoptosis (survival).

BRAF in melanocyte transformation. Expression of mutant BRaf[V600E] protein in cultured human melanocytes induces p16INK4a-dependent cell cycle arrest and non p16INK4a-dependent cell senescence.[42] These observations indicate the presence of a tumor suppressor within this unknown pathway leading to senescence, whose inactivation ought to cooperate with *BRAF* mutations for melanoma progression.[11] The notion that *BRAF* mutation is not sufficient for a full melanocyte neoplastic transformation is also supported by a genetically engineered fish model (see below).

There have also been reports documenting mutations in *RAS* genes in melanocytic tumors. The most frequently mutated member of the family is *NRAS*, while mutations in *HRAS* and *KRAS* have only been found occasionally. Activating point mutations in *NRAS* have been reported in as many as 56% of congenital nevi, 33% of primary melanomas and 26% of metastatic melanoma samples,[43,44] but are rarely found in dysplastic nevi.[44,45] This fact indicates the possible existence of two distinct evolutionary paths to melanoma progression, from benign and dysplastic nevi.[46] In contrast to *BRAF* mutations, *NRAS* mutations associated with melanoma appear to arise as a result of UV damage.[43,47] *NRAS* and *BRAF* activating mutations in melanoma (as also occur in other tumor types) are mutually exclusive, indicating that these genes function in the same cellular growth regulatory pathway.[48] On the other hand, a recent report has found that mutations in *BRAF* are associated with enhanced sensitivity to pharmacological inhibitors of MEK compared to cells harbouring *RAS* mutations. These data suggest that melanoma cells carrying *BRAF* mutations are much more dependent on MEK-ERK signalling than *RAS* mutant cells are.[49]

c-MET and Other Receptor Tyrosine Kinases (RTKs)

Several studies support the notion that aberrant hepatocyte growth factor/scatter factor (HGF/SF) signalling is associated with melanoma progression.[50] Increased expression of *c-Met*, the tyrosine kinase receptor of HGF/SF, has been observed in metastatic melanoma.[51] In addition, gain of the 7q33-qter locus (where *c-MET* is located) has been correlated with late stages of melanoma development.[52,53] Besides to stimulate proliferation and motility of cultured melanocytes, HGF/SF disrupts adhesion between melanocytes and keratinocytes by downregulating the expression of the cell-cell adhesion proteins E-cadherin and desmoglein-1, which could favour deregulated cell proliferation and invasiveness.[54] Interestingly, *c-MET* is a transcriptional target of Mitf, the melanocytic lineage transcription factor.[55] As described below, *MITF* is amplified in malignant melanoma. The causal relationship between *c-Met* signalling and malignant melanoma is supported by in vitro experiments and genetically engineered models.[11] Several reports have also linked overexpression of the epidermal growth factor receptor (EGFR), associated with gains of chromosome 7, to advanced melanoma.[53,56] *EGFR* is often amplified in breast and lung carcinomas and overexpression of this RTK in tumors is thought to result in deregulated kinase activity and malignant transformation.[57] An important effector of oncogenic RTKs is the phosphatydilinositol 3-kinase (PI3K)-Akt pathway that controls cell survival and motility.[58]

PTEN and the PI3K-Akt Pathway

PTEN encodes a lipid and protein phosphatase involved in negative regulation of the PI3K-Akt signalling pathway (Fig. 3). *PTEN* is among the tumor suppressor genes most frequently mutated in cancer. Involvement of *PTEN* in melanoma was suspected because loss-of-heterozygosity (LOH) of 10 q (where *PTEN* is located) occurs in 30-50% of melanomas.[59] The region deleted at 10 q is, however, large and could include other tumor suppressor genes.[31] In addition, somatic mutations in *PTEN* have been found in about 10% of melanomas.[60,61] Loss of *PTEN* leads to hyperphosphorylation of Akt and enhanced cell proliferation and survival. The importance of hyperactivation of the PI3K pathway in melanoma development is further emphasized by the finding of constitutive activation of Akt in more than 60% of melanomas.[62,63] The level of phosphorylated Akt increases dramatically with melanoma invasion and metastasis and appears to correlate adversely with patient survival.[64]

The Misunderstood Role of p53

The proportion of primary and metastatic melanomas containing mutations in the gene encoding p53 (*TP53*) is consistently low (<5%).[46] Although UV light-related *TP53* mutations are frequently observed in other skin tumors (basal cell carcinomas and squamous cell carcinomas), the above observation suggests that UV-induced mutational inactivation of p53 is not involved in melanoma formation. However, several groups have reported relatively high mutation frequencies of *TP53* (in the range of 10-25%) in malignant melanomas (reviewed in ref. 4). The relevance of p53 in melanoma suppression is additionally emphasized in genetic models with mutant mice. The *Tyr-Ras⁺/p53⁺/⁻* mutant mice develop cutaneous melanoma characterized by LOH of the wild-type *p53* allele and retention of *ARF*.[65] As p19Arf and p53 are within the same pathway (Fig. 2), the preferred inactivation of the pathway at the level of Arf, via 9p21 deletion, offers a mechanistic explanation for the pattern of genetic mutation observed in human melanoma.[11]

MITF as an Oncogene Involved in Melanoma Progression

Mitf is a basic helix-loop-helix leucine zipper (b-HLH-Zip) transcription factor essential for melanocyte development (see ref. 66 for a review). When mutated in mice (*Mitf^{mi/mi}* mouse) leads to complete absence of neural crest-derived melanocytes as well as defects in the retinal pigmented epithelium, mast cells and osteoclasts.[67] These data suggest that Mitf is essential for survival and differentiation of melanocytes. In fact, although Mitf plays a crucial role in pigmentation (Fig. 1), the destructive consequences of Mitf deficiency suggest that Mitf is primarily involved in lineage survival. Thus, the phenotype of Mitf-deficient mice is characterized by a complete absence of melanocytes. In humans, mutation of *MITF* causes an autosomal inherited disease, known as

Waardenburg type IIA syndrome, characterized by deafness and white hairlock, arising from melanocyte deficiencies in the eye, forelock and inner ear.[68]

The *MITF* gene has a complex organization. At least nine distinct promoter-exon units direct the synthesis of specific Mitf isoforms that arise by alternative splicing.[69] Transcription factors that regulate *MITF* expression include CREB, SOX10, Tcf/Lef-1 and Mitf itself, among others.[66] As already mentioned, α-MSH binds to MC1R which activates adenylate cyclase, followed by cAMP production (Fig. 1). cAMP leads to phosphorylation CREB transcription factors which in turn activates the *MITF* promoter. Despite of the cAMP-CREB pathway is ubiquitous, *MITF* expression is cell-type specific. This is explained, at least in part, by the obligate cooperativity between CREB and SOX10, which is specific for the neural crest lineage.[70] Tcf/Lef-1, which binds β-catenin at the point end of Wingless-type (Wnt) signalling, links MITF with the Wnt signalling pathway that is crucial for the differentiation of melanocytes from the neural crest.[71-73] In addition, Mitf expression is regulated by posttranslational mechanisms, namely by phosphorylation. Kinases that phosphorylate Mitf include MAPK, ribosomal S6 kinase (RSK), glycogen synthase kinase 3β(GSK3β) and p38.[66] Nevertheless, the role of phosphorylation on Mitf activity is obscure. For example, phosphorylation of Mitf by Erk2 increases recruitment of the transcriptional coactivator p300/CBP, a CREB binding protein and enhances *MITF* transcriptional activity, while simultaneously targets Mitf for ubiquitin-dependent proteolysis.[74,75]

Genomic amplification of *MITF* has been found in 10-20% of primary melanomas with a higher incidence in metastatic melanoma. In this setting, *MITF* amplification correlates with a decrease in 5 years patient survival.[76] This, together with functional studies on immortalized melanocytes that have inactivated the p53 and pRb pathways, in which ectopic overexpression of Mitf complemented BRaf[V600E] to confer soft-agar clonogenic growth,[76] suggest that *MITF* is an oncogene in human melanoma. However, in other cases, Mitf and its targets (*Tyrosinase, TRP-1* and *DCT*) have been found downregulated in advanced melanoma.[66] This suggests that there are distinct subsets of melanoma. In some melanomas (characterized by a particular genetic context, as for example *BRAF* mutation), cell survival is dependent on Mitf,[76] while in others decreased expression of Mitf might provide a growth advantage by diminishing energy and oxidative stress associated with pigment production.[66]

Genetic Models of Melanoma

Most of the genes found to be mutated (or altered) in melanoma patients have been tested in animal models, particularly in mice. Thus, a large number of genetically engineered mouse models have been generated in the last years (see refs. 11, 66 and 77 for recent reviews), the most significant of which are summarized in Table 1. These mouse models have permitted to assess the requirement of genetic interactions between distinct pathways, as well as those with the environment, in order to recapitulate human melanoma disease (Table 1).

One of the first melanoma mouse models was developed by targeted expression of simian virus 40 (SV40) large tumor (T)-antigen to melanocytes under the control of the tyrosinase promoter.[78] The viral T-antigen interacts with host proteins inactivating pRb and p53 functions in a manner reminiscent of *p16Ink4a* and *p19Arf* loss. *Tyr-SV40 T-antigen*[+] transgenic mice developed skin melanomas at low frequency that appeared late on life. In contrast, these mice induced highly aggressive ocular melanomas that originated at a young age.[78] However, when exposed to limited UV radiation shortly after birth, the *T-antigen* transgenic mice developed metastatic skin melanoma.[79,80] Mice with loss of *p16Ink4a* that retain *p19Arf* are predisposed to develop melanoma after initiation with the chemical carcinogen 7,12-dimethylbenz(*a*)anthracene[81] (DMBA). Moreover, treatment with DMBA of *p16INK4a*-deficient mice that were heterozygous for *p19ARF* resulted in increased incidence of cutaneous melanoma that produced frequent metastasis.[82] Similarly, DMBA was able to enhance melanomagenesis in mice harbouring a *Cdk4* mutation that inactivates the pRb pathway, as found in familial melanoma.[32,83] These studies have provided compelling evidence that inactivation of both the pRb and p53 pathways are crucial for development of melanoma. The cooperation between these two pathways and that of PI3K-Akt has been evaluated in compound

Table 1. Genetically engineered melanoma animal models

Genetic Lesions	Afftected Pathways	Carcinogen Exposure	Tumor Phenotype/Comments	References
Mouse Models				
Tyr-SV40 T-Ag⁺	pRb, p53	None	Low penetrance skin melanoma (metastatic eye melanoma)	78
		UV	Short term, neonatal, UV exposure induced melanocytic skin lesions and metastatic melanoma	79, 80
Ink4a⁻/⁻, Arfᶠ/⁺	pRb	DMBA	Low penetrance skin melanoma	81
Ink4a⁻/⁻, Arfᶠ/⁻	pRb, p53	DMBA	Metastatic skin melanoma	82
Int4a⁻/⁻, Arf⁻/⁻, Pten⁺/⁻	pRb, p53, PI3K-Akt	None	Low penetrance skin melanoma	84
Cdk4 (R24C)⁺	pRb	None	Low penetrance skin melanoma	83
		DMBA/TPA	High penetrance skin melanoma, no metastasis	32
Tyr-Ras⁺	MAPK	DMBA/UV	No spontaneous skin tumors without carcinogen; each carcinogen induced melanoma; DMBA was superior to chronic adult UV exposure	87
Tyr-Ras⁺/Ink4a⁻/⁻	pRb, MAPK	None	High penetrance, nonmetastatic skin melanoma	85
		UV	Single, neonatal, UV exposure had no impact in melanoma development	86
Tyr-Ras⁺/Arf⁻/⁻	p53, MAPK	None	High penetrance, nonmetastatic skin melanoma	85
		UV	Single, neonatal, UV exposure accelerated melanomagenesis	86
Tyr-Ras⁺/Trp53⁻/⁻	p53, MAPK	None	High penetrance, nonmetastatic skin melanoma	65
MT-HGF/SF⁺	c-Met, MAPK, PI3K-Akt	None	Low penetrance metastatic skin melanoma	88, 89
		UV	Single, neonatal, UV exposure enhanced melanoma development; chronic adult UV exposure had no effect	90,91
MT-HGF/SF⁺/ Ink4a⁻/⁻, Arf⁻/⁻	c-Met, MAPK, PI3K-Akt, pRb, p53	UV	Both loss of pl6/pl9 function and single, neonatal, UV exposure enhanced melanomagenesis	92
Zebrafish Models				
Braf(V600E)⁺	MAPK	None	Benign nevi	93
Braf(V600E)⁺/	MAPK, p53	None	Melanocytic lesions that	93

continued on next page

Table 1. Continued

Genetic Lesions	Afftected Pathways	Carcinogen Exposure	Tumor Phenotype/Comments	References
Trp53⁻/⁻			progress to invasive melanoma	
Xiphophorus Fish Model				
Xmrk	EGFR, MAPK, PI3K-Akt	None	Spontaneous melanoma	94, 95
		UV	Increased melanoma susceptibility	94, 95

mutant *p16INK4a/p19ARF*-deficient mice heterozygous for *Pten*.[84] These mice developed a wide spectrum of tumor types including melanoma. Furthermore, loss of either *p16Ink4a* or *p19Arf* (or *Trp53*) induced spontaneous skin melanomas with high incidence in transgenic mice expressing a *HRAS* oncogene in melanocytes.[65,85] All these studies suggest that sustained activation of either Ras or PI3K-Akt signalling interact with the pRb and p53 suppressor pathways for melanoma development.

The cooperation between UV irradiation and loss of each of the tumor suppressor genes encoded by the *CDKN2A* locus has also been examined in *HRas⁺* transgenic mice.[86] The results of these studies show that loss of *p19Arf*, but not of *p16Ink4a*, cooperates with UV exposure to accelerate melanoma development. As tumors arising in UV-irradiated *Ras⁺/p19ARF⁻/⁻* mice showed either loss of *p16INK4a* or *Cdk6* amplifications (both leading to disruption of the pRb pathway), these data indicate a joint cooperation between mutations at both p53 and pRb pathways and UV irradiation for UV-induced melanogenesis. Chronic exposure of adult mice with activated *HRas* (harbouring a normal *Cdkn2a* locus) to UV irradiation produced melanoma, but at low efficiency.[87] It is interesting to note that DMBA, a chemical agent of unknown environmental relevance for human melanoma, is most efficient than UV to induce melanoma in different mouse models (Table 1).

Interactions between RTK signalling and UV irradiation have been challenged in the *HGF/SF⁺* transgenic mouse model. These mice develop melanomas, but after long latency periods,[88,89] suggesting that additional genetic alterations are needed for tumor development. A single neonatal dose of UV radiation was sufficient to induce melanoma lesions with high penetrance and short latencies in *HGF/SF⁺* transgenic mice, while chronic UV exposure in adult mice had no effect.[90,91] The response of these mice is in accordance with epidemiological studies in humans suggesting that melanoma is caused by intense intermittent exposure to UV during childhood,[1,2] as mentioned before. The cooperation between neonatal UV irradiation and inactivation of the *Cdnk2a* locus has been further demonstrated in *HGF/SF⁺* transgenic mice. UV-irradiated *HGF/SF⁺/p16Ink4a/p19Arf⁻/⁻* mice exhibited a significant acceleration of melanomagenesis with respect to untreated *HGF/SF⁺/p16Ink4a/p19Arf⁻/⁻* mice and UV-irradiated *HGF/SF⁺/p16Ink4a/p19Arf⁺/⁺* mice.[92]

These genetic models also include animals distinct from the mouse, such as zebrafish and *Xiphophorus* fish. Thus, while there has been no report to date on a *BRaf* transgenic mouse model for melanoma, it has been shown that activating mutations of *BRaf* in zebrafish, which leads only to development of benign nevi, cooperate with inactivation of p53 for melanoma development.[93] In *Xiphophorus* fish, activating mutations in *Xmrk*, the *EGFR* homolog, enhances melanoma susceptibility.[94,95] This observation is interesting, as no activating mutations in *EGFR* have been found in human melanoma. However, it is in agreement with a number of studies in melanoma cell lines demonstrating that sustained activation of the EGFR signalling pathway provides potent autocrine survival signals for *RAS*-driven melanoma tumorigenicity.[11]

Acknowledgements
Work in our laboratory has been funded by the Spanish Ministry of Education (grant SAF2004-04902 to MQ) and Fides and Medical Research Funds (grant PI05626 to PM-D). MP is funded by the company Digna Biotech. PM-D is funded by the "Ramón y Cajal" program.

References
1. Jhappan C, Noonan FP, Merlino G. Ultraviolet radiation and cutaneous malignant melanoma. Oncogene 2003; 22:3099-3112.
2. Hussein MR. Ultraviolet radiation and skin cancer: molecular mechanisms. J Cutan Pathol 2005; 32:191-205.
3. Clark Jr WH, Elder DE, van Horn M. The biologic forms of malignant melanoma. Hum Pathol 1986; 17:443-450.
4. Chudnovski Y, Khavari PA, Adams AE. Melanoma genetics and the development of rational therapeutics. J Clin Invest 2005; 115:813-824.
5. Takata M, Saida T. genetic alterations in melanocytic tumors. J Derm Sci 2006; 43:1-10.
6. Meier F, Satyamoorthy K, Nesbit M et al. Molecular events in melanoma development and progression. Front Biosci 1998; 3:D1005-D1010.
7. Rusciano D. Differentiation and metastasis in melanoma. Crit Rev Oncog 2000; 11:147-163.
8. Healy E, Jordan SA, Budd PS et al. Functional variation of MC1R alleles from red-haired individuals. Hum Mol Genet 2001; 10:397-2402.
9. Palmer JS, Duffy DL, Box NF et al. Melanocortin-1 receptor polymorphisms and risk of melanoma: Is the association explained solely by pigmentation phenotype? Am J Hum Genet 2000; 66:176-186.
10. Daya-Grosjean L, Sarasin A. The role of UV induced lesions in skin carcinogenesis: an overview of oncogene and tumor suppressor gene modifications in xeroderma pigmentosum skin tumors. Mutat Res 2005; 571:43-56.
11. Chin L, Garraway LA, Fisher DE. Malignant melanoma: genetics and therapeutics in the genomic era. Genes Dev 2006; 20:2149-2182.
12. Bertolotto C, Abbe P, Hemesath TJ et al. Microphthalmia gene product as a signal transducer in cAMP-induced differentiation of melanocytes. J Cell Biol 1998; 142:827-835.
13. Price ER, Horstmann MA, Wells AG et al. A-Melanocyte-stimulating hormone signaling regulates expression of micrphtalmia, a gene deficient in Waanderburg syndrome. J Biol Chem 1998; 273:33042-33047.
14. Kadekaro AL, Kanto H, Kavanagh R et al. Significance of the melanocortin 1 receptor in regulating human melanocyte pigmentation, proliferation and survival. Ann NY Acad Sci 2003; 994:359-365.
15. Hussussian CJ, Struewing IP, Goldstein AM et al. Germline p16 mutations in familial melanoma. Nat Genet 1994; 8:15-21.
16. Kamb A, Shattuck-Eidens D, Eeles R et al. Analysis of the p16 gene (CDKN2) as a candidate for the chromosome 9p melanoma susceptibility locus. Nat Genet 1994; 8:23-26.
17. Serrano M, Hannon GJ, Beach D. A new regulatory motif in cell-cycle control causing specific inhibition of cyclin D/CDK4. Nature 1993; 366:704-707.
18. Pomerantz J, Schreiber-Agus N, Liegeois NJ et al. The Ink4a tumor suppressor gene product, p19Arf, interacts with MDM2 and neutralizes MDM2's inhibition of p53. Cell 1998; 92:713-723.
19. Zhang Y, Xiong Y, Yarbrough WJ. ARF promotes MDM2 degradation and stabilizes p53: ARF-INK4a locus deletion impairs both the Rb and p53 tumor suppression pathways. Cell 1998; 92:725-734.
20. Kamijo T, Weber JD, Zambetti G et al. Functional and physical interactions of the ARF tumor suppressor with p53 and Mdm2. Proc Natl Acad Sci USA 1998; 95:8292-8297.
21. Stott FJ, bates S, James MC et al. The alternative product from the human CDKN2A locus, p14(ARF), participates in a regulatory feedback loop with p53 and MDM2. EMBO J 1998; 17:5001-5014.
22. Randerson-Moor JA, Harland M, Williams S et al. A germline deletion of p14(ARF) but not CDNK2A in a melanoma-neural system tumour syndrome family. Hum Mol Genet 2001; 10:55-62.
23. Rizos H, Puig S, Badenas C et al. A melanoma-associated germline mutation in exon 1beta inactivates p14ARF. Oncogene 2001; 20:5543-5547.
24. Hewitt C, Lee WC, Evans G et al. Germline mutation of ARF in a melanoma kindred. Hum Mol Genet 2002; 11:1273-1279.
25. Box NF, Duffy DL, Chen W et al. MC1R genotype modifies risk of melanoma in families segregating CDKN2A mutation. Am J Hum Genet 2001; 69:765-773.
26. van der Velden PA, Sandkuijl LA, Bergman W et al. Melanocortin-1 receptor variant R151C modifies melanoma risk in Dutch families with melanoma. Am J Hum Genet 2001; 69:774-779.
27. Wolfel T, Hauer M, Schneider J et al. A p16INK4a-insensitive CDK4 mutant targeted by cytollytic T- lymphocytes in a human melanoma. Science 1995; 269:1281-1284.

28. Zuo L, Weger J, Yang Q et al. Germ-line mutations in the p16INK4a binding domain of CDK4 in familial melanoma. Nat Genet 1996; 12:97-99.
29. Soufir N, Avril MF, Chompret A et al. Prevalence of p16 and CDK4 germline mutations in 48 melanoma-prone families in France. The French Familial Melanoma Study Group. Hum Mol Genet 1998; 7:209-216.
30. Goldstein AM, Struewing JP, Chidambaram A et al. Genotype-phenotype relationships in US melanoma-prone families with CDKN2A and CDK4 mutations. J Natl Cancer Inst 2000; 92:1006-1010.
31. de Snoo FA, Hayward NK. Cutaneous melanoma susceptibility and progression genes. Cancer Lett 2005; 230:153-186.
32. Sotillo R, Garcia JF, Ortega S et al. Invasive melanoma in cdk4-targeted mice. Proc Nat Acad Sci USA 2001; 98:13312-13317.
33. Eng C, Li FP, Abramson DH et al. Mortality from second tumors amon long-term survivors of retinoblatoma. J Natl Cancer Inst 1993; 85:1121-1128.
34. Fletcher O, Easton D, Anderson K et al. Lifetime risks of common cancers among retinoblastoma survivors. J Natl Cancer Inst 2004; 96:357-363.
35. Goldstein AM, Chan M, harland M et al. High-risk melanoma susceptibility genes and pancreatic cancer, neural system tumors and uveal melanoma accross GenoMEL. Cancer Res 2006; 66:9818-9828.
36. Pollock PM, Harper UL, Hansen KS et al. High frequency of BRAF mutations in nevi. Nat Genet 2003; 33:19-20.
37. Uribe P, Wistuba II, Gonzalez S. BRAF mutation: a frequent event in benign, atypical and malignant melanocytic lesions of the skin. Am J Dermatopathol 2003; 25:365-370.
38. Maldonado JL, Fridlyand J, Patel H et al. Determinants of BRAF mutations in primary melanomas J Natl Cancer Inst 2003; 95:1878-1890.
39. Sebolt-Leopold J, Herrera R. Targeting the mitogen-activated protein kinase cascade to treat cancer. Nat Rev Cancer 2004; 4:937-947.
40. Garnett MJ, Marais R. Guilty as charged: B-RAF is a human oncogene. Cancer Cell 2004; 6:313-319.
41. Kumar R, Angelini S, Snellman E et al. BRAF mutations are common somatic events in melanocytic nevi. J Invest Dermatol 2004; 122:342-348.
42. Michaloglou C, Vredeveld LC, Soengas MS et al. BRAFE600-associated senescence-like cell cycle arrest of human naevi. Nature 2005; 436:720-724.
43. Demunter A, Stas M, Degreef H et al. Analysis of N- and K-ras mutations in the distintinctive tumor progression phases of melanoma. J Inv Dermatol 2001; 117:1483-1489.
44. Papp T, Pemsel H, Zimmermann R et al. Mutational analysis of the N-ras, p53, p16INK4a, CD4 and MC1R genes in human congenital melanocytic naevi. J Med Genet 1999; 36:610-614.
45. Jafari M, Papp T, Kirchner S et al. Analysis of ras mutations in human melanocytic lesions: activation of the ras gene seems to be associated with the nodular type of human malignant melanoma. J Cancer Res Clin Oncol 1995; 121:23-30.
46. Chin L. The genetics of malignant melanoma: lessons from mouse and man. Nat Rev Cancer 2003; 3:559-569.
47. van Elsas A, Zerp SF, van der Flier S et al. Relevance of ultraviolet-induced N-ras oncogene point mutations in development of primary human cutaneous melanoma. Am J Pathol 1996; 149:883-893.
48. Davies H, Bignell GR, Cox C et al. Mutations of the BRAF gene in human cancer. Nature 2002; 417:949-954.
49. Solit DB, Garraway LA, Pratilas CA et al. BRAF mutation predicts sensitivity to MEK inhibition. Nature 2006; 439:358-362.
50. Krasagakis K, Garbe C, Zouboulis CC et al. Growth control of melanoma cells and melanocytes by cytokines. Recent Results Cancer Res 1995; 139:169-182.
51. Natali PG, Nicotra MR, Di Renzo MF et al. Expression of the c-Met/HGF receptor in human melanocytic neoplasms: Demonstration of the relationship to malignant melanoma tumor progression. Br J Cancer 1993; 68:746-750.
52. Wiltshire RN, Duray P, Bittner ML et al. Direct visualization of the clonal progression of primary cutaneous melanoma: Application of tissue microdissection and comparative genomic hybridization. Cancer Res 1995; 55:3954-3957.
53. Bastian BC, LeBoit PE, Hamm H et al. Chromosomal gains and losses in primary cutaneous melanomas detected by comparative genomic hybridization. Cancer Res 1998; 58:2170-2175.
54. Li G, Schaider H, Satyamoorthy K et al. Downregulation of E-cadherin and desmoglein 1 by autocrine hepatocyte growth factor during melanoma development. Oncogene 2001; 20:8125-8135.
55. McGill GG, Haq R, Nishimura EK et al. c-Met expression is regulated by Mitf in the melanocytic lineage. J Biol Chem 2006; 281:10365-10373.

56. Koprowski H, Herlyn M, Balaban C et al. Expression for the receptor for epidermal growth factor correlates with increased dosage of chromosome 7 in malignant melanoma. Somat Cell Mol Genet 11: 297-302.

57. Blume-Jensen P, Hunter T. Oncogenic kinase signalling. Nature 2001; 411:355-365.

58. Vivanco I, Sawyers CL. The phosphatidylinositol 3-kinase-AKT pathway in human cancer. Nat Rev Cancer 2002; 2:499-501.

59. Isshiki K, Elder DE, Guerry D et al. Chromosome 10 allelic loss in malignant melanoma. Genes Chromosomes Cancer 1993; 8:178-184.

60. Guldberg P, thor Straten P, Birck A et al. Disruption of the MMAC1/PTEN gene by deletion or mutation is a frequent event in makignant melanoma. Cancer Res 1997; 57:3660-3663.

61. Tsao H, Zhang X, Benoit E et al. Identification of PTEN/MMAC1 alterations in uncultured melanomas and melanoma cell lines. Oncogene 1998; 16:3397-3402.

62. Dhawan P, Singh AB, Ellis DL et al. Constitutive activation of Akt/protein kinase B in melanoma leads to up-regulation of nuclear factor-kappaB and tumor progression. Cancer Res 2002; 62:7335-7342.

63. Stahl JM, Sharma A, Cheung M et al. Deregulated Akt3 activity promotes development of malignant melanoma. Cancer Res 2004; 64:7002-7010.

64. Dai DL, Martinka M, Li G. Prognostic significance of activated Akt expression in melanoma: a clinicopathologic study of 292 cases. J Clin Oncol 2005; 23:1473-1482.

65. Bardeesy N, Bastian BC, Hezel A et al. Dual inactivation of RB and p53 pathways in RAS-induced melanomas. Mol Cell Biol 2001; 21:2144-2153.

66. Levy C, Khaled M, Fisher DE. MITF: master regulator of melanocyte development and melanoma oncogene. Trends Mol Med 2006; 12:406-414.

67. Steingrimsson E, Copeland NG, Jenkins NA. Melanocytes and the microphthalmia transcription factor network. Annu Rev Genet 2004; 38:365-411.

68. Tassabehji M, Newton VE, Read AP. Waardenburg syndrome type 2 caused by mutations in the human microphthalmia (MITF) gene. Nat Genet 1994; 8:251-255.

69. Hershey CL, Fisher DE. Genomic analysis of the Microphthalmia locus and identification of the MITF-J/Mitf-J isoform. Gene 2005; 347:73-82.

70. Huber WE, Price ER, Widlund HR et al. A tissue-restricted cAMP transcriptional response: SOX10 modulates α-melanocyte-stimulating hormone-triggered expression of microphthalmia-associated transcription factor in melanocytes. J Biol Chem 2003; 278:45224-45230.

71. Dorski RI, Raible DW, Moon RT. Direct regulation of nacre, a zebrafish MITF homolog required for pigment cell formation, by the Wnt pathway. Genes Dev 2000; 14:158-162.

72. Takeda K, Yasumoto K, Takada R et al. Induction of melanocyte-specific microphthalmia-associated transcription factor by Wnt-3a. J Biol Chem 2000; 275:14013-14016.

73. Widlund HR, Horstmann MA, Price ER et al. Beta-catenin-induced melanoma growth requires the downstream target Microphthalmia-associated transcription factor. J Cell Biol 2002; 158:1079-1087.

74. Wu M, Hemesath TJ, Takemoto CM et al. c-Kit triggers dual phosphorylation, which couple activation and degradation of the essential melanocyte factor Mi. Genes Dev 2000; 14:301-312.

75. Price ER, Ding HF, Badalian T et al. Lineage-specific signalling in melanocytes. C-kit stimulation recruits p300/CBP to microphthalmia. J Biol Chem 1998; 273:17983-17986.

76. Garraway LA, Widlund HR, Rubin MA et al. Integrative genomic analyses identify MITF as a lineage survival oncogene amplified in malignant melanoma. Nature 2005; 436:117-122.

77. Merlino G, Noonan FP. Modeling gene-environment interactions in malignant melanoma. Trends Mol Med 2003; 9:102-108.

78. Bradl M, Klein-Szanto A, Porter S et al. malignant melanoma in transgenic mice. Proc natl Acad Sci USA 1991; 88:164-168.

79. Kelsall SR, Mintz B. Metastatic cutaneous melanoma promoted by ultraviolet radiation in mice with transgene-initiated low melanoma susceptibility. Cancer Res 1998; 58:4061-4065.

80. Klein-Szanto AJ, Silvers WK, Mintz B. Ultraviolet radiation-induced malignant skin melanoma in melanoma-susceptible transgenic mice. Cancer Res 1994; 54:4569-4572.

81. Sharpless NE, Bardeesy N, Lee KH et al. Loss of p16Ink4a with retention of p19Arf predisposes mice to tumorigenesis. Nature 2001; 413:86-91.

82. Krimpenfort P, Quon KC, Loonstra A et al. Loss of p16Ink4a confers susceptibility to metastatic melanoma in mice. Nature 2001; 413:83-86.

83. Rane SG, Cosenza SC, Mettus RV et al. Germ line transmission of the Cdk4^{R24C} mutation facilitates tumorigenesis and escape from cellular senescence. Mol Cell Biol 2002; 22:644-656.

84. You MJ, Castrillon DH, Bastian BC et al. Genetic analysis of Pten and Ink4a/Arf interactions in the suppression of tumorigenesis in mice. Proc Natl Acad Sci USA 2002; 99:1455-1460.

85. Sharpless NE, Kannan K, Xu J et al. Boyh products of the mouse Ink4a/Arf locus suppress melanoma formation in vivo. Oncogene 2003; 22:5055-5059.

86. Kannan K, Sharpless NE, Xu J et al. Components of the Rb pathway are critical targets of UV mutagenesis in a murine melanoma model. Prc Natl Acad Sci USA 2003; 100:1221-1225.
87. Broome-Powell M, Gause PR, Hyman P et al. Induction of melanoma in TPras transgenic mice. Carcinogenesis 1999; 20:1747-1753.
88. Otsuka T, Takayama H, Sharp R et al. c-Met autocrine activation induces development of malignant melanoma and acquisition of the metastatic phenotype. Cancer Res 1998; 58:5157-5167.
89. Takayama H, LaRochelle WJ, Sharp R et al. Diverse tumorigenesis associated with aberrant development in mice overexpressing hepatocyte growth factor/scatter factor. Proc Natl Acad Sci USA 1997; 94:701-706.
90. Noonan FP, Otsuka T, Bang S et al. Accelerated ultraviolet radiation-induced carcinogenesis in hepatocyte growth factor/scatter factor transgenic mice. Cancer Res 2000; 60:3738-3743.
91. Noonan FP, Recio JA, Takayama H et al. Neonatal sunburn and melanoma in mice. Nature 2001; 413:271-272.
92. Recio JA, Noonan FP, Takayama H et al. Ink4a/Arf deficiency promotes ultraviolet radiation-induced melanomagenesis. Cancer Res 2002; 62:6724-6730.
93. Patton EE, Widlund HR, Kutok JL et al. BRAF mutations are sufficient to promote nevi formation and cooperate with p53 in the genesis of melanoma. Curr Biol 2005; 15:249-254.
94. Bardeesy N, Wong KK, DePinho RA et al. Animals models in melanoma: Recent advances and future prospects. Adv Cancer Res 2000; 79:123-156.
95. Meierjohann S, Schartl M. From mendelian to molecular genetics: The Xiphophorus melanoma model. Trends Genet 2006; 22:654-661.

CHAPTER 21

p53 Protein and Pathogenesis of Melanoma and Nonmelanoma Skin Cancer

Cara L. Benjamin, Vladislava O. Melnikova
and Honnavara N. Ananthaswamy*

Abstract

The p53 tumor suppressor gene and gene product are among the most diverse and complex molecules involved in cellular functions. Genetic alterations within the p53 gene have been shown to have a direct correlation with cancer development and have been shown to occur in nearly 50% of all cancers. p53 mutations are particularly common in skin cancers and UV irradiation has been shown to be a primary cause of specific 'signature' mutations that can result in oncogenic transformation. There are certain 'hot-spots' in the p53 gene where mutations are commonly found that result in a mutated dipyrimidine site. This review discusses the role of p53 from normal function and its dysfunction in precancerous lesions, nonmelanoma and melanoma skin cancers. Additionally, molecules that associate with p53 and alter its function to produce neoplastic conditions are also explored in this chapter.

Introduction

Skin cancer is the most common type of human cancer with the incidence rapidly rising to an occurrence of 1.2 million new cases each year in the United States. Additionally, 1%-2% of the Australian population is affected with nonmelanoma skin cancer (NMSC) annually. It is estimated that about 70% of NMSCs are induced by ultraviolet (UV) radiation, as a consequence of exposure to sunlight. NMSCs, including squamous cell carcinoma (SCC) and basal cell carcinoma (BCC) are the most frequently diagnosed neoplasm. Epidemiological evidence of chronic over-exposure in sun-exposed areas of the body in persons with outdoor occupations have higher incidence of SCC than does a person who works indoors.[1] Additionally, the face, head, neck, back of the hands and arms are predominant sites for development of NMSCs. It is becoming increasingly clear that solar UV radiation is a major causative factor in the development of NMSC and was the first identified human carcinogen. Sun exposure is currently the leading environmental risk factor for the development of NMSC in humans.[2,3] There are several reviews that discuss evidence showing that solar radiation is strongly implicated in the induction of human skin cancer.[4-7]

Lifestyle changes have occurred over the years that have lead to increased UV exposure. Examples include increased outdoor recreational activities, changes in clothing styles and longevity. UV radiation from sunlight is divided into three major categories separated by wavelength, UVC (200-280 nm), UVB (280-320 nm) and UVA (320-400 nm). UVB may have the potential

*Corresponding Author: Honnavara N. Ananthaswamy—Department of Immunology, The University of Texas M.D. Anderson Cancer Center, P.O. Box 301402, Unit #902, Houston, TX 77030-1903 U.S.A. Email: hanantha@mdanderson.org

Sunlight, Vitamin D and Skin Cancer, edited by Jörg Reichrath. ©2008 Landes Bioscience and Springer Science+Business Media.

to be the most damaging due to its higher energy (and shorter wavelength), but UVA accounts for greater than 90% of the solar radiation that reaches the earth's surface. Although UVA is the predominant component of solar UV radiation to which we are exposed, it was believed to be noncarcinogenic or weakly carcinogenic. However, few studies have demonstrated that wavelengths in the UVA region not only causes aging and wrinkling of the skin, but they have also been shown to cause skin cancer in animals when given in high doses over a long period of time.[8-10] More recently, Agar et al[11] demonstrated that human SCCs harbored UVB type mutations in the upper part of the lesions and UVA type mutations in the lower part of the tumor tissue, suggesting a role for UVA in the pathogenesis of human SCC. Interestingly, UVA radiation has been shown to be involved in the development melanoma in fish.[12,13] In contrast, wavelengths in the UVC region are not present in natural sunlight because they are filtered out by the ozone in the atmosphere. Interestingly, UVC radiation although it is more effective in inducing DNA damage, mutation and cell lethality in vitro, it is not relevant to the problem of skin cancer in humans. UVA and UVB are then responsible for DNA damage, sunburn, mutations, immunosuppression and skin cancer. To counteract carcinogenic effects of UV, epidermal cells activate mechanisms that control cell proliferation, DNA repair and apoptosis.

Activation of p53 tumor suppressor protein occurs in response to variety of cellular stresses including DNA damage, oncogenic stimulation, hypoxia, oxidative stress or telomere shortening and directs cells toward cell cycle arrest or apoptosis depending on the amount of DNA damage. The importance of p53 in tumor suppression is underscored by the fact that any impairment of p53 function brought about by direct mutation, reduced gene dosage or by inactivation of p14ARF activator or over expression of MDM2, a negative regulator of p53 is associated with increased tumor susceptibility. However, many of these mechanisms are inactivated once epidermal keratinocytes accumulate mutations in p53 gene. The purpose of this chapter is to provide an overview of recent advances on the mechanism of p53 functions and its role in the development of melanoma and nonmelanoma skin cancers.

p53 Tumor Suppressor Gene

There are multiple genetic alterations that have been shown to have a direct correlation with cancer development. Majority of these mutations can be found within three categories of genes: proto-oncogenes, tumor suppressor genes, or DNA repair genes. A mutation in one of these groups or any combination can cooperate to induce a neoplastic condition. The proto-oncogenes act as crucial growth regulators in normal cell division, while the tumor suppressor genes act as negative growth regulators. The p53 tumor suppressor gene is involved in the cell cycle arrest and activation of programmed cell death.[14,15] Mutations in the p53 gene have been detected in 50% of all human cancers and in almost all skin carcinomas.[16] p53 was discovered as a cellular protein bound to Simian virus 40 T-antigen-bound cellular protein and codes for a 53-kDa phosphoprotein involved in gene transcription and control of the cell cycle by coordinating transcriptional control of regulatory genes.[17-19] Human p53 is a highly conserved 11 exon gene that is located on the short arm of chromosome 17[20] that is about 20 Kb in size. The p53 protein forms tetramers through interactions between C-terminal regions of the protein. These tetramers can then recognize specific binding sites on target genes and stimulate their activation. Mutant forms of p53 rarely exhibit mutations in the oligomerization region, but rather have mutations in the DNA binding domain.

Majority of carcinomas have missense mutations that produce a full-length protein with altered function. Often the other allele is lost resulting in loss of heterozygosity (LOH), which is particularly high (40-80%) in carcinomas of the colon, lung and bladder.[21] In squamous and basal cell carcinomas of the skin, the frequency of LOH is much lower with a higher proportion of both p53 alleles being independently mutated.[22,23] Mouse skin models have shown that standard chemical initiation/promotion protocols results in LOH, where as repeated carcinogen experiments (like UV exposure) results in independent mutations on both p53 alleles.[24]

The p53 protein is a latent, short-lived sequence-specific DNA-binding transcription factor.[11] Upon activation, p53 protein is phosphorylated at one or more serine residues at N- or C-terminus, translocates into the nucleus, binds to the enhancer/promoter elements of downstream target genes and regulates their transcription. About one hundred proteins are known to be regulated by p53.[12] Genes transcriptionally activated by p53 protein induce cell cycle arrest, DNA repair, apoptosis, inhibition of angiogenesis and metastasis.[13-15]

Cell Cycle Control

The wild-type p53 protein maintains normal growth control and genomic stability by enforcing a G1 cell cycle arrest or inducing apoptosis in response to variety of cellular stresses.[3-5] p53-induced G1 arrest allows the cellular repair pathways to remove possible DNA lesions before the onset of DNA synthesis and mitosis, whereas p53-induced apoptosis eliminates potential progenitors of malignant tumor cells.[6-10] The accumulation of p53 protein after cellular DNA damage causes a cell cycle arrest at the G1/S checkpoint by inducing expression of p21$^{WAF1/CIP1}$ inhibitor of cyclin dependent kinases 4/6.[16-18] p21$^{WAF1/CIP1}$ inactivates the cdk-cyclin complex by binding to Cdk4(6)/Cyclin D or E/Proliferating Cell Nuclear Antigen (PCNA). This causes accumulation of hypophosphorylated pRb and sequestration of E2F transcriptional factor, which is needed for cell cycle progression, thus leading the cell into G1 arrest.[16-17] In addition, p53 is capable of inducing G2/M arrest by up regulating transcription of 14-3-3α, GADD45, Reprimo and B99 and subsequent inhibition of Cdc2 cyclin-dependent kinase.[19-23]

DNA Repair

p53 participates in DNA repair by activating G1/S cell cycle check point and allowing more time for DNA repair,[24] and also by inducing transcriptional activation of several genes known to directly participate in DNA repair.[25] An example is of the transactivation is two xeroderma pigmentosum associated gene products, p48XPE and XPC, which are involved in recognition of DNA damage and among some of the factors involved in Nucleotide Excision Repair (NER).[26-27] A third p53-regulated protein is GADD45, which binds to UV-damaged DNA in vitro.[28] p53 can also regulate DNA polymerase β, which is directly involved in DNA repair synthesis.[29]

Apoptosis

An important protection strategy to escape malignant transformation caused by DNA damage is the activation of the apoptosis pathway. The first group of known pro-apoptotic transcriptional targets of p53 includes: Bcl-2 family members, BAX, PUMA (p53 unregulated modulator of apoptosis), NOXA, p53*AIP1* (p53-regulated Apoptosis-Inducing Protein 1) and PIGa (galectin-7), which bind Bcl-2 protein to antagonize its anti-apoptotic function, localize to the mitochondria, induce cytochrome c release and activate the induction of programmed cell death through the Apaf-1-caspase 9-caspase 3 pathway.[30-34] In addition to regulating Bcl-2 family members, p53 may cause rapid disruption of mitochondria through a mechanism involving up regulation of death receptors FAS, Killer/DR5 and PIDD.[35-39] Death receptor activation results in cleavage of procaspase 8 and release of cytochrome C from mitochondria followed by activation of the Apaf-1-caspase 9-caspase 3 apoptotic pathway. Several other transcriptional targets of wild-type p53 exert pro-apoptotic effects utilizing various mechanisms. This group includes such genes as, Siah E3 ubiquitin ligases and *IGF-BP3* (insulin-like growth factor-binding protein-3).[40-41]

Inhibition of Angiogenesis and Metastasis

As normal cells progress toward malignancy, they must switch to an angiogenic phenotype to attract the nourishing vasculature that they depend on for their growth. Over expression of p53 has been found to inhibit angiogenesis through up regulation of Thrombospondin 1 (*TSP1*), Brain-specific angiogenesis inhibitor 1 (*BAI1*), plasminogen activator inhibitor type 1 (*PAI-1*) and some other angiogenesis inhibitors.[42-44]

Alteration of p53 Function Due to Mutation

Normal functions of wild-type p53 are abrogated by mutations. All mutations identified in tumor-derived p53 gene are point mutations in the DNA-binding domain (amino acids

96-292) resulting in defective binding to promoters containing wild-type p53 response elements PuPuPuCA/TA/TGPyPyPy.[13] Acquisition of point mutations in one allele may be sufficient for transdominant suppression of the wild-type p53, since this molecule functions as a tetramer. p53 deficient cells may thus have an impaired ability to execute cell-cycle arrest, DNA repair and apoptosis.[25,47-48] For example, p53-deficient thymocytes are remarkably resistant to radiation-induced apoptosis.[49-50] Epidermal keratinocytes with mutated p53 are resistant to UV-induced apoptosis[51,52] though this effect may depend on their stage of differentiation.[53] Most of the p53 knockout mice show greatly increased genetic instability and develop malignant diseases by month 6 of age.[54] p53 knockout mice lacking one or both copies of the p53 gene are also increasingly susceptible to UV carcinogenesis.[55]

In addition to the loss of functions, certain p53 mutants have been shown to exert oncogenic features due to acquisition of novel functions that confer proliferative advantage to cells sustaining genetic damage.[5,56-58] Some tumor-derived p53 mutants, when introduced into p53-null cells, promote tumorigenicity and tissue invasiveness, increases frequency of metastasis and resistance to p53-independent apoptosis induced by chemotherapeutic drugs.[59-71] We have recently found that UV-induced mouse p53 mutant proteins are phosphorylated at critical serine residues and accumulate in large amounts in cell nucleus.[72]

Induction of p53 by UV and Biologic Consequences

Solar ultraviolet radiation causes DNA damage, photoperoxidation of lipids, protein crosslinking, sunburn, immunosuppression, photoaging and cancer. p53 protein acts as molecular sensor for the effects of UV radiation by mediating cell cycle arrest and apoptosis, or sunburn, in damaged epidermal keratinocytes.[51,73-75] Numerous studies demonstrated UV-induced activation of p53 protein both in cell cultures and in human and mouse tissues.[53,76-82] Studies by Nelson and Kastan[83] indicated that UV-induced DNA lesions, pyrimidine dimers, when accompanied by excision repair-associated DNA strand breaks, trigger p53 induction. UV radiation causes phosphorylation of the p53 protein at multiple serine residues, including Ser15, Ser20, Ser33, Ser37, Ser46 and Ser392.[84-89] Evidence exists for the involvement of ATM, ATR and p38 ERK1/2 and JNK-1 MAP kinases in phosphorylation of various p53 serine residues in response to UV radiation.[90-93]

Excessive DNA damage induced by UV may trigger apoptosis in a p53-dependent manner.[39,51,94-95] Brash and coworkers demonstrated that UV irradiation of normal mouse skin containing wild-type p53 protein induced the formation of sunburn cells (apoptotic keratinocytes) and that p53-null mice were resistant to UV-induced sunburn cell formation.[51] Our studies in Skh-hr1 mice showed that acute UV exposure induces expression of p53, followed by induction of p21Waf1/Cip1 and apoptosis.[79]

An important finding about p53 was the fact that upon UV irradiation, there is an increased half-life of the p53 protein in murine 3T3 fibroblasts.[25] Typically, wild-type p53 has a relatively short half-life, but stabilization and elevation of p53 protein levels may signify early events in tumorigenesis. This information is important when considering that M1 leukemia cells arrest at the G1-S and G2-M phases of the cell cycle when irradiated.[26-28] Additionally, the levels of p53 induction in human skin is proportional to the level of UVB exposure, although there is no correlation to between UVB-induced p53 levels and erythema.[29] Several DNA damaging agents have been shown to induce p53 and growth arrest,[27,30] but only by those agents that induce strand breaks. Pyrimidine dimmers alone do not trigger p53 induction unless accompanied by excision repair-associated DNA strand breaks.[31]

Evidence for p53 Involvement in NMSC

Role of p53 Tumor Suppressor Gene In NMSC

The p53 tumor suppressor gene is involved in the cell cycle arrest and activation of programmed cell death.[14,15] Individuals with Li-Fraumeni syndrome inherit a mutation in one allele of the p53 gene.[32] These individuals have a high incidence of malignancies including NMSC. This data along with observations that many cancers have a mutated or lost p53 gene, suggests that alterations in either pathway can contribute to neoplastic transformation. Inactivation of the p53 plays an important role in the induction of skin cancer by UV radiation. Mutations in the p53 gene have been detected in 50% of all human cancers and in almost all skin carcinomas.[16]

Analysis of mutations in p53 gene has established an unequivocal connection between UV exposure, DNA damage and skin carcinogenesis. UVB and UVC radiation induces unique types of DNA damage, producing cyclobutane-type pyrimidine dimers (CPD) and pyrimidine (6-4) or pyrimidone (6-4) photoproducts.[33-35] And it has been shown that p53 plays an important role in the protection of cells from DNA-damage from UVB exposure.[28,36] UV-induced DNA damage activates mechanisms for removal of DNA damage, delay in cell cycle progression, DNA repair, or apoptosis by transcriptional activation of p53-related genes, such as p21,[37] MDM2,[38] and Bax. Normally, there is little p53 protein in the cell, but in response to UV damage, high levels of p53 are induced.[29,39] With high levels of p53 protein, there is a G1 arrest, allowing the cellular repair pathway to remove DNA lesions before DNA synthesis and mitosis[28,40] and an increase in apoptosis.[41,42] Therefore, p53 aids in the DNA repair or the elimination of cells that have excessive DNA damage.[15,43]

In UV-induced skin cancer, the frequency of C to T transitions is especially frequent at the trinucleotide sequence 5'-PyCG in the p53 gene.[33] There are several 'hot spot' mutation sites with in the p53 gene. Data collected from Pfeifer et al show that of the most commonly mutated sites in p53, five are mutated dipyrimidine in the sequence context 5'-CCG or 5'-TCG (codons 196, 213, 245, 248 and 282). Additionally, they found only 19 5'-CCG or 5'-TCG transitions in the target sequence occurring between codons 120 and 290.[44] Mouse tumors induced by irradiation with UVB lamps or solar simulators have identified a hotspot mutation at codon 270 of the p53 gene, which correlates to a sequence change from 5'-TCGT to 5'-TTGT.[45] Codon 270 of the mouse p53 gene is the equivalent to codon 273 of the human p53 gene, but there is no dipyrimidine sequence at this location. Codon 270 is methylated at the CpG site and UVB produced the strongest CPD at the 5'-TCG. Time course experiments have shown that the CPD at this sequence persists longer than average, which suggests that the CPD is responsible for the induction of this mutational hotspot in UV-induced skin tumors.[46] In fact CPDs are responsible for majority of mutations induced by UVB irradiation in mammalian cells. Using mammalian cells containing the mutational reporter genes *lacI* and *cII* You et al[47] concluded that CPDs are responsible for at least 80% of the UVB-induced mutations in this model.

p53 Mutations in Human Precancerous Skin Lesions

The mutations in p53 gene appear to be an early genetic change in the development of UV-induced skin cancers. Thousands of p53-mutant cell clones are found in normal-appearing sun-exposed skin.[48-50] There is a high frequency of p53 mutations reported in premalignant actinic keratosis (AK) lesions, which are considered to be preSCCs. In an AK study by Ziegler et al,[23] p53 mutations were found at a 66% frequency and a high proportion of them (23/35) were C→T transition. Nelson et al[51] showed that 8 of 15 (53%) AKs had C→T transition in p53 gene. A study by Campbell et al[52] showed that 40% (8 out of 20) of individuals with Bowen's disease carried p53 mutations as well. Many studies analyzed the p53 mutational spectra in Actinic keratoses and found p53 mutations clustering between amino acids 200 and 280.[51] However, SCCs show the majority of mutations in the hot spot region 241 to 280. Since SCCs develop from AK it would appear as if those AKs possessing mutations in the hot-spot region 241-280 confer a clonal advantage toward the progression to malignancy. Hence, AK displays a diverse spectrum of mutations that may result in local, non-invasive, benign proliferation. The process of malignant conversion may select for those tumor cells that have acquired a mutation in the region 241 to 280. Mutations in this region may be either more effective in disruption of p53 function (loss of function phenotype) or confer oncogenic phenotype to p53 due to gain of function. BCCs appear to have a major mutational hot spot region at 241 to 280 and a minor region at 161-200. Thus, the advantage in acquisition of mutation at 161-200 may be specific for development of BCC.

Recent studies on p53 mutation spectra revealed that noncancerous skin adjacent to tumors harbor p53 gene mutations that are distinct from those present in the skin cancers. This provides molecular evidence that only a subset of UV-induced p53 mutations confer cells with malignant phenotype, while other p53 mutants are not necessarily associated with malignant progression. Ren et al[107] has shown that human epidermal cancer cells and accompanying precursors have identical p53 mutations, which are different from p53 mutations in adjacent areas of clonally expanded nonneoplastic keratinocytes. Kanjilal et al[131] in their study of NMSC of the head and neck and adjacent nonmalignant skin samples, revealed multiple but distinct p53 mutations (C→T transitions at dipyrimidine sequences in 30% of missense mutations) in the two areas. Finally, one report[132] compared multiple NMSCs with and without p53 mutations in the same Xeroderma Pigmentosum (XP) patient and found that the former tend to exhibit more rapidly-growing and/or histologically immature clinical features, suggesting that p53 gene mutations would bring more malignant characteristics to NMSCs.

These findings suggested that p53 mutations may be involved in the malignant conversion of precancerous lesions to SCCs and that mutations in p53 and/or p53 over expression may be used as biomarkers for skin cancer susceptibility. Since that, the presence of UV signature C→T and CC→TT mutations in the p53 gene in human and experimental mouse skin cancers has been well documented.[21,22,53-61]

p53 Mutations in SCC and BCC of the Skin

A number of investigators have detected p53 gene mutations in a large proportion of human squamous cell carcinomas and basal cell carcinomas.[21-23,53-59,62,63] Initial studies by Brash and co-workers[64] revealed p53 mutation in 58% of human SCC. Later studies by Ziegler et al[23] and Rady et al[53] have demonstrated p53 mutations in human BCCs at 56% and 50% frequencies, respectively. Interestingly, Ziegler et al[23] found that 45% of human BCCs contained a second point mutation on the other p53 allele. More recently, Bolshakov et al[58] analyzed 342 tissues from patients with aggressive and nonaggressive BCCs and SCCs for p53 mutations. p53 mutations were detected in 66% BCCs, 38% of nonaggressive BCCs, 35% of aggressive SCCs, 50% of nonaggressive SCCs and 10% of samples of sun-exposed skin. About 71% of the p53 mutations detected in aggressive and nonaggressive BCCs and SCCs were UV signature mutations.[58]

Most recently, Agar et al have examined 8 primary SCCs and 8 premalignant solar keratosis lesions for p53 mutations separately, in basal and suprabasal layers of keratinocytes using laser capture microdissection.[11] They were able to detect UVA-type mutations (A:T→C:G transversions) both in SCCs and SC lesions mostly in the basal germinative layer, which contrasted with a predominantly suprabasal localization of UVB-signature mutations in these lesions.[11] This epidermal layer bias was confirmed by immunohistochemical analyses with a superficial localization of UVB-induced CPD contrasting with the localization of UVA-induced 8-hydroxy-2'-deoxyguanine adducts to the basal epithelial layer. The basal location of UVA- rather than UVB-induced DNA damage and mutation suggests that UVA component of solar radiation is an important carcinogen in the stem cell compartment of the skin.

Analyses of mouse skin cancers induced by UV radiation have provided strong evidence for the involvement of p53 mutation in the pathogenesis of UV-induced murine skin cancer. Analogous to human skin cancers, UV-induced mouse skin cancers also display p53 mutations,[60,61,65,66] although the frequency of mutations and the exons in which they occur differ among mouse strains, for reasons that are not yet clear. For example, in our study, p53 mutations were detected at 70-100% frequency in UV-induced SKH-hr1 and C3H mouse skin tumors, respectively.[61,66] In contrast, 20% of SCC from SKH-1/hr hairless mice and 50% of SCC from BALB/c mice exhibited p53 mutations in another study.[60] Nonetheless, most of the mutations detected in UV-induced mouse skin tumors were C→T and CC→TT transitions at dipyrimidine sites, like those found in human skin cancers and most were located on the nontranscribed DNA strand.

Further evidence for the involvement of mutations in p53 on the development of cancer is supplied by studies on p53 knockout mice. Heterozygous (+/−) and homozygous (−/−) p53 mice have been shown to develop spontaneous tumors of both primary lymphoid malignancies and various sarcomas.[67,68] Ionizing radiation can enhance the frequency of these tumors even with a single dose.[69] Interestingly, these mice failed to develop skin tumors. Chemical induction of skin cancer on these mice did not yield an increase in the frequency of papillomas, but there was a enhanced progression from papillomas to carcinomas compared to wild type mice.[70] Since there is a strong association between UV-induced skin cancers and p53 mutations, studies using congenic p53 mutant mice and UV-irradiation revealed that heterozygous mice had increased susceptibility to skin cancer induction and p53-/- mice were at an even greater risk of developing skin cancer. Tumors in the heterozygous (+/-) mice were predominantly sarcomas, while the tumors from homozygous (-/-) mice were mostly squamous cell carcinomas associated with premalignant lesions resembling actinic keratoses.[71] Point mutations in the p53 gene affect the tumor susceptibility differently than allelic loss. Point mutations are generally associated with early stages of skin tumors, while allelic loss enhances tumor development at high levels of UVB exposure and increases progression of skin tumors to a higher malignancy.[72]

p53 Mutations in NMSC of Patients with Xeroderma Pigmentosum and Renal Allograft Recipients (RAR)

p53 mutations have also been found at high frequencies in skin cancers from patients with the genetic disorder Xeroderma Pigmentosum.[55,56] Studies by Sato et al[56] revealed that 5 of 8 XP skin cancers had p53 mutations and of the 6 mutations seen, 2 were $C\rightarrow T$ transitions and 2 were $CC\rightarrow TT$ double base substitutions. Dumaz et al[55] showed that p53 mutations were present in 17 of 43 (40%) skin cancers from XP patients and 61% of these mutations were tandem $CC\rightarrow TT$ base substitutions.

Immunosuppressed recipients of renal allografts (RAR) are also at much higher risk for skin cancer development. Over-expression of p53 protein and p53 mutations has been detected in large proportion of SCCs and premalignant lesions in RAR patients. In one study, accumulated p53 was present in 41% of premalignant keratoses, 65% of intraepidermal carcinomas and 56% of squamous cell carcinomas from RAR patients.[73] McGregor et al[74] has shown similarly high incidence of p53 mutations in nonmelanoma skin tumors from RAR patients and sporadic NMSC from immune-competent patients: 48% and 63% respectively. 75% of all mutations in transplant patients and 100% mutations in nontransplant tumors were UV-signature mutations. Some evidence suggest that arginine/arginine genotype at a common polymorphism site at p53 codon 72 may confer a susceptibility to the development of NMSC in RAR patients.[75] Finally, some evidence suggest a role for human papillomavirus (HPV) and its p53 protein-inhibitory activity in skin carcinogenesis within the immunosuppressed population.[76]

p53 Mutations Are an Early Event in UV Carcinogenesis in Human and Mouse Skin

Mutations in p53 arise early in UV-induced skin cancer[23,50,52,77] and have been identified in normal sun-exposed skin[48,50] as well as UV-irradiated mouse skin.[78] This differs from other cancers such as colon cancer in that p53 mutations are a late event marking the progression form a late adenoma to a carcinoma[79] as well as with melanoma marking the progression to a higher grade malignancy.[80] Noncancerous skin adjacent to cancerous tumors has been shown to harbor p53 mutations that are different from those contained within the tumor.[49,81] Actinic keratoses carry p53 mutations at about 60% with 89% of them UV signature type mutations. This can suggest that actinic keratoses is a clonal expansion of the cells that already contain the 53 mutation. Recent data investigating the role of clonal expansion suggests that it is more involved than hyperproliferation. Brash et al has shown that UV not only can induce mutations, but that it drives clonal expansion of these cells by inducing apoptosis in surrounding normal cells and creating a micro-environment in need of repopulating. Thus, the repopulation is an enrichment for the death-resistant mutant cells. Using a mouse model that over-expresses Survivin, a molecule that functions in suppressing apoptosis, clonal expansion of mutated cells was suppressed due to the reduced apoptotic death of the surrounding normal cells within the micro-environment.[82]

Mechanisms of Clonal Expansion

Murine model of UV-induced carcinogenesis allowed a unique opportunity for investigating the fate of p53-mutant keratinocytes during various stages of skin cancer development. In skin of hairless mice, p53 mutations induced by chronic UV exposure could be detected by allele-specific PCR as early as one week after initiation of the experiment, with 100% animals incurring p53 mutations after eight weeks of UV treatment.[83] Two-three weeks after beginning the UV treatment, clones of keratinocytes carrying mutant p53 can be visualized using immunohistochemical assays.[77,84,85] As a tumor promoter, UV induces cell proliferation by stimulating the production of various growth factors and cytokines, as well as activation of their receptors.[86-93] Repeated exposure of skin to UV radiation therefore results in clonal expansion of initiated p53-mutant cells.[77,84,85] Brash and colleagues have shown that every successive UVB exposure allows p53-mutant keratinocytes to colonize adjacent epidermal stem-cell compartments without incurring additional mutations.[84] Two mechanisms are believed to contribute to selective expansion of p53-mutant cells: their resistance to UV-induced apoptosis and their proliferative advantage over normal keratinocytes in response to stimulation with UV. Indeed, single UV exposure was shown to stimulate the proliferation of p53-mutant cells while inducing apoptosis in normal keratinocytes in culture and in artificial skin models.[23,94,95] However, chronic UV irradiation of skin quickly induces apoptosis-resistance and stimulates hyperproliferation throughout the epidermis as an adaptive response.[83] The mechanism of selective proliferative advantage of p53-mutant cells is yet unclear, but it may be a critical factor promoting clonal expansion of initiated cells.

One mechanism that may contribute to expansion of initiated keratinocytes is the deregulation of UV-induced Fas/Fas-Ligand mediated apoptosis in skin. Hill et al[96] showed that accumulation of p53 mutations in the epidermis of *FasL* deficient mice occurred at much higher frequency compared with wild-type mice after chronic UV irradiation. Authors concluded that *FasL*-mediated apoptosis is important for skin homeostasis and that the dysreguration of Fas-FasL interactions may be central to the development of skin cancer. Ouhtit et al[83] further found that in skin of chronically irradiated SKH-hr1 mice, the progressive decrease of FasL expression was paralleled by accumulation of p53 mutations and the decrease in a number of apoptotic cells. These findings suggest that chronic UV exposure would induce a loss of FasL expression and a gain in p53 mutations, leading to dysregulation of apoptosis, expansion of mutated keratinocytes and initiation of skin cancer.

While patches of p53-mutant keratinocytes grow in density and size while UV treatment continues, they decline rapidly once the UV exposures are ceased.[77,85,97] Remeynic et al[97] showed that regression of precancerous p53-positive clones occurs due to mechanisms other than antigen-specific immunity, proceeding with similar kinetics in the skin of *Rag1−/−* antigen-specific immunity incompetent mice and their wild-type counterparts. Our preliminary results suggest that elimination of p53-mutated keratinocytes occurs due to normal skin turnover.

Both continued and discontinued regiments of chronic UV treatment ultimately result in skin tumor development with 100% incidence, although the kinetics of tumor occurrence is delayed in the later case.[98] De Gruijl and coworkers have used a mathematical model that relates tumor occurrence to the daily dose of UV and the time needed to contract tumors. This model also offers prediction of skin cancer susceptibility depending on the load of p53-mutated keratinocyte clones in skin.[85] Thus these studies suggest that skin cancer development can be delayed but not abrogated upon further avoidance of exposure to UV.

Inhibition of UV-Induced p53 Mutations Protects Against Skin Cancer in Mice

Our studies have shown that p53 mutations can be detected in UV-irradiated mouse skin months before the gross appearance of skin tumors suggesting that p53 mutations can serve as a surrogate early biological endpoint in skin cancer prevention studies.[78,99] To determine whether there is an association between reduction of UV-induced p53 mutations and protection against skin cancer, sunscreen (SPF-15 to 22) was applied onto the shaved dorsal skin of C3H mice 30 min before each exposure to 4.54 kJ/m^2 of UVB (290-400 nm) radiation. Control mice were treated 5 days/wk with UV only or vehicle + UV. p53 mutation analysis indicated that mice exposed to UV only or vehicle + UV for 16 wk (cumulative exposure to 359 kJ/m^2 of UVB) developed p53 mutations at a frequency of 56-69%, respectively, but less than 5% of mice treated with sunscreens + UV showed evidence of p53 mutations. More importantly, 100% of mice that received a cumulative dose of 1,000 kJ/m^2 of UVB only, or vehicle + UVB developed skin tumors, whereas, the probability of tumor development in all the mice treated with the sunscreens +1,000 kJ/m^2 of UVB was 2% and mice treated with sunscreens +1,500 kJ/m^2 of UVB was 15%. These results demonstrate that the sunscreens used in this study not only protect mice against UV-induced p53 mutations, but also against skin cancer. Because of this association, it was concluded that inhibition of p53 mutations is a useful early biologic endpoint of photoprotection against an important initiating event in UV carcinogenesis.

A Model of UV-Induced Initiation and Progression of Squamous Cell Carcinoma

The best-characterized model of carcinogenesis is that of the UV-induced development of SCC, in which mutation-associated inactivation of p53 tumor suppressor gene plays a critical role.[23,36,64,78,100,101] Analysis of data on gene mutations in human premalignant actinic keratosis (AK) lesions, as well as data from the UV-induced carcinogenesis experiments in mice have suggested that the first step involves acquisition of UV-induced mutations in the p53 by epidermal keratinocytes.[23,100,101] This defect diminishes sunburn cell formation and enhances cell survival allowing retention of initiated, precancerous keratinocytes.[23] Second, chronic exposures to solar UV results in the accumulation of p53 mutations in skin, which confer a selective growth advantage to initiated keratinocytes and allow their clonal expansion, leading to formation of premalignant AK.[23] The expanded cell death-defective clones represent a larger target for additional UV-induced p53 mutations or mutations in other genes, thus enabling progression to carcinomas.

Cellular and Molecular Mechanisms

More recent data investigating the role of p53 in UV-induced skin carcinogenesis has revealed other factors that are important to mention, such as the molecular downstream targets of p53: MDM2, GADD45 and p21CIP/WAF1. Murine double minute 2 (MDM2) protein is a transcriptional target of p53 which binds to the N-terminus of p53 to promote degradation through the ubiquitin-proteasome pathway.[102-105] Under normal cellular circumstances, in the presence of DNA damaging agents, p53 protein is stabilized by inhibition of the Mdm2-mediated p53 ubiquination.[106] Growth arrest and DNA damage-inducible gene 45 (GADD45) is a member of a group of genes induced in response to growth-arrest signals and it is a p53 regulated gene that can suppress cell growth. Loss of GADD45 results in reduced nucleotide excision repair activity.[107] p21CIP/WAF1 is a moderator of p53-mediated cell-cycle arrest, by directly interfering with DNA synthesis by binding to PCNA. Its role is largely unknown, but there are two observations to support its importance. First, the p21CIP/WAF1 promoter has a p53 protein-binding site. Secondly, there is a significant increase in p21CIP/WAF1 mRNA following UVR in cells with intact p53, but not in cells with mutant p53.[108]

Calpains are calcium-dependent cytoplasmic proteases that are involved in various cellular functions, including exocytosis, cell fusion, apoptosis and the differentiation and proliferation of keratinocytes. Inhibition of calpains has been correlated with the enhanced stability of the p53 protein suggesting that the calpain system can also cleave the p53 protein.[109] Several studies have shown that calpains cleave the p53 protein to generate an N-terminally truncated protein.[109,110] In vitro addition of calpastatin, a calpain inhibitor, to reconstructed human epidermis resulted in the total inhibition of proteolysis of p53 and an increase in Mdm2 expression, binding and ultimate stabilization of p53 in response to UV irradiation.[111]

Different Mechanisms for Different Tumor Types

Despite similarly high frequencies of UV-induced p53 mutations in BCCs and SCCs of the skin, some differences exist in the mechanisms of their UV induction. The originating cells may arise from interfollicular basal cells, hair follicles or sebaceous glands, thus from a deeper zone than the SCC ones, which probably means exposure to different doses or wavelengths of UV. Some of the genetic alterations in BCC pathway include those in the sonic hedgehog pathway of oncogenic transformation. Patched gene (PTCH) is a tumor-suppressor gene that encodes for a regulatory protein. Under normal conditions, PTCH conveys extracellular growth regulatory signals to the nucleus. Reifenberger et al has shown that 67% of BCC carry a mutation in the PTCH gene.[112] PTCH mutations are more frequent in BCC and are typically UV-specific C:T transitions and represent earlier events that p53 mutations.[113] Additionally, XP patients have more PTCH mutations than sporadic mutations, which may be associated with allelic loss at chromosome region 9q22.3.[114,115] Nonsense, missense and silent PTCH mutations were found in SCCs from individuals with Gorlin's syndrome or a history of sporadic BCC.[116] Besides mutations in the p53 and PTCH genes, a small subset of SCC and BCC of the skin also carries mutations in INK4a/ARF tumor suppressor gene products and *ras* oncogene.[117]

Tumor necrosis factor-related apoptosis-inducing ligand (TRAIL), is a ubiquitously expressed member of the tumor necrosis factor family that has been found to preferentially induce apoptosis in tumor cells, but not in normal cells.[118] SCC and BCC do not express TRAIL while actinic keratoses and Bowen's disease show reduced levels of TRAIL.[119] Additionally, acute UVB does not alter the levels of TRAIL, but chronic UV as seen in elderly individuals shows a reduction of TRAIL.[119]

Nonmelanoma skin cancers are derived from the keratinocytes that lie within the basal and squamous layers of the epidermis, while melanoma originates from the pigmented melanocytes. There are three lines of evidence that show how different p53 mutations are in NMSC and melanomas. P53 mutations occur more frequently in NMSC with 10-90% versus 1-20% in melanoma.[120] Secondly, mutations in p53 of NMSC are generally C→T and CC→TT transitions at dipyrimidine sites and melanomas display C:G→T:A, suggesting an absence of UV mutational influence.[22] Lastly, p53 mutations are early events in NMSC and late events in melanoma.[23] Ras mutations also differ in NMSC and melanoma. While data has shown that H-ras is more commonly mutated in nonmelanoma skin cancer, a mutationally-activated N-ras contributes to melanomagenesis.[121,122]

Melanoma

Association between UV Exposure and Melanoma

While the relationship between UV exposure and basal cell and squamous cell carcinoma is very clear and well documented, the role of UVR in the induction and progression of melanoma remains unclear. The likelihood of an individual developing melanoma is the result of a combination of inherited or predisposition and exposure to environmental factors relevant to tumorigenesis. Melanocytic lesions do not necessarily appear on the most heavily sun-exposed parts of the body, nor do they correlate with occupational or cumulative exposure to sunlight.[123] Regardless, it is believed that the major risk for melanoma is skin color and skin reaction to sunlight. It has been shown that fair-skinned people who burn only and never tan after sunlight exposure have a relatively higher incidence of melanoma as pigmentation is inversely correlated with the incidence of cutaneous melanoma.[124] A history of childhood sunburn may be sufficient to result in the formation of melanoma in later years,[125] while some studies suggest that recreational activity resulting in adult sunburn is associated with melanoma risk.[125,126]

Genetic Alterations in Melanoma

Numerous studies have shown that multiple genetic alterations contribute to the development of cutaneous melanomas as reviewed by Rees and Healy.[127] The high frequency of UV-induced mutations in the p53 gene of skin carcinomas is not seen in melanoma and occurs in 10-30%

of cultured human melanoma cell lines[128-130] and at 0% or 20-25% of uncultured melanoma tissue.[130-134] Similarly low frequency of p53 mutations has been detected in dysplastic naevi (0-16%) and these mutations include CG to TA transition-type mutations induced by UV irradiation.[132,135] This suggests that p53 mutations may arise as early as in premalignant lesions. However, similar frequency of p53 mutations (0-18%) has also been detected in benign nevi, arguing that p53 mutations play an in significant role in melanoma tumorigenesis.[132,133,136] Some studies report that in metastatic melanoma lesions, p53 mutations are observed at a slightly higher rate, suggesting its role in progression toward metastatic melanoma phenotype. There is recent evidence suggesting that genetic alterations in other genes may play a role in the formation of melanoma. These include genes involved in growth promoting pathway, such as RAS and BRAF as well as growth suppressing pathway, such as INK4a-ARF. Despite the overall low frequency of p53 mutations observed, a complex genetic profile including p16INK4a(ARF) + RAS(BRAF) + p53 mutations shows greater correlation with aggressive disease/poor survival than, for example, the p16INK4a(ARF) + RAS(BRAF) profile.[134]

Alteration in Regulatory Mechanism Upstream of p53 in Melanoma

Linkage analysis has identified *INK4a-ARF* as a melanoma susceptibility gene and inactivation of the *INK4a/ARF* has been identified in approximately 20-30% of familial melanoma[137] and 0-30% of sporadic melanomas in which only half contained UV-signature mutations.[138-144] The *INK4a/ARF* locus encodes two independent bona fide tumor suppressor proteins, which function as growth inhibitors and effectors of cellular senescence: the cyclin dependent kinase (CDK) inhibitor p16^{INK4a} and the p53 activator p14^{ARF} (mouse p19^{Arf}). With respect to melanoma progression, several studies have shown similar frequencies of deletions and LOH (loss of heterozygosity) alterations in matched primary melanomas and metastatic lesions.[145-153] Microsatellite analysis has revealed that LOH occurs frequently in uncultured primary melanoma samples at 6q (31%), 9p (46%), 10q (31%) and 18q (22%), while only one of 32 benign nevi displayed LOH.[154] This benign sample was an atypical melanocytic nevus and had LOH at 9q near the *p16^{INK4a}* gene.[154] This finding suggests that LOH at 9q is an early event in progression to melanoma, but that it may not be sufficient for melanoma initiation. Analogous to human melanomas, spontaneous and carcinogen-induced murine melanomas also displayed inactivating mutations in *p16^{Ink4a}* and *p19^{Arf}* genes.[155] Transgenic mice that have a deleted *p16^{INK4a}*, but retain functional *p19^{ARF}* demonstrate melanomagenesis, which suggests that *p16^{INK4a}* acts as a tumor suppressor gene in mice.[156] A higher rate of spontaneous tumor formation (sarcoma, lymphoma and melanoma) was observed in *p16$^{-/-}$* mice over *p16$^{+/-}$* and *p16$^{+/+}$*.[157] Additionally, the highest rate of tumorigenesis was observed in *p16$^{-/-}$* mice with DMBA-induction, which led to frequent metastasis.[156,157] Recently, analysis of a large number of cases for p16INK4a protein expression by immunohistochemistry demonstrated that p16INK4a is lost in melanoma but not in nevi and that metastatic lesions have a higher frequency of protein loss than primary tumors.[145-151] In addition, the thickness of primary melanoma tumors have been correlated to higher occurrence of allelic loss or protein loss.[148]

Alterations and Expression of Targets Downstream of p53 in Melanoma

Apoptosis protease-activating factor (Apaf-1) acts at the effector stages of apoptotic cascade to mediate p53-dependent cell death. Loss of *Apaf-1* is frequently observed in melanoma and is associated with allelic deletion.[158] The associated defect in apoptosome formation can be linked to melanoma resistance to the toxic effect of chemotherapeutic drugs. Murine double minute 2 (Mdm2) binds p53 to suppress its function and results in p53 degradation. Mdm2 expression is correlated with p53 over-expression and neoplastic phenotype.[159] Mdm2 is regulated by p14^{ARF}, which binds to Mdm2 to restrict it to the nuclear compartment.[160] As mentioned previously, p14^{ARF} is often lost in melanoma and in turn Mdm2 is not confined to the nuclear compartment allowing it to destabilize p53 and the p53-regulated apoptosis pathway is abrogated.[161] GADD45 suppresses growth by blocking the progression from G0 to S phase and GADD expression can be either p53-dependent or –independent.[162] The impact of altered GADD expression in melanoma is not fully elucidated, but it has been shown that GADD expression decreases with tumor thickness giving it a prognostic value.[163] There are other genes downstream of p53 that influence the progression of melanoma including, p21, *Bax* and others. For a review see ref. 164.

Alterations in p53 Isoforms p63 and p73 in Melanoma

Two members of the p53 family were discovered to be structurally similar to p53 with similar ability to induce common downstream targets, but with their own unique functions in genome maintenance and embryonic development. For a review see ref. 175. Knock out models of the p53 family members have revealed the individual functions of each family member. Mice lacking p53 develop early tumors of bone, blood and muscle, but have no defects in embryonic development.[165] Knock out of p73 results in sever defects of the nervous system and runting,[166] while mice lacking p63 have sever development defects including truncated limbs and unstratified epidermis.[167] Analysis of melanoma tumorigenesis and progression revealed increased expression of dNp73 isoform.[168] Investigation of melanomacytic nevi, primary melanoma and metastatic melanoma tissues revealed that increased expression of p73 was associated with the progression from primary melanoma to metastatic desease.[169] Two N terminal splice variants of p73 (p73dex2 and p73dex2/3 which lack exons 2 and/or 3 found in full length p73) were also found to be increased in melanoma and this correlated with aberrantly high levels of p73 and E2F1.[168] E2F1 is a cell cycle regulator known to transactivate expression of p73. The role of E2F1 in melanoma progression is yet to be determined. Melanocyte carcinogenesis model has revealed a very specific and limited expression of p53-family response that is different than the expression profile of cultured keratinocytes resulting in biological differences in apoptotic and cell cycle arrest response.[170] This data suggests that the p53 response to DNA-damage in melanocytes needs further study to understand the differences in the cellular response and conversion to malignancy.

Summary

It is well known that UV radiation present in sunlight is a potent human carcinogen. Epidemiological evidence suggested the role of sunlight in skin cancer and both experimental and molecular evidence has shown that UV-radiation is a significant contributor to its pathology. The mutagenic and carcinogenic effects of UV light can be attributed to the induction of DNA damage and errors in repair and replication. Approximately 80,000 pyrimidine dimers per cell are induced in human epidermis in one hour of sunlight exposure.[171] Fortunately, cells are equipped with a variety of mechanisms that constantly monitor and repair most of the damage inflicted by UV light. However, occasional mistakes in DNA repair and replication can introduce mutations in the genome. Accumulation of several mutations in key genes due to chronic exposure to sunlight can lead to the development of skin cancer. The p53 tumor suppressor gene is a primary target of DNA-damage caused by UV exposure that leads to skin cancer development. p53 is a complex molecule involved in numerous pathways as evidenced by the over 41,000 articles citing p53 with well over 3,000 articles published last year. This chapter provides an overview of some of the complex interactions of p53 and skin cancer. A comprehensive understanding of the role of p53 in the pathogenesis of melanoma and nonmelanoma skin cancer is critical step in progressing toward finding a cure or prevention for these malignancies.

Acknowledgements

Supported by National Cancer Institute grants CA 46523 and U01 CA105345, National Institute of Environmental Health Sciences Center Grant ES07784 and The University of Texas M. D. Anderson Cancer Center institutional core grant CA 16672.

References

1. Vitasa BC, Taylor HR, Strickland PT et al. Association of nonmelanoma skin cancer and actinic keratosis with cumulative solar ultraviolet exposure in Maryland watermen. Cancer 1990; 65(12):2811-2817.
2. Rosso S, Zanetti R, Martinez C et al. The mulicentre south European study 'Helios'. II: Different sun exposure patterns in the aetiology of basal cell and squamous cell carcinomas of the skin. Br J Cancer 1996; 73(11):1447-1454.

3. Armstrong BK, Kricker A. The epidemiology of UV induced skin cancer. J Photochem Photobiol 2001; 63(1-3):8-18.

4. de Gruijl FR. UVA vs UVB. Methods Enzymol 2000; 319:359-366.

5. van der Leun JC, de Gruijl FR. Climate change and skin cancer. Photochem Photobiol Sci 2002; 1:324-326.

6. Matsumura Y, Ananthaswamy HN. Toxic effects of ultraviolet radiation on skin. Toxicol Appl Pharmacol 2004; 195:298-308.

7. Kraemer KH. Sunlight and skin cancer: another link revealed. Proc Natl Acad Sci USA 1997; 94:11-14.

8. Zigman S, Fowler J, Kraus AL. Black light induction of skin tumors in mice. J Invest Dermatol 1976; 67:723-725.

9. Strickland P. Photocarcinogenesis by near ultraviolet (UVA) radiation in Sencar mice. J Invest Dermatol 1986; 87:272-275.

10. de Gruijl FR. p53 mutations as a marker of skin cancer risk: comparasion of UVA and UVB effects. Exp Dermatol 2002; 11(Suppl 1):37-39.

11. Agar NS, Halliday GM, Barnetson RS et al. The basal layer in human squamous tumors harbors more UVA than UVB fingerprint mutations: a role for UVA in human skin carcinogenesis. Proc Natl Acad Sci USA 2004; 101(14):4954-4959.

12. Setlow RB, Woodhead AD, Grist E. Animal model for ultraviolet raditation-induced melanoma: platyfish-swortail hybrid. Proc Natl Acad Sci USA 1989; 86(22):8922-8926.

13. Setlow RB, Grist E, Thompson K et al. Wavelengths effective in induction of malignant melanoma. Proc Natl Acad Sci USA 1993; 90:6666-6670.

14. Hartwell LH, Weinert TA. Checkpoints: controls that ensure the order of cell cycle events. Science 1989; 246(4930):629-634.

15. Lane D. p53, guardian of the genome. Nature 1992; 358:15-16.

16. Basset-Seguin N, Moles JP, Mils V et al. TP53 tumor suppressor gene and skin carcinogenesis. J Invest Dermatol 1994; 103(5 Suppl):102S-106S.

17. Levine AJ, Momand J, Finlay CA. The p53 tumor suppressor gene. Nature 1991; 351:453-456.

18. Vogelstein B, Kinzler KW. p53 function and dysfunction. Cell 1992; 70:523-526.

19. Harris CC. Structure and function of the p53 tumor suppressor gene: clues for rational cancer therapeutic strategies. J Natl Cancer Inst 1996; 88:1442-1455.

20. Lamb P, Crawford L. Characterization of the human p53 gene. Mol Cell Biol 1986; 6:1379-1385.

21. Greenblatt MS, Bennett WP, Hollstein M et al. Mutations in the p53 tumor suppressor gene: clues to cancer etiology and molecular pathogenesis. Cancer Res 1994; 54(18):4855-4878.

22. Ziegler A, Leffell DJ, Kunala S et al. Mutation hotspots due to sunlight in the p53 gene of nonmelanoma skin cancers. Proc Natl Acad Sci USA 1993; 90:4216-4220.

23. Ziegler A, Jonason AS, Leffell DJ et al. Sunburn and p53 in the onset of skin cancer. Nature 1994; 372(6508):730-731.

24. Burns PA, Kemp CJ, Gannon JV et al. Loss of heterozygosity and mutational alterations of the p53 gene in skin tumours of interspecific hybrid mice. Oncogene 1991; 6(12):2363-2369.

25. Maltzman W, Czyzyk L. UV irradiation stimulates levels of p53 cellular tumor antigen in nontransformed mouse cells. Mol Cell Biol 1984; 4:1689-1694.

26. Kastan MB, Onyekwere O, Sidransky D et al. Participation of p53 protein in the cellular response to DNA damage. Mol Cell Biol 1991; 51:6304-6311.

27. Kastan MB, Zhan Q, El-Deiry S et al. A mammalian cell cycle checkpoint pathway utilizing p53 and Gadd45 is defective in ataxia-telangiectasia. Cell 1992; 71:587-597.

28. Kuerbitz SJ, Plunkett BS, Walsh WV et al. Wild-type p53 is a cell cycle checkpoint determinant following irradiation. Proc Natl Acad Sci USA 1992; 89:7491-7495.

29. Healy E, Reynolds NJ, Smith MD et al. Dissociation of erythemia and p53 expression in human skin following UVB irradiation and induction of p53 protein and mRNA following application of skin irritants. J Invest Dermatol 1994; 103:493-499.

30. Fritsche M, Haessler C, Brandner G. Induction of the nuclear accumulation of the tumor supressor gene p53 by DNA damaging agents. Oncogene 1993; 8:307-318.

31. Nelson WG, Kastan MB. DNA starnd breaks: the DNA template alterations that trigger p53-dependent DNA damage response. Mol Cell Biol 1994; 14:1815-1823.

32. Malkin D, Li FP, Strong LC et al. Germ line p53 mutations in a familial syndrome of breast cancer, sarcomas and other neoplasms. Science 1990; 250(4985):1233-1238.

33. Setlow RB, Carrier WL. Pyrimidine dimers in ultraviolet-irradiated DNA's. J. Mol Biol 1966; 17:237-254.

34. Mitchell DL. the relative cytotoxicity of (6-4) photoproducts and cyclobutane dimers in mammalian cells. Photochem Photobiol 1988; 48:51-57.

35. Mitchell DL, Nairn RS. The biology of the 6-4 photoproducts and cyclobutane dimers in mammalian cells. Photochem Photobiol 1989; 49:805-819.
36. Smith ML, Fornace Jr AJ. p53-mediated protective responses to UV irradiation. Proc Natl Acad Sci USA 1997; 94:12255-12257.
37. Brugarolas J, Chandrasekaran C, Gordon JI et al. Radiation-induced cell cylce arrest compormised by p21 deficiency. Nature 1995; 377:552-557.
38. Kamijo t, Weber JD, Zambetti G et al. Functional and physical interactions of the ARF tumorsuppressor with p53 and Mdm2. Proc Natl Acad Sci USA 1998; 95:8292-8297.
39. Hall PA, McKee PH, Menage HP et al. High levels of p53 protein in UV-irradiated normal human skin. Oncogene 1993; 8:203-207.
40. Zahn Q, Carrier F, Fornace Jr AJ. Induction of cellular p53 activity by DNA-damaging agents and growth arrest. Mol Cell Biol 1993; 13:4242-4250.
41. White E. Life, death and the pursuit of apoptosis. Genes Dev 1996; 10:1-15.
42. Yonish-Roauch E, Reznitzky D, Lotem J et al. Wild type p53 induces apoptosis of myeloid leukemic cells that is inhibited by IL-6. Nature 1991; 352:345-347.
43. Levine AJ. p53 the cellular gatekeeper for growth and division. Cell 1997; 88:323-331.
44. Pfeifer GP, You Y-H, Besaratinia A. Mutations induced by ultraviolet light. Mut Res 2005; 571:19-31.
45. Tommasi S, Denissenko MF, Pfeifer GP. Sunlight induces pyrimidine dimers preferentially at 5-methylcytosine bases. Cancer Res 1997; 57:4727-4730.
46. You Y-H, Szabo PE, Pfeifer GP. Cyclobutane pyrimidine dimers form preferentially at the mojor p53 mutational hotspot in UVB-induced mouse skin tumors. Carcinogenesis 2000; 21:2113-2117.
47. You Y-H, Lee DH, Yoon JH et al. Cyclobutane pyrimidine dimers are responsible for the vast majority of mutations induced by UVB irradiation in mammalian cells. J Biol Chem 2001; 276:44688-44694.
48. Nakazawa H, English D, Randell PL et al. UV and skin cancer: specific p53 gene mutation in normal skin as a biologically relevant exposure measurement. proc Natl Acad Sci USA 1994; 91(1):360-364.
49. Ren ZP, Hedrum A, Ponten F et al. Human epidermal cancer and accompanying precursors have identical p53 mutations different from p53 mutations in adjacent areas of clonally expanded nonneoplastic keratinocytes. Oncogene 1996; 12(4):765-773.
50. Jonason AS, Kunala S, Price GL et al. Frequent clones of p53-mutated keratinocytes in normal human skin. Proc Natl Acad Sci USA 1996; 93(24):14025-14029.
51. Nelson MA, Einspahr JG, Alberts DS et al. Analysis of the p53 gene in human precancersous actinic keratosis lesions and squamous cell cancers. Cancer Lett 1994; 85(1):23-29.
52. Campbell C, Quinn AG, Ro YS et al. p53 mutations are common and early events that precede tumor invasion in squamous cell neoplasia of the skin. J Invest Dermatol 1993; 100(6):746-748.
53. Rady P, Scinicariello F, Wagner Jr RF et al. p53 mutations in basal cell carcinomas. Cancer Res 1992; 52(13):3804-3806.
54. Pierceall WE, Mukhopadhyay T, Goldberg LH et al. Mutations in the p53 tumor suppressor gene in human cutaneous squamous cell carcinomas. Mol Carcinog 1991; 4(6):445-449.
55. Dumaz N, Drougard C, Sarasin A et al. Specific UV-induced mutation spectrum in the p53 gene of skin tumors from DNA-repair-deficient Xeroderma pigmentosum patients. Proc Natl Acad Sci USA 1993; 90(22):10529-10533.
56. Sato M, Nishigori C, Zghal M et al. Ultraviolet-specific mutations in the p53 gene in skin tumors in Xeroderma pigmentosum patients. Cancer Res 1993; 53(13):2944-2946.
57. van der Riet P, Karp D, Farmer E et al. Progression of basal cell carcinoma through loss of chromosome 9q and inactivation of a single p53 allele. Cancer Res 1994; 54(1):25-27.
58. Bolshakov S, Walker CM, Strom SS et al. p53 mutations in human aggressive and nonaggressive basal and squamous cell carcinoma. Clin Cancer Res 2003; 9(1):228-234.
59. Stern RS, Bolshakov S, Natataj AJ et al. p53 mutation in nonmelanoma skin cancers occuring in psoralen ultraviolet a-treated patients: evidence for heterogeneity and field cancerization. J Invest Dermatol 2002; 119(2):522-526.
60. Kress S, Sutter C, Strickland PT et al. Carcinogen-specific mutational pattern in the p53 gene in ultraviolet B radiation-induced squamous cell carcinomas of mouse skin. Cancer Res 1992; 52(22):6400-6403.
61. Kanjilal S, Pierceall WE, Cummings KK et al. High frequency of p53 mutations in ultraviolet radiation-induced muring skin tumors: evidence for strand bias and tumor heterogeneity. Cancer Res 1993; 53(13):2961-2964.
62. Pierceall WE, Goldberg LH, Tainsky MA et al. Ras gene mutation and amplification in human non-melanoma skin cancers. Mol Carcinog 1991; 4(3):196-202.
63. Moles JP, Moyret C, Guillot B et al. p53 gene mutations in human epithelial skin cancers. Oncogene 1993; 8(3):583-588.

64. Brash DE, Rudolph JA, Simon JA et al. A role for sunlight in skin cancer: UV-induced p53 mutations in squamous cell carcinoma. Proc Natl Acad Sci USA 1991; 88(22):10124-12128.
65. Dumaz N, van Kranen HJ, de Vries A et al. the role of UV-B light in skin carcinogenesis through the analysis of p53 mutations in squamous cell carcinomas of hairless mice. Carcinogenesis 1997; 18(5):897-904.
66. Ananthaswamy HN, Fourtanier A, Evans RL et al. p53 Mutations in hairless SKH-1 mouse skin tumors induced by a solar simulator. Photochem Photobiol 1998; 67(2):227-232.
67. Donehower LA, Harvey M, Slagle BL et al. Mice deficient for p53 are developmentally normal but susceptible to spontaneous tumours. Nature 1992; 356(6366):215-212.
68. Jacks T, Remington L, Williams BO et al. Tumor spectrum analysis in p53-mutant mice. Curr Biol 1994; 4(1):1-7.
69. Kemp CJ, Wheldon T, Balmain A. p53-deficient mice are extremely susceptible to radiation-induced tumorigenesis. Nat Genet 1994; 8(1):66-69.
70. Kemp CJ, Donehower LA, Bradley A et al. Reduction of p53 gene dosage does not increase initiation or pormotion but enhances malignant progression of chemically induced skin tumors. Cell 1993; 74(5):813-822.
71. Jiang W, Ananthaswamy HN, Muller H et al. p53 protects against skin cancer induction by UV-B radiation. Oncogene 1999; 18:4247-4253.
72. van Kranen HJ, Westerman A, Berg RJW et al. Dose-dependent effects of UVB-induced skin carcinogenesis in hairless p53 knockout mice. Mut Res 2005; 571:81-90.
73. Stark LA, Arends MJ, McLaren KM et al. Accumulation of p53 is associated with tumour progression in cutaneous lesions of renal allograft recipients. Br J Cancer 1994; 70(4):662-667.
74. McGregor JM, Berkhout RJ, Rozycka M et al. p53 mutations implicate sunlight in post-transplant skin cancer irrespective of human papillomavirus status. Oncogene 1997; 15(14):1737-1740.
75. McGregor JM, Harwood CA, Brooks L et al. Relationship between p53 codon 72 polymorphism and susceptibility to sunburn and skin cancer. J Invest Dermatol 2002; 119(1):84-90.
76. Purdie KJ, Pennington J, Proby CM et al. The promoter of a novel human papillomavirus (HPV77) associated with skin cancer displays a UV responsiveness, which is mediated through a consensus p53 binding sequence. EMBO J 1999; 18(19):5359-5369.
77. Berg RJW, van Kranen HJ, Rebel HG et al. Early p53 alterations in mouse skin carcinogenesis by UVB radiation: immunohistochemical detection of mutant p53 protein in clusters of preneoplastic epidermal cells. Proc Natl Acad Sci USA 1996; 93(1):274-278.
78. Ananthaswamy HN, Loughlin SM, Cox P et al. Sunlight and skin cancer: inhibition of p53 mutation in UV-irradiated mouse skin by sunscreens. Nature Med 1997; 3(5):510-514.
79. Fearon ER, Vogelstein B. A genetic model for colorectal tumorigenesis. Cell 1990; 61:759-767.
80. Hussein MR, Haemel AK, Wood GS. Apoptosis and melanoma: molecular mechanisms. J Pathol 2003; 199:275.
81. Kanjilal S, Strom SS, Clayman GL et al. p53 mutations in nonmelanoma skin cancer of the head and neck: molecular evidence for field cancerization. Cancer Res 1995; 55(16):3604-3609.
82. Brash DE, Zhang W, Grossman D et al. Colonization of adjacent stem cell compartments by mutant keratinocytes. Seminars in Cancer Biology 2005; 15:97-102.
83. Ouhtit A, Gorny A, Muller HK et al. Loss of Fas-ligand expression in mouse keratinocytes during UV carcinogenesis. Am J Pathol 2000; 157(6):1975-1981.
84. Zhang W, Remenyik E, Zelterman D et al. Escaping the stem cell compartment: sustained UVB exposure allows p53-mutant keratinocytes to colonize adjacent epidermal proliferating units without incurring additional mutations. Proc Natl Acad Sci USA 2001; 98(24):13948-13953.
85. Rebel H, Mosnier LO, Berg RJ et al. Early p53-positive foci as indicators of tumor risk in ultraviole-exposed hairless mice: kinetics of induction, effects of DNA repair deficiency and p53 heterozygosity. Cancer Res 2001; 61(3):977-983.
86. De Meyts P, Urso B, Christoffersen CT et al. Mechanism of insulin and IGF-I receptor activation and signal transduction specificity. Receptor dimer cross-linking, bell-shaped curves and sustained versus transient signaling. Ann N Y Acad Sci 1995; 766:388-401.
87. Rosette C, Karin M. Ultraviolet light and osmotic stress: activation of the JNK cascade through multiple growth factor and cytokine receptors. Science 1996; 274(5290):1194-1197.
88. Bender K, Blattner C, Knebel A et al. UV-induced signal transduction. J Photochem Photobiol B 1997; 37(1-2):1-17.
89. Kuhn C, Hurwitz SA, Kumar MG et al. Activation of the insulin-linke growth factor- receptor promotes the survival of human keratinocytes following ultraviolet B irradiation. Int J Cancer 1999; 80(3):431-438.
90. Jost M, Kari C, Rodeck U. The EGF receptor—and essential regulator of multiple epidermal functions. Eur J Dermatol 2000; 10(7):505-510.

91. Peus D, Vasa RA, Meves A et al. UVB-induced epidermal growth factor receptor phosphorylation is critical for downstream signaling and keratinocyte survival. Photochem Photobiol 2000; 72(1):135-140.
92. Walterscheid JP, Ullrich SE, Nghiem DX. Platelet-activating factor, a molecular sensor for cellular damage, activates systemic immune suppression. J Exp Med 2002; 195(2):171-179.
93. Coffer PJ, Burgering BM, Peppelenbosch MP et al. UV activation of receptor tyrosine kinase activity. Oncogene 1995; 11(3):561-569.
94. Oda K, Arakawa H, Tanaka T et al. p53AIP1, a potential mediator of p53-dependent apoptosis and its regulation by Ser-46-phosphorylated p53. Cell 2000; 102(6):849-862.
95. Mudgil AV, Segal N, Andriani F et al. Ultraviolet B irradiation induces expansion of intraepithelial tumor cells in a tissue model of early cancer progression. J Invest Dermatol 2003; 121(1):191-197.
96. Hill LL, Ouhtit A, Loughlin SM et al. Owen-Schaub LB. Fas ligand: a sensor for DNA damage critical in skin cancer etiology. Science 1999; 285(5429):898-900.
97. Remenyik E, Wikonkal NM, Zhang W et al. Antigen-specific immunity does not mediate acute regression of UVB-induced p53-mutant clones. Oncogene 2003; 22(41):6369-6376.
98. de Gruijl FR, van der Leun JC. Development of skin tumors in hairless mice after discontinuation of ultraviolet irradiation. Cancer Res 1991; 51(3):979-984.
99. Ananthaswamy HN, Ullrich SE, Mascotto RE et al. Inhibition of solar simulator-induced p53 mutations and protection against skin cancerdevelopment in mice by sunscreens. J Invest Dermatol 1999; 112:763-768.
100. Brash DE, Ziegler A, Jonason AS et al. Sunlight and sunburn in human skin cancer:p53 apoptosis and tumor promotion. J Invest Dermatol Symp Proc 1996; 1(2):136-142.
101. Leffell DJ, Brash DE. Sunlight and skin cancer. Sci Am 1996; 275:52-59.
102. Oliner JD, Pietenpol JA, Thiallingam S et al. Oncoprotein MDM2 conceals the activation domain of tumour suppressor p53. Nature 1993; 362:857-860.
103. Kubbutat MH, Jones SN, Vousden KH. Regulation of p53 stability by Mdm2. Nature 1997; 387:299-303.
104. Haupt Y, Maya R, Kazaz A et al. Mdm2 promotes the rapid degradation of p53. Nature 1997; 387:296-299.
105. Giaccia AJ, Kastan MB. The complexity of p53 modulation emerging patterns from divergent signals. Genes Dev 1998; 12:2973-2983.
106. Weissman AM. Regulating protein degradation by ubiquination. Immunol Today 1997; 18:189-198.
107. Korabiowska M, Brinck U, Betke H et al. Growth arrest DNA damage gene expression in naevi. In Vivo 1999; 13(3):247-250.
108. Hussein MR. Ultraviolet radiation and skin cancer: molecular mechanisms. J Cutan Pathol 2005; 32:191-205.
109. Kubbutat MH, Vousden KH. Proteolytic cleavage of human p53 by calpain: a potent regulator of protein stability. Mol Cell Biol 1997; 17:460-468.
110. Pariat M, Carillo S, Molinari M et al. Proteolysis by calpains: a possible contribution to degradation of p53. Mol Cell Biol 1997; 17:2806-2815.
111. Gelis C, Mavon A, Vicendo P. The Contribution of Calpains in the Downregulation of Mdm2 and p53 Proteolysis in Reconstituted Human epidermis in Response to Solar Irradiation. Photochem Photobiol, 2005.
112. Reifenberger J, Wolter M, Knobbe CB et al. Somatic mutations in the PTCH, SMOH, SUFUH and TP53 genes in sporadic basal cell carcinomas. Br J Dermatol 2005; 152(1):43-51.
113. D'Errico M, Calcagnile A, Canzona F et al. UV mutation signiture in tumor suppressor genes involved in skin carcinogenesis in Xeroderma pigmentosum patients. Oncogene 2000; 19(3):463-467.
114. Daya-Grosjean L, Sarasin A. UV-specific mutation of the human patched gene in basal cell carcinomas from normal individuals and Xeroderma pigmentosum patients. Mut Res 2000; 450:193.
115. de Gruijl FR, van Kranen HJ, Mullenders LH. UV-induced DNA damage, repair, mutations and oncogenic pathways in skin cancer. J Photochem Photobiol 2001; 63:19.
116. Ping XL, Ratner D, Zhang H et al. PTCH mutations in squamous cell carcinoma of the skin. J Invest Dermatol 2001; 116(4):614-616.
117. Matsumura Y, Ananthaswamy HN. molecular mechanisms of photocarcinogenesis. Front Biosci 2002; 7:d765-783.
118. Wiley SR, Schooley K, Smolak PJ et al. Identification and characterization of a new member of the TNF family that induces apoptosis. Immunity 1995; 3:673-682.
119. Stander S, Schwarz T. Tumor necrosis factor-related apoptosis-inducing ligand (TRAIL) is expressed in normal skin and cutaneous inflammatory disease, but not in chronically UV-exposed skin and nonmelanoma skin cancer. Am J Dermatopathol 2005; 27(2):116-121.
120. Rees JL. Genetic alterations in nonmelanoma skin cancer. J Invest Dermatol 1994; 103:747.

121. Kreimer-Erlacher H, Seidl H, Back B et al. High mutation frequency at Ha-ras exons 1-4 in squamous cell carcinomas from PUVA-treated psoriasis patients. Photochem Photobiol 2001; 74(2):323-330.

122. Chan J, Robinson ES, Yeh IT et al. Absence of ras gene mutations in UV-induced malignant melanoma correlates with a dermal origin of melanocytes in Monodelphis domestica. Cancer Lett 2002; 184(1):73-80.

123. Fears TR, Scotto J, Schneiderman MA. Mathematical models of age and ultraviolet effects on the incidence of skin cancer among whites in the United States. Am J Epidemiol 1977; 105(5):420-427.

124. Evans RD, Kopf AW, Lew RA et al. Risk factors for the development of malignant melanoma—I: Review of case-control studies. J Dermatol Surg Oncol 1988; 14(4):393-408.

125. Whiteman DC, Whiteman CA, Green AC. Childhood sun exposure as a risk factor for melanoma: a systematic review of epidemiologic studies. Cancer Causes Control 2001; 12(1):69-82.

126. Elwood JM, Jopson J. Melanoma and sun exposure: an overview of published studies. Int J Cancer 1997; 73(2):198-203.

127. Rees JL, Healy E. Molecular genetic approaches to nonmelanoma and melanoma skin cancer. Clin Exp Dermatol 1996; 21(4):253-262.

128. Volkenandt M, Schlegel U, Nanus DM et al. Mutational analysis of the human p53 gene in malignant melanoma. Pigment Cell Res 1991; 4(1):35-40.

129. Weiss J, Schwechheimer K, Cavenee WK et al. Mutation and expression of the p53 gene in malignant melanoma cell lines. Int J Cancer 1993; 54(4):693-699.

130. Albino AP, Vidal MJ, McNutt NS et al. Mutation and expression of the p53 gene in human malignant melanoma. Melanoma Res 1994; 4(1):35-45.

131. Lubbe J, Reichel M, Burg G et al. Absence of p53 gene mutations in cutaneous melanoma. J Invest Dermatol 1994; 102(5):819-821.

132. Papp T, Jafari M, Schiffmann D. Lack of p53 mutations and loss of heterozygosity in noncultured human melanocytic lesions. J Cancer Res Clin Oncol 1996; 122(9):541-548.

133. Sparrow LE, Soong R, Dawkins HJ et al. p53 gene mutation and expression in naevi and melanomas. Melanoma Res 1995; 5(2):93-100.

134. Hartmann A, Blaszyk H, Cunningham JS et al. Overexpression and mutations of p53 in metastatic malignant melanomas. Int J Cancer 1996; 67(3):313-317.

135. Lee JY, Dong SM, Shin MS et al. Genetic alterations of p16INK4a and p53 genes in sporadic dysplastic nevus. Biochem Biophys Res Commun 1997; 237(3):667-672.

136. Levine AJ, Wu MC, Chang A et al. The spectrum of mutations at the p53 locus. Evidence for tissue-specific mutagenesis, selection of mutant alleles and a "gain of function" phenotype. Ann N Y Acad Sci 1995; 768:111-128.

137. Greene MH. The genetics of hereditary melanoma and nevi 1998 update. Cancer 1999; 86(11 Suppl):2464-2477.

138. Fountain JW, Bale SJ, Housman DE et al. Genetics of melanoma. Cancer Surv 1990; 9(4):645-671.

139. Flores JF, Walker GJ, Glendening JM et al. Loss of the p16INK4a and p15INK4b genes, as well as neighboring 9p21 markers, in sporadic melanoma. Cancer Res 1996; 56(21):5023-5032.

140. Piccinin S, Doglioni C, Maestro R et al. p16/CDKN2 and CDK4 gene mutations in sporadic melanoma development and progression. Int J Cancer 1997; 74(1):26-30.

141. Haluska FG, Hodi FS. Molecular genetics of familial cutaneous melanoma. J Clin Oncol 1998; 16(2):670-682.

142. Monzon J, Liu L, Brill H et al. CDKN2A mutations in multiple primary melanomas. N Engl J Med 1998; 338(13):879-887.

143. Gruis NA, van der Velden PA, Bergman W et al. Familial melanoma; CDKN2A and beyond. J Investig Dermatol Symp Proc 1999; 4(1):50-54.

144. Bishop DT, Demenais F, Goldstein AM et al. Geographical variation in the penetrance of CDKN2A mutations for melanoma. J Natl Cancer Inst 2002; 94(12):894-903.

145. Ghiorzo P, Villaggio B, Sementa AR et al. Expression and localization of mutant p16 proteins in melanocytic lesions from familial melanoma patients. Hum Pathol 2004; 35(1):25-33.

146. Talve L, Sauroja I, Collan Y et al. Loss of expression of the p16INK4/CDKN2 gene in cutaneous malignant melanoma correlates with tumor cell proliferation and invasive stage. Int J Cancer 1997; 74(3):255-259.

147. Pollock PM, Welch J, Hayward NK. Evidence for three tumor suppressor loci on chromosome 9p involved in melanoma development. Cancer Res 2001; 61(3):1154-1161.

148. Cachia AR, Indsto JO, McLaren KM et al. CDKN2A mutation and deletion status in thin and thick primary melanoma. Clin Cancer Res 2000; 6(9):3511-3515.

149. Straume O, Sviland L, Akslen LA. Loss of nuclear p16 protein expression correlates with increased tumor cell proliferation (Ki-67) and poor prognosis in patients with vertical growth phase melanoma. Clin Cancer Res 2000; 6(5):1845-1853.

150. Vuhahula E, Straume O, Akslen LA. Frequent loss of p16 protein expression and high proliferative activity (Ki-67) in malignant melanoma from black Africans. Anticancer Res 2000; 20(6C):4857-4862.
151. Pavey SJ, Cummings MC, Whiteman DC et al. Loss of p16 expression is associated with histological features of melanoma invasion. Melanoma Res 2002; 12(6):539-547.
152. Chang TG, Wang J, Chen LW et al. Loss of expression of the p16 gene is frequent in malignant skin tumors. Biochem Biophys Res Commun 1997; 230(1):85-88.
153. Palmieri G, Cossu A, Ascierto PA et al. Definition of the role of chromosome 9p21 in sporadic melanoma through genetic analysis of primary tumours and their metastases. The Melanoma Cooperative Group. Br J Cancer 2000; 83(12):1707-1714.
154. Healy E, Belgaid CE, Takata M et al. Allelotypes of primary cutaneous melanoma and benign melanocytic nevi. Cancer Res 1996; 56(3):589-593.
155. Melnikova VO, Bolshakov SV, Walker C et al. Genomic alterations in spontaneous and carcinogen-induced murine melanoma cell lines. Oncogene 2004; 23(13):2347-2356.
156. Sharpless NE, Bardeesy N, Lee KH et al. Loss of p16Ink4a with retention of p19Arf predisposes mice to tumorigenesis. Nature 2001; 413(6851):86-91.
157. Krimpenfort P, Quon KC, Mooi WJ et al. Loss of p16Ink4a confers susceptibility to metastatic melanoma in mice. Nature 2001; 413(6851):83-86.
158. Soengas MS, Capodieci P, Polsky D et al. Inactivation of the apoptosis effector Apaf-1 in malignant melanoma. Nature 2001; 409(6817):207-211.
159. Polsky D, Bastian BC, Hazan C et al. HDM2 protein overexpression, but not gene amplification, is related to tumorigenesis of cutaneous melanoma. Cancer Res 2001; 61(20):7642-7646.
160. Stott FJ, Bates S, James MC et al. The alternative product from the human CDKN2A locus, p14(ARF), participates in a regulatory feedback loop with p53 and MDM2. EMBO J 1998; 17(17):5001-5014.
161. Castellano M, Parmiani G. Genes involved in melanoma: an overview of INK4a and other loci. Melanoma Res 1999; 9(5):421-432.
162. Bae I, Smith ML, Sheikh MS et al. An abnormality in the p53 pathway following gamma-irradiation in many wild-type p53 human melanoma lines. Cancer Res 1996; 56(4):840-847.
163. Korabiowska M, Betke H, Kellner S et al. Differential expression of growth arrest, DNA damage genes and tumour suppressor gene p53 in naevi and malignant melanomas. Anticancer Res 1997; 17(5A):3697-3700.
164. Hussein MR, Haemel AK, Wood GS. p53-related pathways and the molecular pathogenesis of melanoma. Eur J Cancer Prev 2003; 12(2):93-100.
165. Donehower LA, Harvey M, Slagle BL et al. Mice deficient for p53 are developmentally normal but susceptible to spontaneous tumours. Nature 1992; 356(6366):215-221.
166. Abraham H, Meyer G. Reelin-expressing neurons in the postnatal and adult human hippocampal formation. Hippocampus 2003; 13(6):715-727.
167. Mills AA, Zheng B, Wang XJ et al. p63 is a p53 homologue required for limb and epidermal morphogenesis. Nature 1999; 398(6729):708-713.
168. Tuve S, Wagner SN, Schittek B et al. Alterations of DeltaTA-p73 splice transcripts during melanoma development and progression. Int J Cancer 2004; 108(1):162-166.
169. Zhang H, Schneider J, Rosdahl I. Expression of p16, p27, p53, p73 and Nup88 proteins in matched primary and metastatic melanoma cells. Int J Oncol 2002; 21(1):43-48.
170. Ariza ME, Broome-Powell M, Lahti JM et al. Fas-induced apoptosis in human malignant melanoma cell lines is associated with the activation of the p34(cdc2)-related PITSLRE protein kinases. J Biol Chem 1999; 274(40):28505-28513.
171. Setlow RB. DNA repair, againg and cancer. Natl Cancer Inst Monogr 1982; 60:249-255.

CHAPTER 22

Apoptosis and Pathogenesis of Melanoma and Nonmelanoma Skin Cancer

Peter Erb,* Jingmin Ji, Erwin Kump, Ainhoa Mielgo and Marion Wernli

Abstract

Skin cancers, i.e., basal cell carcinoma (BCC), squamous cell carcinoma (SCC) and melanoma, belong to the most frequent tumors. Their formation is based on constitutional and/or inherited factors usually combined with environmental factors, mainly UV-irradiation through long term sun exposure. UV-light can randomly induce DNA damage in keratinocytes, but it can also mutate genes essential for control and surveillance in the skin epidermis. Various repair and safety mechanisms exist to maintain the integrity of the skin epidermis. For example, UV-light damaged DNA is repaired and if this is not possible, the DNA damaged cells are eliminated by apoptosis (sunburn cells). This occurs under the control of the p53 suppressor gene. Fas-ligand (FasL), a member of the tumor necrosis superfamily, which is preferentially expressed in the basal layer of the skin epidermis, is a key surveillance molecule involved in the elimination of sunburn cells, but also in the prevention of cell transformation. However, UV light exposure downregulates FasL expression in keratinocytes and melanocytes leading to the loss of its sensor function. This increases the risk that transformed cells are not eliminated anymore. Moreover, important control and surveillance genes can also be directly affected by UV-light. Mutation in the p53 gene is the starting point for the formation of SCC and some forms of BCC. Other BCCs originate through UV light mediated mutations of genes of the hedgehog signaling pathway which are essential for the maintainance of cell growth and differentiation. The transcription factor Gli2 plays a key role within this pathway, indeed, Gli2 is responsible for the marked apoptosis resistance of the BCCs. The formation of malignant melanoma is very complex. Melanocytes form nevi and from the nevi melanoma can develop through mutations in various genes. Once the keratinocytes or melanocytes have been transformed they re-express FasL which may allow the expanding tumor to evade the attack of immune effector cells. FasL which is involved in immune evasion or genes which govern the apoptosis resistance, e.g., Gli2 could therefore be prime targets to prevent tumor formation and growth. Attempts to silence these genes by RNA interference using gene specific short interfering RNAs (siRNAs) or short hairpin RNAs (shRNAs) have been functionally successful not only in tissue cultures and tumor tissues, but also in a mouse model. Thus, siRNAs and/or shRNAs may become a novel and promising approach to treat skin cancers at an early stage.

Introduction

The incidence of both melanoma and nonmelanoma (basal cell and squamous cell carcinoma) skin cancers has been raising over the last decades. Since 1985, basal cell carcinoma (BCC) rates have increased by 35%, squamous cell carcinoma (SCC) by even 133%. According to the World

*Corresponding Author: Peter Erb—Institute for Medical Microbiology, University of Basel, Basel, Switzerland. Email: peter.erb@unibas.ch

Sunlight, Vitamin D and Skin Cancer, edited by Jörg Reichrath. ©2008 Landes Bioscience and Springer Science+Business Media.

Health Organization between 2 and 3 million nonmelanoma and over 130,000 melanoma skin cancers globally occur each year. One in every three diagnosed cancers is skin cancer. In USA, every fifth citizen may develop skin cancer in his/her lifetime according to the Skin Cancer Foundation. In Australia, according to a report of the National Cancer Control Initiative (NCCI 2003), the rates for treated BCC and SCC were 893 and 295 per 100,000 in 2002, respectively. Concerning melanoma, the American Cancer Society reported that this skin tumor represented 3% of all cancers and 1% of all cancer deaths in 2005 with a 12-fold increase in incidence since 1935. The lifetime risk to develop melanoma is 1 in 75 in USA and 1 in 25 in Australia. Only 14% of patients with metastatic melanoma survive for five years. Altogether, skin cancers belong worldwide to the most frequent malignancies.

The risk to develop skin cancers is usually based on constitutional and inherited factors combined with environmental factors, mainly exposition to UV light through sun exposure. This is aggravated by the fact that ozon levels are getting lower and therefore more UV radiation reaches the earth increasing the risk for skin cancer development. The WHO estimates that a 10% decrease of ozon level will result in an additional number of 300,000 nonmelanoma and 4,500 melanoma skin cancer per year.

While SCC and melanoma bear the risk to metastasize, BCC does usually not. The reason why BCC does not metastasize but SCC and melanoma can metastasize is still unclear. Therapeutically, it is therefore mandatory to treat skin cancers as early as possible, in the case of melanoma or SCC to prevent the tumor to spread, for BCC to prevent invasive growth. Surgery to remove the primary tumor is the most frequent treatment. Other treatment forms include chemotherapy, cryotherapy, radiation, or topical treatment, e.g., with imiquimod (for BCC). Despite the variety of treatment possibilities, there is a need for more simple and efficient therapeutical options including modifiers of biological responses and gene therapy.

In each multicellular organism homeostasis determines whether cells remain quiescent, divide, differentiate or die by apoptosis. Cell division as well as cell death by apoptosis are crucial to precisely control cell numbers and tissue size. Cancer cells often exhibit defective cell regulatory and apoptotic mechanisms allowing them to develop in an uncontrolled way. The various cancers may make use of these mechanisms in a different way. Apart from the fact that the formation of all skin cancers is a very complex multistage process, the underlying mechanisms are understood in general context, but there are many gaps when looking in molecular details. However, it is evident that restoring the disordered apoptotic and cell regulatory processes may be a new and promising way to cure skin cancers.

Pathogenesis of Nonmelanoma Skin Cancer

Among the skin cancers the pathogenesis of BCC is currently perhaps the best understood one. BCC derives from undifferentiated pluripotent keratinocytes presumably located in the basal layer of the hair follicles. SCC seems to originate from keratinocytes possibly located in the suprabasal layer of the epidermis.

Sunlight and its underlying UVB (290-315 nm) radiation has two major effects, it suppresses the immune response in the skin and it can initiate transformation of skin epidermal cells. Upon UV exposure keratinocytes upregulate the RANK ligand (receptor activator of NF-kB ligand) which induces the proliferation of regulatory T-cells (Tregs).[1] Tregs are then able to suppress the physiological immune responses in the skin. Thus, the immune response is locally reduced. Concerning the transforming potential, UVA (315-400 nm) has been shown to be less effective than UVB. However, UVA, together with UVB radiation, may accelerate carcinogenesis. UV light is known to induce DNA breaks in exposed cells.[2] Most DNA breaks or local DNA damages are repaired by the *p53* tumor suppressor gene which is regarded as the "guardian of the genome".[3] If DNA repair is not possible, the DNA damaged keratinocytes must be eliminated. This occurs by apoptosis (so called 'sunburn cells') and takes place either under the control of the *p53* gene or, as recently reported, via the BH3-only protein Noxa, a member of the bcl-2 family.[4] FasL—Fas interaction has been found to play an important role for the formation of sunburn cells[5] and thus for the removal of dangerously altered cells. Certain individuals have inherited a lower DNA repair capacity and for that reason, not only have a higher risk to develop skin cancers, they indeed develop a greater number of skin tumors. For example, persons with Xeroderma pigmentosum, an autosomal recessive disorder, which is characterized by extreme sun sensitivity, develop multiple skin cancers on sun-exposed parts of their body due to such a defective DNA repair mechanism. The risk of BCC and SCC formation is more than 1000-fold increased in these patients.

Unfortunately, the 'guardian of the genome', the *p53* gene can be itself mutated by UV irradiation. As a consequence, uncontrolled cell proliferation and loss of apoptosis of the DNA damaged cells can occur with the high risk of BCC or SCC formation. Mutations in the *p53* gene are detected in about 56% of BCC[6] and in >90% of SCC.[7] The important role for *p53* inactivation in skin carcinogenesis is further supported by the observation that homozygous or heterozygous *p53* knockout mice develop skin tumors much earlier than wild-type mice upon UV irradiation.[8] For SCC formation the *p53* mutation is a major pathway. Following further solar UV exposure, *p53* mutations accumulate and allow the clonal expansion of affected keratinocytes leading to the formation of premalignant actinic keratosis. Depending on environmental factors and the state of the immune system actinic keratosis can regress or further develop into invasive SCC.

For BCC formation, an additional mechanism beside *p53* mutation is known. Thus, mutations can occur in certain genes of the hedgehog (HH) signaling pathway, the *patched (ptch)* or *smoothened (Smo)* genes which control transcription via the downstream *Gli* genes. The HH signaling pathway is very essential during embryogenesis. It regulates cell proliferation, tissue formation and differentiation but also apoptosis.[9] Although the HH signaling pathway is less important after embryogenesis, it remains active in some adult organs including the skin where it regulates keratinocytic stem cell proliferation and maintenance. Due to its broad activity the HH signaling pathway bears an oncogenic risk if deregulated. Indeed, different malignancies have been linked to overactivated HH signaling. *Ptch* gene mutations were originally found in patients with basal cell nevus syndrome or Gorlin syndrome.[10,11] Basal cell nevus syndrome is an autosomal dominant disorder characterized by the development of multiple BCCs at an early age, of medulloblastomas and meningiomas and skeletal abnormalities. Most tumors where *ptch* is inactivated display a truncating mutation in one allele and deletion of the other allele. In sporadic BCC, 30-40% *ptch* mutations are found. Ptch is the transmembrane receptor for the HH protein family.[10-12] If the Hedgehog peptides are absent, ptch inhibits Smo, another transmembrane protein functioning as a G-protein coupled-like receptor and prevents it to signal. In this situation, the Gli proteins are retained in the cytoplasm being bound to microtubules via a protein complex comprised of Costal2, SuFu and an adapter protein Fused. This makes the Gli proteins sensitive to cleavage through protein kinases PKA, CK1α and GSK-3β, resulting in a c-terminally truncated form of Gli which translocates to the nucleus and acts as a repressor of HH target genes. In the reverse situation, when the HH peptides bind to and inactivate *ptch*, *smo* exerts its activity leading to a hyperphosphorylation of the proteins bound to the complex with Gli. This allows full length Gli proteins to dissociate from the microtubules and to translocate to the nucleus where they bind to and induce transcription of HH target genes (Fig. 1).

Thus, loss-of-function mutations of *ptch* or gain-of-function mutations of *Smo* are often associated with BCC development, because these mutations result in a continuous overactivation of the Gli transcription factors. The direct link between human BCC and Gli activation has also been verified in animal studies. Transgenic mice overexpressing Gli1 or Gli2 in cutaneous keratinocytes develop BCC-like tumors.[13] In human, three Gli genes exist, *Gli1, Gli2* and *Gli3.* They code for large (>1000 amino acids) 5-finger Zinc finger transcription factors which bind DNA target sequences with the last three zinc fingers.[14] They have partially redundant and partially distinct functions, they activate different target genes and presumably act in a combinatorial manner. While Gli1 possesses only an activation domain, Gli2 and Gli3 contain both activation and repression domains. Gli1 and Gli2 are transcriptional activators of HH signaling, some of their regulatory functions are distinct, others are overlapping.[15] Gli3 is a transcriptional repressor of HH genes and is itself repressed in response to HH signals.[16,17] Among other targets, *ptch* is a gene that is

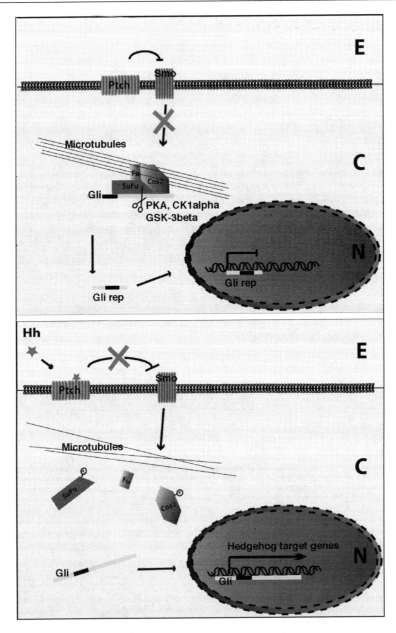

Figure 1. Overview over the Hedgehog signaling pathway inactive (top) or active (bottom). In the absence of the Hedgehog signal peptide (Hh), Smoothened (Smo) is inhibited by Patched (Ptch). In this situation Gli is retained in the cytosol bound to the cytoskeleton via a protein complex and gets processed by protein kinases, giving rise to a repressive form of Gli (c-terminally truncated). When Hh binds and inactivates Ptch, Smo is released, becomes active and signals to the protein complex, leading to hyperphosphorylation of the latter, followed by its disintegration. Full length Gli loosens its hold to the cytoskeleton and now translocates to the nucleus where it acts as a transcriptional activator. (E: Extracellular space; C: Cytosol; N: Nucleus).

transcriptionally repressed by Gli3 which thereby exerts a negative feedback loop of the HH signal itself. High expression of Gli1 and Gli2 is frequently found in human BCCs.[18-20] All available data so far show that Gli2 seems to be the primary positive transducer of HH signaling. Indeed, *Gli1* knockout mice are viable and have no obvious defects whereas *Gli2* knockout mice are not viable and are defective in the very same aspects as HH knockout mice.[21-23] Moreover, hair follicle development is dependent on Gli2, but not on Gli1.[24] The link between Gli2 overexpression and BCC formation is partially revealed and will be addressed below in more detail.

Pathogenesis of Melanoma

Melanocytes located in the basal layer of the epidermis form multiple contacts with keratinocytes.[25] Upon adhesion keratinocytes control the growth of melanocytes and the expression of surface receptors. Most melanomas arise within the epidermis escaping the control of keratinocytes. The progression of normal melanocytes to melanoma is very complex. Melanocytes proliferate and can form nevi. Subsequently, out of the nevi dysplasia, hyperplasia, invasion and metastasis can develop.[26] In this process numerous molecular events are taking place, many are the result of gene mutations.

Mutations of the *NRAS* or *BRAF* genes cause abnormal constitutive activation of the serine-threonine kinases in the ERK-MAPK pathway stimulating melanoma cell growth.[27-29] Blocking NRAS and BRAF suppresses melanoma cell growth in vitro.[30,31] Mutation in the *CDKN2A* or *PTEN* genes is another molecular step towards development of melanoma. In 25-40% of familial melanoma inactivated *CDKN2A* due to a gene defect is found,[32] while *PTEN* gene mutations occur in 25-50% of nonfamilial melanoma.[33] Especially, lesions in the *CDKN2A* gene increase the probability of dysplastic nevi to become malignant. Alternative splicing of exons within the *CDKN2A* gene yields the tumor-suppressor protein ARF (alternate reading frame) which arrests cell cycle and promotes cell death after DNA damage via p53 accumulation.[34] Mutation in *CDKN2A* gene therefore prevents the recruitment of ARF. Indeed, immortalization of cells often occurs with loss of either ARF or p53.

PTEN which encodes a phosphatase acts via phosphatidylinositol phosphate (PIP$_3$) and AKT, a protein kinase B. In the absence of PTEN, PIP$_3$ and AKT levels rise increasing cell proliferation and prolonging cell survival through the inactivation of the Bcl-2 antagonist BAD.[35]

The development, differentiation and maintenance of melanocytes is regulated by MITF (microphthalmia-associated transcription factor).[36] In addition, MITF function leads to melanocyte pigmentation. Mice without functional MITF are albinos because they lack melanocytes. Development from nevus to melanoma is accompagnied by decreased or absent pigmentation.[37] MITF amplification is frequently seen in melanomas with a poor prognosis and is associated with resistance to chemotherapy.[38] In vitro, overexpression of MITF and BRAF transforms primary melanocytes suggesting that MITF is an oncogene. MITF is therefore a potential target for therapy.

Finally, invasion and spread of melanoma are consequences of alterations in cell adhesion. In this context, cadherins and integrins are of significance. Cadherins are important to sustain cell-to-cell contacts, to provide the link with the actin cytoskeleton and to induce signaling via β-catenin which is linked to the WNT (wingless-type mammary tumor virus integration-site family) pathway. Alterations in cadherin expression affects the interaction of melanoma cells with the environment and alters β-catenin signaling. Integrins mediate cell contact with components of the extracellular matrix, i.e., laminin, collagen and fibronectin.[39] Melanoma growth is associated with the expression of αVβ3 integrin which in turn increases the expression of the anti-apoptotic 6cl-2.[40,41]

A comprehensive review featuring the many possible pathways of the progression from melanocyte to melanoma has been recently published.[42]

The question arises why the immune system fails to successfully combat the tumor. This is an enigma because many tumor antigens have been identified on human melanomas, e.g., antigens encoded by cancer-germline genes (e.g., the various MAGE genes) or encoded by differentiation genes (Melan-A/Mart-1, gp100/pMel,17 TRP-1, TRp-2 and others) or antigens resulting from point mutations (e.g., CDK4) (reviewed by).[43] Patients usually build a T-cell response against their melanoma, but the T-cells soon become ineffective. This is most likely due to local immunosuppressive processes at the tumor sites, e.g., by the development of T-cell anergy and by the acquisition of apoptosis resistance of the tumor. The local immunosuppression may also be responsible for the failure of vaccination with tumor-specific antigens in most patients.[43]

Apoptosis Resistance of Skin Cancer

A major feature of skin cancers is their sophisticated way to evade cell death and to prevent their destruction by the immune system. Two important pathways exist. Firstly, skin cancer cells actively defend themselves against immune effector cells via the expression of death-ligands (see below). Secondly, skin cancer cells acquired mechanisms to inhibit the intrinsic and extrinsic cell death program, i.e., apoptosis. In mammalian cells, both extrinsic and intrinsic apoptotic pathways are dependent on the activity of a defined set of enzymes, the caspases. Caspases are proteases with a cysteine residue that cleave other proteins behind an aspartic acid residue. Twelve caspases have so far been identified, among them are initiator and effector caspases. Initiator carnases (8 and 9) activate effector caspases by cleaving their inactive pro-forms. Effector carnases (3, 6 and 7) in turn cleave other proteins within the cell and mediate the apoptotic process. The extrinsic pathway is mediated by death ligands and their receptors all belonging to the TNF- or TNF-receptor (TNF-R) family. Two ligands, Fas-ligand (FasL) and TRAIL and their corresponding receptors,

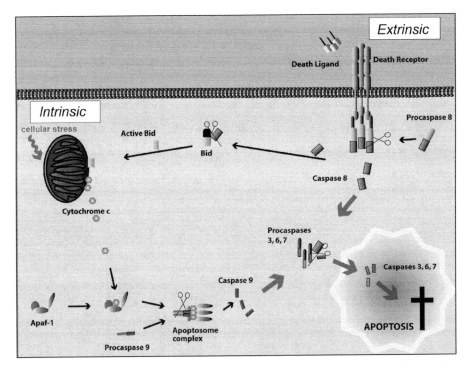

Figure 2. Extrinsic and intrinsic apoptotic pathways. In the extrinsic apoptotic pathway death ligands bind to the death receptors activating initiator caspases which in turn activate effector caspases. In the intrinsic apoptotic pathway cell stress of any kind leads to pore formation of mitochondria and the release of cytochrome c which forms together with Apaf-1 and procaspase 9 the apoptosome complex and activates caspase 9. Effector caspeses are then activated and mediate the apoptotic processes. Both the extrinsic and intrinsic apoptotic pathways are linked by bid, which is cleaved and activated by caspase 8. For details refer to the text.

Fas or TRAIL-receptors (TRAIL-Rs), are of particular importance (reviewed in).[44] For FasL, one Fas-receptor and one Fas-decoy receptor (DcR3) exist, for TRAIL, five TRAIL-Rs have been identified, TR1 (DR4) and TR2 (DR5) are functional receptors, while TR3 (DcR1) and TR4 (DcR2) are decoy receptors. The fifth receptor is the soluble osteoprotegerin, a regulator of osteoclastogenesis.[45] All death receptors have a similar intracellular region, called the death domain (DD) which is required for signal transmission. Upon binding of the ligand, the death receptor is trimerized and its cytoplasmic domain undergoes a conformational change. These two events make the cytoplasmic tail of the death receptor available for the binding of an adaptor molecule, FADD (Fas Associated Death Domain), which then recruits procaspase 8.[46,47] Procaspase 8 binds to FADD via its death effector domains (DEDs). Upon binding it undergoes autocatalysis resulting in active caspase 8, which subsequently cleaves the effector caspase 3 (beside other caspases). Caspase 3 now becomes activated and initiates apoptosis. The intrinsic death pathway is mitochondrial-dependent. It takes place in response to cell stress of any kind including oxidative stress, DNA damage or other insults. This leads to pore-formation followed by disintegration of the mitochondrial membranes resulting in the release of cytochrome c from the mitochondria. Cytochrome c together with Apaf1 cleave procaspase 9 to active caspase 9 which then cleaves and activates the effector caspase 3 with the consequence of apoptosis initiation (Fig. 2).

Apoptosis is a tightly regulated and balanced process which includes different pro- and anti-apoptotic molecules. Inhibition of the extrinsic apoptosis can be mediated by the decoy receptors which block the death-inducing activity of the ligands, or by other apoptosis-inhibitors such as IAPs (inhibitors of apoptosis), survivin or cellular Flice Inhibitory Protein (cFlip). cFlip, a structural homolog of carnate 8, binds to the death domains (DD) of FADD and prevents the recruitment of procaspase 8, thereby blocking caspase 8-mediated apoptosis. The intrinsic apoptotic pathway is executed by the members of the bcl-2 family. Different members of the bcl-2 family can

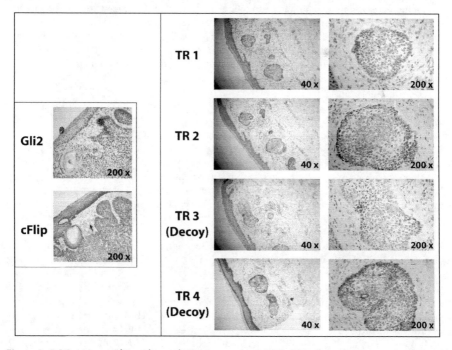

Figure 3. BCC express Gli2, cFlip and TRAIL-receptors (TR). Gli2 and cFlip expression is found in the epidermis layer as well as in the BCC nodules. TR1 is very weakly if at all expressed, whereas TR2 is strongly expressed in BCC. The decoy receptor TR4 is also very strongly expressed in BCC and may compete the activity of TRAIL.

function oppositely. For example, bax and bak induce while bcl-2 and bcl-xL inhibit apoptosis.[48] Both the extrinsic and the intrinsic pathways are linked by bid.[49] Bid, a pro-apoptotic member of the 6cl-2 family, is cleaved and activated by caspase 8. It then translocates to the mitochondrial membrane where it forms pores together with the pro-apoptotic bax leading to the disintegration of the membrane, the release of cytochrome c and the activation of caspase 9. As it will be discussed later, BCC cells increase their apoptosis resistance by controlling the anti-apoptotic molecules bcl-2 and cFlip via Gli2

Most cancer cells have either defective apoptotic mechanisms or actively block apoptosis, allowing them to develop in an uncontrolled way. Therefore, trying to restore apoptosis is a promising approach to treat cancers. In fact, some therapies (e.g., chemotherapy or radiation) already function in this way.[50]

Skin Cancers May Use Death Ligands for Their Protection

Melanoma cells have been found to express FasL,[51] whereas Fas,[52] TRAIL and TRAIL-Rs are not or to a variable amount expressed.[53-55] Melanoma progression has been shown to be associated with downregulation of Fas and upregulation of FasL[56] as well as a decreased expression of TRAIL-Rs.[57] Moreover, lack of Fas expression in malignant melanomas has been linked to poor prognosis.[58]

Nonmelanoma skin cancers strongly express FasL, but not its receptor Fas.[59-61] TRAIL expression has been found by some authors,[61] but not by others.[62] The differing data might mainly arise from the reagents used to detect TRAIL. TRAIL-Rs seem to be variably expressed. In some BCC we found a strong expression of TR2 (DR5) and decoy receptor TR4 (DcR2), but weak or no expression of TR1 (DR4) and decoy receptor TR3 (DcR1) (Fig. 3).

The high expression of FasL strongly suggests that it is used by the nonmelanoma and melanoma cells for immune evasion, by killing attacking effector cells via FasL-Fas interaction. Although there is so far no direct proof for such a mechanism, indirect evidence supports such an assumption. Firstly, immune effector cells, which are as effectors highly activated, express Fas. Secondly, FasL expressed on nonmelanoma skin cancers has been shown to be functional and to kill Fas-positive target cells in vitro.[59,61] Thirdly, infiltrating immune effector cells are hardly found in BCCs indicating that they are not able to invade the tumor.[59] Fourthly, autocrine secretion of FasL was reported to shield uveal melanomas from Fas-mediated killing by cytotoxic effector cells.[63]

Thus, FasL seems to be 'missused' by the tumor cells for their protection as its biological role is clearly a different one. FasL is expressed in the normal skin epidermis, especially in the basal layer and it does not only prevent the influx of inflammatory cells from the dermis, it also eliminates DNA-damaged cells (sunburn cells) which have the potential to transform.[5] Chronic exposure to UV light downregulates FasL in epidermal cells which now lack their protection allowing DNA-damaged cells to survive and to transform into tumor cells. In the unfortunate case that the many other inbuild safeguards are overcome as well and/or genetic predisposition exists, skin cancer may develop. Once formed, the tumor cells switch back to the original epidermal expression pattern, i.e., they again express FasL, this time with the purpose to protect the tumor cells. The molecular mechanism governing this re-expression of FasL is unknown.

However, FasL expression on skin cancers might be an interesting target for future treatment. From a therapeutical view, when tumor cells are forced to downregulate FasL, they might become accessible to the immune response.

Whether skin cancers also use TRAIL for immune evasion remains unclear. TRAIL and TRAIL-Rs are rather considered as anti-tumor agents. Indeed, cancer cells are more sensitive to TRAIL-induced apoptosis than nontransformed cells[64] and TRAIL is mostly unable to induce apoptosis in normal cells.[65] Possible explanations are that normal cells might be protected by TRAIL decoy-receptors which compete with TRAIL-Rs for binding of TRAIL[66] and/or high expression of cFlip and/or high NF-kB activation.[67] Thus, it is rather unlikely that the tumor cells use TRAIL as an immune escape mechanism. Therefore, TRAIL might be therapeutically used. Indeed, melanoma cells are reported to be sensitive to TRAIL-mediated apoptosis provided they express TR1

(DR4) and they are resistant if they lack DR4.[68,69] Whether this also holds true for nonmelanoma skin cancers has not been reported. We found that BCC cells expressing high DR5 and low DR4 were also rather resistant to TRAIL-mediated killing in vitro (unpublished observation). Thus, if the cancer cells express the appropriate receptors or can be induced to express them, they might become promising targets for treatment. Attempts into this direction provide some hope.[70-72]

Attempts to Break the Apoptosis-Inducing and -Resisting Properties of Skin Cancers

As already mentioned, melanoma and nonmelanoma skin cancers strongly express FasL on their cell surface. Using this death ligand the tumor cells may counteract the attack of Fas-bearing immune effector cells, thereby supporting their immune evasion. Thus, it is possible that inhibiting FasL expression may make these tumors susceptible to immune effector cells preventing their growth or even leading to their regression.

Downregulation of FasL has been successfully achieved by RNA interference (RNAi) which is a sequence-specific post-transcriptional gene silencing process using short double-stranded RNA of 21-23 nucleotides of length, so called small interfering RNAs (siRNAs).[73] FasL-downregulation with specific antisense oligonucleotides was also shown to be possible,[74] but the siRNA approach is more efficient. Although gene silencing very reliably works in vitro, its application in vivo is more difficult. One of the largest obstacle of the siRNA technology in vivo is the siRNA delivery into tissues. However, we recently showed that siRNA duplexes can be indeed efficiently transfected ex vivo in BCC tissues paving the way for their in vivo application.[73] Appropriate transfection of human BCC tissues showed that Rhodamin-labeled siRNA duplexes can be detected in all parts of the tissue. Using confocal microscopy, we were able to demonstrate that the siRNA complexes entered the cells within the BCC tissues. Moreover, the transfected siRNA duplexes were functional and induced specific FasL gene silencing of about 70% which is similar as in cultured cells. A disadvantage of this treatment is that the transfection has to be regularly repeated as the siRNAs are used up for their gene silencing job. As a possible solution, plasmids containing shRNA (short hairpin RNA) cassettes could be used. ShRNAs continuously produce siRNAs and therefore maintain the gene silencing process. While this approach shows very promising results in a mouse model (unpublished results), its in vivo application in humans might still have ethical constraints. A similar treatment scheme could be envisaged for SCC and even melanoma at least for the primary tumors, which have not yet metastasized, although this has not yet been tried.

Whether in vivo FasL downregulation alone would make skin cancers susceptible to the immune response and lead to regression is, however, an open question, because it is known that tumor cells are also resistant to apoptosis. Thus, additional treatments may be necessary to overcome this resistance. At least for BCC, breaking the apoptosis resistance seems to be a very promising treatment approach. As mentioned before, in most sporadic BCC the hedgehog signaling pathway and its downstream mediator Gli2 is involved. What is the contribution of high Gli2 expression to BCC formation? In gene chip analysis it was tested which genes are up- or downregulated if Gli2 expression is high. Among several genes two were found to play a prominent anti-apoptotic role, bcl-2[75] and cFlip (manuscript submitted). Thus, Gli2 overexpression leads to the upregulation of bcl-2 and cFlip thereby increasing apoptosis-resistance. This could be proven using a tetracycline (tet)-inducible Gli2 keratinocytic cell line (HaCat NHis-Gli2)[75] but also directly in BCC tissues (Fig. 3). We found, that these cells and BCC cells were resistant to TRAIL-mediated apoptosis when Gli2 expression was high and that downregulation of either Gli2 or cFlip using specific siRNA made the cells sensitive to apoptosis (manuscript submitted). Thus, in BCC a prime target for intervention is Gli2 or the downstream *bcl*-2 and/or cFlip genes. Further strong support for the key role of Gli2 for tumor formation comes from mouse studies where BCC-like tumors showed a highly retarded growth if Gli2 expression was in vivo downregulated (manuscript submitted).

As in SCC and melanoma the Gli-pathway is not involved, cFlip and/or bcl-2 might be direct interventional targets. In most human melanoma cell lines cFlip was found to be strongly expressed[76] and overexpression of cFlip by transfection rendered these cell lines more resistant to

FasL- or TRAIL-mediated apoptosis. Moreover, TRAIL-resistance of melanoma could be reversed by UV-irradiation which was shown to downregulate cFlip expression.[77] Downregulation of cFlip, bcl-2 or IAPs (inhibitors of apoptosis)[78,79] using specific siRNAs also strongly reduced apoptosis resistance of melanoma cells. In head-and-neck squamous cell carcinoma a synergistic cytotoxicity was observed when the cells were treated with cisplatin followed by TRAIL. Interestingly, the synergism was related to Flip-short cleavage, but not to Flip-long cleavage.[80] However, all these experiments have been done with cell lines and not with tumor tissues.

Conclusions

The formation of skin cancers is an extremely complex biological process from which we usually only see rather narrow aspects of our scientific interest. Still, many pieces of the puzzle contributed from various research disciplines may eventually lead to an overall picture. This is necessary for an efficient treatment. There are different therapeutical options already available, but the success rate is still not optimal at least not for malignant melanoma and for metastasizing and advanced tumor stages. Gene silencing by RNA interference may become a new and promising approach. However, two major prerequisites are necessary for its success. The in vivo delivers of the siRNAs or shRNAs have to be improved and to become more efficient and the right target genes have to be identified. While the former is a mere technical and therefore resolvable matter, the latter requires a clear and concise understanding of the biological mechanisms of tumor formation. Our attempts to reverse apoptosis resistance by targeting Gli2 in cell lines, BCC tissues ex vivo and in a transgenic mouse model in vivo provides the proof of concept that such an approach may be therapeutically feasible. Skin tumors which are rather easily accessible due to its location are particular good targets for the gene silencing approach.

Acknowledgements

This work was supported by the Swiss National Science Funds grant nr. 3100A0-111368/1 and the Oncosuisse grant nr. 01630-02-2005.

References

1. Loser K, Mehling A, Loeser S et al. Epidermal RANKL controls regulatory T-cell numbers via activation of dendritic cells. Nat Med 2006; 12(12):1372-1379.
2. Grossman D, Leffell DJ. The molecular basis of nonmelanoma skin cancer: new understanding. Arch Dermatol 1997; 133(10):1263-1270.
3. Levine AJ. p53, the cellular gatekeeper for growth and division. Cell 1997; 88:323-331.
4. Naik E, Michalak EM, Villunger A et al. Ultraviolet radiation triggers apoptosis of fibroblasts and skin keratinocytes mainly via the BH3-only protein Noxa. J Cell Biol 2007; 176(4):415-424.
5. Hill LL, Ouhtit A, Loughlin SM et al. Fas ligand: A sensor for DNA damage critical in skin cancer etiology. Science 1999; 285(5429):898-900.
6. Soehnge H, Ouhtit A, Ananthaswamy ON. Mechanisms of induction of skin cancer by UV radiation. Front Biosci 1997; 2:D538-D551.
7. Ziegler A, Jonason AS, Leffell DJ et al. Sunburn and p53 in the onset of skin cancer [see comments]. Nature 1994; 372(6508):773-776.
8. Jiang W, Ananthaswamy HN, Muller HK et al. p53 protects against skin cancer induction by UV-B radiation. Oncogene 1999; 18(29):4247-4253.
9. Cohen MM, Jr. The hedgehog signaling network. Am J Med Genet 2003; 123A(1):5-28.
10. Hahn H, Wicking C, Zaphiropoulous PG et al. Mutations of the human homolog of Drosophila patched in the nevoid basal cell carcinoma syndrome. Cell 1996; 85(6):841-851.
11. Johnson RL, Rothman AL, Xie J et al. Human homolog of patched, a candidate gene for the basal cell nevus syndrome. Science 1996; 272(5268):1668-1671.
12. Stone DM, Hynes M, Armanini M et al. The tumour-suppressor gene patched encodes a candidate receptor for Sonic hedgehog. Nature 1996; 384(6605):129-134.
13. Grachtchouk M, Mo R, Yu S et al. Basal cell carcinomas in mice overexpressing Gli2 in skin. Nat Genet 2000; 24(3):216-217.
14. Pavletich NP, Pabo CO. Crystal structure of a five-finger GLI-DNA complex: new perspectives on zinc fingers. Science 1993; 261(5129):1701-1707.
15. Eichberger T, Sander V, Schnidar H et al. Overlapping and distinct transcriptional regulator properties of the GLI1 and GLI2 oncogenes. Genomics 2006; 87(5):616-632.

16. Marigo V, Johnson RL, Vortkamp A et al. Sonic hedgehog differentially regulates expression of GLI and GLI3 during limb development. Dev Biol 1996; 180(1):273-283.
17. Lee J, Platt KA, Censullo P et al. Gli1 is a target of Sonic hedgehog that induces ventral neural tube development. Development 1997; 124(13):2537-2552.
18. Dahmane N, Lee J, Robins P et al. Activation of the transcription factor Gli1 and the Sonic hedgehog signalling pathway in skin tumours. Nature 1997; 389(6653):876-881.
19. Nilsson M, Unden AB, Krause D et al. Induction of basal cell carcinomas and trichoepitheliomas in mice overexpressing GLI-1. Proc Natl Acad Sci USA 2000; 97(7):3438-3443.
20. Sheng H, Goich S, Wang A et al. Dissecting the oncogenic potential of Gli:2 deletion of an NH(2)-terminal fragment alters skin tumor phenotype. Cancer Res 2002; 62(18):5308-5316.
21. Chiang C, Litingtung Y, Lee E et al. Cyclopia and defective axial patterning in mice lacking Sonic hedgehog gene function. Nature 1996; 383(6599):407-413.
22. Ding Q, Motoyama J, Gasca S et al. Diminished Sonic hedgehog signaling and lack of floor plate differentiation in Gli2 mutant mice. Development 1998; 125(14):2533-2543.
23. Park HL, Bai C, Platt KA et al. Mouse Gli1 mutants are viable but have defects in SHH signaling in combination with a Gli2 mutation. Development 2000; 127(8):1593-1605.
24. Mill P, Mo R, Fu H et al. Sonic hedgehog-dependent activation of Gli2 is essential for embryonic hair follicle development. Genes Dev 2003; 17(2):282-294.
25. Haass NK, Smalley KS, Li L et al. Adhesion, migration and communication in melanocytes and melanoma. Pigment Cell Res 2005; 18(3):150-159.
26. Clark WH, Jr., Elder DE, Guerry Dt et al. A study of tumor progression: the precursor lesions of superficial spreading and nodular melanoma. Hum Pathol 1984; 15(12):1147-1165.
27. Albino AP, Nanus DM, Mentle IR et al. Analysis of ras oncogenes in malignant melanoma and precursor lesions: correlation of point mutations with differentiation phenotype. Oncogene 1989; 4(11):1363-1374.
28. Davies H, Bignell GR, Cox C, et al. Mutations of the BRAF gene in human cancer. Nature 2002; 417(6892):949-954.
29. Omholt K, Platz A, Kanter L et al. NRAS and BRAF mutations arise early during melanoma pathogenesis and are preserved throughout tumor progression. Clin Cancer Res 2003; 9(17):6483-6488.
30. Eskandarpour M, Kiaii S, Zhu C et al. Suppression of oncogenic NRAS by RNA interference induces apoptosis of human melanoma cells. Int J Cancer 2005; 115(1):65-73.
31. Hingorani SR, Jacobetz MA, Robertson GP et al. Suppression of BRAF(V599E) in human melanoma abrogates transformation. Cancer Res 2003; 63(17):5198-5202.
32. Thompson JF, Scolyer RA, Kefford RF. Cutaneous melanoma. Lancet 2005; 365(9460):687-701.
33. Wu H, Goel V, Haluska FG. PTEN signaling pathways in melanoma. Oncogene 2003; 22(20):3113-3122.
34. Sharpless E, Chin L. The INK4a/ARF locus and melanoma. Oncogene 2003; 22(20):3092-3098.
35. Cantley LC, Neel BG. New insights into tumor suppression: PTEN suppresses tumor formation by restraining the phosphoinositide 3-kinase/AKT pathway. Proc Natl Acad Sci USA 1999; 96(8):4240-4245.
36. Hodgkinson CA, Moore KJ, Nakayama A et al. Mutations at the mouse microphthalmia locus are associated with defects in a gene encoding a novel basic-helix-loop-helix-zipper protein. Cell 1993; 74(2):395-404.
37. Salti GI, Manougian T, Farolan M et al. Micropthalmia transcription factor: a new prognostic marker in intermediate-thickness cutaneous malignant melanoma. Cancer Res 2000; 60(18):5012-5016.
38. Garraway LA, Widlund HR, Rubin MA et al. Integrative genomic analyses identify MITF as a lineage survival oncogene amplified in malignant melanoma. Nature 2005; 436(7047):117-122.
39. Kuphal S, Bauer R, Bosserhoff AK. Integrin signaling in malignant melanoma. Cancer Metastasis Rev 2005; 24(2):195-222.
40. Danen EH, Ten Berge PJ, Van Muijen GN et al. Emergence of alpha 5 beta 1 fibronectin- and alpha v beta 3 vitronectin-receptor expression in melanocytic tumour progression. Histopathology 1994; 24(3):249-256.
41. Petitclerc E, Stromblad S, von Schalscha TL et al. Integrin alpha(v)beta3 promotes M21 melanoma growth in human skin by regulating tumor cell survival. Cancer Res 1999; 59(11):2724-2730.
42. Miller AJ, Mihm Jr MC. Melanoma. N Engl J Med 2006; 355(1):51-65.
43. Boon T, Coulie PG, Van den Eynde BJ et al. Human T-cell responses against melanoma. Annu Rev Immunol 2006; 24:175-208.
44. Bhardwaj A, Aggarwal BB. Receptor-mediated choreography of life and death. J Clin Immunol 2003; 23(5):317-332.
45. Emery JG, McDonnell P, Burke MB et al. Osteoprotegerin is a receptor for the cytotoxic ligand TRAIL. J Biol Chem 1998; 273(23):14363-14367.

46. Nagata S. Fas ligand-induced apoptosis. Annu Rev Genet 1999; 33:29-55.
47. Krammer PH. CD95's deadly mission in the immune system. Nature 2000; 407(6805):789-795.
48. Kirkin V, Joos S, Zornig M. The role of Bcl-2 family members in tumorigenesis. Biochim Biophys Acta 2004; 1644(2-3):229-249.
49. Li HL, Zhu H, Xu CJ et al. Cleavage of BID by caspase 8 mediates the mitochondrial damage in the Fas pathway of apoptosis. Cell 1998; 94(4):491-501.
50. Friesen C, Fulda S, Debatin KM. Cytotoxic drugs and the CD95 pathway. Leukemia 1999; 13(11):1854-1858.
51. Hahne M, Rimoldi D, Schroter M et al. Melanoma cell expression of Fas(Apo-1/CD95) ligand: implications for tumor immune escape [see comments]. Science 1996; 274(5291):1363-1366.
52. Igney FH, Krammer PH. Death and anti-death: Tumor resistance to apoptosis. Nat Rev Cancer 2002; 2(4):277-288.
53. Griffith TS, Chin WA, Jackson GC et al. Intracellular regulation of TRAIL-induced apoptosis in human melanoma cells. J Immunol 1998; 161(6):2833-2840.
54. Zhang XD, Franco A, Myers K et al. Relation of TNF-related apoptosis-inducing ligand (TRAIL) receptor and FLICE-inhibitory protein expression to TRAIL-induced apoptosis of melanoma. Cancer Res 1999; 59(11):2747-2753.
55. McCarthy MM, DiVito KA, Sznol M et al. Expression of Tumor Necrosis Factor-Related Apoptosis-Inducing Ligand Receptors 1 and 2 in Melanoma. Clin Cancer Res 2006; 12(12):3856-3863.
56. Soubrane C, Mouawad R, Antoine EC et al. A comparative study of Fas and Fas-ligand expression during melanoma progression. Brit J Dermatol 2000; 143(2):307-312.
57. Zhuang L, Lee CS, Scolyer RA et al. Progression in melanoma is associated with decreased expression of death receptors for tumor necrosis factor-related apoptosis-inducing ligand. Human Pathology 2006; 37(10):1286-1294.
58. Helmbach H, Rossmann E, Kern MA et al. Drug-resistance in human melanoma. Int J Cancer 2001; 93(5):617-622.
59. Buechner SA, Wernli M, Harr T et al. Regression of basal cell carcinoma by intralesional interferon-alpha treatment is mediated by CD95 (Apo-1/Fas)-CD95 ligand-induced suicide. J Clin Invest 1997; 100(11):2691-2696.
60. GutierrezSteil C, WroneSmith T, Sun XM et al. Sunlight-induced basal cell carcinoma tumor cells and ultraviolet-B-irradiated psoriatic plaques express Fas ligand (CD95L). J Clin Invest 1998; 101(1):33-39.
61. Bachmann F, Buechner SA, Wernli M et al. Ultraviolet light downregulates CD95 ligand and trail receptor expression facilitating actinic keratosis and squamous cell carcinoma formation. J Invest Dermatol 2001; 117(1):59-66.
62. Stander S, Schwarz T. Tumor necrosis factor-related apoptosis-inducing ligand (TRAIL) is expressed in normal skin and cutaneous inflammatory diseases, but not in chronically UV-exposed skin and nonmelanoma skin cancer. Am J Dermatopathol 2005; 27(2):116-121.
63. Hallermalm K, De Geer A, Kiessling R et al. Secretion of Fas Ligand Shields Tumor Cells from Fas-Mediated Killing by Cytotoxic Lymphocytes. Cancer Res 2004; 64(18):6775-6782.
64. Ashkenazi A, Dixit VM. Apoptosis control by death and decoy receptors. Curr Opin Cell Biol 1999; 11(2):255-260.
65. LeBlanc HN, Ashkenazi A. Apo2L/TRAIL and its death and decoy receptors. Cell Death Differentiation 2003; 10(1):66-75.
66. Zhang XD, Nguyen T, Thomas WD et al. Mechanisms of resistance of normal cells to TRAIL induced apoptosis vary between different cell types. Febs Lett 2000; 482(3):193-199.
67. Schneider P, Thome M, Burns K et al. TRAIL receptors 1 (DR4) and 2 (DR5) signal FADD-dependent apoptosis and activate NF-kappa B. Immunity 1997; 7(6):831-836.
68. Kim K, Fisher MJ, Xu SQ et al. Molecular determinants of response to TRAIL in killing of normal and cancer cells. Clin Cancer Res 2000; 6(2):335-346.
69. Kurbanov BM, Fecker LF, Geilen CC et al. Resistance of melanoma cells to TRAIL does not result from upregulation of antiapoptotic proteins by NF-[kappa]B but is related to downregulation of initiator caspases and DR4. Oncogene 2006.
70. Thomas WD, Hersey P. TNF-related apoptosis-inducing ligand (TRAIL) induces apoptosis in Fas ligand-resistant melanoma cells and mediates CD4 T-cell killing of target cells. J Immunol 1998; 161(5):2195-2200.
71. Walczak H, Miller RE, Ariail K et al. Tumoricidal activity of tumor necrosis factor-related apoptosis-inducing ligand in vivo [see comments]. Nat Med 1999; 5(2):157-163.
72. Kagawa S, He C, Gu J et al. Antitumor activity and bystander effects of the tumor necrosis factor-related apoptosis-inducing ligand (TRAIL) gene. Cancer Res 2001; 61(8):3330-3338.
73. Ji J, Wernli M, Mielgo A et al. Fas-ligand gene silencing in basal cell carcinoma tissue with small interfering RNA. Gene Ther 2005; 12(8):678-684.

74. Ji J, Wernli M, Buechner S et al. Fas ligand downregulation with antisense oligonucleotides in cells and in cultured tissues of normal skin epidermis and basal cell carcinoma. J Invest Dermatol 2003; 120(6):1094-1099.
75. Regl G, Kasper M, Schnidar H et al. Activation of the BCL2 promoter in response to Hedgehog/GLI signal transduction is predominantly mediated by GLI2. Cancer Res 2004; 64(21):7724-7731.
76. Bullani RR, Huard B, Viard-Leveugle I et al. Selective Expression of FLIP in Malignant Melanocytic Skin Lesions 2001; 117(2):360-364.
77. Zeise E, Weichenthal M, Schwarz T et al. Resistance of Human Melanoma Cells Against the Death Ligand TRAIL Is Reversed by Ultraviolet-B Radiation via Downregulation of FLIP. J Investig Dermatol 2004; 123(4):746-754.
78. Chawla-Sarkar M, Bae SI, Reu FJ et al. Downregulation of Bcl-2, FLIP or IAPs (XIAP and survivin) by siRNAs sensitizes resistant melanoma cells to Apo2L/TRAIL-induced apoptosis. Cell Death Differ 2004; 11(8):915-923.
79. Ivanov VN, Hei TK. Sodium arsenite accelerates TRAIL-mediated apoptosis in melanoma cells through upregulation of TRAIL-R1/R2 surface levels and downregulation of cFLIP expression. Experimental Cell Research 2006; 312(20):4120-4138.
80. Young-Ho Kim YJL. Time sequence of tumor necrosis factor-related apoptosis-inducing ligand (TRAIL) and cisplatin treatment is responsible for a complex pattern of synergistic cytotoxicity. Journal of Cellular Biochemistry 2006; 98(5):1284-1295.

CHAPTER 23

Treatment of Melanoma and Nonmelanoma Skin Cancer

Knuth Rass* and Wolfgang Tilgen

Abstract

The incidence of skin cancer is increasing in Caucasian populations worldwide. Treatment approaches for Nonmelanoma skin cancer (NMSC) are predominantly curative and surgery can be regarded as standard of care. Nevertheless, novel and less invasive topical therapy modalities like photodynamic therapy or local immune modifiers are in progress.

In contrast to NMSC, the mortality of melanoma has not changed considerably over the last years and decades. Melanoma survival mainly depends on primary tumor thickness underlining the importance of primary and secondary prevention by avoidance or early detection of the disease. The chance to cure melanoma patients is steadily decreasing with tumor stage. As the prognosis in distant metastatic disease is still poor, except for single situations therapy approaches are palliative and accompanied by an optimal supportive care of the patients concerned. Albeit removal of localized metastases is currently the most effective approach in metastatic melanoma, chemo- and chemoimmunotherapy has to be regarded as standard treatment in most of the cases.

Novel and promising therapeutic options accrue from growing insights in tumor biology and immunology. Not only in melanoma, development and application of targeted therapies currently attract the most attention in the treatment of advanced tumors. First clinical experiences with those antiproliferative, antiangiogenic and proapoptotic agents reveal only moderate antitumoral activity in melanoma, so that future efforts aim at defining more effective combination strategies using chemo-, targeted and vaccination therapy approaches.

Melanoma

Introduction

The incidence of malignant melanoma in Caucasian populations is steadily increasing worldwide, whereas mortality is leveling off. This phenomenon is explained by a decrease of the mean tumor thickness and probably a success from information and prevention strategies.[1] Once a melanoma has developed, survival mainly depends on Breslow's tumor thickness and the occurrence of regional or distant metastases (Table 1).[2] Therefore the most crucial requirement to cure the disease is early detection of thin primary tumors.

The treatment modalities of melanoma can be subdivided into surgical procedures, adjuvant and palliative therapy approaches.

*Corresponding Author: Knuth Rass—Clinic for Dermatology, Venerology and Allergology, The Saarland University Hospital, 66421 Homburg/Saar, Germany. Email: knuth.rass@uks.eu

Sunlight, Vitamin D and Skin Cancer, edited by Jörg Reichrath. ©2008 Landes Bioscience and Springer Science+Business Media.

Table 1. *Melanoma survival rates depending on AJCC classification[11]*

Pathologic Stage	TNM	Breslow-Thickness	Ulceration	No. of Pos. Nodes	Nodal Size	Distant Metastases	5-Year-Survival
IA	T1a	≤1 mm	No	–	–	–	95%
IB	T1b	≤1 mm	Yes or Level IV,V	–	–	–	91%
	T2a	1.01-2.0 mm	No	–	–	–	89%
IIA	T2b	1.01-2.0 mm	Yes	–	–	–	77%
	T3a	2.01-4.0 mm	No	–	–	–	79%
IIB	T3b	2.01-4.0 mm	Yes	–	–	–	63%
	T4a	>4.0 mm	No	–	–	–	67%
IIC	T4b	>4.0 mm	Yes	–	–	–	45%
IIIA	N1a	Any	No	1	Micro	–	70%
	N2a	Any	No	2-3	Micro	–	63%
IIIB	N1a	Any	Yes	1	Micro	–	53%
	N2a	Any	Yes	2-3	Micro	–	50%
	N1b	Any	No	1	Macro	–	59%
	N2b	Any	No	2-3	Macro	–	46%
IIIC	N1b	Any	Yes	1	Macro	–	29%
	N2b	Any	Yes	2-3	Macro	–	24%
	N3	Any	Any	>3	Any	–	27%
IV	M1a	Any	Any	Any	Any	Skin, soft tissue	19%
	M1b	Any	Any	Any	Any	Lung	7%
	M1c	Any	Any	Any	Any	Other visceral and/or elevated LDH	10%

Surgical Procedures

Management of the Primary Tumor

In the last three decades the surgical therapy of primary melanoma has changed considerably. As wide excisions with up to 5 cm margins, en bloc resections including the draining lymphatic vessels and prophylactic lymph node dissections have been usual up to the 1980's, those strategies have been overcome by controlled clinical trials revealing no advantage due to survival or avoiding local recurrences.[3,4] The other way round, it has been demonstrated for primary tumors with ≥2.0 mm tumor thickness that further reductions of the safety distance to 1 cm versus 3 cm might be disadvantageous.[5] Nowadays, complete excision with safety margins from 0.5 cm (Insitu-melanoma), 1 cm (tumor thickness <2.0 mm) and 2 cm (tumor thickness ≥2.0 mm) is recommended as standard treatment for primary melanoma patients.[6]

Since nodal staging by sentinel lymph node biopsy (SNB) has been implemented into primary care of melanoma in the last few years, adjuvant elective lymph node dissection (ELND) is not longer provided. Furthermore the missing benefit of ELND has been demonstrated in several randomized trials that were not able to show any survival advantage in melanoma patients compared with delayed lymph node dissection in case of clinical evident metastases.[7]

As SNB status has been figured out to be an important prognostic factor in melanoma—the detection of micrometastasis is associated with a worse prognosis—SNB has become a routine diagnostic tool in melanomas with a tumor thickness ≥1.0 mm in many countries worldwide.[1,8,9] If SNB is positive, a completing lymph node dissection is recommended to date for all patients concerned, even though the necessity of ELND for micrometastatic sentinel status (tumor cell complexes <2 mm in diameter) is currently under investigation in randomized trials.

However, the therapeutic value of the SNB approach is discussed controversially, because a significant survival advantage, similar to ELND, could not be clearly demonstrated in a large randomized multicenter trial and effective adjuvant systemic therapies for patients suffering from micrometastatic disease are lacking so far.[10]

Management of Locoregional Metastases

Locoregional metastatic spread defines stage III melanoma with satellite, intransit and/or regional lymph node metastases (Table 1). The 10 year survival rates for macrometastatic disease range between 15% and 48% implicating a curative treatment option that can be realized by complete surgical removement of skin or subcutaneous metastases and/or lymph node dissection respectively.[11] Where tumor resection is unfeasible, different palliative strategies have to be discussed, for example isolated limb perfusion with melphalan +/− TNFalpha, intralesional injection of interleukin-2, cryosurgery, radiotherapy, systemic chemotherapy or chemoimmunotherapy (see below).

Management of Distant Metastases

At the stage of distant metastatic melanoma the treatment modalities are predominantly palliative, but again, surgery of localized metastases is currently the most effective approach in stage IV as numerous studies implicate.[12] The main requirements for a potentially curative approach are complete resectability of the metastases (R0 situation), an adequate performance status of the patient and a slow tumor progression, which can be estimated by re-evaluating the tumor dimensions after 2-3 cycles of chemotherapy if applicable. Certainly the surgical risk has to be taken into account and should not exceed the expected benefit for the patient.

As it is crucial to assess the tumor extent before performing metastasis surgery as sensitive as possible, staging with 18-fluorodeoxyglucose positron emission tomography (FDG-PET) and paticularly FDG-PET/CT will presumably gain in importance as diagnostic tool in this situation.[13,14]

The most convenient constellation for surgery in stage IV would be one metastasis at one site (isolated skin, distant lymph node, lung, liver, brain metastasis etc.). For an example, it has been shown that the 5 year survival rate in patients suffering from resectable lung metastases can be increased threefoldly compared with all patients in stage M1b (22 vs 6,7%).[15] The resection of metastatic disease followed by vacciniation with melanoma associated peptides could be even more successful with a previously reported median OS of 3.8 years and a 5 year survival rate of 45% in 41 stage IV patients; 46% of them had visceral disease.[16]

Palliative removal of metastases aims on the other hand at symptom control and life quality in situations, where complete resectability is impossible, other treatment options are not available or not immediately helpful. Important indications for palliative surgery are for instance resection of stigmatizing and function-limiting skin metastases, symptomatic brain metastases, bleeding or obstructing bowel metastases, lymph node and soft tissue metastases, which injure nerves or blood vessels.

Adjuvant Therapy

The goal of adjuvant treatment approaches is to avert a progression of high-risk tumors. In melanoma, the risk of recurrence, progression and death is most of all enhanced with an increase of Breslow's tumor thickness and an occurrence of regional or distant metastases. In general, adjuvant therapies are recommended for stage II (tumor thickness ≥1.5 mm) and stage III melanoma (after removal of locoregional/nodal metastases). For surgically resected stage IV disease, no evidence for prophylactic treatment approaches exists.

Immunotherapy

Interferon α (IFN α) can be basically regarded as standard of care in the adjuvant treatment of intermediate and high-risk melanoma patients beyond surgery as it is approved for stage II and III of the disease by the US and European authorities. Two types of IFN α (2a and 2b) are established in melanoma therapy, which are slightly different in the carbohydrate components without displaying significant differences in their effectiveness. Several adjuvant trials have been carried out to examine, if IFN α is superior to clinical observation and some are still ongoing in order to find out ideal dosages and treatment durations. However, the results of the studies published so far are inconsistent with respect to overall and disease-free survival and generated some controversies. All relevant and below mentioned studies are summarized in Table 2.

Basically, two IFN α treatment strategies can be distinguished: Low-dose IFN α (LDI) being in favor for stage II melanoma and the more toxic High-dose IFN α (HDI) is preferred for stage III disease. An intermediate dose approach showed no evidence due to distant-metastasis-free and overall survival in a recent trial and is currently not recommended.[17] At present, some studies were conducted to prove an efficacy of modified, i.e., pegylated IFN α. As relevant data are not published so far, the future role of pegylated interferons in melanoma can not be anticipated by now.

For stage II melanoma only two relevant randomized controlled trials (RCT) are available.[18,19] They both demonstrated a significant prolongation of recurrence-free survival by LDI treatment over periods of 12 to 18 months, but a statistically significant survival benefit has not been attained.

As only one study so far could demonstrate a significant better disease-free and overall survival in stage III melanoma patients treated with LDI (published as abstract),[20] the majority of trials revealed no effectivity in stage III disease (Table 2).[21-23] Three published RCTs on HDI, conducted by the Eastern Cooperative Oncology Group (ECOG 1684, 1690, 1694), with a treatment duration of 12 months reported a significant benefit for recurrence-free survival and two of these trials showed an improved overall survival (OS), whereas the third one did not.[23-25] One study with a short treatment period of 12 weeks could not detect any survival benefit.[26]

A recent systematic review on adjuvant therapies for high-risk melanoma patients with IFN α, levamisole, vaccine, or chemotherapy evaluated data from 37 RCTs, two meta-analyzes and one systematic review.[27] Another overview on diagnosis and treatment of melanoma calculated 11 RCTs on adjuvant IFN α therapy with 4878 patients based on two meta-analyses.[1] With regard to IFN α the following issues can be concluded:

- HDI as well as LDI significantly improve recurrence-free survival with a risk reduction ranging between 20-30% (Odds ratio 0.78 [0.68-0.90]; p < 0.0001); these effects are stronger for HDI, especially in stage III melanoma
- The effects of IFN α (all dose regimens) on OS are not significant with a minor risk reduction of 10% (Odds ratio 0.90 [0.81-1.02]; p = 0.09)
- HDI improves OS yielding a slightly significant risk ratio for 2-year death of 0.85 [0.73-0.99; p = 0.03]
- Side effects of HDI occur frequently and mainly concern constitutional and neurologic symptoms, myelosuppression and hepatotoxicity. Adverse events may force to a dose reduction or treatment delay in up to 59% of the patients concerned.[24]

Thus, to date only a minority of patients gained a real survival advantage from an adjuvant IFN α therapy. That's the reason, why IFN α is not supplied in some European countries outside clinical trials. Furthermore, those patients responding to IFN α are not yet well characterized due to disease stage, tumor characteristics and individual factors. With respect to the large numbers needed to treat to probably save one life from melanoma and to the considerable therapy costs, this will be one urgent and challenging issue to be solved in the future.

Other adjuvant immunotherapeutic approaches like nonspecific immune stimulation (e.g., BCG, C. parvum, Transfer factor, Megestrol, Levamisol, GM2-ganglioside, Iscador, melanoma oncolysate), other cytokines (Interferon γ, Interleukin 2) and specific vaccination approaches revealed either no significant impact on recurrence-free and OS, or have not precede the experimental

Table 2. Adjuvant treatment with interferon α (≥12 months). Randomized, observation-controlled studies in stage II and III melanoma

Author	Stage (UICC 1992)	Treatment Schedule	Patients	Disease-Free Survival	Overall Survival
Kirkwood et al 1996[24]	IIB-IIIB	20 MU/m² d1-5 for 4 weeks 10 MU/m² tiw for 48 weeks	143 vs 137	p = 0.0023	p = 0.0237
Grob et al 1998[18]	IIA-IIB	3 MU tiw for 18 months	244 vs 255	p = 0.035	p = 0.059
Pehamberger et al 1998[19]	IIA-IIB	3 MU tiw for 12 months	154 vs 157	p = 0.02	not available
Kirkwood et al 2000[23]	IIB-IIIB	20 MU/m² d1-5 for 4 weeks 10 MU/m² tiw for 48 weeks	215 vs 212	p = 0.03	not significant
		3 MU tiw for 24 months	215 vs 212	n.s.	n.s.
Cascinelli et al 2001[21]	IIIB	3 MU tiw for 36 months	218 vs 209	n.s.	n.s.
Garbe et al 2004[20]	IIB	3 MU tiw for 24 months	146 vs 147	p = 0.018	p = 0.0045
Hancock et al 2004[22]	IIB-IIIB	3 MU tiw for 24 months	338 vs 336	n.s.	n.s.
Eggermont et al 2005[17]	IIB-IIIB	10 MU d1-5 for 4 weeks 10 MU tiw for 12 months	553 vs 279	n.s. (DMFS)	n.s.
		10 MU d1-5 for 4 weeks 5 MU tiw for 24 months	556 vs 279	n.s. (DMFS)	n.s.

MU = million units.
DMFS = Distant metastasis-free survival.

phase so far.[27-29] But it should be noted on the other hand that a significant survival benefit from an adjuvant melanoma vaccine trial has been reported previously, which depends on the patient's HLA-status.[30] This observation again puts the focus on an "individualized" treatment approach.

Chemotherapy

Nearly all cytotoxic agents and combinations displaying palliative effects in metastatic melanoma have been tested in adjuvant settings predominantly in the 1980's and 1990's. In a recent meta-analysis RCT's on systemic adjuvant chemotherapy in melanoma showed no survival benefit compared to untreated control patients [risk ratio 0.94; p = 0.3], while cytostatic drugs obviously enhance morbidity.[27,28]

The combination of cytotoxic and immunogenic substances (DTIC and IFN α) seems to be as ineffective. Preliminary results from a recent trial conducted by the German Dermatologic Cooperative Oncology Group (DeCOG) give evidence, that the impact of IFN α on OS in stage II and III melanoma patients was even abolished by the addition of dacarbazine.[20]

Prophylactic locoregional adjuvant chemotherapy in melanoma located at the extremities can be performed by isolated limb perfusion (ILP) under hyperthermia. ILP is able to significantly reduce the incidence of recurrent in-transit metastases, but fails to influence the OS compared to observation as well.[31] With respect to the invasiveness and considerable toxicity of ILP, this approach should be restricted to unresectable locoregional metastases.

Palliative Treatment

The prognosis of metastatic melanoma (Fig. 1) mainly depends on tumor extent and affected organ systems [M1a (skin/lymph node) > M1b (lung) > M1c (other visceral organs or elevated LDH)]. The median OS in stage IV disease ranges between 7-9 months, the 10-year-survival rates between 2.5% (M1c) and 15.7% (M1a).[11]

Palliative treatment of metastatic malignant melanoma is based on the three established columns of chemo-(immuno-)therapy, tumor surgery and radiation therapy. The aims of palliative treatment approaches consist in survival prolongation, delaying tumor progression, relieving tumor associated symptoms or at least providing life quality as long as possible.

So far, all applied treatment options did not attain a significant impact on OS in patients with distant melanoma metastases, whereas few individuals who respond to therapy or can be treated by surgery might develop long lasting remissions and thus clearly have a surivival benefit.[12,32]

The choice of a certain treatment strategy in advanced melanoma should be generally adapted to the performance status, tumor associated symptoms, affected organs, localisation and amount of metastases and progression dynamics. Whenever possible and reasonable with respect to the restrictions mentioned above, metastases should be removed surgically. In all other cases the application of cytotoxic drugs, immunogenic approaches and radiotherapy comes to the fore.

Due to the fact that these treatment options have only a limited prospect of success, new approaches that can be generated from an increasing molecular and immunological knowledge, like targeted therapies or vaccine strategies, are urgently needed and currently under investigation. Those approaches target pathogenetically important pathways in the tumor cell and/or peritumoral stroma or augment antitumor immune responses (Fig. 2).

Chemotherapy and Biochemotherapy

The application of cytostatic drugs alone or in combination with cytokines (IFN α, IL-2) can be regarded as standard of care in metastatic melanoma, especially if a surgical approach is not feasible.[33-35] Even though randomized placebo-controlled trials are missing in metastatic melanoma, chemotherapy with single dacarbazine (DTIC) is established as first-line therapy over the last three decades.[36] Two previously published randomized phase III trials on first-line DTIC reported objective response rates (OR) between 5,5-7,5% and median survival rates from 9.3-9.7 months in stage IV patients without brain metastases (n > 400) [Schadendorf 2006; Bedikian 2006].[37,38] From these humbling results it can be concluded that the antitumoral effects of DTIC are rather limited.

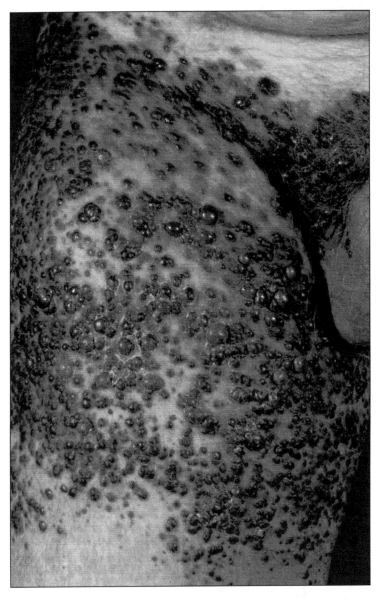

Figure 1. Patient presenting with multiple cutaneous melanoma metastases on his right groin and thigh.

The alkylating prodrug temozolomide (TMZ) shares its active metabolite (MTIC) with DTIC, but has the advantage to penetrate the blood-brain barrier and is orally applicable, so that a complete outpatient treatment is feasible. The activity and toxicity of TMZ is similar to DTIC. A large phase III study comparing first-line DTIC (250 mg/m², d1-5, q3w) versus TMZ (200 mg/m², d1-5, q4w) in metastatic melanoma demonstrated a significant impact on progression-free survival and a trend to a prolonged survival in favour for TMZ.[39] Currently TMZ, which is approved for primary brain tumors, is tested in a randomized trial on an extended, escalated dose schedule

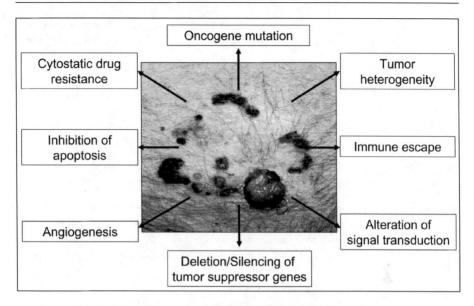

Figure 2. Molecular mechanisms of tumor progression in malignant melanoma.

versus DTIC by the European Organisation for Research and Treatmenf of Cancer (EORTC) to achieve an approval for melanoma.

Further cytostatic substances with antitumoral effects in metastatic melanoma are amongst others vinca alkaloids, nitrosourea derivates, platin compounds and taxanes (Table 3). With respect to overall survival none of these drugs has been proved superior to DTIC in phase III trials.[40]

Fotemustine, an alkylating substance from the nitrosourea group has to be highlighted for its activity in melanoma and its ability to pass the blood-brain barrier, so that another substance especially for brain-metastasized patients is availabe. A randomized phase III study comparing fotemustine with DTIC showed significantly higher response rates and trends towards prolonged OS and time to occurrence of brain metastases.[41] Fotemustine is approved for melanoma only in few European countries.

A more effective opportunitiy to enhance remission rates in melanoma up to 45% consists in combining several cytostatics. Polychemotherapy regimens might be indicated in situations, where an efficient tumor response is needed (tumor associated symptoms, high tumor burden etc.), or as second-line treatment after failure of monochemotherapy. However, RCTs have failed so far to demonstrate a survival advantage for polychemotherapy over single-agent treatment.[42]

Table 3. Palliative monochemo- and immunotherapies: treatment regimens and objective response rates (OR)[34]

Drug	Treatment Schedule	OR
Dacarbazine	250 mg/m² iv d1-5, q3w or q4w	12-18%
Dacarbazine	800-1200 mg/m² iv d1, q3w or q4w	5-23%
Temozolomide	150-200 mg/m² po d1-5, q4w	14-21%
Fotemustine	100 mg/m² iv d1,8,15 after 5 w rest: d1, q3w	7-24%
Interferon-alpha	9-18 MU/m² sc tiw continuously	13-25%
Interleukin-2	6 MU/kg iv 3 times daily d1-5 up to 14 single doses, q2w	16-22%

As combination regimens are more frequently accompanied by toxic side effects, the probability of adverse events and the potential of tumor remissions should be balanced with patients' performance status and life expectancy.

Polychemotherapies usually applied in metastatic melanoma are for instance the CVD-, BHD-, BOLD- and Dartmouth(DBCT)-regimens (Table 4).

In order to therapeutically use the immunogenicity of melanoma cells, cytokines have been introduced in the palliative treatment as well. IL-2 and IFN α have been applied as single-agents and are now usually combined with cytostatics (so called biochemotherapy); schedules and treatment efficacies of cytokines are listed in tables 3 and 4. Response rates and survival times are comparable with those achievable by single-agent chemotherapy.[40] However, immunotherapy can cause significantly more severe side effects, especially high dose IL-2. Similar to polychemotherapy approaches objective response rates are improvable up to 60% by adding cytokines to cytostatics.[43,44]

Table 4. Palliative polychemo- and chemoimmunotherapies: treatment regimens and objective response rates (OR)[34]

Drug	Treatment Schedule		OR
CVD 1	DTIC	450 mg/m² iv d1+8	24-45%
	Vindesine	3 mg/m² iv d1+8	
	Cisplatin	50 mg/m² iv d1+8	
	q3w or q4w		
CVD 2	DTIC	250 mg/m² iv d1-5	
	Vindesine	3 mg/m² iv d1	
	Cisplatin	100 mg/m² iv d1	
	q3w or q4w		
BHD	BCNU	150 mg/m² iv d1 odd cycles	13-30%
	Hydroxyurea	1500 mg/m² po d1-5	
	DTIC	150 mg/m² iv d1-5	
	q4w		
DTIC (TMZ)	DTIC	850 mg/m² iv d1	14-28%
+ Interferon-alpha	(or TMZ	150 mg/m² po d1-5)	
	IFN-α2a/b	3 MU/m² d1-5 sc, w1	
	IFN-α2a/b	5 MU/m² tiw, w2-4,	
	q4w		
BOLD	Bleomycin	15 mg iv d1+4	22-40%
	Vincristine	1 mg/m² iv d1+5	
	CCNU	80 mg/m² po d1	
	DTIC	200 mg/m² iv d1-5	
	q4w – q6w		
DBCT	DTIC	220 mg/m² iv d1-3	19%[42]
	BCNU	150 mg/m² iv d1 odd cycles	
	Cisplatin	25 mg/m² iv d1-3	
	Tamoxifen	2 × 10 mg po/d	
	q3w or q4w		
"Legha"	DTIC	800 mg/m² iv d1	48%[32]
	Vinblastine	1,5 mg/m² iv d1-4	
	Cisplatin	20 mg/m² iv d1-4	
	IL-2	9 MU/m² iv d1-4	
	IFN-α2a/b	9 MU sc d1-5,7,9,11,13	
	q3w		

But again, the advantage in favor of biochemotherapy in terms of OR is not translatable into better OS, as recently demonstrated by several phase III trials on biochemotherapy.[32,45,46] Without an impact on OS, cytokines substantially augment the antitumor activity of chemotherapy, but at the expense of considerable toxicity and impairment of quality of life. Severe and potentially life threatening complications by cytokine therapies have been reported, like fatal rhabdomyolysis or capillary leak syndrome.[47,48] Therefore, at this moment biochemotherapy cannot be recommended as standard first-line therapy for metastatic melanoma.[35]

A fundamental cause of the limited efficacy of cytotoxic drugs in advanced melanoma patients has to be seen in chemoresistance mechanisms of the tumor, as shown by in vitro studies on metastatic melanoma cell lines.[49] In this regard, the most crucial factor seems to be resistance against chemotherapy induced apoptosis. Tumor cells display heterogeneous sensitivities to different cytostatic drugs in vitro. One strategy to overcome chemoresistance consists in performing in vitro chemosensitivity tests to pretherapeutically predict the individual antitumor activity. Recent data from a phase II trial on an ATP-based luminescence viability assay in advanced melanoma patients demonstrated multicenter feasibility and a survival benefit for chemosensitive patients.[50]

Besides resistance against apoptosis, tumor cells are able to develop effective repair mechanisms to eliminate chemotherapy induced DNA damage. A novel approach to enhance the antitumoral activity of cytotoxic drugs is the addition of so called chemosensitizers, which inhibit DNA repair or antiapoptotic pathways in the tumor cell. The alkylating cytostatic effect of TMZ is attributed to methylation of O^6-guanine. This DNA damage can be diminished by an upregulation of the repair enzyme O^6-methylguanine-DNA-methyltransferase (MGMT) in tumor cells. The co-application of TMZ with pseudosubstrates competing with methylated DNA strands for the MGMT binding site might attenuate chemoresistance against TMZ. MGMT inhibitors like O^6-benzylguanine and lomeguatrib in combination with TMZ are currently under investigation in early phase clinical trials and the optimum dosage and application duration of these molecules still needs to be defined.[51-53]

Another approach to abrogate resistance to TMZ relies on the pharmacological inhibition of Poly(ADP-Ribose) Polymerase-1 (PARP-1), a component of the base excision repair system; preclinical studies with the PARP-1 inhibitor GPI 15427 showed efficacy as chemosensitizer on cerebral tumors.[54]

Radiotherapy

Melanoma cell lines exhibit a nearly total resistance to ionizing radiation in vitro as older investigations in melanoma cell lines revealed.[55] However, this observation is not completely translatable to the biological behaviour of melanoma cells in vivo. Radiation of lentigo maligna melanoma for instance is an established alternative treatment with curative intention, if complete resectability is not feasible or reasonable in view of the predominantly elderly patients. In contrast to this, melanoma metastases are characterized by an even worse response to radiotherapy, so that other treatment options generally should be prefered in metastatic melanoma (surgery, chemotherapy). With the objective of controlling tumor growth and symptoms, the use of radiation therapy in advanced melanoma can be considered in the following situations anyway:

- Whole brain radiation—disseminated brain metastases[56]
- Gamma knife (stereotactic) radiosurgery—single brain metastases (up to 3(-5) lesions measuring ≤3cm in diameter); radiosurgery improves survival and is associated with a high local control rate and minimal morbidity[57,58]
- Bone metastases—to avoid fractures and/or to treat metastatic bone pain[59]
- Irradiation of irresectable soft tissue, lymph node or visceral metastases, which injure blood vessels or nerves or cause unmanageable pain[59]
- Adjuvant radiotherapy after incomplete surgical resections (R1, R2 situations)[60]

Experimental Approaches

Vaccination Therapy

Over the last decades tumorimmunological mechanisms—antitumor response and tumor escape—have been intensively investigated. Malignant melanoma can be regarded as an immunogenic tumor, because melanoma cells express specific cancer antigens, wich are able to induce specific immune responses with tumor infiltrating lymphocytes (TILs). Furthermore melanoma is responsible to cytokine therapies, as mentioned above. This is one reason, why several different specific and immune modulating therapy approaches have been developed. Vaccination approaches are impressive owing to their specificity for tumor cells and their low toxicity in contrast to cytostatic agents. On the other hand it is difficult to establish standardized vaccines for a broad use, the technical effort and costliness at least for autologous approaches might be disadvantageous and tumor material is not always accessible if required. Nevertheless the optimization of vaccination strategies due to different adjuvants, ways of application (intradermal, subcutaneous, intramuscular, intravenous, intranodal etc.) and combination schedules with immunmodulating substances, targeted approaches or chemotherapy will be pursued.[61]

It can be distinguished between autologous and allogeneic tumor-cell-based approaches with or without gene modifications, peptide-, DNA- and glycolipid-vaccines and cell-based vaccines with activated autologous immune competent cells (Dendritic cells, adoptive T-cell transfer).[62] The proof of principle for several antitumoral vaccination strategies in melanoma has been shown in smaller studies; for a review see reference 40. However, as antitumor immune responses are considered as surrogate parameter correlating per se with a favorable prognosis, the value and significance of small nonrandomized studies are discussed controversially.[63] Until now, RCT's on adjuvant or palliative melanoma treatment could not demonstrate a survival benefit for vaccinated patients compared with standard of care in each situation (i.e., observation, interferons, DTIC).[25,38,64] On the other hand one ot these trials on metastatic melanoma impressively demonstrated that patients with defined HLA-haplotypes (HLA-A2+, C3+, B44-) gain a significant survival benefit, if treated with peptide-pulsed dendritic cells versus DTIC: the median survival in this subgroup analysis was almost doubled (20.8 vs 11.1 months).[38] This promising observation implies further prospective randomized investigations with appropriately selected patients.

The vaccination field of metastatic melanoma is currently focussed on how to make immune responses more efficient, especially by circumventing immune tolerance. The induction of regulatory T-lymphocytes is an essential sequence of cellular immunity that averts autoimmune reactivity, but also weakens the antitumor activity of vaccines. One strategy to overcome tolerance consists in administration of a lymphodepleting chemotherapy followed by autologous adoptive T-cell transfer with heterogenous TILs. An OR of 51% has been reported with this approach in a phase I study of 35 patients.[65]

The termination of immune responses particularly depends on CTL-associated antigen (CTLA-4) expression on activated T-cells, which binds to B7 on antigen presenting cells and thus inihibits the costimulatory signalling via CD28 / B7. By inhibiting the inhibitor with monoclonal anti-CTLA-4 antibodies [ipilimumab (MDX-010) and ticilimumab (CP-675,206)] more effective immune repsonses can be generated (Fig. 3).[66] This approach has been recently introduced into the treatment of metastatic melanoma: A phase II study showed an OR of 21% by the administration of MDX-010 combined with a gp100 peptide vaccine.[67] As expected, a major problem of CTLA-4 blockade is the frequent occurance of autimmune reactions (43% CTC grade III/IV in the above mentioned study), especially colitis, hypophysitis and hepatitis, which can be therapy limiting and even life-threatening. On the other hand autoimmunity seems to correlate with tumor regression and thus should be tolerated to a certain extent under intensive treatment monitoring.[68] The value of anti-CTLA-4 antibodies for metastatic melanoma in combination with other vaccination regimens or chemotherapeutics has to be awaited, as several first-line phase III studies are currently ongoing.

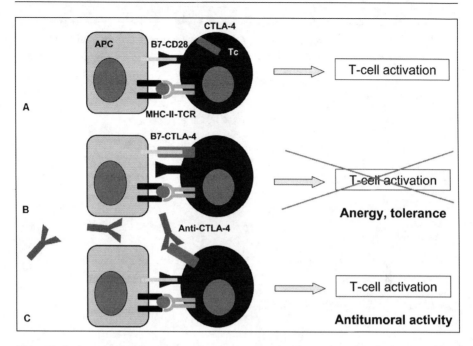

Figure 3. Improvement of antitumoral immune response by CTLA-4 blockade. A) Antigen presenting cells (APC) stimulate T-cells (Tc) by presenting tumor specific peptides on MHC class II molecules on their surface. The specific recognition of the T-cell receptor (TCR) and costimulatory signaling via B7-CD28 binding leads to an immune response against the tumor antigen. Activated T-cells in turn induce CTLA-4 to abrogate the immune response later on. B) The inhibitory CTLA-4 molecule displays a higher affinity to B7 and thus displaces CD28; the result is T-cell inactivation and induction of tolerance. C) By application of anti-CTLA-4 antibodies the inhibition of T-cell responses can be restored.

Further innovative approaches to enhance antitumor immune responses focus on stimulation of components of the innate immune system via so called toll-like receptors (TLR). TLR binding oligonucleotides or bacterial CpG motifs are acting as unspecific immune modifiers and probably have the potential to induce tumor regressions as single agents or vaccine adjuvants.[69] An activity of TLR binding oligonucleotides on metastatic melanoma has been recently demonstrated in a phase II study.[70]

Targeted Therapy

Targeted therapy has currently to be regarded as the most innovative field in the treatment of cancer, as several targeting substances have been developed and approved over the last few years, particularly for colon, breast, renal and lung cancer, myeloid leukemia and plasmocytoma. Targeted therapy comprises substances, which inhibit or modulate target molecules inside or outside the tumor cell. Those target molecules are defined to play an important role for tumor pathogenesis (cell growth and proliferation, inhibition of apoptosis, angiogenesis and metastasis) for instance by genetic or epigenetic alterations of tumor suppressor gene expression or by activating oncogene mutations. Concerning malignant melanoma targeted therapy approaches are still experimental, but raise great expectations. Several molecules with different targets have already entered clinical phase III trials on patients with metastatic melanoma (Table 5).[71,72]

Important mechanisms in the pathogenesis of malignant melanoma, which are accessible to targeted therapies, include:

- Growth regulation/proliferation (e.g., Ras/Raf/MEK/ERK signaling pathway),

Table 5. *Selection of targeted therapies under clinical investigation in malignant melanoma [modified according to ref. 72]*

Substance Group	Therapeutic Agent	Target(s)	Administration
Tyrosine kinase inhibitors (Small molecules)	(1) Bay 43-9006 (Sorafenib)	Raf, MEK, VEGFR-2, -3, PDGFR, EGFR, p38, Flt-3, c-kit	po
	(2) SU11248 (Sunitinib)	VEGFR-2, PDGFR, Flt-3, c-kit	po
	(3) STI-571 (Imatinib)	Bcr/Abl, c-kit, PDGFR	po
	(4) OSI-774 (Erlotinib)	EGFR	po
	(5) ZD1839 (Geftinib)	EGFR	po
	(6) SU5416 (Semaxinib)	VEGFR-1, VEGFR-2	iv twice weekly
Humanized antibodies	(7) Anti-VEGF (Bevacizumab)	VEGF	iv q2w
	(8) C225 (Cetuximab)	EGFR	iv q1w
	(9) MEDI-522 (Vitaxin)	αVβ3 Integrin	iv q1w
Antisense molecules	(10) bcl-2 antisense (Oblimersen)	bcl-2 mRNA	iv 5x / cycle q3w
m-TOR inhibitors	(11) CCI-779 (Temsirolimus)	Mammalian target of rapamycin, PTEN/PI3K/Akt signaling	iv 1x week.
Farnesyl transferase inhibitors	(12) R115777 (Tipifarnib)	RAS	po
Proteasome inhibitors	(13) PS-341 (Bortezomib, Velcade®)	NF-κB	iv 4x / cycle q3w

- Tumor angiogenesis (e.g., by upregulation of VEGF secretion),
- Resistance to apoptosis (e.g., by induction of the apoptosis inhibitor bcl-2) and
- Chemoresistance (e.g., by induction of the DNA repair enzyme MGMT, see above).

Hence different intra- and extracellular molecules inside the tumor stroma (tumor cell, endothelial cell, interstitium and blood circulation) can serve as targets for an antitumoral therapy (Fig. 4).

Growth Modulating Substances/Signal Transduction Pathway Inhibitors

Proliferation of tumor cells is mediated amongst others by mitogen-activated protein kinase signaling (MAPK = Ras/Raf/MEK/ERK). Somatic mutations of BRAF (V599E), which entail a constitutive activation of MAPK signaling, can be frequently found in melanoma in up to 65% of the cases.[73] Sorafenib (BAY 43-9006) as an orally applicable "multi kinase inhibitor" interacts with wild-type B-Raf, with the V599E mutant, with Raf-1, VEGFR-2, PDGFRβ and other receptor tyrosine kinases involved in tumor progression and angiogenesis.[74] When administered as a single agent, sorafenib diplays only moderate activity in the treatment of advanced melanoma, but

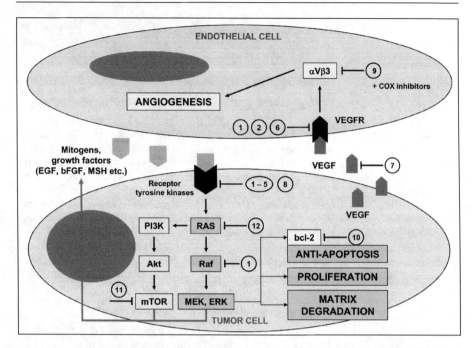

Figure 4. Pathogenetically important mechanisms for tumor progression of malignant melanoma. Relevant target molecules of tumor and endothelial cells accessible to targeted therapy approaches are characterized. The numbers fit to the therapeutic agents listed in table 5. αVβ3 = proangiogenic integrin. Akt = murine v-akt oncogene homologue. Bcl-2 = B-cell-lymphoma/leukemia-2 mRNA. bFGF = basic fibroblast growth factor. EGF = Epidermal growth factor. ERK = extracellular signal-regulated kinase. MEK = mitogen-activated protein kinase kinase (MAP2K). mTOR = mammalian target of rapamycin. MSH = melanocyte stimulating hormon. PI3K = phosphatidylinositol-3 kinase. Raf = raf murine sarcoma viral oncogene homologue. RAS = rous avian sarcoma homologue. VEGF = vascular endothelial growth factor. VEGFR = VEGF receptor.

has the capability to induce sustained disease stabilizations in melanoma and other solid tumors as well.[75] As Sorafenib has been already approved for the second-line treatment of metastatic renal cell carcinoma, several phase II/III trials on stage IV melanoma are currently conducted to support antitumoral activity in combination with cytotoxic drugs (DTIC, temozolomide, carboplatin/paclitaxel).

Further presently investigated molecules with probable activity in melanoma targeting MAPK or phosphoinositol-3-kinase/Akt signaling are the farnesyl transferase inhibitor tipifarnib (R115777) and mTOR inhibitors like temsirolimus (CCI-779).[71,72] However, CCI-779 revealed only limited effects on metastastatic melanoma as single agent.[76] That's why current strategies rather place emphasis on combination of different targeting drugs with each other or with cytostatics.[77]

The tyrosine kinase inhibitors imatinib, erlotinib and geftinib interact with the signaling of different growth factor receptors on tumor cells (c-kit, PDGFR, EGFR). The single substance activity on metastatic melanoma again seems to be rather weak, whereas even imatinib mesylate, which is approved for myeloid leukemia, gastrointestinal stromal tumors and dermatofibrosarcoma protuberans, revealed notable toxicities in a high-dose phase II study.[78] However, a restriction on patients revealing activating c-kit mutations was not provided in this trial, so that further investigations correlating the treatment outcome of imantinib with the individual mutational status of c-kit might be reasonable in melanoma patients.[79] In contrast to imatinib, the side effect profile of erlotinib seems to be more convenient, but data from clinical trials on melanoma are missing so far.

Antiangiogenic Substances

Tumor cells have the ability to generate endothelial growth factors and to escape control mechanisms of vascular homeostasis. Metastases from malignant melanoma are characterized by a tumor stroma plenty of blood vessels, so that antiangiogenic approaches seem to make sense.

Thalidomide and lenalidomide (CC-5013) display antiangiogenic and immune modulating features, though the precise mode of action of these drugs has not been unravelled so far. Several phase II studies on metastatic melanoma reveal a favourable tolerability of thalidomide and anti-tumor activity in combination with cytotoxic drugs. An OR of 32% was recently reported for the combination of thalidomide and TMZ in a phase II trial in patients with metastatic melanoma without brain metastases.[80] Furthermore it's interesting to note that thalidomide clearly reduces CTC grade III/IV myelosuppression effects of TMZ as demonstrated by a randomized trial with 181 stage IV melanoma patients.[81] On the other hand thalidomide seems to considerably enhance the risk for thromboembolic events in melanoma patients metastatic to the brain.[82]

Further substances with antiangiogenic activity currently investigated in palliative melanoma treatment target the endothelial growth factor VEGF and its signaling pathway. Bevacizumab, a humanized monoclonal antibody directed against VEGF, is approved for combination therapy of colon carcinoma due to a significant survival benefit.[83] Several clinical trials are currently in progress to verify an activity of bevacizumab in metastatic melanoma in combination with chemotherapy, IFN-α, sorafenib, imatinib, erlotinib and temsirolimus.

The predominantly antiangiogenic tyrosine kinase inhibitors semaxinib and sunitinib are further candidates for melanoma treatment as early clinical data suggest.[84,85]

VEGF upregulates the alpha v beta 3 (αVβ3) integrin expression, which is involved in proangiogenic mechanisms. MEDI-522 (Vitaxin), a humanized monoclonal antibody directed against αVβ3 and the human monoclonal anti-integrin (αVβ3, αVβ5) antibody CNTO-95 are further substances currently tested alone or in combination with DTIC in metastatic melanoma.[86] A preliminary analysis of a randomized open-label study comparing Vitaxin +/– DTIC showed a better overall survival for the MEDI-522 single-agent group, although objective tumor responses were not observed in the single-agent group.[87]

The acitivity of COX-2 inhibitors like rofecoxib on malignant melanoma, particularly on skin metastases as previously reported, seems to depend predominantly on antiangiogenic effects via inhibition of αVβ3 as well.[88,89]

Proapoptotic Substances

Chemoresistance in melanoma is attributed to a deficiency of the tumor cells to undergo apoptosis and is connected with an overexpression of the antiapoptotic Bcl- 2 (B-cell leukemia-lymphoma 2) protein, which blocks the mitochondrial release of cytochrome C.[90] In order to overcome apoptosis deficiency and thus enhance chemosensitivity in melanoma an antisense approach has been developed to inhibit Bcl-2 protein translation.[91] The activity of this antisense oligonucleotide (oblimersen) in metastatic melanoma has recently been investigated in combination with DTIC in a large randomized phase III study. The combination of oblimersen/DTIC revealed a significantly better progression free survival and OR compared to DTIC alone, whereas the survival difference was not significant (9.0 vs 7.8 months, p = 0.077).[37] However, in a post-hoc subgroup analysis, patients with normal LDH levels showed a significant survival benefit in favor of oblimersen/DTIC. Other regimens with oblimersen are currently being studied.

Several further approaches to restore apoptosis are in clinical progress, for instance blockage of members of the "inhibitor of apoptosis protein" (IAP) and the "X-linked IAP" (XIAP) families by small molecules targeting the IAP survivin or by XIAP antisense nucleotides.[71,92] Inhibitors of the proteasome, an important multienzyme complex, which is frequently deregulated in tumor cells, display proapoptotic and antiangiogenic effects by reducing p53 and I-κB degradation; the latter effect averts translocation of transcription factor NF-κB from cytoplasm to nucleus.[93,94] The antitumor effectivity of proteasome inhibitor bortezomib (PS-341), which is less active as single agent in metastatic melanoma, is presently beeing investigated in combination with TMZ and carboplatin/paclitaxel.[71,72]

From the hitherto experiences with targeted molecular therapeutics—not only in melanoma —can be concluded, that the characterization of pathogenetically relevant molecular mechanisms in tumors offer a plenty of targets available for a more or less specific antitumor therapy. However, with respect to melanoma a significant single-agent activity of targeting molecules has not been proven so far. Therefore, one future task in metastatic melanoma treatment will consist in proceeding with combination regimens with other targeting, immune modulating or cytostatic agents. Similar to vaccination therapies, an increase in antitumor effectivity can be presumably achieved by a more directed selection of patients due to specific expression patterns or mutations of tumor targets.

Nonmelanoma Skin Cancer

Introduction

The most common epithelial tumors of the skin—basal cell carcinoma (BCC) and squamous cell carcinoma (SCC)—are set up in contrast to malignant melanoma and thus summarized as nonmelanoma skin cancers (NMSC). NMSC's are also increasing in incidence in the recent decades, approximately 80% are BCCs.[95] Several factors are considered responsible for the growing risk to develop NMSCs besides well-defined genetical disorders (xeroderma pigmentosum, basal cell nevus syndrome): cumulative exposure to ultraviolet light, increased life expectancy and number of patients, who are immunosuppressed, particularly organ transplant recipients.[96,97]

NMSCs can be easily treated with a curative intention in most cases even in early stages. Thus, the timely and complete removal of the tumor has to be aspired in general. The standard treatment of NMSCs is complete excision of the tumor with histographic control of the excision margins where required (see below). Other local approaches can be considered in defined indications: cryotherapy, radiotherapy, photodynamic therapy, topical immune-modifiers, cytotoxic drugs and laser therapy. These techniques share the disadvantage of a missing immediate histopathological control of the therapeutic success and the subsequent risk of higher recurrence rates. Most of the latter treatment options, with the exception of radiotherapy, are restricted to superficial BCCs, nodal BCCs with a limited invasion depth and precancerous lesions like Bowen's disease and actinic keratoses. Thus, the treatment choice depends on tumor size, invasion depth, localization, clinical behaviour, histopathological type and growth pattern, as well as on individual attributes like age and clinical performance status. The cosmetic outcome of each approach is an important factor for the patient and should be considered as far as the cure rates of the competing techniques do not significantly differ from each other.

Basal Cell Carcinoma

In contrast to SCC, BCCs reveal a more benign behaviour: while potentially invading deeper layers of the skin, muscle, cartilage and bone structures, BCCs virtually do not metastasize. Hence, it is not surprising that the treatment options for BCC are more comprehensive compared to SCC.

Surgical removal of BCCs (i.e., excision with 3-5 mm safety margin) has to be regarded as standard therapy and can be performed with conventional histology or micrographic control of the resection margins, the so called Mohs micrographic surgery (MMS). As conventional histology is afflicted with a slightly higher 5 year-recurrence rate compared to MMS (3%-14% vs 1%-10%), MMS is recommended for large-sized (>2 cm), morphea-type and recurrent BCCs and for cosmetically sensitive locations, especially the face.[98] Surgical alternatives for superficial and localized nodular BCCs consist in shave excision and curettage with or without electrodesiccation of the wound ground. The latter approach in fact is convenient for the medical practitioner but is clearly accompanied by more recurrences compared with conventional surgery.[99]

Cryotherapy is an effective treatment option as well for primary and recurrent BCCs showing 5-year recurrence rates of 4%-17%.[98,100] Commonly, cryosurgery should be restricted to tumors with well-defined borders and patients need to be informed about the expected side-effects, pain, scarring and dyspigmentations. Cryosurgery is performed with two freeze-thaw cycles of 30 seconds each. The cosmetic outcome of cryosurgery might be worse compared with surgical excision.[101]

Expedient indications for radiation therapy of BCCs are mainly large-sized tumors in difficult locations, extensive recurrent tumors and BCCs in elderly patients.[102] Recurrence rates of X-ray treated BCCs are reported to be 7.4% for primaries and 9.5% for recurrent BCCs at 5 years.[103] As radiotherapy is afflicted with less favourable cosmetic results and an occurance of secondary malignancies in the radiation field after several decades, this treatment option is basically not suitable for younger patients (<50 years) and contraindicated in patients genetically disposed to skin cancer (e.g., xeroderma pigmentosum).

The mechanisms of action of topical photodynamic therapy (PDT) are based on the local application of photosensitizing precursors [methyl aminolevulinate (MAL), 5-aminolevulinic acid (ALA)], which are converted into photoactive porphyrins predominantly by the neoplastic tissue. After an incubation time of at least 3 hours tumor areas are treated with red light in sufficient energy doses. Hereupon, the excited protoporphyrin IX induces cytotoxic free radicals and singulet oxygen molecules with the result of tumor cell apoptosis and necrosis.[104] Treatment with PDT is typically associated with local reactions (burning pain, swelling, erythema and edema), so that cooling with different techniques should be applied.

PDT is recommended as an effective and reliable treatment option for superficial BCCs and nodular BCCs less than 2 mm in depth and outside the so-called H zone of the face (region with high risk BCCs due to deep tumor invasion). It offers advantages particularly for large, extensive and multiple lesions with excellent cosmetic outcomes.[105] Certainly, RCTs demonstrate better cosmetic results of PDT compared to excision and to cryosurgery. But on the other hand BCC recurrence rates after PDT are ranging between 14% and 38% at 4- and 5-year follow-ups in prospectively designed trials (for a review see ref. 106). The only available RCT of PDT vs conventional surgery in nodular BCC with 101 treated lesions revealed 2-year recurrence rates of 19% (PDT) vs 4% (surgical excision).[106] This trend for higher recurrence rates with PDT in BCC compared to surgery should implicate further controlled studies with larger patient cohorts and longer follow up intervals. Even if PDT is repeatable in case of recurrence, the critical issues of thoroughly monitoring PDT treated patients over longer periods, the potential development of hardly recognizable deep invading recurrent tumors, PDT costs and missing long term results of RCTs have to be opposed to the cosmetic aspects.

Other topical approaches to treat superficial BCCs are 5-fluorouracil (5-FU), which is approved as chemical ablative agent for many years and imiquimod, a topical immune-modulating drug that was at first approved for the treatment of genital warts and later on for actinic keratoses and superficial BCCs.

There are only limited data available on 5-FU revealing 5-year recurrence rates between 6% and 21% in superficial BCCs, comparable with cryotherapy. As local administration of 5-FU generates severe skin reactions, scarring and dyspigmentation, this approach is basically not indicated for resectable tumors and PDT as well as imiquimod achieve better cosmetic results.

Imiquimod displays antitumoral effects via binding to cell surface Toll-like receptors on macrophages and other cells, which in turn induces synthesis and secretion of proinflammatory cytokines like IFN α and tumor necrosis factor-α. Concerning BCC, it has been shown that imiquimod cream additionally causes Fas receptor (FasR) induction and FasR mediated apoptosis.[107] Imiquimod has to be applied once daily on 5 consecutive days per week over 6 weeks. Dose-related side effects (erythema, crusting and erosions) indicate an antitumoral activity and are generally well tolerated. The histopathological clearance rates at 12 weeks post-treatment range between 76% in nodular BCCs (off-label) and 82% in superficial BCCs. The cosmetic outcome has been assessed to be excellent (for a review see ref. 98). However, long-term and comparative data for imiquimod are also not available so far. Its indication for BCC is therefore difficult to define. Provided that a good patient's compliance is on hand, imiquimod might be a useful treatment approach for large-sized and multilocular superficial BCCs comparable to PDT.[108]

The mentioned treatment options for BCC offer many advantages and disadvantages. A paucity of comparative studies of BCC treatment has to be noticed. Regarding the low recurrence risk of surgical excision with or without micrographic histopathology, this approach has to be regarded as standard of care for BCC. Resectability and individual factors (age, compliance, importance attached to cosmetic outcome) have to be considered for the use of alternative methods as described.

Squamous Cell Carcinoma

As squamous cell carcinomas (SCC) exhibit the potential to metastasize depending on tumor localization (mouth, scalp, ears, genital region, mucous membranes and recurrent tumors), invasion depth and differentiation (histopathological grading), complete surgical removal is the treatment of first choice. Analogous to BCCs Mohs micrographic surgery is recommended for recurrent SCCs, SCCs in problematic regions and desmoplastic SCC.

In cases of unresectability or patient's refusal to surgery, radiotherapy is an effective alternative treatment option, as SCCs are predominantly radiosensitive.[102] Tumor control rates by radiotherapy are stated to range between 70-100%.[109-110] Due to possible cartilage radionecrosis, SCCs at the ears an tip of the nose should be generally treated by surgery. As far as possible, radiotherapy has to be avoided in immunocompromised patients and those suffering from DNA repair defects (xeroderma pigmentosum, see above).

Alternative treatment approaches are appropriate and approved solely for precancerous lesions (Actinic keratoses (AK), Bowen's disease): e.g., cryotherapy, PDT, imiquimod, 5-FU and diclofenac sodium gel.[111] Those topical treatments are particularly attractive for extensive fields of precancerous lesions ("field cancerization"). Regarding AK, the competing approaches show complete clearance rates in 50%-60% (diclofenac sodium, imiquimod), 70% (cryotherapy) and up to a maximum of 80%-90% (5-FU, PDT) of the treated lesions.[112-115] Advantages and disadvantages of these techniques for BCC treatment have been described in detail and accordingly apply for the treatment of precancerous lesions. Due to effectiveness and cosmetic outcome, PDT seems to be the most favourable approach for field cancerized patients by now. But again, RCTs comparing these novel therapies with each other are largely missing.

Lymph node metastases are treated by complete lymph node dissection. Radiotherapy is recommended for irresectable or incompletely dissected lymph node metastases (R1, R2) possibly in combination with chemotherapy.[116]

The occurrence of visceral metastases of SCCs is a rare event (~2%), but is connected with a very poor prognosis. Mainly affected are elderly patients, so that the application of aggressive chemotherapy regimens is not feasible in many cases. Though remission rates up to 80% are reported for polychemotherapy approaches in metastatic SCC, a significant survival prolongation can not be expected. Thus, the application of single-agent or polychemotherapy regimens has to be regarded as palliative approach. Mostly applied cytostatic substances are methotrexate, cisplatin, 5-fluorouracil, bleomycin and combinations with cisplatin and 5-FU or doxorubicine.[117-118]

Concluding Remarks

In contrast to the highly effective treatment options for NMSC with a curative approach by surgery in the majority of cases, the therapeutic efficacy in melanoma utterly depends on early recognition of superficial tumors, which highlights the basic importance to advance with prevention strategies. For melanoma skin cancer, especially the metastatic disease, there still is a gap between our progress in knowledge about the biological and molecular behaviour of the tumor on the one hand and the hitherto missing therapeutical benefit from these insights on the other. Thus, in all fields of melanoma and nonmelanoma skin cancer, great efforts are being made to develop more effective treatment modalities or to optimize the available approaches. Although standard treatment in metastatic melanoma did not change since decades, the presently growing spectrum of potential therapeutic targets in melanoma and the multitude of promising agents currently tested in clinical trials give hope that the therapeutical deadlock can be broken in the future. Along with improved vaccination strategies, the fascinating targeted therapy approaches currently attract the most attention in advanced melanoma treatment. Linked to these efforts, great importance might be placed on defining the most effective ways of how to combine available antitumoral agents and treatment strategies adapted to patients' characteristics and the individual tumor expression profile.

References

1. Garbe C, Eigentler TK. Diagnosis and treatment of cutaneous melanoma: state of the art 2006. Melanoma Res 2007; 17:117-127.
2. Balch CM, Soong SJ, Gerschenwald JE et al. Prognostic factors analysis of 17.600 melanoma patients: validation of the American Joint Committee on Cancer melanoma staging system. J Clin Oncol 2001; 19:3622-3634.
3. Ringborg U, Andersson R, Eldh J et al. Resection margins of 2 versus 5 cm for cutaneous malignant melanoma with a tumor thickness of 0.8 to 2.0 mm: randomized study by the Swedish Melanoma Study Group. Cancer 1996; 77:1809-1814.
4. Veronesi U, Cascinelli N, Adamus J et al. Thin stage I primary cutaneous malignant melanoma. Comparison of excision with margins of 1 or 3 cm. N Engl J Med 1988; 318:1159-1162.
5. Thomas JM, Newton-Bishop J, A'Hern R et al. Excision margins in high-risk malignant melanoma. N Engl J Med 2004; 350:757-766.
6. Hauschild A, Rosien F, Lischner S. Surgical standards in the primary care of melanoma patients. Onkologie 2003; 26:218-222.
7. Cascinelli N, Morabito A, Santinami M et al. Immediate or delayed dissection of regional nodes in patients with melanoma of the trunk: A randomised trial. Lancet 1998; 351:793-796.
8. Gershenwald JE, Thompson W, Mansfield PF et al. Multi-institutional melanoma lymphatic mapping experience: the prognostic value of sentinel lymph node status in 612 stage I or II melanoma patients. J Clin Oncol 1999; 17:976-982.
9. Morton DL, Wen DR, Wong JH et al. Technical details of intraoperative lymphatic mapping for early stage melanoma. Arch Surg 1992; 127:392-399.
10. Morton DL, Thompson JF, Cochran AJ et al. Sentinel-node biopsy or nodal observation in melanoma. N Engl J Med 2006; 355:1307-1317.
11. Balch CM, Buzaid AC, Soong SJ et al. Final version of the American Joint Committee on Cancer staging system for cutaneous melanoma. J Clin Oncol 2001; 19:3635-3648.
12. Wong SL, Coit DG. Role of surgery in patients with stage IV melanoma. Curr Opin Oncol 2004; 16:155-160.
13. Reinhardt MJ, Joe AY, Jaeger U et al. Diagnostic performance of whole body dual modality 18F-FDG-PET/CT imaging for N- and M-staging of malignant melanoma: experience with 250 consecutive patients. J Clin Oncol 2006; 24:1178-1187.
14. Stas M, Stroobants S, Dupont P et al 18-FDG-PET scan in the staging of recurrent melanoma: additional value and therapeutic impact. Melanoma Res 2002; 12:479-490.
15. Leo F, Cagini L, Rocmans P et al. Lung metastases from melanoma: when is surgical treatment warranted? Br J Cancer 2000; 83:569-572.
16. Tagawa ST, Cheung E, Banta W et al. Survival Analysis after resection of metastatic disease followed by peptide vaccines in patients with stage IV melanoma. Cancer 2006; 106:1353-1357.
17. Eggermont AMM, Suciu S, MacKie R et al. Postsurgery adjuvant therapy with intermediate doses of interferon alfa 2b versus observation in patients with stage IIb/III melanoma (EORTC 18952): randomised controlled trial. Lancet 2005; 366:1189-1196.
18. Grob JJ, Dreno B, de la Salmoniere P et al. Randomised trial of interferon alpha-2a as adjuvant therapy in resected primary melanoma thicker than 1.5 mm without clinically detectable node metastases. French Cooperative Group on Melanoma. Lancet 1998; 351:1905-1910.
19. Pehamberger H, Soyer HP, Steiner A et al. Adjuvant interferon alfa-2a treatment in resected primary stage II cutaneous melanoma. Austrian Malignant Melanoma Cooperative Group. J Clin Oncol 1998; 16:1425-1429.
20. Garbe C, Hauschild A, Linse R et al. Adjuvant treatment of patients with cutaneous melanoma and regional node metastasis with low dose interferon- or interferon- plus DTIC versus observation alone. Preliminary evaluation of a randomised multicenter DeCOG trial. 5th International Conference on the Adjuvant Therapy of Malignant Melanoma, Abstract booklet, 2004; No I-21, p. 14.
21. Cascinelli N, Belli F, MacKie RM et al. Effect of long-term adjuvant therapy with interferon alpha-2a in patients with regional node metastases from cutaneous melanoma: a randomised trial. Lancet 2001; 358:866-869.

22. Hancock BW, Wheatley K, Harris S et al. Adjuvant interferon in high-risk melanoma: the AIM HIGH Study—United Kingdom Coordinating Committee on Cancer Research randomized study of adjuvant low-dose extended-duration interferon alfa-2a in high-risk resected malignant melanoma. J Clin Oncol 2004; 22:53-61.
23. Kirkwood JM, Ibrahim JG, Sondak VK et al. High- and low-dose interferon alfa-2b in high-risk melanoma: first analysis of intergroup trial E1690/S9111/C9190. J Clin Oncol 2000; 18:2444-2458.
24. Kirkwood JM, Strawderman MH, Ernstoff MS et al. Interferon alfa-2b adjuvant therapy of high-risk resected cutaneous melanoma: the Eastern Cooperative Oncology Group Trial EST 1684. J Clin Oncol 1996; 14:7-17.
25. Kirkwood JM, Ibrahim JG, Sosman JA et al. High-dose interferon alfa-2b significantly prolongs relapse-free and overall survival compared with the GM2-KLH/QS-21 vaccine in patients with resected stage IIB-III melanoma: results of intergroup trial E1694/S9512/C509801. J Clin Oncol 2001; 19:2370-2380.
26. Creagan ET, Dalton RJ, Ahmann DL et al. Randomized, surgical adjuvant clinical trial of recombinant interferon alfa-2a in selected patients with malignant melanoma. J Clin Oncol 1995; 13:2776-2783.
27. Verma S, Quirt I, McCready D et al. Systematic review of systemic adjuvant therapy for patients at high risk for recurrent melanoma. Cancer 2006; 106:1431-1442.
28. Mohr P, Weichenthal M, Hauschild A. Adjuvant therapy in melanoma. Onkologie 2003; 26:227-233.
29. Tilgen W. Malignant melanoma: current therapeutic concepts. Onkologie 1995; 18:534-547.
30. Sondak VK, Sosman J, Unger JM et al. Significant impact of HLA class I allele expression on outcome in melanoma patients treated with an allogeneic melanoma cell lysate vaccine. Final analysis of SWOG-9035 [abstract 7501]. Proc Am Soc Clin Oncol 2004; 14S:22.
31. Koops HS, Vaglini M, Suciu S et al. Prophylactic isolated limb perfusion for localized, high-risk limb melanoma: results of a multicenter reandomized phase III trial. European Organization for Research and Treatment of Cancer Malignant Melanoma Cooperative Group Protocol 18832, the World Health Organization Melanoma Program Trial 15 and the North American Perfusion Group Southwest Oncology Group-8593. J Clin Oncol 1998; 16:2906-2912.
32. Eton O, Legha SS, Bedikian AY et al. Sequential biochemotherapy versus chemotherapy for metastatic melanoma: results from a phase III randomized trial. J Clin Oncol 2002; 20:2045-2052.
33. Gogas HJ, Kirkwood JM, Sondak VK. Chemotherapy for metastatic melanoma: time for a change? Cancer 2007; 109:455-464.
34. Rass K, Tadler D, Tilgen W. Therapy of malignant melanoma. First-, second- and pathogenesis-oriented third-line therapies. Hautarzt 2006; 57:773-784.
35. Sasse AD, Sasse EC, Clark LG et al. Chemoimmunotherapy versus chemotherapy for metastatic malignant melanoma. Cochrane Database Syst Rev 2007 (1):CD005413.
36. Eggermont AMM, Kirkwood JM. Re-evaluating the role of dacarbazine in metastatic melanoma: what have we learned in 30 years? Eur J Cancer 2004; 40:1825-1836.
37. Bedikian AY, Millward M, Pehamberger H et al. Bcl-2 antisense (oblimersen sodium) plus dacarbazine in patients with advanced melanoma: The Oblimersen Melanoma Study Group. J Clin Oncol 2006; 24:4738-4745.
38. Schadendorf D, Ugurel S, Schuler-Thurner B et al. Dacarbazine (DTIC) versus vaccination with autologous peptide-pulsed dendritic cells (DC) in first-line treatment of patients with metastatic melanoma: a randomized phase III trial of the DC study group of the DeCOG. Ann Oncol 2006; 17:563-570.
39. Middleton MR, Grob JJ, Aaronson N et al. Randomized phase III study of temozolomide versus dacarbazine in the treatment of patients with advanced metastastatic melanoma. J Clin Oncol 2000; 18:158-66.
40. Danson S, Lorigan P. Improving outcomes in advanced malignant melanoma—Update on systemic therapy. Drugs 2005; 65:733-743.
41. Avril MF, Aamdal S, Grob JJ et al. Fotemustine compared with dacarbazine in patients with disseminated malignant melanoma: a phase II study. J Clin Oncol 2004; 22:1118-25.
42. Chapman PB, Einhorn LH, Meyers ML et al. Phase III multicenter randomized trial of the Dartmouth regimen versus dacarbazine in patients with metastatic melanoma. J Clin Oncol 1999; 17:2745-2751.
43. Huncharek M, Caubet JF, McGarry R. Single-agent DTIC versus combination chemotherapy with or without immunotherapy in metastatic melanoma: a meta-analysis of 3273 patients from 20 randomized trials. Melanoma Res 2001; 11:75-81.
44. Legha SS, Ring S, Bedikian A et al. Treatment of metastatic melanoma with combined chemotherapy containing cisplatin, vinblastine and dacarbazine (CVD) and biotherapy using interleukin-2 and interferon-alpha. Ann Oncol 1996; 7:827-835.
45. Bajetta E, Del Vecchio M, Nova P et al. Multicenter phase III randomized trial of polychemotherapy (CVD regimen) versus the same chemotherapy (CT) plus subcutaneous interleukin-2 and interferon-alpha2b in metastatic melanoma. Ann Oncol 2006; 17:571-577.

46. Kaufmann R, Spieth K, Leiter U et al. Temozolomide in combination with Interferon-alfa versus Temozolomide alone in patients with advanced metastatic melanoma: A randomized, Phase III, multicenter study from the Dermatologic Cooperative Oncology Group. J Clin Oncol 2005; 23:9001-9007.

47. Reinhold U, Hartl C, Hering R et al. Fatal rhabdomyolysis and multiple organ failure associated with adjuvant high-dose interferon alfa in malignant melanoma. Lancet 1997; 349:540-541.

48. Thompson JF, Scolyer RA, Kefford RF. Cutaneous melanoma. Lancet 2005; 365:687-701.

49. Serrone L, Hersey P. The chemoresistance of human malignant melanoma: an update. Melanoma Res 1999; 9:51-58.

50. Ugurel S, Schadendorf D, Pföhler C et al. In vitro drug sensitivity predicts response and survival after individualized sensitivity-directed chemotherapy in metastatic melanoma: a multicenter phase II trial of the Dermatologic Cooperative Oncology Group. Clin Cancer Res 2006; 12:5454-5463.

51. Quinn JA, Desjardins A, Weingart J et al. Phase I trial of temozolomide plus O_6-benzylguanine for patients with recurrent or progressive malignant glioma. J Clin Oncol 2005; 23:7178-87.

52. Ranson M, Middleton MR, Bridgewater J et al. Lomeguatrib, a potent inhibitor of O_6-alkylguanine-DNA-alkyltransferase: phase I safety, pharmacodynamic and pharmacokinetic trial and evaluation in combination with temozolomide in patients with advanced solid tumors. Clin Cancer Res 2006; 12:1577-84.

53. Ranson M, Hersey P, Thompson D et al. Randomized trial of the combination of lomeguatrib and temozolomide compared with temozolomide alone in chemotherapy naïve patients with metastatic cutaneous melanoma. J Clin Oncol 2007; 25:2540-2545.

54. Tentori L, Leonetti C, Scarsella M et al. Brain distribution and efficacy as chemosensitizer of an oral formulation of PARP-1 inhibitor GPI 15427 in experimental models of CNS tumors. Int J Oncol 2005; 26:415-22.

55. Barranco S, Romsdahl M, Humphrey R. The radiation response of human malignant melanoma cells grown in vitro. Cancer Res 1971; 31:830.

56. Isokangas OP, Muhonen T, Kajanti M et al. Radiation therapy of intracranial malignant melanoma. Radiother Oncol 1996; 38:139-144.

57. Buchsbaum JC, Shu JH, Lee SY et al. Survival by radiation therapy oncology group recursive partitioning analysis class and treatment modality in patients with brain metastases from malignant melanoma. Cancer 2002; 94:2265-2272.

58. Mathieu D, Kondziolka D, Cooper PB et al. Gamma knife radiosurgery in the management of malignant melanoma brain metastases. Neurosurgery 2007; 60:471-481.

59. Kirova YM, Chen J, Rabarijaona LI et al. Radiotherapy as palliative treatment for metastatic melanoma. Melanoma Res 1999; 9:611-613.

60. Ballo MT, Strom EA, Zagars GK et al. Adjuvant irradiation for axillary metastases from malignant melanoma. Int J Radiat Oncol Biol Phys 2002; 52:964-972.

61. Belardelli F, Ferrantini M, Parmiani G et al. International Meeting on Cancer Vaccines: How can we enhance efficacy of therapeutic vaccines? Cancer Res 2004; 64:6827-6830.

62. Schuler-Thurner B, Schuler G. Vaccination therapy of melanoma. J Dtsch Dermatol Ges 2005; 3:630-645.

63. Sosman JA, Weeraratna AT, Sondak VK. When will melanoma vaccines be proven effective? J Clin Oncol 2004; 22:387-389.

64. Sondak VK, Liu PY, Tuthill RJ et al. Adjuvant immunotherapy of resected, intermediate-thickness node-negative melanoma with an allogeneic tumor vaccine. Overall results of a randomized trial of the Southwest Oncology Group. J Clin Oncol 2002; 20:2058-2066.

65. Rosenberg SA, Dudley ME. Cancer regression in patients with metastatic melanoma after the transfer of autologous antitumor lymphocytes. Proc Natl Acad Sci USA 2004; 101(Suppl. 2):14639-14645.

66. Wolchok JD, Saenger YM. Current topics in melanoma. Curr Opin Oncol 2007; 19:116-120.

67. Phan GQ, Yang J, Sherry RM et al. Cancer regression and autoimmunity induced by cytotoxic T-lymphocyte-associated antigen 4 blockade in patients with metastatic melanoma. Proc Natl Acad Sci USA 2003; 100:8372-8377.

68. Attia P, Phan GQ, Maker AV et al. Autoimmunity correlates with tumor regression in patients with metastatic melanoma treated with Anti-Cytotoxic T-Lymphocyte Antigen-4. J Clin Oncol 2005; 23:6043-6053.

69. Schneeder A, Wagner C, Zemann A et al. CpG motifs are efficient adjuvants for DNA vaccines. J Invest Dermatol 2004; 123:371-379.

70. Pashenkov M, Goëss G, Wagner C et al. Phase II trial of a toll-like receptor 9-activating oligonucleotide in patients with metastatic melanoma. J Clin Oncol 2006; 24:5716-24.

71. Becker JC, Kirkwood JM, Agarwala SS et al. Molecular targeted therapy for melanoma. Current reality and future options. Cancer 2006; 107:2317-2327.

72. Sosman JA, Puzaniv I. Molecular targets in melanoma from angiogenesis to apoptosis. Clin Cancer Res 2006; 12(Suppl. 7):2376-2383.
73. Davies H, Bignell GR, Cox C et al. Mutations of the BRAF gene in human cancer. Nature 2002; 417:949-954.
74. Wilhelm SM, Carter C, Tang L et al. BAY 43-9006 exhibits broad spectrum oral antitumour activity and targets the RAF/MEK/ERK pathway and receptor tyrosine kinases involved in tumour progression and angiogenesis. Cancer Res 2004; 6:7099-7109.
75. Strumberg D, Richly H, Hilger RA et al. Phase I clinical and pharmacokinetic study of the novel Raf kinase and vascular endothelial growth factor receptor inhibitor BAY 43-9006 in patients. J Clin Oncol 2005; 23:965-72.
76. Margolin K, Longmate J, Baratta T et al. CCI-779 in metastatic melanoma: a phase II trial of the California Cancer Consortium. Cancer 2005; 104:1045-8.
77. Thallinger C, Poeppl W, Pratscher B et al. CCI-779 plus cisplatin is highly effective against human melanoma in a SCID mouse xenotranplantation model. Pharmacology 2007; 79:207-13.
78. Wyman K, Atkins MB, Prieto V et al. Multicenter phase II trial of high-dose imatinib mesylate in metastatic melanoma. Cancer 2006; 1006:2005-2011.
79. Curtin JA, Busam K, Pinkel D et al. Somatic activation of KIT in distinct subtypes of melanoma. J Clin Oncol 2006; 24:4340-6.
80. Hwu WJ, Krown SE, Menell JH et al. Phase II study of temozolomide plus thalidomide for the treatment of metastatic melanoma. J Clin Oncol 2003; 21:3351-3356.
81. Danson S, Lorigan P, Arance A et al. Randomized phase II study of temozolomide given every 8 hours or daily with either interferon alfa-2b or thalidomide in metastatic malignant melanoma. J Clin Oncol 2003; 21:2551-2557.
82. Krown SE, Niedzwiecki D, Hwu WJ et al. Phase II study of temozolomide and thalidomide in patients with metastatic melanoma in the brain: high rate of thromboembolic events (CALGB 500102). Cancer 2006; 107:1883-1890.
83. Hurwitz H, Fehrenbacher Novotny W et al. Bevacizumab plus irinotecan, fluorouracil and leucovorin for metastatic colorectal cancer. N Engl J Med 2004; 350:2335-2342.
84. Chow LQ, Eckhardt SG. Sunitinib: from rational design to clinical efficacy. J Clin Oncol 2007; 25:884-96.
85. Peterson AC, Swiger S, Stadler WM et al. Phase II study of thr Flk-1 tyrosine kinase inhibitor SU5416 in advanced melanoma. Clin Cancer Res 2004; 10:4048-4054.
86. Tucker GC. Alpha v integrin inhibitors and cancer therapy. Curr Opinion Investig Drugs 2003; 4:722-731.
87. Hersey P, Sosman J, O'Day S et al. A phase II, randomized, open label study evaluating the antitumor activity of MEDI-522, a humanized monoclonal antibody directed against the human alpha v beta 3 (avb3) integrin +/− dacarbazine in patients with metastatic melanoma. Proc Am Soc Clin Oncol 2005: Abstract 7570.
88. Dormond O, Foletti A, Paroz C et al. NSAIDs inhibit alpha V beta 3 integrin-mediated and Cdc42/Rac-dependent endothelial-cell spreading, migration and angiogenesis. Nat Med 2001; 7:1041-1047.
89. Lejeune FL, Monnier Y, Rüegg C. Complete and long-lasting regression of disseminated multiple skin melanoma metastases under treatment with cyclooxygenase-2 inhibitor. Melanoma Res 2006; 16:263-265.
90. Helmbach H, Kern MA, Rossmann E et al. Drug resistance towards etoposide and cisplatin in human melanoma cells is associated with drug-dependent apoptosis deficiency. J Invest Dermatol 2002; 118:923-932.
91. Jansen B, Schlagbauer-Wadl H, Brown BD et al. Bcl-2 antisense therapy chemosensitizes human melanoma in SCID mice. Nat Med 1998; 4:232-234.
92. Hu Y, Cherton-Horvat G, Dragowska V et al. Antisense oligonucleotides targeting XIAP induce apoptosis and enhance chemotherapeutic activity against human lung cancer cells in vitro and in vivo. Clin Cancer Res 2003; 9:2826-2836.
93. Amiri KI, Horton LW, LaFleur BJ et al. Augmenting chemosensitivity of malignant melanoma tumours via proteasome inhibition: implication for bortezomib (VELCADE, PS-341) as a therapeutic agent for malignant melanoma. Cancer Res 2004; 64:4912-4918.
94. Baldwin AS. Control of oncogenesis and cancer therapy resistance by the transcription factor NF-κB. J Clin Invest 2001; 107:241-246.
95. Katalinic A, Kunze U, Schafer T. Epidemiology of cutaneous melanoma and nonmelanoma skin cancer in Schleswig-Holstein, Germany: incidence, clinical subtypes, tumour stages and localization (epidemiology of skin cancer). Br J Dermatol 2003; 149:1200-1206.
96. Boukamp P. Nonmelanoma skin cancer: what drives tumor development and progression? Carcinogenesis 2005; 26:1657-1667.

97. Rass K. UV damage and DNA repair in basal cell and squamous cell carcinomas. In: Reichrath J, ed. Molecular Mechanisms of Basal Cell and Squamous Cell Carcinomas. Georgetown: Landes Bioscience 2006:18-30.

98. Ceilly RI, Del Rosso JQ. Current modalities and new advances in the treatment of basal cell carcinoma. Int J Dermatol 2006; 45:489-498.

99. Rodriguez-Vigil T, Vazquez-Lopez F, Perez-Oliva N. Recurrence rates of primary basal cell carcinoma in facial risk areas treated with curettage and electrodesiccation. J Am Acad Dermatol 2007; 56:91-95.

100. Thissen MR, Neumann MH, Schouten LJ. A systematic review of treatment modalities for primary basal cell carcinomas. Arch Dermatol 1999; 135:1177-1183.

101. Thissen MR, Nieman FH, Ideler AH et al. Cosmetic results of cryosurgery versus surgical excision for primary uncomplicated basal cell carcinomas of the head and neck. Dermatol Surg 2000; 26:759-764.

102. Panizzon RG. Dermatologic radiotherapy. Hautarzt 58:701-712.

103. Silverman MK, Kopf AW, Gladstein AH et al. Recurrence rates of treated basal cell carcinomas. Part 4: X-ray therapy. J Dermatol Surg Oncol 1992; 18:549-554.

104. Noodt BB, Berk K, Stokke T et al. Apoptosis and necrosis induced with light and 5-aminolaevulinic acid-derived protoporphyrin IX. Br J Cancer 1996; 74:22-29.

105. Braathen LR, Szeimies RM, Basset-Seguin N et al. Guidelines on the use of photodynamic therapy for nonmelanoma skin cancer: an international consensus. J Am Acad Dermatol 2007; 56:125-143.

106. Rhodes LE, de Rie M, Enstrom Y et al. Photodynamic therapy using topical methyl aminolevulinate vs surgery for nodular basal cell carcinoma: results of a multicenter randomized prospective trial. Arch Dermatol 2004; 140:17-23.

107. Berman B, Sullivan T, De Araujo T et al. Expression of Fas-receptor on basal cell carcinomas after treatment with imiquimod 5% cream or vehicle. Br J Dermatol 2003; 149(Suppl. 66):59-61.

108. Stockfleth E, Trefzer U, Garcia-Bartels C et al. The use of Toll-like receptor-7 agonist in the treatment of basal cell carcinoma: an overview. Br J Dermatol 2003; 149(Suppl. 66):53-56.

109. Locke J, Karimpour S, Young G et al. Radiotherapy for epithelial skin cancer. Int J Radiat Oncol Biol Phys 2001; 51:748-755.

110. McCord MW, Mendenhall WM, Parsons JT et al. Skin cancer of the head and neck with clinical perineural invasion. Int J Radiat Oncol Biol Phys 2000; 47:89-93.

111. Schmook T, Stockfleth E. Current treatment patterns in nonmelanoma skin cancer across Europe. J Dermatolog Treat 2003; 14(Suppl. 3):3-10.

112. Freeman M, Vinciullo C, Francis D et al. A comparison of photodynamic therapy using topical methyl aminolevulinate (Metvix) with single cycle cryotherapy in patients with actinic keratosis: a prospective, randomized study. J Dermatolog Treat 2003; 14:99-106.

113. Szeimies RM, Gerritsen MJ, Gupta G et al. Imiquimod 5% cream for the treatment of actinic keratosis: results from a phase III, randomized, double-blind, vehicle-controlled, clinical trial with histology. J Am Acad Dermatol 2004; 51:547-555.

114. Tanghetti E, Werschler P. Comparison of 5% 5-fluorouracil cream and 5% imiquimod cream in the management of actinic keratoses on the face and scalp. J Drugs Dermatol 2007; 6:144-147.

115. Wolf JE, Taylor JR, Tschen E et al. Topical 3.0% diclofenac in 2.5% hyaluronan gel in the treatment of actinic keratoses. Int J Dermatol 2001; 41:371-372.

116. Mendenhall NP, Million RR, Cassisi NJ. Parotid area lymph node metastases from carcinoma of the skin. Int J Radiat Oncol Biol Phys 1985; 11:707-714.

117. Guthrie TH Jr, Porubsky ES et al. Cisplatin-based chemotherapy in advanced basal and squamous cell carcinomas of the skin: results in 28 patients including 13 patients receiving multimodality therapy. J Clin Oncol 1990; 8:342-346.

118. Khansur T, Kennedy A. Cisplatin and 5-fluorouracil for advanced locoregional and metastatic squamous cell carcinoma of the skin. Cancer 1991; 67:2020-2032.

INDEX